Continence

Continence

Current Concepts and Treatment Strategies

Edited by

Gopal H. Badlani
Wake Forest University Baptist Medical Center, Winston Salem, NC, USA

G. Willy Davila
Cleveland Clinic Florida, Weston, FL, USA

Martin C. Michel
Academic Medical Center, Amsterdam, The Netherlands

Jean J.M.C.H. de la Rosette
Academic Medical Center, Amsterdam, The Netherlands

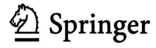 Springer

Editors
Gopal H. Badlani, MD
Department of Urology
Wake Forest University
Baptist Medical Center
Winston Salem, NC, USA

G. Willy Davila, MD
Department of Gynecology
Cleveland Clinic Florida
Weston, FL
USA

Martin C. Michel, MD, MAE
Department of Pharmacology and Pharmacotherapy
Academic Medical Center
University of Amsterdam
Amsterdam
The Netherlands

Jean J.M.C.H. de la Rosette, MD, PhD
Department of Urology
Academic Medical Center
University of Amsterdam
Amsterdam
The Netherlands

ISBN: 978-1-84996-616-0   e-ISBN: 978-1-84628-734-3
DOI: 10.1007/978-1-84628-734-3

British Library Cataloguing in Publication Data

Printed on acid-free paper

Springer Science+Business Media
springer.com

Foreword

Urinary incontinence and pelvic prolapse have affected the quality of many lives over the years. Only recently, however, has increased attention to these areas led to a better understanding of the epidemiology, pathophysiology, and newer approaches to treatment, both from the pharmacological and device standpoint. This text is a step forward in bringing these new innovations together in a comprehensive and well-organized manner. The editors have chosen an international group of authors who are highly regarded in their fields, and these authors have in turn provided details in an easy to read format. The editors themselves have provided a diversity of expertise from the fields of urology, urogynecology, pharmacology, and minimally invasive approaches. This combination is unique. The latest concepts in epidemiology, anatomy, and pathophysiology are presented in the first two parts on the book. Stress incontinence is totally reviewed from the standpoint of all types of conservative, minimally invasive, and not so minimally invasive therapies. Urinary urgency incontinence likewise is reviewed from the same standpoints, including a separate section on contemporary views regarding the use of intradetrusor or suburothelial botulinum toxin injections. The section on pelvic organ prolapse includes a thorough discussion of biomaterials, as well as complete discussions of conservative and surgical management of the various forms of prolapse. Male urinary incontinence is included as a separate part of the book, and there are two parts devoted to "special situations and socioeconomic considerations." The special situations include fistulas, postradiation incontinence, recurrent incontinence, voiding dysfunction after surgery, and the multioperated patient with recurrent incontinence and/or prolapse; the socioeconomic issues include the economic impacts of urinary incontinence and prolapse and a well-thought out contribution on community awareness and education. All in all, this is a complete package, unique in the field, and I recommend it to any audience interested in the topic.

Alan J. Wein, MD, PhD (Hon)
Professor and Chair
Division of Urology
University of Pennsylvania Health System
and
Chief of Urology
Hospital of the University of Pennsylvania

Preface

When we first met to consider a proposal to put together a book on urinary incontinence and pelvic organ prolapse, the obvious question was "why another book." The answer was not easy but a need was perceived based on the tremendous changes in our understanding and the way we practice today compared to even 5 years ago, let alone when we were in training. The radical changes were initiated by the infusion of new pharmaceutical agents in bladder-driven incontinence and by the more recent device-driven approaches to the urethral incontinence in female and male population. The emerging field of kits for the pelvic organ prolapse is further fueling the interest. Journal articles reflect individual reports, reviews, and meta-analysis data; however, to a reader a comprehensive book offers a resource for reference, an aid to understanding for new practitioners entering the field, or an expansion of the horizons and/or a substantiation of their reasons for practice in the field for the more experienced practitioners. We hope that this effort of many international stars will fulfill these needs.

We have made a great effort to put together authors who are progressive in their thoughts and are willing to reflect the changes from established patterns. This in no way minimizes the efforts of others in the past, for it is upon their shoulders that we climb in order to see farther.

There is one individual who toiled to make this effort possible. Kaytan Amrute was the glue that binds this book, so to this young individual, who is just beginning his journey in the field of urogynecology, the four of us express our deep gratitude.

Individually, we would like to thank our families who give up so much of their time to allow us to put in this effort. We list their names jointly, as the four of us remain bound together by this book.

Gopal Badlani, MD
G. Willy Davila, MD
Martin C. Michel, MD, MAE
Jean J.M.C.H. de la Rosette, MD, PhD

Acknowledgments

For all their help and support during the long editorial process, Dr. Badlani would like to thank his hard-working colleague Kaytan Amrute; G. Willy Davila would like to thank Kristin Dunn; Martin C. Michel would like to thank Karla Dabekaussen-Peters; and Jean J.M.C.H. de la Rosette would like to thank Sonja van Rees Vellinga.

This book is dedicated to our family members who give up so much!

GB: Charu, Pooja and Chirag
WD: Carolyn, Claudia, Daniel and Will
MM: Martina and Liesel
JD: Pilar

Gopal H. Badlani, MD
G. Willy Davila, MD
Martin C. Michel, MD, MAE
Jean J.M.C.H. de la Rosette, MD, PhD

Contents

Contributors

Baharak Amir, BSc, MD
Department of Obstetrics and Gynecology, IWK
Health Center, Dalhousie University, Halifax, NS,
Canada

Kaytan V. Amrute, MD, FACOG
Department of Obstetrics and Gynecology, Jacobi
Medical Center, Bronx, NY, USA

Apostolos Apostolidis, MD
2nd Department of Urology, Papageorgiou
Hospital, Aristotle University of Thessaloniki,
Thessaloniki, Greece

Rodney A. Appell, MD, FACS
Professor and *Chief*
Division of Voiding Dysfunction and Female
Urology, The Scott Department of Urology, Baylor
College of Medicine, Houston, Texas, USA

Walter Artibani, MD
Professor of Urology and *Chief*
Department of Oncological and Surgical Sciences,
Urology Clinic, University of Padova, Padova, Italy

Sarit O. Aschkenazi, MD
Department of Obstetrics and *Gynecology,*
Evanston Continence Center, Evanston Hospital–
Northwestern University, Evanston, IL, USA

Gopal H. Badlani, MD
Professor and *Vice Chair*
Department of Urology, Wake Forest University
Baptist Medical Center, Winston Salem, NC, USA

Matthew A. Barker, MD
Department of Obstetrics and Gynecology, Good
Samaritan Hospital, Cincinnati, OH, USA

Alfred E. Bent, MD
Head, Division of Gynecology and *Professor*
Department of Obstetrics and Gynecology, IWK
Health Center, Dalhousie University, Halifax, NS,
Canada

Daniel Biller, MD
Department of Obstetrics and Gynecology,
Vanderbilt University, Nashville, TN, USA

Jerry G. Blaivas, MD
Department of Urology, Weill Medical College,
Cornell University, New York, NY, USA

Kari Bø, PhD
Professor, PT and *Exercise Scientist*
Department of Sports Medicine, Norwegian School
of Sport Sciences, Oslo, Norway

Linda Cardozo, MD FRCOG
Professor of Urogynaecology
Department of Urogynaecology, King's College
Hospital, London, UK

David Castro-Diaz, MD, PhD
Professor of Urology / Consultant Urologist
Department of Urology, University Hospital of the
Canary Islands, Tenerife, Spain

Emily Cole, MD
Department of Urologic Surgery, Vanderbilt
University Medical Center, Nashville, TN, USA

Craig V. Comiter, MD
Associate Professor
Department of Urology, Stanford University School
of Medicine, Stanford, CA, USA

Jean J.M.C.H. de la Rosette, MD, PhD
Professor and *Chairman*
Department of Urology, Academic Medical Center,
University Hospital, Amsterdam, The Netherlands

Anurag K. Das, MD, FACS
Assistant Professor of Surgery
Division of Urology, Beth Israel Deaconess
Medical Center, Harvard Medical School, Boston,
MA, USA

Prokar Dasgupta, MSc(Urol), MD, DLS,
FRCS(Urol), FEBU
Consultant Urological Surgeon
and *Hon. Senior Lecturer*
Department of Urology, Guy's Hospital, London,
UK

G. Willy Davila, MD
Chairman, Department of Gynecology
Head, Section of Urogynecology and
Reconstructive Pelvic Surgery
Cleveland Clinic Florida, Weston, FL, USA

Ananias C. Diokno, MD, FACS
Executive Vice President and *Chief Medical Officer*
William Beaumont Hospitals, Royal Oak, MI, USA

Roger R. Dmochowski, MD
Professor
Department of Urologic Surgery, Vanderbilt
University Medical Center, Nashville, TN, USA

Clare J. Fowler, MB, BS, MSc, FRCP
Department of Uro-Neurology, National Hospital
for Neurology and Neurosurgery, London, UK

Sergio Fumero, MD
Department of Urology, University Hospital of the
Canary Islands, Tenerife, Spain

Gamal M. Ghoniem, MD, FACS
Head, Section of Voiding Dysfunction, Female
Urology and Reconstruction
Clinical Professor of Surgery/Urology NSU,
OSU and USF
Chairman of Medical Student Education
Department of Urology, Cleveland Clinic Florida,
Weston, FL, USA

Ali S. Goezen, MD
Department of Urology, SLK Kliniken Heilbronn,
Teaching Hospital University, Heidelberg, Germany

Meidee Goh, MD, MPH
Huron Valley Urology Associates, Ypsilanti, MI,
USA

Howard B. Goldstein, DO, MPH
Department of Female Pelvic Medicine and
Reconstructive Surgery, UMDNJ-Robert Wood
Johnson Medical School, Cooper University
Hospital, Camden, NJ, USA

Brooke H. Gurland, MD
Staff Physician, Department of Colon & Rectal
Surgery, Center for Functional Bowel Disorder,
The Cleveland Clinic Foundation, 9500 Euclid
Avenue-Desk A30, Cleveland, OH, USA

Eric A. Hurtado, MD
Fellow
Division of Female Voiding Dysfunction
and Female Urology, The Scott Department
of Urology, Baylor College of Medicine, Houston,
Texas, USA

Mickey M. Karram, MD
Department of Obstetrics and Gynecology, Good
Samaritan Hospital, Cincinnati, OH, USA

Vik Khullar, BSc, MD, MRCOG, AKC
Consultant Urogynaecologist
Department of Urogynaecology, St. Mary's
Hospital, Imperial College, London, UK

Rajeev Kumar, MD
Associate Professor of Urology
All India Institute of Medical Sciences, New Delhi,
India

Carolyn F. Langford, DO
Clinical Associate Urology
Department of Urology, Cleveland Clinic Florida,
Weston, FL, USA

M. Pilar Laguna, MD, PhD, FEBU
Department of Urology, Academic Medical Center,
University Hospital, Amsterdam, The Netherlands

Marie Carmela M. Lapitan, MD, FPUA, FPCS
Clinical Associate Professor
College of Medicine,
University of the Philippines, Manila
Research Assistant Professor
National Institutes of Health–Manila,
University of the Philippines, Manila
Consultant
Division of Urology, Department of Surgery,
Philippine General Hospital,
University of the Philippines, Manila
Philippines

Gil Levy, MD
Director, Center for Pelvic Floor Dysfunction and
Reconstructive Surgery
Chief, Division of Urogynecology and
Reconstructive Surgery
Department of Obstetrics and Gynecology,
Maimonides Medical Center, Brooklyn, NY, USA
Director, Division of Female Pelvic Medicine and
Reconstructive Surgery
Department of Obstetrics and Gynecology, Staten
Island University Hospital, Staten Island, NY, USA
Assistant Professor of Obstetrics and Gynecology
State University of New York (SUNY Downstate),
NY, USA

Lawrence R. Lind, MD, FACOG, FACS
*Co-Chief of Urogynecology and Pelvic
Reconstructive Surgery*
Division of Urogynecology, Department of
Obstetrics and Gynecology, North Shore–LIJ
Health System, Great Neck, NY, USA

Martin C. Michel, MD, MAE
Professor
Department of Pharmacology and
Pharmacotherapy, Academic Medical Center,
University Hospital, Amsterdam, The Netherlands

Drogo K. Montague, MD
Professor of Surgery and *Director*
Center for Genitourinary Reconstruction,
Department of Urology, Glickman Urological and
Kidney Institute, Cleveland Clinic Foundation,
Cleveland, OH, USA

Ajay Nehra, MD, FACS
Professor of Urology
Mayo Clinic College of Medicine, Rochester, MN,
USA

Diane K. Newman, MSN, ANP-BC, CRNP,
FAAN, BCIA-PMDB
Co-Director, Penn Center for Continence and
Pelvic Health
Director, Clinical Trials
Division of Urology, Department of Surgery,
University of Pennsylvania Medical Center,
Philadelphia, PA, USA

Victor W. Nitti, MD
Professor and Vice Chairman
Director of Female Pelvic Medicine and
Reconstructive Surgery, Department of Urology,
NYU Langone Medical Center, New York, NY,
USA

Jørgen Nordling, MD
Professor of Urology
Department of Urology, Herlev Hospital,
University of Copenhagen, Denmark

Giacomo Novara, MD, FEBU
Consultant Urologist
I.R.C.C.S. Istituto Oncologico Veneto (I.O.V.),
Department of Oncological and Surgical Sciences,
Urology Clinic, University of Padova,
Padova, Italy

Matthias Oelke, MD, FEBU
Vice-Chairman
Department of Urology, Hannover Medical School,
Hannover, Germany

Dennis J.A.J. Oerlemans, MD
Department of Urology, University Hospital of
Maastricht, Maastricht, The Netherlands

Priya Padmanabhan, MD
Fellow
Female Pelvic Medicine and Reconstructive
Surgery, Vanderbilt University School of Medicine,
Nashville, TN, USA

Demetri C. Panayi, MB.BS(Lon), BSc(Hons),
MRCOG
Subspecialty Trainee Urogynaecology
Department of Urogynaecology, St. Mary's
Hospital, Imperial College, London, UK

Jill Maura Rabin, MD
Department of Obstetrics and Gynecology,
Division of Urogynecology, Long Island Jewish
Medical Center, New Hyde Park, NY, USA

Jens J. Rassweiler, MD
Professor of Urology
Department of Urology, SLK-Kliniken Heilbronn
GmbH, Teaching Hospital University, Heidelberg,
Germany

Ardeshir R. Rastinehad, DO
Smith Institute for Urology, North Shore LIJ
Health System, Long Island, New York USA

Dudley Robinson, MD, MRCOG
Consultant Urogynaecologist
Department of Urogynaecology, King's College
Hospital, London, UK

Jan-Paul Roovers, MD, PhD
Department of Gynaecology and Obstetrics,
Academic Medical Center, University Hospital,
Amsterdam, The Netherlands

Matthew P. Rutman, MD
Assistant Professor
Department of Urology, Columbia University
Medical Center, New York, NY, USA

Arun Sahai, BSc(Hons), MRCS(Eng)
Specialist Registrar in Urology
Department of Urology, Guy's Hospital, London,
UK

Peter K. Sand, MD
Department of Obstetrics and Gynecology,
Evanston Continence Center, Evanston Hospital–
Northwestern University, Evanston, IL, USA

Walter Scheitlin, MD
Department of Urology, SLK Kliniken Heilbronn,
Teaching Hospital University, Heidelberg, Germany

Mohammad Shamim Khan, FRCS(Urol), FEBU
Consultant Urological Surgeon
Department of Urology, Guy's Hopsital, London,
UK

Petros Sountoulides, MD, FEBU
Department of Urology, Academic Medical Center,
University Hospital, Amsterdam, The Netherlands

Mary M.T. South, MD
Urogynecology and Pelvic Reconstructive Surgery,
Department of Obstetrics and Gynecology,

University of Cincinnati College of Medicine,
Cincinnati, OH, USA

Christian Stock, MD
Department of Urology, SLK Kliniken Heilbronn,
Teaching Hospital University, Heidelberg, Germany

Lynn Stothers, MD, MHSc, FRCSC
Associate Professor of Surgery
Associate Member,
Department of Health Care and Epidemiology
Associate Member, Department of Pharmacology
Director of Research, Bladder Care Centre
Department of Urologic Sciences, Bladder Care
Centre, University of British Columbia, Vancouver,
BC, Canada

Dogu Teber, MD
Department of Urology, SLK Kliniken Heilbronn,
Teaching Hospital University,
Heidelberg, Germany

Peter Tsakiris, MD
Department of Urology, Academic Medical Center,
University Hospital, Amsterdam,
The Netherlands

Philip E.V. Van Kerrebroeck, MD, PhD
Department of Urology, University Hospital
Maastricht, Maastricht, The Netherlands

George D. Webster, MD
Department of Urology, Duke University Medical
Center, Durham, NC, USA

Kristene E. Whitmore, MD
*Division Chief of Female Pelvic Medicine and
Reconstructive Surgery, and Urology*
Drexel University College of Medicine,
Hahnemann University Hospital, Pelvic and Sexual
Health Institute, Philadelphia, PA, USA

Harvey A. Winkler, MD, FACOG
Co-Chief of Urogynecology and Pelvic
Reconstructive Surgery
Division of Urogynecology, Department of
Obstetrics and Gynecology, North Shore–LIJ
Health System, Great Neck, NY, USA

Part I
Introduction

Chapter 1
Epidemiology of Urinary Incontinence

Marie Carmela M. Lapitan

Urinary incontinence (UI) is one of the priority health issues recognized by the World Health Organization. An understanding of the epidemiology of this condition effectively leads to a better appreciation of its importance and its impact on the population and the health care delivery system. The past two decades have seen intensified research on the prevalence of UI and the identification of its determinants.

The synthesis of the published literature on the epidemiology of UI is complex because of the differences in the definitions of UI used, the population types included, and the methodology used [1]. For the definition used, variance may be in the severity or in the interval measured. The influence of restrictions in the definition of UI insofar as severity, frequency, and duration of the leakage is apparent when comparing prevalence rates of UI established in epidemiological studies to those in clinical trials on treatment for UI, wherein rates in the former are often higher than in the latter. Particularly for surveys and cross-sectional studies, the design and wording of the questionnaires, response rates, and the timing of the study in relation to potential confounders, such as pregnancy, childbirth, prostatectomy, and stroke can influence the results. Advertising for incontinence medications and products to the public in recent years also has been identified as influential in increasing the reported prevalence of UI by increasing the willingness of women to disclose the condition [2].

Notwithstanding these issues, this chapter aims to discuss the prevalence, incidence, and remission rates of UI in a comprehensive and cohesive manner,

integrating all available information on the topic. It also seeks to elaborate on potential risk factors for the development of UI.

Prevalence of UI in the General Population

Urinary incontinence is increasingly recognized as a prevalent condition worldwide. Surveys performed in large cohorts of community-dwelling persons involving both men and women in all age groups report overall prevalence rates ranging from 5 to 69%, with a majority of the studies citing the prevalence between 25 and 45% among women and 1 and 9% among men.

The 3rd International Consultation on Incontinence generated a comprehensive report on the overall prevalence of adult women and men in the general population. The epidemiology committee of the Consultation cited a median prevalence range of 20–30% for young women, 30–40% for women in the middle age group, and 30–50% in the elderly [3]. Among men, prevalence rates from 3 to 39% have been cited, with increasing rates as the study population ages.

A significant difference is found between the prevalence of UI among males and females. Aggazzotti reported that the prevalence of UI was significantly higher in women than in men (59.8% vs. 39.2%) [4]. Such a difference in prevalence was particularly apparent with increasing age. Women had an almost twofold risk of being incontinent (OR = 1.95 95% CI 1.24–3.06). In a survey of a

Japanese community with 1,836 respondents, Ueda and co-workers had found that women with UI were five times more common as men [5]. In a survey of nursing home residents, Nelson et al. established that the male gender was a protective factor in the occurrence of UI [OR = 0.8 (0.7–1.0)] [6].

Prevalence of UI According to Type

Stress urinary incontinence (SUI), commonly defined in the epidemiological literature as the presence of involuntary leakage during periods of exertion such as laughing, sneezing, and coughing, is the most prevalent type in population-based trials, occurring 40–50% of the time [5, 7, 8]. It is the type of incontinence that predominates among women, accounting for as much as 65% of all types on UI in women. Studies including women of all ages cite SUI as the type of UI among 33–50% of the incontinent population [9–12]. Its rate in women is highest in the young and middle-age group. Thereafter, there is a relative decrease with increasing age. Among elderly women, the proportion of SUI declines, at times with rates approaching the other types. In contrast, SUI is found to be the least common type in men, with reported prevalence rates limited to less than 10% across all age groups.

Urgency urinary incontinence (UUI) is frequently defined as involuntary urine leakage associated with a sudden desire to urinate and failing to reach the toilet in time. It is one of the components of the overactive bladder (OAB), which includes symptoms such as urgency, nocturia, and frequency. Approximately one third of patients diagnosed to have OAB present with UUI [13].

The overall prevalence of UUI across both sexes and all age groups in the general population is 20–40%. It is consistently found to be the predominant UI type among men, accounting for 40–80% of all UI types [5, 14–16]. Among women, the proportion with UUI is noted to be from 11 to 25%. Such proportion increases beyond age 60 years [17–19].

Incidence and Remission Rates

Recent years have seen an increase in the number of studies performed to determine the incidence and remission rates of UI. Longitudinal studies performed on varied populations showed annual incidence rates ranging from 0.9 to 10%. The MRC Incontinence Team followed up with more than 39,000 people aged 40 years and above to establish a 6.3% annual incidence rate for incontinence. Studies that focused on SUI cited incidence rates of 3.8–8.1% [20, 21]. In a study of an older population, Thom found a slightly higher incidence among women compared to men (17.5 per 1,000 women vs. 12.2 per 1,000 men) [19]. For both men and women, incidence increased with age. However, incidence plateaus at age 40–50 years among females [22].

Remission rates have been reported to be at 2.9–6.8% annually [22, 23]. Remission rates decrease with age and with severity. Compared to UUI, SUI has been found to have higher remission rates [22]. Data from the MESA study suggest that remission rates among men are higher compared to women [24, 25], in congruence with the finding of the MRC Incontinence study [20].

Prevalence in Specific Populations

UI Among the Elderly in Communities and in Long-Term Care Facilities

The elderly in long-term care facilities are reported to have higher prevalences of UI. Giorgiou et al. reported prevalence rates of UI in nursing homes and long-term wards as twice that of residential homes (70 and 71% vs. 34%, respectively) [26]. Studies including residents in nursing homes in the United States, Italy, and Japan showed UI prevalence rates ranging from 54 to 72% [4, 6, 27]. Landi and co-workers studied more than 5,000 frail elderly under a home-care program and found an overall prevalence of 51% with similar rates between males (49%) and women (52%) [28].

Pregnancy-Related and Postpartum UI

Pregnant and postpartum women are a special group with high prevalence rates of UI. Pregnancy-associated UI generally is viewed as a transient condition attributed to the many physiological changes in the woman's body such as fluctuating hormone levels, increased urine production, and changes in the position and relations of the pelvic structures brought about by the enlarging uterus occurring during gestation. On the other hand, the development of UI in the postpartum period is thought to be a consequence of the alterations in the pelvic floor anatomy after childbirth and is believed to be persistent in a proportion of women.

A review of the published literature on the topic by Mason revealed pregnancy-associated UI prevalence rates ranging from 27 to 67% [29]. A population-based survey of 1,874 adult women revealed an overall prevalence of pregnancy-associated UI of 16.6% [30]. In an interview of 525 postpartum women within 3 days of their delivery, 59.5% admitted to experiencing UI during the pregnancy [31]. This figure is very similar to the 59% prevalence in 717 women on their 34th week of gestation reported by Mason and co-workers [29]. Chaliha prospectively studied 549 women through their first pregnancy and delivery and found the prevalence of SUI and UUI during pregnancy to be 8.0 and 35.7%, respectively [32].

After delivery, a proportion of women will continue to experience UI, and a few will develop de novo incontinence in the postpartum period. The literature review of Mason cited postpartum incontinence prevalence rates ranging from 5.8 to 42.6% [29]. The wide range of rates may be due to the differences in the timing of the survey and the definition of UI used. In a prospective study of more than 500 pregnant women up to 12 months postpartum, Burgio and co-workers showed UI prevalence rates of 11.4, 9.3, 10.5, and 13.25% at 6 weeks, 3, 6, and 12 months postpartum, respectively [31]. Mason found a postpartum UI prevalence of 31% at 8 weeks [29]. Chaliha's group reported 2.2 and 12.4% of patients reporting SUI and UUI, respectively, in the postnatal period [32].

Many studies related pregnancy UI and postpartum UI. The population-based survey of Foldspang reported that UI during pregnancy predicted the occurrence of postpartum UI, age-adjusted OR = 9.2 (95% CI 6.5–13.0) for the first childbirth and OR = 12.3 (95% CI 7.6–19.9) for the second childbirth [30]. Attributable risk for persistent UI after delivery by pregnancy UI was 56.1–67.6%. The prospective study by Burgio et al. showed a twofold increase in the risk for postpartum UI for women who experienced incontinence during pregnancy (OR = 2.1, 95% CI 1.29–3.45) [31]. The 5-year longitudinal study of Viktrup demonstrated

that UI during the first pregnancy was independently associated with long-lasting SUI after 5 years (OR = 3.8, 95% CI 1.9–7.5) [21]. In the same study, SUI in the postpartum period was associated with greater odds for persistent SUI (OR = 4.5, 95% CI 2.5–13.2). The risk of long-lasting SUI and UUI was found to be related to the time of onset and the duration of the incontinence after pregnancy and delivery in a "dose–response-like" manner.

Multivariate analyses of several factors to determine their association with postpartum UI have been performed. Higher parity was associated with increased likelihood for SUI following delivery [29]. Vaginal delivery was found to be a consistent predictor of postpartum UI in three studies, with odds ratios ranging from 1.2 to 3.6 [21, 30, 31]. Correlated with this observation, caesarean delivery was noted to be associated with lower rates of postpartum UI [33, 34]. Forceps delivery and the performance of an episiotomy were other obstetric factors found to be independent predictors of postpartum UI [21, 31, 34].

Smoking (OR = 1.91, 95% CI 1.20–3.45) and BMI (OR = 1.15, 95% CI 1.03–1.28) also were found to be significantly associated with postpartum UI [31]. Hvidman, on the other hand, did not find the same association with BMI [33].

Postprostatectomy Incontinence

Postprostatectomy incontinence is a distinctive form of male UI. The accepted incidence of UI following transurethral resection of the prostate is 1%. Higher figures are reported after radical prostatectomy with overall prevalence ranging from 5 to 62%, with most studies citing rates between 10 and 30%. This very wide range of prevalence rates may be explained by the same factors cited to be responsible for the variation in the prevalence of UI in the general population. In addition, rates also are found to be influenced by the basis of the diagnosis. Rates based on the symptoms reported by patients are generally 2–3× higher than those based on physicians' observations. Several studies have demonstrated that doctors underestimate postprostatectomy UI by as much as 75% [35–37].

Incontinence rates are observed to progressively decline from the time of catheter removal after prostatectomy and they plateau 1–2 years postoperation [38–42]. Thus, it is important to emphasize that studies presenting postprostatectomy incontinence rates should have a minimum followup of 1 year to establish true and reliable rates.

Modifications in the techniques of radical prostatectomy have been developed primarily to minimize the complication of UI. The variations associated with lower incontinence rates include the perineal (vs. the abdominal) approach [43, 44] and the preservation of neurovascular bundle [45, 46]. Bladder neck preservation affords earlier return to continence compared to bladder neck resection, although continence rates at 1 year postoperation do not significantly differ between the two techniques [47].

Age at time of prostatectomy may be a significant factor associated with the occurrence of postoperative UI [40, 43, 45, 46, 48]. Catalona's work has shown that the risk for postprostatectomy UI doubles for every 10 years of age beginning at age 40 years. Horie, however, noted that rather than absolutely affecting likelihood of developing UI, age determined the rate at which continence would be achieved [39]. Older men were found to take a longer time to achieve continence. On the other hand, two studies found no relation between age and postprostatectomy UI prevalence [35, 49].

Risk Factors

Age

Increasing age is found consistently to be associated with increasing likelihood for UI. Aggazzotti reported that the risk of UI increased by 1.34 times every 5 years (OR 1.34, 95% CI 1.02–1.51) in the general population [4]. Astudy on the elderly by Brown and co-workers found similar odds for each 5 years of advancing age (OR 1.3, 95% CI 1.2–1.5) [50]. A study by Nelson et al. found a more modest association (OR 1.03, 95% CI 1.02–1.04) [6].

An almost linear correlation between age and risk for UI is found among men. For women, however, a somewhat different pattern has emerged from several studies [12, 51, 52]. A peak in the prevalence of UI among women in the range of 30–36% is seen during the middle ages of 50–60 years. A second peak is found in older age greater than 65 years.

Race and Ethnicity

Evidence is increasing on the effect of race in the prevalence of UI. Several studies have established race as a significant predictor for UI [53, 54] and a significant association between race and the type of UI (see Table 1.1). Specifically, Caucasian whites were found to be at a higher risk for SUI compared to African-Americans and Asians. Brown and co-workers found Caucasians nearly 3× at risk for SUI compared to nonwhites (RR 2.8, 95% CI 1.6–5.0) [55].

Urodynamic findings of lower maximal urethral closing pressures and lower resting and straining urethral angles found among Caucasians compared to African-Americans support this difference in prevalence [56, 57]. Howard and co-workers compared white and black nulliparous women using urodynamics and MRI of the pelvic floor [58]. They found that blacks had 21% greater urethral volume measured by MRI. Blacks also were noted to have 29% higher mean urethral closure pressure and 14% higher mean maximum urethral closure

TABLE 1.1. Studies comparing odds ratio for urinary incontinence among women of different races.

Study	Odds ratio (95% CI)				
	Blacks	Hispanics	Asians	Caucasians	Non-whites
Danforth 2006 [60]	0.49 (0.4–0.6)	Not significant	0.57 (0.46–0.72)	Reference	
Lewis 2005 [59]	0.46 (0.38–0.56)	0.69 (0.52–0.92)	Not studied	Reference	
Grodstein 2003 [61]	0.39 (0.31–0.50)	0.75 (0.56–1.00)	0.79 (0.61–1.02)	Reference	
Nygaard 2003 [80]	Severe UI 0.30 (0.19–0.46)	Severe UI 0.29 (0.15–0.53)	Not studied	Reference	
	Mild UI 0.42 (0.31–0.56)	Mild UI 0.50 (0.34–0.74)			
Melville 2005 [12]				Reference	0.68 (0.54–0.86)
Brown 1999 [55]				2.8 (1.6–5.0)	Reference

pressure, suggesting greater urethral sphincter capacity. There also was 17% greater levator ani muscle cross-sectional area at the level of the midurethra and 24% greater pelvic floor muscle strength.

Correlated with this finding was the report of Melville that indicated nonwhites to be 32% less prone to have UI (RR 0.68, 95% CI 0.54–0.86) [11]. The Health and Retirement Study, which investigated older women in Florida, likewise reported 54% (RR 0.46, 95% CI 0.38–0.56) and 31% (RR 0.69, 95% CI 0.52–0.92) lesser risk of UI among blacks and Hispanics, respectively [59]. The Nurses' Health Study found a similar trend among blacks (RR 0.49, 95% CI 0.4–0.6) but did not find any lesser risk for Hispanics [60]. One study even cited Hispanics having the highest age-adjusted UI prevalence compared to the other racial groups (Hispanics, whites, blacks, Asian-Americans: 38, 30, 25, 19%, respectively) [54]. Asians also were protected against UI by 43% (RR 0.57, 95% CI 0.46–0.72) [60]. An earlier report of the Nurses' Health Study in 2003 showed similar findings [61].

A higher risk of UUI was found in African-Americans [53]. Duong explained this as a result of the lower MCC in the urodynamic studies of black women. On the other hand, Sze found similar rates of UUI among blacks, whites, and Hispanics (19% vs. 16% vs. 16%, $p = 0.214$) [62].

No evidence was found to demonstrate any the effect of race on UI prevalence among men, as all studies on the topic have been limited to women.

Parity

One of the most consistent determinants of UI in women is parity. Partial denervation of the pelvic floor muscle resulting from pudendal nerve damage during childbearing is theorized to be responsible for the association between UI and parity. The results of several observational studies on UI prevalence among women support such an association.

In a population-based survey of elderly women, Brown et al. found 30% higher odds for parous women to report UI compared to nulliparous women [50]. Similarly, Hagglund and co-workers found that UI was more common among those who have given birth to one child (27% vs. 23%, $p < 0.001$) and among those who had two children

(42% vs. 23%, $p < 0.001$) compared to nulliparous women [51]. In the Nurses' Health Survey, increasing odds for UI was found with each additional birth [60]. Ushiroyama, in a study of 3,046 post-menopausal women who consulted at a gynecology clinic, found a significantly higher prevalence among the parous women, particularly those who have given birth to three to four children [63].

Mode of Delivery and Other Obstetrical Factors

One of the more controversial factors being studied as a predictor of UI in women is the mode of child delivery. Vaginal birth has been closely linked with UI in women and several pathophysiological mechanisms have been proposed to justify such an association. These include tissue damage resulting in impaired bladder neck support and the myogenic changes of the levator ani muscles, including fibrosis. During caesarean delivery, the female pelvis is spared from these insults.

Foldspang, in a study of women in the Danish registry, noted increased prevalence of UI among women who had given birth vaginally compared to those who did not (22.9% vs. 9.0%) [30]. He also noted UI immediately following vaginal childbirth (OR = 4.3, 95% CI 3.3–5.7) and incontinence during pregnancy (OR = 2.2, 95% CI 1.2–4.1) as strong predictors of long-term SUI.

Although a majority of studies lendsupport to the adverse effect of vaginal delivery on a woman's continence, the impact of caesarean delivery on the risk for UI is not certain. Several papers have shown that caesarean delivery is protective [34, 64], with a lesser risk for UI among those who had caesarean deliveries compared to those who delivered vaginally.

Farrell prospectively studied 484 primaparous women and noted higher risk of UI at 6 months for patients who had spontaneous vaginal delivery compared to those who had caesarean delivery (RR 2.1, 95% CI 1.1–3.7), for patients who had forceps delivery compared to those who had spontaneous vaginal delivery (RR 1.5, 95%CI 1.0–2.3), and for patients who had caesarean delivery (RR 3.1, 95% CI 1.7–5.9) [34]. Caesarean delivery protected against UI (RR 0.6, 95% CI 0.3–1.0).

In a prospective study of more than 700 pregnant women, Mason found no significant difference in the prevalence of SUI in women who had a normal vaginal delivery compared to those who had an instrumental delivery [29]. There was a significant reduction, however, in the prevalence of SUI in women who had a caesarean section.

McKinnie, in contrast, noted that those who delivered by caesarean section exclusively did not have a significantly different UI prevalence from those who had one vaginal delivery [65]. As some women who had had a caesarean section reported symptoms of SUI, it appears that the protective effect is not absolute. It is suggested that the protective effect of caesarean delivery may be only for the short term, so that the longer the interval from delivery to survey, the difference in UI was not significant [66]. Wilson et al. found that the protective effect of caesarean delivery is lost after three deliveries [64].

Other obstetric techniques (episiotomy, forceps, perineal suturing) were not associated with UI in the multivariate analysis of several studies [30, 32]. In contrast, Viktrup noted episiotomy during the first delivery doubled the risk of having persistent SUI 5 years after the delivery (OR 2.0, 95% CI 0.9–4.1) [21]. Vacuum extraction, on the other hand, was associated with increased odds of nearly 3× (OR 2.9, 95% CI 1.1–7.7).

Menopause

There is conflicting evidence from cross-sectional surveys on the association between menopause and UI in women. Some studies report a significant association [67, 68], while others do not [54, 69].

Prospective longitudinal studies present more consistent evidence. The Melbourne Women's Midlife Health Project prospectively studied the association of problems with control of urine and the menopausal transition over 7 years. It found that becoming menopausal was not associated with increased incidence of UI [70]. A survey by Chen and co-workers of 1,253 randomly selected women in the community yielded a similar conclusion that storage dysfunctions, including UI, were not affected by the pre- to postmenopausal transition, but rather are closely associated with aging changes [71].

Hysterectomy

Hysterectomy may cause damage to the urethral and bladder supportive structures or to the pelvic nerve plexus, which in turn may lead to UI. Indeed, Brown and co-workers reported 40% higher odds (OR 1.4, 95% CI 1.1–1.6) [55] for hysterectomized elderly women to report UI than those who were not. Similar odds were reported by Danforth (OR 1.23, 95% CI 1.13–1.33) [60].

As a contrasting point, hysterectomy was not found to be associated with UI by Holtendahl and co-workers, who offered the explanation that hysterectomy removes the weight of the uterus and so may diminish pressure on urethra-supporting structures [72].

Obesity

Numerous studies have investigated the relationship of UI occurrence and obesity or increased body mass index (BMI). The stress placed on the pelvic floor by the abdominal contents is the primary factor identified in the pathophysiology of incontinence among overweight people. Richter reported a striking 66.9% prevalence of UI among 180 morbidly obese women awaiting weight loss surgery [73]. The Health and Retirement study demonstrated that women with increased BMI had a greater risk for mild (OR 1.17, 95% CI 1.07–1.27) and severe UI (OR 1.44, 95% CI 1.26–1.64) [59]. Brown reported obesity as having a 16% attributable risk proportion for UI, with those who havehigher BMI having increased odds of 1.6 (OR 1.6, 95% CI 1.4–1.7) [50].

Cognitive and Functional Impairment

Particularly in the older population, limits in cognition and functional impairment have been associated with higher occurrences of UI. In a study of community-dwelling frail elderly people, Landi demonstrated limitations in activities of daily living (ADL) to be independent predictors of UI in both men and women [28]. Urinary incontinence was found to be 2–5× more likely in those with impairments in ADL. A survey of Mexican-Americans 65 years and older showed a significant association between UI and impaired ADL (OR 1.4, 95% CI 1.0–2.0) [17]. A similar relationship was reported by Holroyd-Leduc (OR 1.31, 95% CI 1.05–1.63) [74]. The elderly persons who had suffered a stroke were 27–37% more likely to be found to be incontinent [28]. Among stroke patients, those with moderate to severe paresis were 3× more at risk of having UI (OR 3.1, 95% CI 0.9–10.4) than those with mild to no paresis [75].

The prevalence of UI increases significantly with a worsening of mental status. Several studies in the elderly population have shown that those with impaired cognition had increased odds of having incontinence. A comprehensive study of stroke patients by Jorgensen demonstrated a tendency for older people with UI to have lower Mini-Mental State Examination (MMSE) scores (OR 2.8, 95% CI 0.9–8.6) [76]. A survey of nursing home residents by Nelson demonstrated a 50% increased likelihood for those with dementia to have UI (OR 1.5, 95% CI 1.2–1.7) [6]. Aggazzotti stated that nursing home residents lacking mental orientation had an almost fourfold increased risk (OR 3.61, 95% CI 2.42–5.39) [4]. Landi showed that for the frail elderly living in the community, both men and women with higher cognitive performance scale scores (i.e. greater impairment) were 2–6× more likely to have UI [28]. Elderly females suffering from delirium were found to have 66% higher odds of being incontinent (OR 1.66, 95% CI 1.31–2.11) [54].

Smoking

Smoking is one of the factors for UI occurrence found in several studies. The repeated stress on the pelvic floor with chronic coughing associated with smoking is believed to be the reason for this finding. A survey of more than 1,500 Mexican-American women of 65 years and older demonstrated a more than twofold increase in the prevalence of UI among smokers (OR 2.1, 95% CI 1.5–2.8) [17]. The SWAN study [2] found current smokers to have a greater likelihood of moderate to severe incontinence (OR 1.38, 95% CI 1.04–1.82). The Nurses Health Study reported very similar odds ratio (OR 1.34, 95% CI 1.25–1.45) [60]. A study on postpartum women found smoking to be a strong predictor of UI, with smokers at 3× higher odds (OR 2.9, 95% CI 1.37–3.85) of having UI 1 year after childbirth [31].

Estrogen–Hormone Replacement

Elderly women on oral estrogens were found to be 90% more likely to report UI than those who were not (OR 1.9, 95% CI 1.5–2.4). A similar risk (OR 2.0, 95% CI 1.3–3.1) was found in 1,584 women surveyed by Jackson and co-workers [76]. Samuelsson found women on estrogen replacement therapy almost 3× at risk of having UI (OR 2.9, 95% CI 1.4–5.9) [22]. Hagglund found higher estrogen use in women more than 50 years of age with UI compared to those without [51]. The Melbourne Women's Midlife Health Project also showed a higher prevalence of UI among women receiving hormone replacement therapy compared to those who did not (23% vs. 15%) [70].

The strongest evidence in literature relating hormone replacement with UI in women is seen in the placebo-controlled clinical trials on estrogen replacement on menopausal women. After 3 years of hormone replacement, significant differences in the prevalence of UI were noted between those receiving estrogen (28.1% vs. 19.1%) and combination estrogen–progesterone (25.5% vs. 14.1%) compared to the respective placebo groups [77]. A 3-year trial using estrogen as the standard comparator for a drug for osteoporosis among menopausal women showed a significantly higher UI rate in the group receiving estrogen compared to the placebo group (7.0% vs. 1.3%) [78].

Depression

Using data from a large population-based survey, the Health and Retirement Survey found that depression was significantly associated with the prevalence of UI [11, 71, 79–81]. Women with severe incontinence were 80% more likely to be depressed (OR 1.82, 95% CI 1.26–2.63), whereas for women with mild incontinence the risk of depression was 40% higher compared to those with no incontinence (OR 1.41, 95% CI 1.06–1.87). In a survey of nuns, Buchsbaum found a strong association between UI and depression (OR 2.96, 95% CI 1.21–7.55) [79].

Diabetes Mellitus

Physiological, microvascular, and neurological complications of diabetes mellitus may result in changes that impair the function for the continence mechanism. Several studies have reported consistent results supporting this, citing 20–63% increase in risk for UI among diabetics compared to nondiabetics.

The large-scale longitudinal Nurses' Health Study showed that diabetics were 28% more at risk (RR 1.28, 95% CI 1.18–1.39) of having UI than those who were not diabetic [81]. It also showed a 21% higher chance of developing incident UI (RR 1.21, 95% CI 1.03–1.43) associated with diabetes mellitus. The Health and Retirement Study, which surveyed more than 10,000 women aged 50–90 years, found an impressive 63% greater risk of having UI among insulin-requiring diabetics (RR 1.63, 95% CI 1.28–2.09) and a more modest 20% increase in chance among non–insulin-requiring diabetics compared to nondiabetics [59]. The SWAN study showed a 53% greater likelihood of UI among diabetics (OR 1.55, 95% CI 1.12–2.10) [2].

Caffeine and Alcohol Intake

The impact of consumption of caffeine and alcohol on the occurrence of UI has been the subject of few studies. The ability of caffeine to produce an excitatory effect on the detrusor smooth muscle and induce a transient contraction has been cited as the possible mechanism to explain the significant association between detrusor instability and high caffeine intake [82]. The EPICONT study had found that tea drinkers were slightly at a higher risk for all types of UI. On the other hand, coffee had no effect on UI risk [83]. A community survey of nearly 5,000 Chinese women over 20 years of age showed a significant relationship between alcohol consumption and SUI (OR 4.7, 95% CI = 1.1–20.2) [84]. However, the majority of the epidemiological surveys in the rest of the published literature have not found any association between coffee, tea, or alcohol intake and UI [9, 11, 55].

Help Seeking for Incontinence

Despite high prevalence rates of UI, less than 30% of affected people seek consultation [2, 5, 8–10, 12, 52, 63]. Women, compared to men, were more likely to discuss the problem with their doctor [8]. Severity of incontinence was strongly associated with the likelihood of seeking help from a health care provider. Those suffering from UUI were more likely to seek consult [63].

Impact of UI on the Quality of Life

Urinary incontinence, though not life-threatening, is acknowledged to be of considerable burden to the affected individuals and their families. Incontinence sufferers reported more physical discomfort, were more worried about their health, were more troubled and more frequently were hindered in their social activities compared to individuals who did not suffer from incontinence. More severe UI was significantly associated with higher BII scores, i.e., lower quality of life [85]. Lower quality of life scores [86] and lower SF36 scores [7] were found among individuals with UI. Kocak reported that incontinence had a severe impact on the quality of life in 12% of those with the condition [9].

Urinary Incontinence and Mortality

Several studies involving the older population did not find UI to be significantly associated with either 2- or 6-year mortality rates [24, 25, 59]. Likewise, a study on more than 7,000 community-dwelling people aged 70 years and above failed to show UI to be an independent predictor of mortality (OR 0.90, 95% CI 0.67–1.21). Instead, UI was found to be marker of frailty [87]. Nakanishi, on the other hand, found that severe incontinence increased the risk for mortality even after adjustment for potential confounders [88].

Conclusion

Urinary incontinence is a common condition affecting the entire adult population, although certain groups are identified as having higher prevalence rates. These include the elderly, pregnant and postpartum women, andmen who underwent prostatectomy. Several risk factors have been associated with an increased likelihood of UI occurrence, including age, parity, smoking, obesity, hormone therapy with estrogens, diabetes mellitus, depression, and cognitive and functional impairment. Urinary incontinence impacts greatly on the quality of life and may be a signal of poor health status, particularly in the elderly.

References

1. Hampel C, Artibani W, Espuna M, et al. Understanding the burden of stress urinary incontinence in Europe: A qualitative review of the literature. Eur Urol 2004; 46:15–27.

2. Sampselle C, Harlow S, Skurnick J, et al. Urinary incontinence predictors and life impact in ethnically diverse perimenopausel women. Obstet Gynecol 2002; 100(6):1230–1238.

3. Hunskaar S, Burgio K, Clark A, et al. Epidemiology of urinary and faecal incontinence and pelvic organ prolapse. In: Abrams P, Cardozo L, Khoury S, Wein A, editors. Incontinence 3rd edn. Paris: Health Publication, 2005:255–312.

4. Aggazzotti G, Pesce F, Grassi D, et al. Prevalence of urinary incontinence among institutionalized patients: A cross-sectional epidemiologic study in a midsized city in northern Italy. Urology 200; 56(2):245–249.

5. Ueda T, Tamaki M, Kageyama S, et al. Urinary incontinence among community dwelling people aged 40 years or older in Japan: Prevalence risk factors, knowledge and self-perception. Int J Urol 2000; 7:95–103.

6. Nelson R, Fumer S, Jesudason V. Urinary incontinence in Wisconsin skilled nursing facilities: Prevalence and associations in common with fecal incontinence. J Aging Health 2001; 13(4):539–47.

7. Roe B, Doll H. Prevalence of urinary incontinence and its relationship with health status. J Clin Nur 2000; 9(2):178–87.

8. Muscatello DJ, Rissel C, Szonyi G. Urinary symptoms and incontinence in an urban community: Prevalence and associated factor in older men and women. Intern Med J 2001;31:151—160.

9. Kocak I, Okyay P, Dundar M, et al. Female urinary incontinence in the west of Turkey: Prevalence, risk factors and impact on quality of life. Eur Urol 2005; 48:634–641.

10. Hunskaar S, Lose G, Sykes D, et al. The prevalence of urinary incontinence in woman in four European countries. BJU Int 2004; 93:324–330.

11. Melville J, Katon W, Delaney K, et al. Urinary incontinence in US women: A population-based study. Arch Intern Med 2005; 165:537–542.

12. Hannestad Y, Rortviet G, Sandvik H, Hunskaar S. A community-based epidemiological survey of female urinary incontinence. J Clin Epidemiol 2000; 53:1150–1157.

13. Tubaro A. Defining overactive bladder: Epidemiology and burden of disease. Urology 2004; 64(6 Suppl):2–6.

14. Damian J, Martin-Moreno JM, Lobo F, et al. Prevalence of urinary incontinence among Spanish older people living at home. Eur Urol 1998; 34(4):333–338.

15. Diokno A, Brock B, Brown M, et al. Prevalence of urinary incontinence and other urological symptoms in the noninstitutionalized elderly. J Urol 1986; 136(5):1022–1025.

16. Schulman C, Claes H, Matthis J. Urinary incontinence in Belgium: A population-based epidemiological survey. Eur Urol 1997; 32(3):315–320.

17. Espino D, Palmer R, Miles T, et al. Prevalence and severity urinary incontinence in elderly Mexican-American woman. J Am Geriatr Soc 2003; 51: 1580–1586.

18. Jackson S, Scholes D, Boyko E, et al. Urinary incontinence and diabetes in postmenopausal women. Diabetes Care 2005; 28:1730–1738.

19. Thom D. Variation in estimate of urinary incontinence prevalence in the community: Effects of difference in definition, population characteristics and study type. J Am Geriatr Soc 1998; 46(4):1–15.

20. Dallosso H, Matthews R, McGrother C, et al. Diet as a risk factor for the development of stress urinary incontinence: A longitudinal study in women. Eur J Clin Nutrition 2004; 58:920–926.

21. Viktrup L, Lose G. The risk of stress incontinence 5 years after first delivery. Am J Obstet Gynecol 2001; 185(1):1–10.

22. Samuelsson E, Arne Victor F.T, Svardsudd K. Five-year incidence and remission rates of female urinary incontinence in a Swedish population less than 65 years old. Am J Obstet Gynecol 2000; 183(3):1–12.

23. Moller LA, Lose G, Jorgensen T. Incidence and remission rates of lower urinary tract symptoms at one year in women aged 40–60: Longitudinal study. BMJ 2000; 320:1429–1432.

24. Herzog AR, Diokno AC, Brown MB, et al. Two-year incidence, remission, and change patterns of urinary incontinence in noninstitutionalized older adults. J Gerontol 1990; 45(2):M67–M74

25. McGrother C, Resnick M, Yalla S, et al. Epidemiology and etiology of urinary incontinence in the elderly. World J Urol 1998; 16:S3–S9.

26. Giorgiou A, Potter J, Brocklehurst J. Measuring the quality of urinary continence care in long term care facilities: An analysis of outcome indicators. Age Ageing 2001; 30:63–66.

27. Toba K, Ouchi Y, Orimo H, et al. Urinary incontinence in elderly inpatients in Japan: A comparison between general and geriatric hospitals. Aging 1996; 8(1):47–54.

28. Landi F, Cesari M, Russo A, Onder G, et al. Potentially reversible risk factors and urinary incontinence in frail older people living in community. Age Ageing 2003; 32:194—199.

29. Mason L, Glenn S, Walton I, et al. The prevalence of stress incontinence during pregnancy and following delivery. Midwifery 1999; 15:120—128.

30. Foldspang A, Hvidman L, Mommsen S, et al. Risk of postpartum urinary incontinence associated with pregnancy and mode of delivery. Acta Obstet Gynecol Scand 2004; 83:923–927.

31. Burgio K, Zyczynski H, Locher J, et al. Urinary incontinence in the 12-month postpartum period. Obstet Gynecol 2003; 102:1291–1298.

32. Chaliha C, Kalia V, Stanton S, et al. Antenatal prediction urinary and fecal incontinence. Obstet Gynecol 1999; 94(5):689–694.

33. Hvidman L, Foldspang A, Mommsen A, et al. Postpartum urinary incontinence. Acta Obstet Gynecol Scand 2003; 82:556–563.

34. Farrell S, Allen V, Baskett T. Parturition and urinary incontinence in primiparas. Obstet Gynecol 2001; 97(3):350–356.

35. Donnellan S, Duncan H, MacGregor, et al. Prospective assessment of incontinence after radical retropubic prostatectomy: Objective and subjective analysis. Urology 1997; 49:225–230.

36. Ojdeby G, Claezon A, Brekkan E, et al. Urinary incontinence and sexual impotence after radical prostatectomy. Scand J Urol Nephrol 1996; 30:473–477.

37. McCammon K, Kolm P, Main B, et al. Comparative quality of life analysis after radical prostatectomy or external beam radiation for localized prostate cancer. Urology 1999; 54:509–516.

38. Walsh P, Marschke P, Ricker D, et al. Patient-reported urinary continence and sexual function after anatomic radical prostatectomy. Urology 2000; 55:58–61.

39. Horie S, Tobisu K, Fujimoto H, et al. Urinary incontinence after non–nerve-sparing radical prostatectomy with neoadjuvant androgen deprivation. Urology 1999; 53:561–567.

40. Goluboff ET, Saidi JA, Mazer S, et al. Urinary continence after radical prostatectomy: The Columbia experience. J Urol 1998; 159:1276–1280.

41. Lowe BA. Comparison of bladder neck preservation to bladder neck resection in maintaining post-prostatectomy urinary incontinence. Urology 1996; 48:889–893.

42. Weldon VE, Tavel FR, Neuwirth H. Continence, potency and morbidity after radical perineal prostatectomy. J Urol 1997; 158:1470–145.

43. Gray M, Petroni G, Theodorescu D. Urinary function after radical prostatectomy: A comparison of the retropubic and perineal approaches. Urology 1999; 53:881–891.

44. Bishoff JT, Motley G, Optenberg SA, et al. Incidence of fecal and urinary incontinence following radical perineal and retropubic prostatectomy in a national population. J Urol 1998; 160:454–458.

45. Eastham JA, Kattan MW, Rogers E, et al. Risk factors for urinary incontinence after radical prostatectomy. J Urol 1996; 156:1707–1713.

46. Van Kampen M, De Weerdt W, Van Poppel H, et al. Prediction of urinary continence following radical prostatectomy. Urol Int 1998; 60:80–84.

47. Poon M, Ruckle H, Bamshad DBR, et al. Radical retropubic prostatectomy: Bladder neck preservation versus reconstruction. J Urol 2000; 163:194–198.

48. Catalona WJ, Carvalhal GF, Mager DE, Smith DS. Potency, continence and complication rates in 19,870 consecutive radical retropubic prostatectomies. J Urol 1999; 162:433–438.

49. Kao TC, Garner D, Foley J, et al. Multicenter patient self-reporting questionnaire on impotence, incontinence and stricture after radical prostatectomy. J Urol 2000; 163:858–864.

50. Brown J, Seeley D, Fong J, et al. Urinary incontinence in older women: Who is at risk? Obstet Gynecol 1996; 87(5):715–721.

51. Hagglund D, Olsson H, Lepper J. Urinary incontinence: An unexpected large problem among young females. Results from a population-based study. Family Practice 1999; 16(5):506–509.

52. Lagace E, Hansen W, Hickner J. Prevalence and severity of urinary incontinence in ambulatory adult. An UPRnet study. J Fam Pract 1993; 6(6):610–614.

53. Graham C, Mallett V. Race as a predictor of urinary incontinence and pelvic organ prolapse. Am J Obstet Gynecol 2001; 185(1):1–8.

54. Thom D, Van den Eeden S, Ragins A, et al. Differences in prevalence of urinary incontinence by race/ethnicity. J Urol 2006; 175(1):259–264.

55. Brown J, Grady D, Ouslander J, et al. Prevalence of urinary incontinence and associated risk factors in postmenopausal women. Obstet Gynecol 1999; 94(1):66–70.

56. Duong T, Korn A. A comparison of urinary incontinence among African-American, Asian, Hispanic, and white women. Am J Obstet Gynecol 2001; 184(6):1083–1086.

57. Mattox TF, Bhatia NN The prevalence of urinary incontinence or prolapse among white and Hispanic women. Am J Obstet Gynecol 1996; 174(2):646–648.

58. Howard D, Delancey J, Tunn R, et al. Racial differences in the structure and function of the stress urinary continence mechanism. Obstet Gynecol 2000; 95(5):713–717.

59. Lewis C, Schrader R, Many A, et al. Diabetes and urinary incontinence in 50- to 90-year-old women: A cross-sectional population-based study. Am J Obstet Gynecol 2005; 193:2154–2158.

60. Danforth K, Townsend M, Lifford K, et al. Risk factors for urinary incontinence among middle-aged women. Am J Obstet Gynecol 2006; 194:339–345.

61. Grodstein F, Fretts R, Lifford K, et al. Association of age, race, and obstetric history with urinary symptoms

among women in the Nurses' Health Study. Am J Obstet Gynecol 2003; 189(2):428–434.

62. Sze E, Jones W, Ferguson J, et al. Prevalence of urinary incontinence symptoms among black, white and hispanic women. Obstet Gynecol 2002; 99(4):572–575.

63. Ushiroyama T, Ikeda A, Ueki M. Prevalence, incidence and awareness in the treatment of menopausal urinary incontinence. Maturitas 1999; 33:127–132.

64. Wilson PD, Herbison R, Herbison G, et al. Obstetric practice and the prevalence of urinary incontinence 3 months after delivery. Br J Obstet Gynecol 1996; 103:154–161.

65. McKinnie V, Swift SE, Wang W, et al. The effect of pregnancy and mode of delivery on the prevalence of urinary and fecal incontinence. Am J Obstet Gynecol 2005; 193:512–518.

66. MacLennan AH, Taylor AW, Wilson DH, et al. The prevalence of pelvic floor discorders and their relationship to gender, age, parity and mode of delivery. Br J Obstet Gynecol 2000; 107(12):1460–1470.

67. Vinker S, Kaplan B, Nakar S, et al. Urinary incontinence in women: Prevalence, characteristics and effect on quality of life. A primary care clinic study. Isr Med Assoc J 2001; 3(9):663–668.

68. Kuh D, Cardozo L, Hardy R. Urinary incontinence in middle aged women: Childhood enuresis and other lifetime risk factors in a British prospective cohort. J Epidemiol Commun Health 1999; 53(8):453–458.

69. Dolan L, Casson K, McDonald P, Ashe R. Urinary incontinence in Northern Ireland: A prevalence study. BJU Int 1999; 83:760–766.

70. Sherburn M, Guthrie J, Dudley E, et al. Is incontinence associated with menopause? Obstet Gynecol 2001; 98(4):628–633.

71. Chen YC, Chen GD, Hu SW, et al. Occurrence of storage and voiding dysfunction affected by menopausal transition or associated with the normal ageing process. Menopause 2003; 10(3):203–208.

72. Holtendahl K, Hunskaar S. Prevalence, 1-year incidence and factors associated with urinary incontinence: A population based study of women 50–74 years of age in primary care. Maturitas 1998; 28:205–211.

73. Richter H, Burgio K, Clements R, et al. Urinary and anal incontinence in morbidly obese women considering weight loss surgery. Obstet Gynecol 2005; 106(6):1272–1277.

74. Holroyd-Leduc J, Mehta K, Covinsky K. Urinary incontinence and its association with death, nursing home admission and functional decline. J Am Geriatr Soc 2004; 52:712–718.

75. Jorgensen L, Engstad T, Jacobsen B. Self-reported urinary incontinence in noninstitutionalized long-term stroke survivors: A population-based study. Arch Phys Med Rehab 2005; 86:416–420.

76. Jackson S, Scholes D, Boyko E, et al. Urinary incontinence and diabetes in postmenopausal women. Diabetes Care 2005;18:1730—1738.

77. Hendrix S, Cochrane B, Nygaard I, et al. Understanding the burden of stress urinary incontinence in Europe: A qualitative review of the literature. Eur Urol 2004; 46:15–27.

78. Goldstein S, Johnson S, Watts, et al. Incidence of urinary incontinence in postmenopausal women treated with raloxifene or estrogen. Menopause 2005; 12(2):160–164.

79. Buchsbaum G, Chin M, Glantz C, Guzick D. Prevalence of urinary incontinence and associated risk factors in a cohort of nuns. Obstet Gynecol 2002; 100(2):226–229.

80. Nygaard I, Turvey C, Burn T, et al. Urinary incontinence and depression in middle-aged United States women. Obstet Gynecol 2003;101:49–56

81. Lifford K, Curhan G, Hu F, et al. Type 2 diabetes mellitus and risk of developing urinary incontinence. J Am Geriatr Soc 2005; 53:1851–1857.

82. Arya, L, Myers D, Jackson N. Dietary caffeine intake and the risk for detrusor instability: A case-control study. Obstet Gynecol 2000; 96:85–89.

83. Hannestad YS, Rortveit G, Daltveit AK, Hunskaar S. Are smoking and other lifestyle factors associated with female urinary incontinence? The Norwegian EPINCONT Study. Br J Obstet Gynecol 2003; 110(3):247–254.

84. Song, YF, Zhang WJ, Song J, Xu B.Prevalence and risk factors of urinary incontinence in Fuzhou Chinese women. Chin Med J (Engl) 2005; 118(11):887–892.

85. Vandoninck V, Bemelmans B, Mazzetta C, et al. The prevalence of urinary incontinence in community-dwelling married women: A matter of definition. BJU Int 2004; 94(9):1291–1295.

86. Araki I, Beppu M, Kajiwara M, et al. Prevalence and impact of generic quality of life of urinary incontinence in Japanese working women: Assessment by ICI-Q questionnaire and SF-36 health survey. Urology 2005; 66:88–93.

87. Holroyd-Leduc J, Mehta K, Covinsky K. Urinary incontinence and its association with death, nursing home admission and functional decline. J Am Geriatr Soc 2004;52:712–718.

88. Nakanishi N, Tatara K, Shinsho F, et al. Mortality in relation to urinary and faecal incontinence in elderly people living at home. Age Ageing 199; 28:301–306.

Part II
Current Concepts on Anatomy and Physiology

Chapter 2
Neurophysiology of Micturition: What's New?

Apostolos Apostolidis and Clare J. Fowler

Central Control of Micturition

The apparently simple repertoire of bladder function comprising the storage and periodic elimination of urine is under the complex regulatory control of a neural system that involves three sets of peripheral nerves (the T11–L2 originating sympathetic hypogastric nerves, the S2–S4 originating parasympathetic pelvic nerves and the sacral somatic pudendal nerves) [1–3], the sacral spinal cord, and the higher brain centers located in the brain stem, diencephalon, and cerebral cortices. The central nervous system centers not only allow for the perception of bladder fullness but also determine the "correctness" implicated in the social part of the micturition act and coordinate the activities of the striated and smooth muscles involved in the micturition reflex. Such coordination is achieved via a series of locally organized reflexes that use all these types of peripheral nerves, interneurons, and vesical parasympathetic ganglia to convey inhibitory and excitatory input to maintain a reciprocal relationship between the bladder and the urethral outlet [4].

Animal experiments in the cat have shown that in spinal health, sensory stimuli associated with the sensation of bladder fullness ascend via the spinal cord to an integrative brain center—the periaquaeductal grey (PAG)—and are relayed to the pontine micturition center (PMC), which promotes micturition via excitatory parasympathetic outflow to the bladder [5, 6]. In humans, the use of functional imaging technology such as single photon emis-

sion computerized tomography (SPECT), positron emission tomography (PET) [7–12], and functional magnetic resonance imaging (fMRI) [13] confirmed that the PAG and the PMC are key centers in the supraspinal control of micturition and continence. In addition to the former centers, areas such as the anterior cingulate gyrus, the prefrontal cortex, and the insula appear to be involved in the perception of a full versus empty bladder. One study reported that activation of the medial premotor cortex, basal ganglia, and cerebellum may be involved in continence in health [13], whereas another study showed the thalamus was also activated when the bladder was full [11]. A schematic representation of possible connections between the brain areas that appear to be involved in micturition control is given in Fig. 2.1 (adapted from [14]).

Functional imaging techniques are now being applied in pathological conditions. Women with urinary retention due to a primary disorder of urethral sphincter relaxation (Fowler's syndrome) had activation of cortical regions without midbrain or brain stem activity, in contrast to control subjects [12]. Activity in the latter two areas was normalized following sacral nerve stimulation [12]. Increased activation of cortical areas but with a weak activation of the orbitofrontal cortex was seen in patients with idiopathic detrusor overactivity (IDO) on filling as opposed to strong activation of the orbitofrontal cortex seen in control subjects [15]. Activation of the primary motor cortex, the cerebellum, and the cingulate gyrus also was seen in patients with urgency incontinence during the first hours of sacral

17

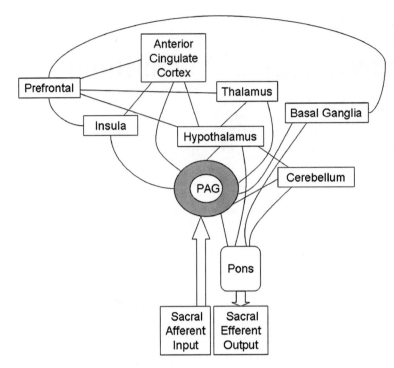

FIG. 2.1. Schematic representation of possible connections and interactions existing among various brain structures thought to be involved in micturition control (as in reference [14]). The exact direction of interactions has yet to be clarified. PAG = Periaqueductal gray

neuromodulation [16]. The significance of these findings are being further investigated in light of results from anxiety provocation studies showing activation of similar areas in the prefrontal, cingulate, and insular regions [17]. Similarly, studies on the effect of distraction on painful conditions showed activation of the PAG and the prefrontal, cingulate, and thalamic areas [18].

Reflex Mechanisms Involved in Micturition Control

The bladder and the urethral sphincters exhibit excitatory and inhibitory interactions via a series of reflexes that are either organized at a spinal level or have a more complicated central organization involving spinal and spinobulbospinal pathways. Reflexes promoting urine storage are served by sympathetic and somatic (pudendal) nerves that mediate efferent input to the urethral sphincter and inhibitory input to the bladder, whereas reflexes promoting micturi-

tion are served by parasympathetic nerves mediating efferent input to the detrusor and inhibitory input to the urethral sphincters [19].

Evidence to support the presence of such reflexes in humans has been provided by urodynamic studies [20]. During filling cystometry, a low detrusor pressure is maintained until micturition threshold is reached, in parallel with an increase in urethral electromyographic activity. It is thought that parasympathetic afferent firing from the bladder during filling activates the external urethral sphincter via a synapse with sacral interneurons, which results in stimulation of the pudendal urethral efferents (the "guarding reflex"). In addition, in some species a sympathetically mediated reflex is believed to inhibit detrusor contraction and promote urethral smooth muscle contraction during bladder filling [4, 21]. When micturition threshold is reached and voiding is initiated, urethral sphincter activity ceases first, followed by a rise in detrusor pressure due to detrusor contraction and flow of urine. Micturition is further promoted by a bladder-to-bladder excitatory reflex and a bladder-to-urethral sphincter inhibitory reflex, which are activated when the bladder is full [4, 21].

The role of interneurons at various levels of the spinal cord appears to be central in the regulation of reflex activity, serving as integrating areas of afferent projections from both the bladder and the urethra [4, 21]. Using interneuronal pathways, pudendal afferent activity from the urethral sphincter and also from other urogenital sites can inhibit the excitatory parasympathetic outflow to the bladder. In support, stimulation of pudendal afferents has been shown to successfully suppress the sensation of urgency [22] and improve urodynamic parameters [23] in patients with IDO and urgency incontinence. Similarly, peripheral afferent stimulation (tibial nerve) effectively controlled symptoms of overactive bladder [24]. It has been recently proposed that a bladder–sphincter–bladder reflex pathway in which the bladder-to-external urethral sphincter excitatory reflex activates the urethral sphincter-to-bladder inhibitory reflex via interneuronal synapses facilitates urine storage [4]. Inhibition of excitatory interneurons and preganglionic parasympathetic neurons are proposed as additional mechanisms contributing to suppression of bladder activity and urine storage. It is possible that such augmented inhibitory pathways constitute part of the mechanism by which urinary retention occurs in women with primary disorder of urethral sphincter relaxation (Fowler's syndrome). In contrast, activation of excitatory interneurons and preganglionic parasympathetic neurons contributes to maintenance of bladder activity until completion of bladder emptying. At the same time, activation of interneurons by bladder afferents stimulates parasympathetic efferent inhibitory activity to the urethral smooth muscle.

The complete explanation for the surprising observation that sacral nerve stimulation (SNS) is effective in the treatment of both refractory detrusor overactivity [21] and urinary retention [25] remains to be discovered. However, activation of the bladder–sphincter–bladder reflex pathway now is proposed as a possible mechanism by which SNS suppresses detrusor contraction in conditions of bladder overactivity [4, 21]. In women with urinary retention, however, the initial pathophysiology is different, i.e., an upregulated sphincter–bladder reflex. Restoration of bladder sensation

and reactivation of activity in brain areas receiving afferent input from the bladder suggests that, in these cases, SNS suppresses inhibitory interneurons and releases the bladder from that augmented sphincter–bladder reflex.

In addition to the spinal control of the micturition reflexes, various areas of the brain are believed to regulate reflex activity. In the cat, stimulation of a lateral pontine area known as "the urine storage center" results in an increase in sphincter EMG activity and inhibition of detrusor smooth muscle activity. Stimulation of a medial pontine area considered to be the "PMC" results in inhibition of sphincter EMG activity and increase in detrusor smooth muscle activity. In addition, Onuf's nucleus, which is involved in the regulation of the activity of sphincter motoneurons, receives projections from bulbospinal pathways. Research into the neurotransmitters involved in these pathways (norepinephrine, serotonin) has demonstrated facilitatory glutamatergic excitatory transmission to the sphincter motoneurons, and this resulted in the development of oral pharmacotherapy (duloxetine) for the treatment of stress urinary incontinence [26].

Peripheral Control of Micturition

Bladder sensation is conveyed by two types of afferent axons: the myelinated Aδ-fibers, which are sensitive to mechanical stimuli, e.g., distension, stretch, and the primarily nociceptive, unmyelinated C-fibers. The latter have a high mechanical threshold and do not normally respond to bladder distension but do respond to noxious stimuli, such as chemical irritation and cooling. Thus, in conditions of health, it is the Aδ-fibers that convey information about bladder filling, whereas C-fibers remain largely quiescent. Afferent nerve endings form a dense network in the bladder suburothelium (Fig. 2.2), with occasional fibers penetrating the basal lamina to appear in close apposition to urothelial cells. The efferent parasympathetic input, mediated by acetylcholine (ACh) receptors in the bladder wall, results in contraction of the detrusor muscle [19].

Detrusor overactivity is the most common urodynamic abnormality in suprasacral lesions; it occurs in patients with spinal cord injury or multiple sclerosis, and therefore it is referred to as

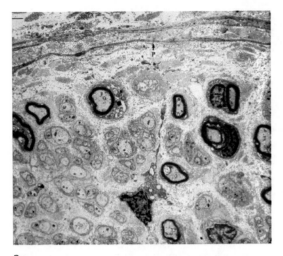 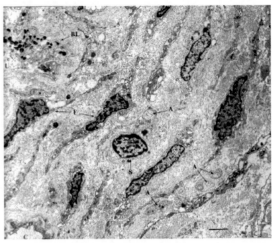

a   b

F<small>IG</small>. 2.2. Electron micrographs of the lamina propria space of the human bladder (courtesy of Professor D.N. Landon, Institute of Neurology, University College London). Bladder biopsies were obtained via a flexible cystoscope, fixed in 3% glutaraldehyde in 0.1 M Na cacodylate buffer, and processed routinely for transmission electron microscopy. Ultrathin sections were obtained from the midpoint of each biopsy specimen. (**a**) Image of a section through part of the nerve close to the inner surface of the detrusor muscle, showing small myelinated and unmyelinated axons and their Schwann cells surrounded by a thin perineurial sheath (P). (**b**) Image of a section though the superficial aspect of the lamina propria, showing the base of the urothelium (U), its basal lamina (BL), beneath which are layers of flattened fibroblasts (F) and collagen fibrils. Among the latter structures, Schwann cells (S) and unmyelinated axons (A) can be identified. Scale = 2 μm in both (**a**) and (**b**)

neurogenic detrusor overactivity (NDO). Animal studies have proposed that spinal NDO is related to the emergence of an aberrant C-fiber–driven sacral spinal reflex [27]. Following the disruption of the spinobulbospinal pathways, capsaicin-sensitive C-fiber afferents in the suburothelium undergo plastic changes, including hypertrophy related to an increase in neurofilament content, and increased excitability associated with elevated expression of tetrodotoxin-sensitive Na^{2+} channels [19], consequently becoming sensitive to mechanical stimuli (mechanosensitive). Such changes lead to increased afferent firing to the spinal cord during bladder distension, followed by increased parasympathetic input to the bladder, and thus detrusor overactivity.

Such animal observations became the basis for the use of deafferenting neurotoxins, such as capsaicin (CAPS) and resiniferatoxin (RTX), in the treatment of lower urinary tract symptoms (LUTS). Clinical and basic research results from these studies provided evidence for activation of a similar, C-fiber–mediated spinal reflex in humans with spinal NDO [19, 27]. Immunohistochemical

studies of the suburothelium of patients with spinal NDO using general neuronal markers such as PGP9.5 [28] and S100 [29] demonstrated increased suburothelial innervation in patients compared to controls. Intravesical application of either CAPS or RTX reduced the suburothelial nerve fiber density in patients who responded to treatment, suggesting a pathophysiological role of the augmented suburothelial nerve network in neurogenic overactive bladders [28, 29].

Immunohistochemical studies also have confirmed the presence of sensory receptors in suburothelial nerves, such as the capsaicin or vanilloid receptor [transient receptor potential vanilloid 1 (TRPV1)] and the ATP-gated purinergic receptor $P2X_3$ (Fig. 2.3), both of which have been associated with normal bladder mechanosensation in animal experiments [32–34]; TRPV1-deficient ($^{-/-}$) mice display enhanced short-term voluntary urination and increased frequency of non-voiding contractions on urodynamics, increased cystometric capacity, and inefficient voiding [32]. The $P2X_3^{-/-}$ mice exhibit increased cystometric capacity and

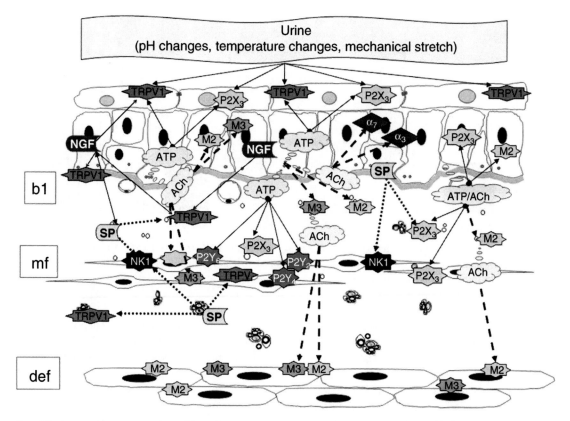

FIG. 2.3. A cartoon representation of identifiable ultrastructural components of the human bladder wall with known or proposed locations of receptors and sites of release of neuropeptides and growth factors thought to be involved in bladder mechanosensation, as updated from relevant figures in references [30] and [31]. Abbreviations: bl = basal lamina of urothelium; mf = myofibroblast layer; det = detrusor muscle, see also [30] for more detailed explanation of ultrastructural elements. It has been proposed that the urothelial–suburothelial pathways of bladder mechanosensation are served by a complex system of interactions between the release of neurotransmitters and actions on respective receptors located on these structural constituents. All connections identified by *arrows* (see [31] for *arrow* identification) are thought to be upregulated in detrusor overactivity. Identification of receptors, neuropeptides and neurotransmitters: TRPV1 – transient receptor potential vanilloid 1; $P2X_3$ – ionotropic purinergic receptor type 3; $P2Y_2/P2Y_4/P2Y_6$ – metabotropic purinergic receptors types 2, 4, and 6; M2/M3 – muscarinic acetylcholine receptors types 2 and 3; α_3/α_7 – nicotinic acetylcholine receptors types 3 and 7; NK1 – neurokinin receptor type 1 (SP receptor); SP – Substance P; NGF – Nerve growth factor; ACh – acetylcholine; ATP – adenosine triphosphate

decreased frequency of voiding [33]. Patients with NDO and, to a lesser degree, those with IDO were found to have increased TRPV1- and $P2X_3$-immunoreactive (-IR) suburothelial innervation compared to controls [28, 35, 36] (Fig. 2.4). Intravesical instillations of RTX in NDO patients resulted in dramatic decreases of TRPV1- and $P2X_3$-IR fibers only in clinical responders [28, 35] and produced significant improvements in LUTS and urodynamic parameters in some patients with IDO [37]. As previous preclinical research had

characterized CAPS and RTX as C-fiber toxins, the findings in human studies were considered to provide further evidence for a role of the suburothelial C-fiber afferents expressing TRPV1 and/or $P2X_3$ in the pathophysiology of NDO and IDO.

It recently was proposed that the TRPV1 located in synaptic vesicles in DRG neurons is coexpressed and interacts with proteins active in exocytosis, such as synaptotagmin and snapin, a colocalization that extends to the nerve axons [38]. The presence of $P2X_3$ in terminal afferent boutons with complex

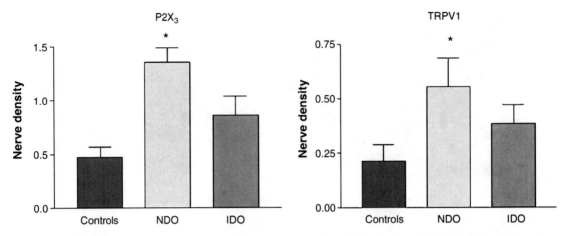

FIG. 2.4. Suburothelial nerve immunoreactivity to the sensory receptors P2X$_3$ (*left*) and TRPV1 (*right*) was found to be significantly increased in patients with NDO (* signifies a statistical *P* value of less than 0.05) and, to a lesser, statistically non-significant degree, in patients with IDO when compared to control subjects

synaptic properties [39] and its colocalization with TRPV1 in the CNS have been shown [40], and there is indirect evidence for colocalization with TRPV1 in bladder suburothelial afferents [28, 35].

Further to its role in normal and pathological sensation of bladder fullness, the capsaicin receptor TRPV1 also is known to be a thermal receptor activated by temperatures higher than 43°C. In the same superfamily of transient receptor potential (TRP) channels, another five thermoreceptors have been identified, with distinct temperature thresholds [41]. A bladder-cooling reflex has been described in animals and humans, which is thought to be mediated by C-fiber afferents [42–44]. A receptor sensitive to low temperatures and menthol that possibly mediates this reflex recently was identified and cloned: the TRPM8 receptor [45, 46]. Its presence was shown in suburothelial fiberlike structures of both fine and thicker caliber in the human bladder [47]. TRPM8 immunoreactivity was significantly increased in fine-caliber axons in patients with IDO compared to controls and the numbers of immunoreactive axons and fibers correlated significantly with frequency scores in those patients [47]. As intravesical instillation of menthol was shown to decrease threshold activation of C-fibers [43], these findings were proposed as a partial explanation for increased frequency in IDO patients [47]. Interestingly, no correlation was found with urgency scores.

Immunohistochemistry also has demonstrated the presence of the sensory neuropeptides substance

P (SP) and calcitonin gene-related peptide (CGRP) in suburothelial afferents [48, 49]. Substance P has been shown to colocalize with glutamate in primary afferent terminals [50], whereas all SP-IR fibers contain colocalized CGRP [49] and SP and CGRP are found on more than 90% of TRPV1-immunoreactive fibers that traverse the rat bladder wall [51]. Women with IDO were found to have increased density of suburothelial SP- and CGRP-immunoreactive fibers compared to controls [49], while treatment with intravesical vanilloids resulted in marked decrease of TRPV1, SP, and CGRP immunoreactivity in the bladder wall of rats [52]. Several animal studies support an association between SP-CGRP and bladder sensation; SP levels in the rat bladder were found to inversely correlate to the micturition threshold [52, 53]. Increased SP and CGRP content of spinalized rat bladders was significantly reduced after capsaicin application and was associated with a decrease in urodynamic-proven DO [54]. Increasing evidence suggests a role of these neuropeptides also in human bladder sensation, with urinary levels of SP correlating with degree of urgency or bladder pain [55–57].

Both SP and CGRP appear to be involved in LUT neuromodulation via complex central and peripheral interactions (Fig. 2.3). Neurotrophic factors such as the nerve growth factor (NGF) and the glial-derived neurotrophic factor (GDNF) regulate the expression of TRPV1 and P2X$_3$, respectively, via modulation of nociceptive dorsal root ganglion cells expressing SP and CGRP [58, 59]. Substance P also can induce directly the expression of NGF [60] and has been shown to activate the nonselective cation TRP channels via a G-protein–coupled/phospholipase C (PLC) pathway in afferent neurons [61]. Experimental data on ganglion neurons have suggested that SP, ATP, and ACh activate nonselective cation channels by a common intracellular metabolic process [62]. In turn, activation of TRPV1 on small afferent nerves, as through vanilloid application, promotes vesicular release of SP and CGRP via an ATP-P2Y–mediated pathway [63]. Further, SP has been associated with sensitization of the $P2X_3$ and heteromeric $P2X_{2/3}$ receptors to the action of ATP via protein-kinase-C–mediated phosphorylation [64].

Ultrastructural studies have shown that suburothelial nerves are packed with both clear and dense-cored vesicles, whose contents have not been identified yet (Fig. 2.5). The presence of SP has been reported in large granular synaptic vesicles in axon terminals of the rat LUT [65] and human bladder [48], and CGRP was found to colocalize with SP in synaptic vesicles in peripheral sensory nerves [66].

However, traditionally, clear vesicles are believed to contain ACh in cholinergic nerve endings [67, 68]. In addition, the association of clear vesicles with large, dense-cored vesicles also is known to occur in cholinergic nerves [69], whose terminals are reported to release ACh and ATP or a related purine [70, 71]. The presence of muscarinic ACh receptors (MAChRs) in nerve fibers in the suburothelium and mainly the detrusor recently has been demonstrated in human overactive and painful bladders [72] (Fig. 2.3). This study also has claimed the presence of MAChRs types 2 and 3 in suburothelial cells with long bipolar processes, thought to be myofibroblastlike [72]. Immmunoreactivity for both types of MAChRs in these suburothelial cells was found to be increased in IDO bladders compared to controls. Furthermore, a shift was noted in mediation of detrusor contractions in NDO bladders from M3AChRs to M2AChRs, implying a possible functional role for M2AChRs in bladder disease states [73]. In health, despite the M2AChRs outnumbering the M3AChRs by a ratio of 3:1, in vitro experiments have shown that detrusor contractions are mediated by the M3AChRs [74]. Activation of muscarinic type 1 receptors may facilitate the release of other transmitters; the facilitatory mechanisms were found to be enhanced in the rat overactive bladder [75].

Muscarinic receptors also have been identified in the human bladder urothelium [72, 76], which represents the main nonneuronal source of ACh release during bladder filling [77] (Fig. 2.3). Urothelial release of ACh increases with detrusor stretch [77]. It was proposed that in health a basal release of ACh from the urothelium during bladder filling acts on smooth muscle cells' MACh receptors to regulate bladder tone or even on MACh receptors in suburothelial nerves [77]. However, the presence of functional muscarinic receptors in the urothelium implies a possible autocrine role for urothelially released ACh, and a yet unidentified urothelium-derived inhibitory factor has been shown to be released upon stimulation of muscarinic receptors [76]. Moreover, functional nicotinic ACh receptors (nAChRs) recently were identified in the rat bladder urothelium [78] (Fig. 2.3). Two opposing nicotinic signaling pathways appear to exist: an inhibitory one mediated by type α_7 nAChRs and an excitatory one mediated by type α_3 nAChRs. It was proposed that activation of these pathways by ACh released by the urothelium takes place at different phases of bladder filling, urine storage being facilitated by activation of the inhibitory α_7 nAChRs, while voiding is promoted by activation of the excitatory α_3 nAChRs [78].

In addition to TRPV1 and $P2X_3$ [79–82], the urothelium also was found to express TRPM8 [47] and neurotrophic factors (NGF) [83] and to release tachykinins [84], prostaglandins [85], NO [86, 87], and ATP [88], further evidence for a possible interaction with the suburothelial nerves (Fig. 2.3). The urothelium was shown to be the main source of ATP release in response to bladder stretch [89]; it was proposed that ATP released in such manner would bind to suburothelial $P2X_3$, thus initiating signaling for the perception of bladder fullness [39]. In support of this hypothesis it was shown that suburothelial afferents in $P2X_3^{-/-}$ mice displayed a significant delay and increased threshold of activation by P2X agonists [34]. A proposed nociceptive role for ATP [90] and a significant reduction in nociceptive behavioral responses noted in $P2X_3^{-/-}$ mice after injection of ATP and formalin [33] was taken as further evidence for the presence of urotheliosuburothelial sensory pathways. ATP release from the urothelium appears to be partly due to vesicular exocytosis [91]. Acetylcholine was found to interact

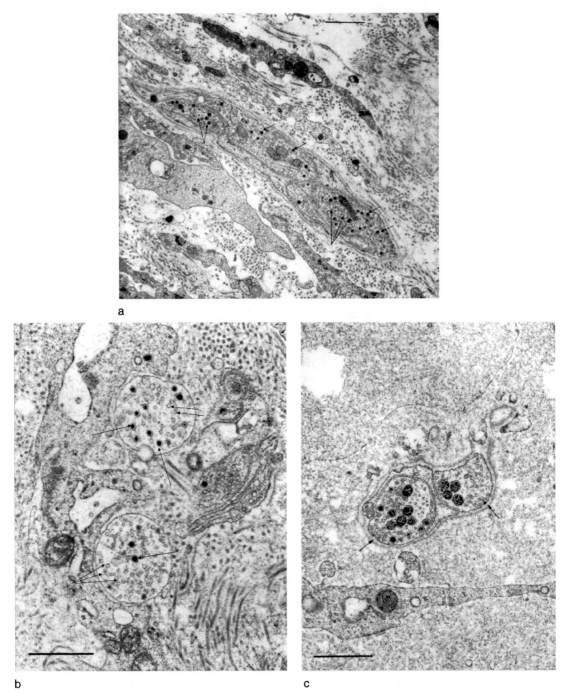

a

b   c

FIG. 2.5. Electron micrographs of unmyelinated suburothelial nerves of the human bladder lamina propria space containing clear and dense-cored vesicles (courtesy of Professor D.N. Landon, Institute of Neurology, University College London). Bladder biopsies were obtained via a flexible cystoscope, fixed in 3% glutaraldehyde in 0.1 M Na cacodylate buffer, and processed routinely for transmission electron microscopy. Ultrathin sections were obtained from the midpoint of each biopsy specimen. (**a**) An oblique section through unmyelinated nerves containing several axons filled with clear and dense-cored vesicles (*arrows*), in between layers of fibroblast processes. (**b**) A transverse section through unmyelinated axon varicosities packed with clear and dense-cored vesicles (*arrows*) in close contact with portions of fiboblasts and myofibroblasts. (**c**) An example of axonal varicosity of an unmyelinated nerve with *arrows* identifying clear vesicle release sites. Scale = 1μm. in all photos

with ATP, significantly increasing its release both in normal and pathological bladder conditions [91]. The presence of $P2X_3$ receptors in the urothelium may imply an autocrine role for ATP.

A reciprocal interaction also may exist between ATP and TRPV1. In animal experiments, TRPV1 was found to act as an initiator for urothelial ATP release and as a mediator of hypotonically evoked ATP release [32]. In cultured cells expressing TRPV1, ATP-potentiated TRPV1 responses through activation of metabotropic P2Y1 receptors via a G-protein–coupled dependent pathway [92]. Importantly, when these cells expressed both TRPV1 and Gq/11-coupled MACh receptors, extracellular application of ACh significantly increased the magnitude of currents evoked by either capsaicin or protons [92], supporting the hypothesis that there is involvement of G-protein–coupled signaling in TRPV1 sensitization and also suggesting an interaction between the cholinergic and the TRPV1 sensory pathway.

Further findings suggest the presence of a urothelio-suburothelial functional syncitium with a crucial role in bladder pathophysiology (Fig. 2.3). An increased basal urothelial release of ACh during bladder filling has been proposed as exciting afferent nerves in the suburothelium and within the detrusor, increasing detrusor smooth muscle tone, and contributing to detrusor overactivity [77]. It was suggested, therefore, that anticholinergics mainly act during the storage phase to produce an increase in bladder capacity and decrease in urgency [93]. Distension-evoked (?co-) release of ACh from the urothelium was found to increase significantly with age, providing a possible explanation for the increased rate of DO in the elderly [77]. In addition, continuing studies in human IDO bladders show that the muscarinically mediated inhibitory influence of the urothelium on the detrusor that was recently identified in health is suppressed in these patients [76]. Finally, ATP release from the urothelium during stretch was found to be significantly increased in conditions of spinal NDO [94, 95].

TRVP1 urothelial levels have been shown to be increased in patients with NDO and to be reduced in responders to intravesical RTX [81]. This decrease was in parallel with a decrease in suburothelial TRPV1; thus it was proposed that a functional consortium exists between urothelial

and suburothelial TRPV1 that allows the perception of mechanical and irritant stimuli by the bladder, a function mediated by the release of ATP from the urothelium [32]. Similarly, an increase in urothelial cell $P2X_3$ immunoreactivity was found in a mixed population of NDO and IDO patients in comparison with controls. Unexpectedly, intradetrusor injections of BoNT/A did not reduce urothelial expression of either $P2X_3$ or TRPV1 despite a dramatic decrease in suburothelial receptor levels in patients who responded to treatment [36]. These results indicate differences in the mechanisms of action among various neurotoxins applied intravesically and further highlight our inadequate knowledge of the complex pathways involved in intrinsic bladder reflexes.

Ultrastructural studies of the human bladder suburothelium recently established the presence of a nexus of myofibroblasts attaching to each other and in close apposition to vesicle-packed unmyelinated nerve fibers (Fig. 2.6). Other investigators identified a suburothelial network of interstitial cells bearing some myofibroblastic morphological characteristics, which were extensively linked by connexin 43-containing gap junctions [96] or were immunoreactive for c-kit, TRPV channels, and nNOS [97].

Electrophysiological experiments have shown that a subpopulation of human bladder suburothelial cells possessing some myofibroblastic morphological and immunohistochemical characteristics have high membrane capacitance, show spontaneous spikes of electrical activity, and respond to ATP by an increase in intracellular Ca^{2+} sufficient to activate contractile proteins and generation of an inward current [98]. Such characteristics together with the presence of the connexin 43-containing gap junctions support the hypothesis that the myofibroblasts/interstitial cells and their closely associated axonal varicosities could function collectively as a bladder stretch receptor [99]. Intracellular electrical signaling could pass from cell to cell enabled by their high membrane capacitance, while contraction of that cell layer could exert stretch-dependent activation of the sensory nerves [98]. Similarly, guinea pig suburothelial vimentin-positive cells, thought to be myofibroblasts, were shown to respond to ATP in a manner similar to the activation of ATP-gated P2Y receptors [100]. Subsequently, it was shown

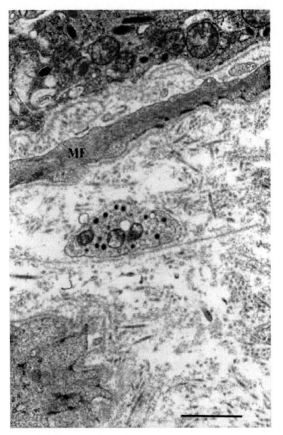

FIG. 2.6. Electron micrograph of the lamina propria space of the human bladder presenting an example of a myofibroblast (MF) adjacent to an unmyelinated axonal varicosity rich in clear and dense-cored vesicles (courtesy of Professor D.N. Landon, Institute of Neurology, University College London). Bladder biopsies were obtained via a flexible cystoscope, fixed in 3% glutaraldehyde in 0.1 M Na cacodylate buffer, and processed routinely for transmission electron microscopy. Ultrathin sections were obtained from the midpoint of each biopsy specimen. Scale = 1 μm

in single-cell immunohistochemical experiments that these cells may express a variety of purinergic receptors, including $P2X_3$, $P2Y_2$, and $P2Y_4$, but mainly the $P2Y_6$ subtype [100] (Fig. 2.3). Further electrophysiological findings from guinea pig suburothelial "myofibroblasts" show that cell pair formation greatly enhances their functional properties, such as the inward current generated in response to exogenous ATP (C. Fry, personal communication). However, our ultrastructural study of the guinea pig bladder suburothelium reveals that

only a small proportion (1.2%) of suburothelial cells possess human myofibroblastic characteristics (A. Pullen, personal communication), suggesting that the guinea pig bladder may not be an entirely appropriate model for the study of human myofibroblasts. Nevertheless, the properties of this strategically positioned cell layer (Fig. 2.3) constitute an exciting novel area of research; their role in human bladder physiology and disease states warrants further investigation.

Neurophysiological Basis of the Painful Bladder

There is increasing evidence for a role of abnormal afferent activity in the pathophysiology of the painful bladder syndrome [(PBS) previously interstitial cystitis (IC)]. Bladder afferents in cats with feline IC showed increased firing in response to various levels of intravesical pressure compared to normal cats, suggesting increased mechanoreceptor sensitivity in this condition [101]. In addition, the presence of an abnormally permeable urothelium [102] has been proposed, exposing suburothelial afferents to the chemical irritants of urine. In support of this hypothesis, high concentrations of intravesical KCl almost could abolish afferent neural activity in cats with feline IC [101], whereas lower concentrations of KCl are thought to cause bladder pain via depolarization of suburothelial afferents [103].

Stretch-evoked ATP release from urothelial cells is increased in patients with IC compared to controls [104]. In addition, $P2X_3$ expression was upregulated in the urothelium of IC patients [105] and stretch of cultured urothelial cells from IC bladders resulted in higher $P2X_3$ expression compared to stretch of "normal" cells [106]. Increased numbers of SP-immunoreactive fibers have been found in the suburothelium of IC patients in comparison to controls [107], while SP receptor-encoding mRNA was found to be increased within the vascular endothelium of IC bladders [108]. Women with IC have increased mean urine concentration of SP compared to age-matched controls, which correlated significantly with urinary frequency and urgency in those treated with dimethylsulfoxide (DMSO) [56]. Also, decrease in urine SP levels after epidural anesthesia was accompanied by successful pain control in IC patients [57]. In support of neuroplastic changes in IC bladders, NGF immunoassay levels were found to be increased in such bladders, with increased NGF immunoreactivity localizing in the bladder urothelium, but not in the muscular component of the biopsies [83]. Moreover, significant attenuation of pain and urgency in IC patients treated with intravesical instillation of alkalinized lidocaine, which is known to have an inhibitory effect on neurite regeneration and synapse formation [109], suggested modulation of bladder afferents [110].

Furthermore, in patients with urgency-frequency due to increased bladder sensation (previously "bladder hypersensitivity"), a condition thought by some to be a precursor of PBS/IC, a short-lived decrease in pain was noted following treatment with intravesical RTX, suggesting a pathophysiological role for TRPV1-expressing suburothelial afferents [111, 112]. Indeed, a recent study of patients with PBS/IC showed increased suburothelial TRPV1-positive nerve density in comparison with controls, which correlated significantly with pain scores in these patients [113]. However, a multicenter placebo-controlled trial of various doses of intravesical RTX in patients with PBS/IC showed no additional benefit on pain above the placebo effect [114], suggesting more complex pathophysiological mechanisms involved in PBS/IC or yet unidentified gaps between basic research findings and clinical applications.

PBS/IC also is characterized by evidence of long-standing inflammation. Increased urinary levels of mast cell mediators have been found in these patients [115] and mast cells often are found in close apposition to nerve fibers. These can be activated by SP and carbachol [116], suggesting a neuroimmunomodulatory role. Increased mast cell count in the urothelium/suburothelium has been reported in PBS/IC, although not consistently [117]. Detrusor mastocytosis now is proposed as a diagnostic criterion for IC [118]. Interestingly, novel findings demonstrate that detrusor smooth muscle cells from patients with PBS/IC express and release a variety of factors that are involved in the regulation of the development, function, and signaling of mast cells [119]. A constitutive and cytokine-induced production of chemokines and cytokines from such detrusor smooth muscle cells now has been shown [120]. Together these findings suggest that in PBS/IC the detrusor may play

a significant role in the inflammatory process by contributing to the infiltration of mast cells into the bladder interstitium.

The sensory bladder pathways involved in PBS/IC are being extensively investigated. Recently, M2AChR immunoreactivity was reported to be increased in suburothelial myofibroblastlike cells in patients with PBS [72], a finding that may be associated with the local anesthetic action attributed to certain anticholinergics. Increased expression of the bradykinin B1 receptor was found in cultured urothelial cells of a rat model of cyclophosphamide-induced cystitis. Activation of the receptor resulted in initiation of the micturition pathway, a response that was attenuated by P2 receptor antagonists, implying involvement of purinergic signaling pathways in bradykinin-induced micturition [121].

Neurophysiological Basis of Urgency

Urinary urgency is a pathological sensation, distinct from the normal sensation of even strong desire to void and is the defining symptom of the overactive bladder syndrome [122]. The pathophysiology of urgency is not fully understood but is assumed to be due to aberrant afferent activity; peripheral afferent neuromodulation has been used successfully to suppress the sensation of urgency and urge incontinence [22, 24]. When urgency occurs in the context of DO, it is thought that pathologically sensitive bladder stretch-sensing receptors may give rise to afferent activity, which causes both reflex detrusor contractions and— provided the spinal cord is sufficiently preserved— ascends as a barrage to consciousness, perceived as "urgency."

Understanding urgency now is seen as a central goal for reaching an effective treatment of DO. Several reports suggested a role of the afferents in the pathophysiology of human DO-associated urgency and incontinence [22, 123, 124]. In this respect, at a cellular level a recent study showed an association between suburothelial P2X$_3$ and, to a lesser degree, TRPV1 and the pathological sensation of urgency: in patients with intractable DO who were successfully treated with intradetrusor injections of botulinum toxin type A (BoNT/A), posttreatment changes in quantified sensation of urgency from their bladder diaries correlated significantly with respective changes in $P2X_3$ receptor levels in suburothelial nerve fibers. A trend for correlation was found for changes in TRPV1 receptor levels [36].

In a further study of the natural history of the decline of urgency following BoNT/A bladder injections, we found that urgency and associated incontinence were markedly improved as soon as day 2 postinjection, whereas a significant reduction in frequency only occurred on day 4, suggesting different pathophysiological mechanisms regulating these symptoms [125]. In support of such a hypothesis, TRPM8 receptor levels in suburothelial, presumably afferent, nerve fibers did not correlate with urgency scores in either IDO or PBS/IC patients, while a significant positive correlation was seen with frequency scores [47].

In a mixed population of patients with IDO or PBS/IC, M2AChR and M3AChR immunoreactivity in a population of suburothelial cells was found to correlate significantly with urgency scores [72], the latter measured with a recently designed pelvic pain/urgency/frequency (PUF) questionnaire [126]. However, DO-associated urgency may be fundamentally different to the urgency seen in PBS/IC. Nevertheless, this finding appears to be in keeping with the proposed mechanism of action of anticholinergics in the decrease of urgency in the overactive bladder [127].

As urgency now is identified as the most bothersome of the symptoms of the overactive bladder syndrome with significant effect on patients' quality of life, it has understandably become a prime target for the pharmaceutical industry.

Acknowldgments. Funding. A. Apostolidis: Pfizer Inc Independent Research Grant; C.J. Fowler: Pfizer Inc Independent Research Grant, Allergan Ltd Unrestricted Educational Health Grant, and Multiple Sclerosis Society of Great Britain and Northern Ireland Research Grant.

References

1. de Groat WC, Booth AM, Yoshimura N. Neurophysiology of micturition and its modification in animal models of human disease. In: Maggi CA, ed. The autonomic nervous system, Vol. 3, Nervous control of the urogenital system. London: Harwood Academic Publishers, 1993:227–290.

2. Chai TC, Steers WD. Neurophysiology of micturition and continence. Urol Clin North Am 1996;23:221–236.

3. Yoshimura N, de Groat WC. Neural control of the lower urinary tract. Int J Urol 1997;4:111–125.

4. de Groat WC. Integrative control of the lower urinary tract: Preclinical perspective. Br J Pharmacol 2006;147(Suppl 2):S25–40.

5. Blok BF, Holstege G. Direct projections from the periaqueductal grey to the pontine micturition centre (M-region). An antegrade and retrograde tracing study in the cat. Neurosci Lett 1994;166:93–96.

6. Blok BF, de Weerd H, Holstege G. Ultrastructural evidence for a paucity of projections from lumbosacral cord to the pontine micturition centre or M-region in the cat: A new concept for the organization of the micturition reflex with the periaqueductal grey as central relay. J Comp Neurol 1995;359:300–309.

7. Blok BF, Willemsen AT, Holstege G. A PET study on brain control of micturition in humans. Brain 1997;120(Pt 1):111–121.

8. Blok BF, Sturms LM, Holstege G. Brain activation during micturition in women. Brain 1998;121(Pt 11):2033–2042.

9. Nour S, Svarer C, Kristensen JK, et al. Cerebral activation during micturition in normal men. Brain 2000;123(Pt 4):781–789.

10. Athwal BS, Berkley KJ, Hussain I, et al. Brain responses to changes in bladder volume and urge to void in healthy men. Brain 2001;124(Pt 2):369–377.

11. Matsuura S, Kakizaki H, Mitsui T, et al. Human brain region response to distention or cold stimulation of the bladder: A positron emission tomography study. J Urol 2002;168(5):2035–2039.

12. Dasgupta R, Critchley HD, Dolan RJ, Fowler CJ. Changes in brain activity following sacral neuromodulation for urinary retention. J Urol 2005;174(6):2268–2272.

13. Zhang H, Reitz A, Kollias S, et al. An fMRI study of the role of suprapontine brain structures in the voluntary voiding control induced by pelvic floor contraction. Neuroimage 2005;24(1):174–180.

14. Kavia RB, Dasgupta R, Fowler CJ. Functional imaging and the central control of the bladder. J Comp Neurol 2005;493(1):27–32.

15. Griffiths D, Derbyshire S, Stenger A, Resnick N. Brain control of normal and overactive bladder. J Urol 2005;174(5):1862–1867.

16. Blok B, Groen J, Veltman D, Bosch R. Brain plasticity and urge incontinence: PET studies during the first hours of sacral neuromodulation. Neurourol Urodyn 2003;22:490.

17. Rauch SL, Savage CR, Alpert NM, et al. Probing striatal function in obsessive-compulsive disorder: A PET study of implicit sequence learning. J Neuropsychiatry Clin Neurosci 1997;9(4):568–573.

18. Valet M, Sprenger T, Boecker H, et al. Distraction modulates connectivity of the cingulo-frontal cortex and the midbrain during pain—An fMRI analysis. Pain 2004;109(3):399–408.

19. Yoshimura N. Bladder afferent pathway and spinal cord injury: Possible mechanisms inducing hyperreflexia of the urinary bladder. Prog Neurobiol 1999;57:583–606.

20. Morrison J, Birder L, Craggs M, et al. Neural control. In: Abrams P, Cardozo L, Khoury S, Wein A, eds. Incontinence. New Jersey: Health Publications; 2005:363–422.

21. Leng WW, Chancellor MB. How sacral nerve stimulation neuromodulation works. Urol Clin North Am 2005;32(1):11–18.

22. Oliver S, Fowler CJ, Mundy A, Craggs M. Measuring the sensations of urge and bladder filling during cystometry in urge incontinence and the effects of neuromodulation. Neurourol Urodyn 2003;22:7–16.

23. Aguirre OA. Acute pudendal nerve stimulation improves cystometric volumes in urge incontinent patients. Int Urogynecol J Pelvic Floor Dysfunct 2006;17(Suppl. 2):S125 (Abstract 13).

24. Congregado RB, Pena OXM, Campoy MP, et al. Peripheral afferent nerve stimulation for treatment of lower urinary tract irritative symptoms. Eur Urol 2004;45:65–69.

25. Dasgupta R, Wiseman OJ, Kitchen N, Fowler CJ. Long-term results of sacral neuromodulation for women with urinary retention. BJU Int 2004;94(3):335–337.

26. Michel MC, Oelke M. Duloxetine in the treatment of stress urinary incontinence. Women's Health 2005;1(3):345–358.

27. de Groat WC, Kawatani M, Hisamitsu T, et al. Mechanisms underlying the recovery of urinary bladder function following spinal cord injury. J Auton Nerv Syst 1990;30(Suppl):S71–77.

28. Brady CM, Apostolidis A, Harper M, et al. Parallel changes in bladder suburothelial vanilloid receptor TRPV1 (VR1) and pan-neuronal marker PGP9.5 immunoreactivity in patients with neurogenic detrusor overactivity (NDO) following intravesical resiniferatoxin treatment. BJU Int 2004;93:770–776.

29. Dasgupta P, Chandiramani VA, Beckett A, et al. The effect of intravesical capsaicin on the suburothelial innervation in patients with detrusor hyper-reflexia. BJU Int 2000;85(3):238–245.

30. Fowler CJ, Harper M, Fry CH. Voiding and the sacral reflex arc: Lessons from capsaicin instillation. Scand J Urol Nephrol 2002;Suppl 210:46–50.

31. Apostolidis A, Dasgupta P, Fowler CJ. Proposed mechanism for the efficacy of injected botulinum toxin in the treatment of human detrusor overactivity. Eur Urol 2006;49(4):644–650.

32. Birder LA, Nakamura Y, Kiss S, et al. Altered urinary bladder function in mice lacking the vanilloid receptor TRPV1. Nat Neurosci 2002;5(9):856–860.

33. Cockayne DA, Hamilton SG, Zhu Q-M, et al. Urinary bladder hyporeflexia and reduced pain-related behaviour in P2X3-deficient mice. Nature 2000;407:1011–1015.

34. Vlaskovska M, Kasakov L, Rong W, et al. P2X3 knock-out mice reveal a major sensory role for urothelially released ATP. J Neurosci 2000;21(15):5670–5677.

35. Brady C, Apostolidis A, Yiangou Y, et al. P2X3-immunoreactive nerve fibres in neurogenic detrusor overactivity and the effect of intravesical resiniferatoxin (RTX). Eur Urol 2004;46:247–253.

36. Apostolidis A, Popat R, Yiangou Y, et al. Decreased sensory receptors P2X3 and TRPV1 in suburothelial nerve fibres following intra-detrusor injections of botulinum toxin for human detrusor overactivity. J Urol 2005;174:977–83.

37. Silva C, Ribeiro MJ, Cruz F. The effect of intravesical resiniferatoxin in patients with idiopathic detrusor instability suggests that involuntary detrusor contractions are triggered by C-fiber input. J Urol 2002;168(2):575–579.

38. Morenilla-Palao C, Planells-Cases R, Garcia-Sanz N, Ferrer-Montiel A. Regulated exocytosis contributes to protein kinase C potentiation of vanilloid receptor activity. J Biol Chem 2004;279:25665–25672.

39. Burnstock G. Purine-mediated signalling in pain and visceral perception. Trends Pharmacol Sci 2001;22:182–188.

40. Guo A, Vulchanova L, Wang J, et al. Immunocytochemical localization of the vanilloid receptor 1 (VR1): Relationship to neuropeptides, the P2X3 purinoceptor and IB4 binding sites. Eur J Neurosci 1999;11(3):946–958.

41. Montell C. Physiology, phylogeny, and functions of the TRP superfamily of cation channels. Sci STKE 2001;2001(90):RE1.

42. Geirsson G. Evidence of cold receptors in the human bladder: Effect of menthol on the bladder cooling reflex. J Urol 1993;150(2 Pt 1):427–430.

43. Lindstrom S, Mazieres L. Effect of menthol on the bladder cooling reflex in the cat. Acta Physiol Scand 1991;141(1):1–10.

44. Fall M, Lindstrom S, Mazieres L. A bladder-to-bladder cooling reflex in the cat. J Physiol 1990;427:281–300.

45. Peier AM, Moqrich A, Hergarden AC, et al. A TRP channel that senses cold stimuli and menthol. Cell 2002;108(5):705–715.

46. McKemy DD, Neuhausser WM, Julius D. Identification of a cold receptor reveals a general role for TRP channels in thermosensation. Nature 2002;416(6876):52–58.

47. Mukerji G, Yiangou Y, Corcoran SL, et al. Cool and menthol receptor TRPM8 in human urinary bladder disorders and clinical correlations. BMC Urol 2006;6:6.

48. Wakabayashi Y, Tomoyoshi T, Fujimiua M, et al. Substance P-containing axon terminals in the mucosa of the human urinary bladder: Pre-embedding immunohistochemistry using cryostat sections for electron microscopy. Histochemistry 1993;100:401–407.

49. Smet PJ, Moore KH, Jonavicius J. Distribution and colocalization of calcitonin gene-related peptide, tachykinins, and vasoactive intestinal peptide in normal and idiopathic unstable human urinary bladder. Lab Invest 1997;77:37–49.

50. De Biasi S, Rustioni A. Glutamate and substance P coexist in primary afferent terminals in the superficial laminae of spinal cord. Proc Natl Acad Sci USA 1988;85:7820–7824.

51. Cruz F. Vanilloid receptor and detrusor instability. Urology 2002;59(5 Suppl 1):51–60.

52. Avelino A, Cruz F. Peptide immunoreactivity and ultrastructure of rat urinary bladder nerve fibers after topical desensitization by capsaicin or resiniferatoxin. Auton Neurosci 2000;86(1–2):37–46.

53. Maggi CA, Gepetti P, Santicioli P, et al. The correlation between sensory-efferent functions mediated by the capsaicin-sensitive neurons and substance P content of the urinary bladder of the rat. Neurosci Lett 1987;76:351–356.

54. Shaker HS, Tu LM, Kalfopoulos M, et al. Hyperreflexia of the urinary bladder: Possible role of the efferent function of the capsaicin sensitive primary afferents. J Urol 1998;160(6 Pt 1):2232–2239.

55. Crowe R, Moss HE, Chapple CR, et al. Patients with lower motor spinal cord lesion: A decrease of vasoactive intestinal polypeptide, calcitonin gene-related peptide and substance P, but not neuropeptide Y and somatostatin-immunoreactive nerves in the detrusor muscle of the bladder. J Urol 1991;145:600–604.

56. Kushner L, Chiu PY, Brettschneider N, et al. Urinary substance P concentration correlates with urinary frequency and urgency in interstitial cystitis patients treated with intravesical dimethyl sulfoxide and not intravesical anesthetic cocktail. Urology 2001;57 (6 Suppl 1):129.

57. Sukiennik A, Carr DB, Bonney I, et al. The effect of short-term epidural local anesthetic blockade on urinary levels of substance P in interstitial cystitis. Anesth Analg 2004;98:846–850.

58. Priestley JV, Michael GJ, Averill S, et al. Regulation of nociceptive neurons by nerve growth factor and glial cell line derived neurotrophic factor. Can J Physiol Pharmacol 2002;80:495–505.

59. Donnerer J, Amann R, Schuligoi R, Skofitsch G. Complete recovery by nerve growth factor of neuropeptide content and function in capsaicin-impaired sensory neurons. Brain Res 1996;741(1–2):103–108.

60. Burbach GJ, Kim KH, Zivony AS, et al. The neurosensory tachykinins substance P and neurokinin A directly induce keratinocyte nerve growth factor. J Invest Dermatol 2001;117:1075–1082.

61. Oh EJ, Gover TD, Cordoba-Rodriguez R, Weinreich D. Substance P evokes cation currents through TRP channels in HEK293 cells. J Neurophysiol 2003;90:2069–2073.

62. Ito K, Rome C, Bouleau Y, Dulon D. Substance P mobilizes intracellular calcium and activates a nonselective cation conductance in rat spiral ganglion neurons. Eur J Neurosci 2002;16:2095–2102.

63. Huang H, Wu X, Nicol GD, et al. ATP augments peptide release from rat sensory neurons in culture through activation of P2Y receptors. J Pharmacol Exp Ther 2003;306(3):1137–1144.

64. Paukert M, Osteroth R, Geisler HS, et al. Inflammatory mediators potentiate ATP-gated channels through the P2X(3) subunit. J Biol Chem 2001;276(24):21077–21082.

65. Persson K, Johansson K, Alm P, et al. Morphological and functional evidence against a sensory and sympathetic origin of nitric oxide synthase-containing nerves in the rat lower urinary tract. Neuroscience 1997;77(1):271–281.

66. Gulbenkian S, Merighi A, Wharton J, et al. Ultrastructural evidence for the coexistence of calcitonin gene-related peptide and substance P in secretory vesicles of peripheral nerves in the guinea pig. J Neurocytol 1986;15(4):535–542.

67. Burnstock G. The changing face of autonomic neurotransmission. Acta Physiol Scand 1986;126(1):67–91.

68. Parsons SM, Prior C, Marshall IG. Acetylcholine transport, storage, and release. Int Rev Neurobiol 1993;35:279–390.

69. Gabella G. Structure of the intramural nerves of the rat bladder. J Neurocytol 1999;28(8):615–637.

70. Gabella G. The structural relations between nerve fibres and muscle cells in the urinary bladder of the rat. J Neurocytol 1995;24(3):159–187.

71. Hoyle CH, Burnstock G. Postganglionic efferent transmission in the bladder and urethra. In: Maggi CA, ed. Nervous control of the urogenital system. Chur, Switzerland: Harwood Academic Publishers, 1993:349–381.

72. Mukerji G, Yiangou Y, Grogono J, et al. Localization of M2 and M3 muscarinic receptors in human bladder

disorders and their clinical correlations. J Urol 2006;176(1):367–373.

73. Pontari MA, Braverman AS, Ruggieri MR, Sr. The M2 muscarinic receptor mediates in vitro bladder contractions from patients with neurogenic bladder dysfunction. Am J Physiol Regul Integr Comp Physiol 2004;286(5):R874–880.

74. Chess-Williams R, Chapple CR, Yamanishi T, et al. The minor population of M3-receptors mediate contraction of human detrusor muscle in vitro. J Auton Pharmacol 2001;21(5–6):243–248.

75. Somogyi GT, Zernova GV, Yoshiyama M, et al. Frequency dependence of muscarinic facilitation of transmitter release in urinary bladder strips from neurally intact or chronic spinal cord transected rats. Br J Pharmacol 1998;125:241–246.

76. Chess-Williams R. Muscarinic receptors of the urinary bladder: Detrusor, urothelial and prejunctional. Auton Autacoid Pharmacol 2002;22:133–145.

77. Yoshida M, Miyamae K, Iwashita H, et al. Management of detrusor dysfunction in the elderly: Changes in acetylcholine and adenosine triphosphate release during aging. Urology 2004;63(Suppl 3A):17–23.

78. Beckel JM, Kanai A, Lee SJ, et al. Expression of functional nicotinic acetylcholine receptors in rat urinary bladder epithelial cells. Am J Physiol Renal Physiol 2006;290(1):F103–110.

79. Birder LA, Kanai AJ, de Groat WC, et al. Vanilloid receptor expression suggests a sensory role for urinary bladder epithelial cells. Proc Natl Acad Sci USA 2001;98(23):13396–13401.

80. Lazzeri M, Vannucchi G, Zardo C, et al. Immunohistochemical evidence of vanilloid receptor 1 in normal human urinary bladder urothelium. Eur Urol 2004;46:792–799.

81. Apostolidis A, Brady CM, Yiangou Y, et al. Capsaicin receptor TRPV1 in the urothelium of neurogenic human bladders and the effect of intravesical resiniferatoxin. Urology 2005;65:400–405.

82. Elneil S, Skepper JN, Kidd EJ, et al. Distribution of P2X(1) and P2X(3) receptors in the rat and human urinary bladder. Pharmacology 2001;63(2):120–128.

83. Lowe EM, Anand P, Terenghi G, et al. Increased nerve growth factor levels in the urinary bladder of women with idiopathic sensory urgency and interstitial cystitis. Br J Urol 1997;79:572–577.

84. Lecci A, Maggi CA. Tachykinins as modulators of the micturition reflex in the central and peripheral nervous sytem. Regul Pept 2001;101:1–18.

85. Badawi AF, Habib SL, Mohammed MA, et al. Influence of cigarette smoking on prostaglandin synthesis and cyclooxygenase-2 gene expression in human urinary bladder cancer. Cancer Invest 2002;20(5–6):651–656.

86. Birder LA, Apodaca G, De Groat WC, Kanai AJ. Adrenergic- and capsaicin-evoked nitric oxide release from urothelium and afferent nerves in urinary bladder. Am J Physiol 1998;275(2 Pt 2):F226–229.

87. Moon A. Influence of nitric oxide signalling pathways on pre-contracted human detrusor smooth muscle in vitro. BJU Int 2002;89:942–949.

88. Ferguson DR, Kennedy I, Burton T. ATP is released from rabbit urinary bladder epithelial cells by hydrostatic pressure changes – a possible sensory mechanism? J Physiol 1997;505:503–511.

89. Kumar V, Chapple CR, Chess-Williams R. Characteristics of adenosine triphosphate release from porcine and human normal bladder. J Urol 2004;172:744–747.

90. Kennedy C, Leff P. Painful connection for ATP. Nature 1995;377:385–386.

91. Birder LA, Barrick SR, Roppolo JR, et al. Feline interstitial cystitis results in mechanical hypersensitivity and altered ATP release from bladder urothelium. Am J Physiol Renal Physiol 2003;285(3):F423–429.

92. Tominaga M, Wada M, Masu M. Potentiation of capsaicin receptor activity by metabotropic ATP receptors as a possible mechanism for ATP-evoked pain and hyperalgesia. Proc Natl Acad Sci USA 2001;98(12):6951–6956.

93. Andersson KE. Antimuscarinics for treatment of overactive bladder. Lancet Neurol 2004;3:47–53.

94. Khera M, Somogyi GT, Kiss S, et al. Botulinum toxin A inhibits ATP release from bladder urothelium after chronic spinal cord injury. Neurochem Int 2004;45:987–993.

95. Yoshida M, Inadome A, Masunaga K, et al. Non-neuronal acetylcholine and ATP releases from isolated normal and neurogenic human bladder. Neurourol Urodyn 2004;23(5/6):503–504 (A73).

96. Sui GP, Rothery S, Dupont E, et al. Gap junctions and connexin expression in human suburothelial interstitial cells. BJU Int 2002;90:118–129.

97. Ost D, Roskams T, Van Der Aa F, deRidder D. Topography of the vanilloid receptor in the human bladder: More than just the nerve fibers. J Urol 2002;168:293–297.

98. Sui GP, Wu C, Fry CH. Electrical characteristics of suburothelial cells isolated from the human bladder. J Urol 2004;171(2 Pt 1):938–943.

99. Wiseman OJ, Fowler CJ, Landon DN. The role of the human bladder lamina propria myofibroblast. BJU Int 2003;91:89–93.

100. Wu C, Sui GP, Fry CH. Purinergic regulation of guinea pig suburothelial myofibroblasts. J Physiol 2004;559(Pt 1):231–243.

101. Roppolo JR, Tai C, Booth AM, et al. Bladder Adelta afferent nerve activity in normal cats and cats with feline interstitial cystitis. J Urol 2005;173(3):1011–1015.

102. Keay S, Zhang CO, Shoenfelt JL, Chai TC. Decreased in vitro proliferation of bladder epithelial cells from patients with interstitial cystitis. Urology 2003;61(6):1278–1284.

103. Parsons CL, Stein PC, Bidair M, Lebow D. Abnormal sensitivity to intravesical potassium in interstitial cystitis and radiation cystitis. Neurourol Urodyn 1994;13(5):515–520.

104. Sun Y, Keay S, De Deyne PG, Chai TC. Augmented stretch activated adenosine triphosphate release from bladder uroepithelial cells in patients with interstitial cystitis. J Urol 2001;166(5):1951–1956.

105. Tempest HV, Dixon AK, Turner WH, et al. P2X2 and P2X3 receptor expression in human bladder urothelium and changes in interstitial cystitis. BJU Int 2004;93:1344–1348.

106. Sun Y, Chai TC. Up-regulation of P2X3 receptor during stretch of bladder urothelial cells from patients with interstitial cystitis. J Urol 2004;171:448–452.

107. Pang X, Marchand J, Sant GR, et al. Increased number of substance P positive nerve fibres in interstitial cystitis. Br J Urol 1995;75(6):744–750.

108. Marchand JE, Sant GR, Kream RM. Increased expression of substance P receptor-encoding mRNA in bladder biopsies from patients with interstitial cystitis. Br J Urol 1998;81(2):224–228.

109. Onizuka S, Takasaki M, Syed NI. Long-term exposure to local but not inhalation anesthetics affects neurite regeneration and synapse formation between identified lymnaea neurons. Anesthesiology 2005;102(2):353–363.

110. Parsons CL. Successful downregulation of bladder sensory nerves with combination of heparin and alkalinized lidocaine in patients with interstitial cystitis. Urology 2005;65(1):45–48.

111. Lazzeri M, Beneforti P, Spinelli M, et al. Intravesical resiniferatoxin for the treatment of hypersensitive disorder: A randomized placebo controlled study. J Urol 2000;164(3 Pt 1):676–679.

112. Apostolidis A, Gonzales GE, Fowler CJ. Effect of intravesical resiniferatoxin (RTX) on lower urinary tract symptoms, urodynamic parameters, and quality of life of patients with urodynamic increased bladder sensation. Eur Urol 2006.

113. Mukerji G, Yiangou Y, Agarwal SK, Anand P. Transient receptor potential vanilloid receptor subtype 1 in painful bladder syndrome and its correlation with pain. J Urol 2006;176(2):797–801.

114. Payne CK, Mosbaugh PG, Forrest JB, et al. Intravesical resiniferatoxin for the treatment of interstitial cystitis: A randomized, double-blind, placebo controlled trial. J Urol 2005;173(5):1590–1594.

115. Sant GR, Theoharides TC. The role of the mast cell in interstitial cystitis. Urol Clin North Am 1994;21(1):41–53.

116. Spanos C, el-Mansoury M, Letourneau R, et al. Carbachol-induced bladder mast cell activation: Augmentation by estradiol and implications for interstitial cystitis. Urology 1996;48(5):809–816.

117. Theoharides TC, Kempuraj D, Sant GR. Mast cell involvement in interstitial cystitis: A review of human and experimental evidence. Urology 2001;57(6 Suppl 1):47–55.

118. Nordling J, Anjum FH, Bade JJ, et al. Primary evaluation of patients suspected of having interstitial cystitis (IC). Eur Urol 2004;45(5):662–669.

119. Bouchelouche K, Andresen L, Alvarez S, et al. Interleukin-4 and -13 induce the expression and release of monocyte chemoattractant protein 1, interleukin-6 and stem cell factor from human detrusor smooth muscle cells: Synergy with interleukin-1beta and tumor necrosis factor-alpha. J Urol 2006;175(2):760–765.

120. Bouchelouche K, Alvarez S, Horn T, et al. Human detrusor smooth muscle cells release interleukin-6, interleukin-8, and RANTES in response to proinflammatory cytokines interleukin-1beta and tumor necrosis factor-alpha. Urology 2006;67(1):214–219.

121. Chopra B, Barrick SR, Meyers S, et al. Expression and function of bradykinin B1 and B2 receptors in normal and inflamed rat urinary bladder urothelium. J Physiol 2005;562(Pt 3):859–871.

122. Abrams P, Cardozo L, Fall M, et al. The standardisation of terminology of lower urinary tract function: Report from the Standardisation Subcommittee of the International Continence Society. Neurourol Urodyn 2002;21:167–178.

123. Everaert K, De Ridder D, Baert L, et al. Patient satisfaction and complications following sacral nerve stimulation for urinary retention, urge incontinence and perineal pain: A multicenter evaluation. Int Urogynecol J Pelvic Floor Dysfunct 2000;11(4):231–235; discussion 236.

124. Silva C, Silva J, Ribeiro MJ, et al. Urodynamic effect of intravesical resiniferatoxin in patients with neurogenic detrusor overactivity of spinal origin: Results of a double-blind randomized placebo-controlled trial. Eur Urol 2005;48(4):650–655.

125. Kalsi V, Apostolidis A, Gonzales G, et al. The decline of urgency following intradetrusor botulinum neurotoxin type A (BoNT/A) injections for detrusor overactivity (DO): Preliminary results. Eur Urol 2006;49(Suppl. 1):A798.

126. Parsons CL, Dell J, Stanford EJ, et al. Increased prevalence of interstitial cystitis: Previously unrecognized

urologic and gynecologic cases identified using a new symptom questionnaire and intravesical potassium sensitivity. Urology 2002;60(4):573–578.

127. Andersson KE, Yoshida M. Antimuscarinics and the overactive detrusor – which is the main mechanism of action? Eur Urol 2003;43(1):1–5.

Chapter 3
Continence: Bladder Neck versus Mid-Urethra

Matthias Oelke and Jan-Paul Roovers

Introduction

Urinary incontinence is a common medical and social problem of women of all age groups. Up to 28% of women younger than 60 years of age and up to 35% older than 60 years suffer from urinary incontinence [1, 2]. Of all incontinence types, women are predominantly afflicted by stress urinary incontinence, with an estimated proportion of about 60% [2]. Women with stress urinary incontinence report about a varying amount of urinary leakage during physical activity, coughing, sneezing, laughing, or straining. Basically, urinary incontinence occurs when the intravesical pressure rises above the urethral pressure. In stress urinary incontinence, intra-abdominal pressure is transmitted to the bladder and exceeds urethral pressure, which leads to passive urinary leakage through the urethra. Therefore, urethral closure insufficiency is responsible for stress urinary incontinence. Understanding the continence mechanisms and the underlying causes of urethral closure insufficiency helps to restore continence.

Strategies for the treatment of stress urinary incontinence have been established, and later, concepts have been developed to explain the successful outcome. However, much of the discussion is speculation, theory, and hypothesis [3]. The efficacy of the chosen treatment seems to support the individual theory. Today, two concepts are widely accepted and used in clinical practice. However, these concepts seem to compete with each other. The key question in the discussion of the concepts is related to the part of the urethra that is assumed to be responsible for urethral closure and continence: is it the bladder neck or midurethra?

Anatomy of the Female Lower Urinary Tract and Continence Mechanisms

The urinary bladder is located in the pelvis at the caudal site of the abdominal cavity and surrounded by fatty tissue. The urethra has a total length of about 4–5 cm and reaches from the bladder neck to the external meatus. The bladder neck is located above the level of the inferior margin of the symphysis and lies on the endopelvic fascia. The endopelvic fascia is attached to the levator ani muscle at both sides of the urethra and contraction of the levator ani muscle leads to simultaneous elevation of the bladder neck [4]. The urethral wall consists of a mucosal lining, underneath a submucosal cushion of blood vessels embedded in connective tissue and elastic fibers, and a longitudinal and circular layer of smooth muscle cells [5]. The urethra runs nearly parallel to the axis of the anterior vaginal wall and is closely attached to the surrounding vaginal tissue. The posterior wall of the urethra is supported by the fibromuscular vaginal tissue, which is connected to the pelvic bones via the pubovaginal portion of the levator ani muscle and the longitudinal muscle of the anus. The urethra is attached to the posterior site of the symphysis by the pubourethral ligaments.

Accumulations of muscle cells exist around the urethra. The bladder neck is densely surrounded by smooth muscle cells (internal urethral sphincter, 0–15th percentile of the urethra) that are innervated by sympathetic nerve fibers coming from the level Th11–L2 of the spinal cord [3, 4]. The distal part of the proximal and midurethra is surrounded by striated muscle cells (20–60th percentile of the urethra); this rhabdomyosphincter (external urethral sphincter) is innervated by the pudendal nerves, which leave the spinal cord at the level S2–S4.

The following mechanisms are believed to contribute to female urinary continence ("stress continence control system" [4]):

1. Smooth and striated muscle cells in and around the urethra close the urethral lumen (active sphincteric system).
2. The length of the urethra and urethral wall tension (collagen and elastic fibers, mucosa and submucosal cushion of blood vessels in the urethral wall) guarantee additional positive pressure in the urethra in the resting position (passive sphincteric system or urethral wall factor) [6].
3. Pressure transmission from the abdominal cavity to the proximal urethra (passive pressure transmission) [7].
4. Activation of the coughing reflex via the pudendal nerve leads to a fast contraction of the urethral rhabdomyosphincter and pelvic floor before and during vesical pressure increase (active pressure transmission) [7, 8].
5. Posterior urethral wall support by fibromuscular tissue of the anterior vaginal wall and the tendinous arch of the pelvic fascia (hammock system) [9].
6. Ventral kinking of the urethra during contraction of the levator ani muscle, longitudinal muscle of the anus, and the hammock muscle pulls the vagina and bladder base back- and downward and presses the urethra against the pubic bone (integral theory) [10].

Bladder Neck: Intrinsic Sphincter Deficiency, Urethral Hypermobility, and the "Hammock Hypothesis"

The active and passive sphincteric systems, active and passive pressure transmissions, as well as the "hammock hypothesis" (points 1–5, above) support the concept that the bladder neck and proximal urethra are responsible for urinary continence. Sphincters guarantee that the urethral lumen is watertightly closed in the filling phase of the bladder and, together with the surrounding tissue, give structural support to keep the proximal urethra from moving during abdominal pressure increase. Anatomical or functional damage of the sphincteric systems may cause an insufficient approximation of the urethral lumen. Two causes were identified for sphincteric insufficiency:

- In intrinsic sphincter deficiency (ISD), the urethral sphincters are too weak to close the urethral lumen. Urinary leakage may be associated with a minimal increase in intravesical pressure or even may be gravitational. Patients with this type of incontinence have a low leak point pressure during coughing or straining (<60 cm H_2O) and a low urethral closure pressure at rest in urethral pressure profilometry (<20 cm H_2O) [11, 12]. During video-urodynamic investigation, the bladder neck and proximal urethra, regardless of the anatomic position, are open at rest.
- In urethral hypermobility, the sphincters remain strong in the resting position but become insufficient during stress situations. Patients with this type of incontinence have a pathological cotton swab (Q-tip) test (difference of the urethrovesical angle *from the horizontal plane* $>30°$), whereas the leak point pressure (>60 cm H_2O) and the urethral closure pressure at rest remain high (>20 cm H_2O) [13, 14]. A loss of the anchoring system of the bladder neck and proximal urethra is believed to cause urethral hypermobility, leading to insufficiency of pressure transmission to the proximal urethra. During video-urodynamic investigation, the bladder neck and proximal urethra are closed at rest but open and descend during stress.

Based on these two distinct findings, a classification system of stress urinary incontinence consisting of five subtypes has been established (Table 3.1) [15–17]. Types 0 – IIb refer to urethral hypermobility and type III refers to ISD. Ultrasound investigations demonstrated that the rhabdomyosphincter is significantly thicker in continent than incontinent women and significantly thicker in women with urethral hypermobility than ISD [18].

The hammock system is a supportive anatomical structure that can explain closure of the bladder

TABLE 3.1. Classification of stress urinary incontinence based on the concept of urethral hypermobility and intrinsic sphincter deficiency.

Incontinence type	Description
Type O	The patient has a typical history of stress incontinence, which, however, cannot be reproduced during clinical or urodynamic investigation. The bladder neck and proximal urethra are closed at rest and situated at or above the inferior end of the symphysis. The bladder neck and proximal urethra descend and open during stress. Failure to demonstrate urinary incontinence may be due to momentary voluntary contraction of the external urethral sphincter during the examination
Type I	The bladder neck is closed at rest and located above the inferior margin of the symphysis. The bladder neck and proximal urethra open and descend less than 2 cm during stress, and urinary incontinence is apparent during periods of increased abdominal pressure. There is a small or no cystocele
Type IIa	The bladder neck is closed at rest and located above the inferior margin of the symphysis. The bladder neck and proximal urethra open during stress and a rotational descent is observed (cystourethrocele)
Type IIb	The bladder neck is closed at rest and situated at or below the inferior margin of the symphysis. During stress, there may or may not be further descent but the proximal urethra opens and urinary leakage occurs
Type III	The bladder neck and proximal urethra are open at rest. The proximal urethra does not function as a sphincter anymore

neck and proximal urethra during abdominal pressure increase [9]. According to this hypothesis, the bladder neck and proximal urethra lie in a position where they can be compressed against a backboard and sealed during abdominal pressure increase. The hammock consists of the anterior vaginal wall and the surrounding connective tissue that are connected with the pelvic bones via the pubovaginal portion of the levator ani muscle and the tendinous arch of the pelvic fascia. If the hammock system is intact but in a more caudal position, continence still may be maintained. The stability of the supporting layers and muscles therefore are responsible for continence during stress situations. Laxity of the hammock would give less resistance during abdominal pressure increase and lead to urinary incontinence. DeLancey described this system like a water hose: stepping on the hose would stop the water flow if the hose would lie on a firm, noncompliant ground [4, 9]. The results after anterior colporrhaphy support this hypothesis. In a prospective randomized trial comparing the outcome of three different operation techniques 37% of women reported to be dry 5 years after colporraphy [19].

Midurethra: The Integral Theory

The integral theory (6) supports the concept that the midurethra is responsible for urinary continence. The integral theory is a complex musculoelastic concept whereby muscle forces pull on the vaginal tissue to open and close the urethra [10, 20]. This theory adds a dynamic extrinsic mechanism – contractions of specific pelvic floor muscles – to the concept of urethral closure. Closure of the urethra occurs when three muscle forces interact together, pulling the vagina simultaneously to the dorsal, caudal, and ventral direction. The levator ani muscle contracts and pulls the vagina and the attached bladder base and urethra to the dorsal direction, the longitudinal muscle of the anus contracts and pulls the vagina to a caudal direction, and the so-called "hammock muscle" contracts and pulls the vagina to the ventral direction. As a result of the muscle contractions, the upper urethra moves to a horizontal and the lower urethra to a vertical position, causing kinking of the midurethra and closure of the urethral lumen. Mechanical obstruction of the urethral lumen occurs only during muscle contraction; this effect was named "dynamic mid-urethral knee angulation" or "iris effect" [21, 22]. Possible mechanisms of damage of this system during childbirth with regard to urinary incontinence, prolapse, and voiding disorders were described [23]. Laxity of any of the involved muscles or ligaments prevents the urethra, vagina, and bladder base from stretching, and therefore weakens the transmission of muscular forces, leading to urinary incontinence. Application of a forceps on one side of the vagina at the midurethral area can control supine urine loss while coughing by preventing abnormal descent and funneling of the bladder base (midurethral one-sided Bonney test) [20].

Efficacy of Surgical Therapies

Superiority of one continence concept could be proved by direct comparison of the efficacy of operations that are based on the individual theory. Treatment of urethral hypermobility is possible with suspension operations such as the retropubic urethropexy (Burch operation) [24]. During the Burch operation, the lateral parts of the anterior vaginal wall are connected with the ipsilateral Cooper's ligament using nonresorbable sutures [25]. Suspension operations aim to elevate and fix the bladder neck in order to avoid (excessive) movement [24, 26]. Restoration of pubourethral ligament support and treatment of insufficient urethral kinking is possible with the tension-free vaginal tape (TVT) operation [27]. During the operation, a polypropylene tape is implanted via an anterior colpotomy at the level of the midurethra, causing stabilization of the posterior urethral wall, kinking of the urethra during abdominal pressure increase, and intermittent mechanical compression of the urethra between implant and symphysis [22, 27]. Until August 2006, five randomized studies have been published that compared the results of the Burch urethropexy with the TVT operation (Table 3.2). Even though the studies have a limited follow up and continence results might change after a longer

period, no significant differences with regard to efficacy have been found. Differences of continence results of one operation technique are caused by using different continence definitions.

Conclusions

Concepts aim to explain the mechanisms of urinary continence. The bladder neck and midurethra have become the center of interest. Clinical, urodynamic, and radiological signs seem to support the individual theory. However, many women have risk factors for urinary incontinence (e.g., overweight, childbirth, hysterectomy, advanced age), urethral hypermobility, a low urethral closure pressure, laxity of the anterior vaginal wall, or cystourethrocele without being incontinent [14, 33]. Furthermore, no strict relationship exists between the degree of urethral hypermobility and the severity of stress incontinence [33, 34]. Additionally, urethral hypermobility or ISD after midurethral operations and urethral closure pressure after bladder neck operations remain unchanged; nevertheless, these women become continent [21, 35–37]. Obviously, insufficiency of one mechanism can be compensated for by others. Therefore, continence seems to be produced by several mechanisms. However, damage of one part of the continence system may be more severe than damage of other parts.

Randomized studies demonstrated that operation techniques (suspension operations vs. TVT) are equally effective in restoring continence in 65–90% of patients. Surgical restoration of one part of the continence mechanism at the level of the bladder

TABLE 3.2. Prospective randomized trials comparing the efficacy of the bladder neck suspension (Burch urethropexy) and midurethral operation [tension-free vaginal tape (TVT)].

Publication	Follow up (months)	Patients (n)	Continence (%)	p-Value between operations
Ward and Hilton [28]	6	Burch: 128	65	0.83
		TVT: 150	73	
Bai et al. [29]	12	Burch: 33	88	>0.05
		TVT: 31	87	
Wang and Chen [30]	12–36 (median 22)	Burch: 41	88	1.0
		TVT: 49	90	
Liapis et al. [31]	24	Burch: 35	86	>0.05
		TVT: 36	84	
Ward and Hilton [32]	24	Burch: 175	87	0.64
		TVT: 169	85	

No Significant differences with regard to the Continence results were found

neck or midurethra compensates for the existing loss of urethral support and functions by creating new areas for urethral compression. However, some women remain incontinent after the operation, indicating that reconstruction of the individual system was wrong or not sufficient enough to restore continence [38, 39]. Consequently, it is hypothesized to choose an operation based on the other continence concept after failed primary surgery. This strategy is clinical reality; however, it remains to be proved in randomized studies.

References

1. Thom D. Variation in estimates of urinary incontinence prevalence in the community: Effects of differences in definition, population characteristics, and study type. J Am Geriatr Soc 1998; 46:473480.
2. Hunskaar S, Burgio K, Diokno A et al. Epidemiology and natural history of urinary incontinence in women. Urology 2003; 62(Suppl 4A):1623.
3. DeLancey JO. Stress urinary incontinence: Where are we now, where should we go? Am J Obstet Gynecol 1996; 175:311319.
4. DeLancey JO, Ashton-Miller JA. Pathophysiology of adult urinary incontinence. Gastroenterology 2004; 126(Suppl 1): S23–S32.
5. Strohbehn K, Quint LE, Prince MR, et al. Magnetic resonance imaging anatomy of the female urethra: A direct histologic comparison. Obstet Gynecol 1996; 88:750756.
6. Zinner NR, Sterling AM, Ritter RC. Role of inner urethral softness and urinary continence. Urology 1980; 16:115–117.
7. Enhörning G. Simultaneous recording of intravesical and intraurethral pressure. Acta Chir Scand 1961; 276(Suppl):168.
8. Kamo I, Cannon TW, Conway DA, et al. The role of bladder-to-urethral reflexes in urinary continence mechanisms in rats. Am J Physiol Renal Physiol 2004; 287:F434–F441.
9. DeLancey JO. Structural support of the urethra as it relates to stress urinary incontinence: The hammock hypothesis. Am J Obstet Gynecol 1994; 170:1713–1720.
10. Petros PE, Ulmsten UI. An integral theory of female urinary incontinence. Experimental and clinical considerations. Acta Obstet Gynecol Scand Suppl 1990; 153:731.
11. McGuire EJ, Fitzpatrick CC, Wan J, et al. Clinical assessment of urethral sphincter function. J Urol 1993; 150:1452–1454.
12. Summitt RL, Bent AE, Ostergard DR, et al. Stress incontinence and low urethral closure pressure. Correlation of preoperative urethral hypermobility with successful suburethral sling procedures. J Reprod Med 1990; 35:877–880.
13. Crystle CD, Charm LS, Copeland WE. Q-tip test in stress urinary incontinence. Obstet Gynecol 1972; 38:313315.
14. Bergman A, McCarthy TA, Ballard CA, et al. Role of the Q-tip test in evaluating stress urinary incontinence. J Reprod Med 1987; 32:273275.
15. Green TH. The problem of stress urinary incontinence in female: An appraisal of its current status. Obstet Gynecol Surv 1968; 23:603634.
16. McGuire EJ, Lytton B, Pepe V, et al. Stress urinary incontinence. Obstet Gynecol 1976; 47:255264.
17. Blaivas JG, Olsson CA. Stress incontinence: Classification and surgical approach. J Urol 1988; 139:727731.
18. Kondo Y, Homma Y, Takahashi S, et al. Transvaginal ultrasound of urethral sphincter at the midurethra in continent and incontinent women. J Urol 2001; 165:149152.
19. Bergman A, Elia G. Three surgical procedures for genuine stress incontinence: Five-year follow-up of a prospective randomized study. Am J Obstet Gynecol 1995; 173:6671.
20. Petros PE, Ulmsten UI. An integral theory and its method for the diagnosis and management of female urinary incontinence. Scand J Urol Nephrol Suppl 1993; 153:193.
21. Lo TS, Wang AC, Horng SG, et al. Ultrasonograhic and urodynamic evaluation after tension free vagina tape procedure (TVT). Acta Obstet Gynecol Scand 2001; 80:6570.
22. Dietz HP, Wilson PD. The "iris effect": How two-dimensional and three-dimensional ultrasound can help us understand anti-incontinence procedures. Ultrasound Obstet Gynecol 2004; 23:267271.
23. Petros PP, Ulmsten U. An anatomical classification. A new paradigm for management of female lower urinary tract dysfunction. Eur J Obstet Gynecol Reprod Biol 1998; 80:8794.
24. Creighton SM, Clark A, Pearce JM, et al. Perineal bladder neck ultrasound: Appearances before and after continence surgery. Ultrasound Obstet Gynecol 1994; 4:428433.
25. Burch JC. Urethrovaginal fixation to Cooper's ligament for the correction of stress incontinence, cystocele and prolapse. Am J Obstet Gynecol 1961; 81:281290.
26. Viereck V, Bader W, Krauss T, et al. Intra-operative introital ultrasound in Burch colposuspension reduces post-operative complications. BJOG 2005; 112:791796.

27. Ulmsten U, Henriksson L, Johnson P, et al. An ambulatory surgical procedure under local anesthesia for treatment of female urinary incontinence. Int Urogynecol J Pelvic Floor Dysfunct 1996; 7:8185.
28. Ward K, Hilton P. Prospective multicentre randomised trial of tension-free vaginal tape and colposuspension as primary treatment for stress incontinence. BMJ 2002; 325:6770.
29. Bai SW, Sohn WH, Chung DJ, et al. Comparison of the efficacy of Burch colposuspension, pubovaginal sling, and tension-free vaginal tape for stress urinary incontinence. Int J Gynaecol Obstet 2005; 91:246251.
30. Wang AC, Chen MC. Comparison of tension-free vaginal taping versus modified Burch colposuspension on urethral obstruction: A randomized controlled study. Neurourol Urodyn 2003; 22:185190.
31. Liapis A, Bakas P, Creatsas G. Burch colposuspension and tension-free vaginal tape in the management of stress urinary incontinence in women. Eur Urol 2002; 41:469473.
32. Ward KL, Hilton P. A prospective multicenter randomized trial of tension-free vaginal tape and colposuspension for primary urodynamic stress incontinence: Two-year follow-up. Am J Obstet Gynecol 2004; 190:324331.
33. Fleischmann N, Flisser AJ, Blaivas JG, et al. Sphincteric urinary incontinence: Relationship of vesical leak point pressure, urethral mobility and severity of incontinence. J Urol 2003; 169:9991002.
34. Cross CA, Cespedes RD, McGuire EJ. Treatment results using pubovaginal slings in patients with large cystoceles and stress incontinence. J Urol 1997; 158:431–434.
35. Atherton MJ, Stanton SL. A comparison of the bladder neck movement and elevation after TVT and colposuspension. BJOG 2000; 107:13661370.
36. Klutke JJ, Carlin BI, Klutke CG. The tension-free vaginal tape procedure: Correction of stress incontinence with minimal alteration in proximal urethral mobility. Urology 2000; 55:512514.
37. Lukacz ES, Luber KM, Nager CW. The effects of the tension-free vaginal tape on proximal urethral position: A prospective, longitudinal observation. Int Urogynecol J Pelvic Floor Dysfunct 2003; 14:179184.
38. Paick JS, Ku JH, Shin JW, et al. Tension-free vaginal tape procedure for urinary incontinence with low Valsalva leak point pressure. J Urol 2004; 172:13701373.
39. O"Connor RC, Nanigian DK, Lyon MB, et al. Early outcomes of mid-urethral slings for female stress incontinence stratified by Valsalva leak point pressure. Neurourol Urodyn 2006; 25: 685–688.

Chapter 4
Pelvic Floor: Three-Dimensional Surgical Anatomy

Ardeshir R. Rastinehad and Gopal H. Badlani

Introduction

For many surgeons, the anatomy of the pelvic floor has been the foundation for the advancement of novel techniques in the treatment of incontinence and prolapse of the pelvic organs. From the early descriptions of pelvic floor dysfunction (Ebers Papyrus, 1550 BC) to present-day medical literature, the techniques are founded on the basic understand of three-dimensional pelvic anatomy. This chapter will serve as the basis to understand, treat, and develop new techniques in the ongoing efforts to treat these disease processes.

In a historical prospective on female prolapse, Legendre and Bistien (1858) first investigated the tendency of prolapse of the uterus by applying traction. Mengert repeated their initial studies in an attempt to further determine which of the pelvic ligaments provided the primary support to the uterus. By applying 1 kg weight to the uterus, the pelvic ligaments were systematically cut. He reported that when the parametrial and paravaginal tissues were cut and the round ligaments were left intact, the cervix easily prolapsed.

Bony Pelvis

The bony pelvis consists of sacrum, coccyx, and paired bones of the pubis, ischium, and the ilium. The pelvis is divided into the true (below the arcuate line) and the false pelvis. The pelvis is the foundation from which the pelvic support is derived (Fig. 4.1). The sciatic foramen is formed medially by the sacrum, laterally by the ischium, superiorly by the ilium, and is divided into the greater and lesser sciatic foramen by the sacrospinous ligament. The internal pudendal vessels and nerve traverses the greater and lesser sciatic foramen in close proximity (inferior) to the ischial spine. The pudendal canal is bound medially by the fascia of the obturator internus and laterally by its corresponding muscle, and lines the lateral wall of the ischioanal fossa.

Obturator Foramen

The obturator foramen (OF) is the result of the fusion of the pubic bone and the ischium. The anatomy of the OF allows surgeons to approach the female urethra from the lateral aspect, as opposed to the traditional suprapubic approach. The OF is traversed by the obturator nerve artery and vein, all at the most inferiolateral aspect, via the obturator canal (Figs. 4.2–4.4). The OF is covered medially and laterally by the obturator internus/externus, respectively. Using cadaveric dissections, the transobturator needle was an average of 2.3 cm inferior-medial to the obturator canal. The needle was passed through the gracilis, adductor brevis, obturator externus, and obturator membrane, and beneath or through the obturator internus muscle and periurethral endopelvic connective tissue [1].

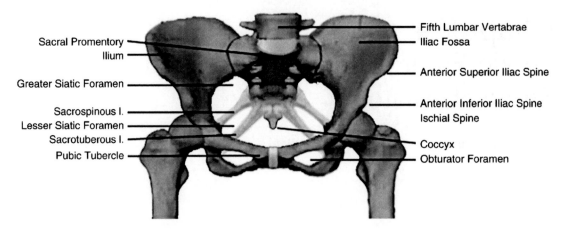

FIG. 4.1. Bony pelvis

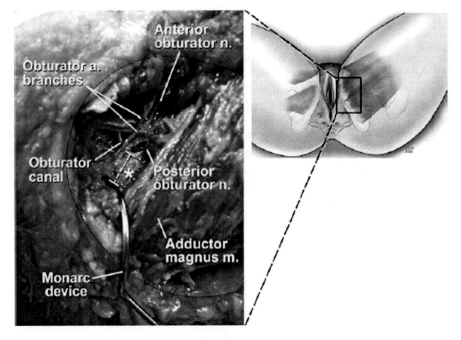

FIG. 4.2. Anatomical dissection of the path of the transobturator sling. Published by Whiteside and Walters (reproduced with permission) [1]

Soft Tissues of the Pelvis

The tendinous arch (arcus tendineus) is a condensation of the medial fascia of the obturator internus muscle, spanning from the posterior aspect of the pubic ramus to the ischial spine (Fig. 4.5). The arcus tendineus is the origin of the pelvic diaphragm (levator ani and coccygeus muscle (Fig. 4.6). The levator ani is considered to be the true muscular floor of the pelvis and is composed of the pubococcygeus, ischiococcygeus, and puborectalis muscles. The levator ani muscle forms a U-shaped hiatus through which the urethra, rectum, and in the female the vagina traverse (Fig. 4.7). The coccygeus and piriformis muscles are the remaining paired muscles that complete the pelvic floor.

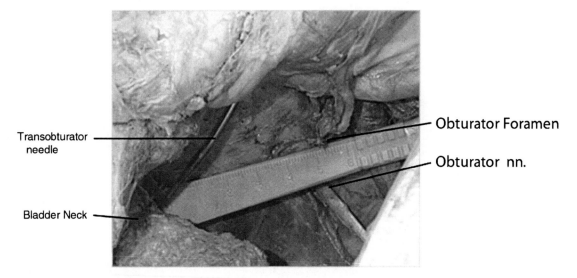

FIG. 4.3. Cadaveric dissection of the endopelvic fascia and right lateral pelvic fossa, including the obturator foramen. The scalpel handle measures the distance from the obturator foramen to the path of the transobturator needle

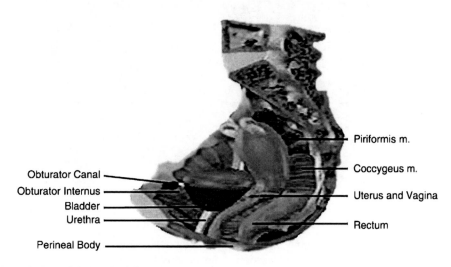

FIG. 4.4. Lateral view of the hemipelvis

The levator ani muscles have a baseline resting tone, similar to other postural muscles [2]. They are composed of type I and type II fibers [3]. The contraction of the levator ani closes the urogenital hiatus by compressing the vagina, rectum, and urethra, displacing the pelvic contents in a cephalad direction. This shifts the strain of the pelvic contents to the muscles from the ligamentous supports and also eliminates potential spaces through which pelvic contents could herniate [2].

Endopelvic Fascia

Endopelvic fascia is an extension of the transversalis fascia [4], which drapes on the pelvic floor. The endopelvic fascia is the result of the ingrowth of splanchnic mesoderm. The endopelvic fascia, which lies immediately beneath the peritoneum, is a viscerofascial layer that interconnects various pelvic organs [4]. DeCaro et al. analyzed the pelvic viscera of cadaveric females, describing the traditional subdivisions of the endopelvic fascia

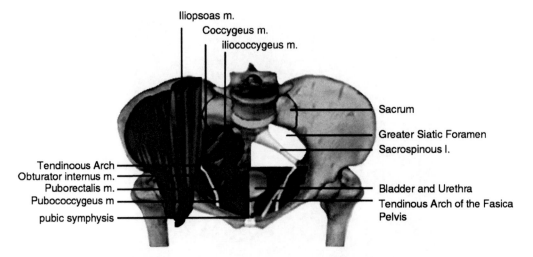

FIG. 4.5. Four-layer artistic interpretation of the pelvis, from the bony ligamentous structures progressing through the deep and superficial musculature

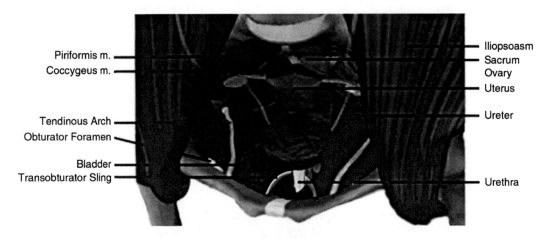

FIG. 4.6. Three-dimensional rotation of the pelvis, anteriorly denoting the path of transobturator needle

(cardinal, uterosacral, urethropelvic, and pubourethral ligaments) as one continuous condensation (3D network) of areolar tissue, with smooth muscle cells surrounding pelvic neurovasculature and no true demarcation between the "ligaments"[5]. Therefore, the strength provided by the endopelvic fascia is due to the entire fascia, not the individual ligaments appreciated during surgical dissection (Figs. 4.8 and 4.9).

Cardinal ligaments give support to the uterus, cervix, and upper vagina by attaching to the pelvic side wall. As described previously, the "ligaments" contain divisions of the hypogastric vessels, which supply the uterus and upper vagina. In conjunction with the uterosacral ligaments, they maintain the position of the cervix and vagina over the levator plate by restricting the downward and outward movements [4]. Uterosacral ligaments are formed by the medial aspect of the endopelvic fascia, spanning from the cervix and upper vagina to the sacrum. The combined uterosacral and cardinal ligaments are the paracolpium, which attach to the vagina, and the parametrium, which attach to the uterus. Urethropelvic ligaments are an anterior medial condensation of the endopelvic fascia, which combines with fibers from the pubococcygeus muscle to span the area from the anterior aspect of the tendinous arc to the anterior vaginal wall, bladder neck, and proximal urethra [4]. This portion of the pelvic floor is the main musculofascial support for the bladder, neck, and proximal urethra. The pubourethral ligament attaches the

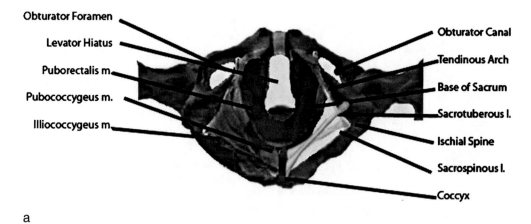

a

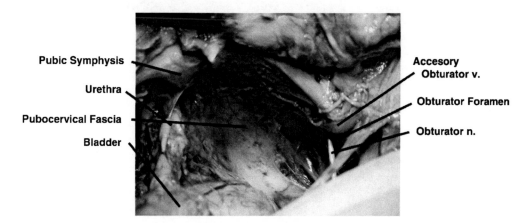

b

FIG. 4.7. Vaginal view of (a) levator ani muscle and bony pelvis with (b) MRI correlation

FIG. 4.8. Lateral pelvic view of endopelvic fascia and associated structures

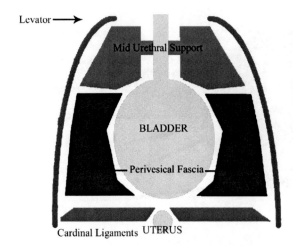

FIG. 4.9. A diagram representing the corresponding fascial support of the bladder, urethra, and uterus. Adapted from four-defect repair of grade 4 cystocele [6]

mid-urethra to the inferior surface of the pubic symphysis. The pubourethral ligaments are analogous to the puboprostatic ligaments in the male. The pubourethral ligaments, in conjunction with the pubourethralis muscle, prevent the rotational decent of the proximal urethra [2].

The fascia of the bladder has two divisions: the perivesical fascia on the vaginal side and the endopelvic fascia on the abdominal side. This provides the posterior support to the bladder and bladder neck. DeLancey described the pelvic fascial support in three distinct functional levels. Level I, upper portion, consists of long sheets endopelvic fascia attaching the vagina to the pelvic wall. Level II, paracolpium, attaches the vagina laterally and more directly to the pelvic walls and stretches the vagina between the bladder and the rectum. The pubocervical fascia is composed of the anterior vaginal wall and directly supports the bladder. Posteriorly, the vaginal wall and the endopelvic fascia form the restraining layer that prevents the formation of a rectocele. Level III, the distal vagina, the walls are directly anchored to the surrounding structures without any intervening paracolpium (Figs. 4.10 and 4.11) [7].

The bladder is a hollow viscus organ used for the temporary storage of urine. While empty, the bladder resides within the true pelvis; during filling, the bladder is displaced anteriorly and superiorly into the preperitoneal space. The bladder neck is located ~3cm posterior to the pubic symphysis

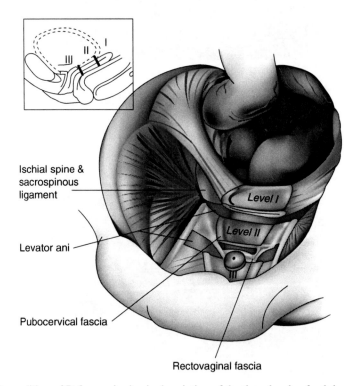

FIG. 4.10. Artist's rendition of DeLancey's classic description of the three levels of pelvic support [8]

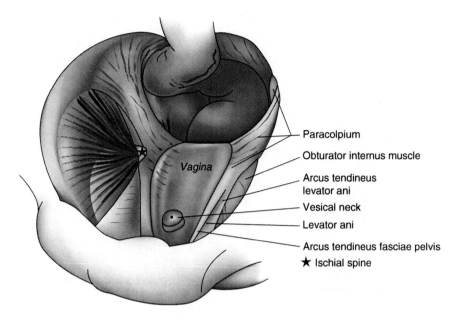

Paracolpium

Obturator internus muscle

Arcus tendineus
levator ani

Vesical neck

Levator ani

Arcus tendineus fasciae pelvis

★ Ischial spine

Vagina

FIG. 4.11. Artist's rendition of the vagina and supportive structures which have been extirpated, including the bladder, which was removed above the bladder neck. The paracolpium extends along the lateral aspects of the vagina [8]

and is supported by the endopelvic fascia. The urachus anchors the bladder dome to the anterior abdominal wall.

Yucel and Baskin proposed a three-component mechanism to male/female continence: the detrusor, trigone, and urethral muscles. These components were of a distinctly different muscular origin. Also, the levator ani muscles do not converge ventrally to the urethra; therefore, their role in continence is questioned [9]. This contrasts the previous theories relating to urethral sphincter development, which postulated a continuation of the trigone and bladder musculature in the formation of the urethral sphincter [10]. The smooth muscle of the urethra, surrounding rhabdosphincter, and periurethral striated muscle of the levator ani are the distinct components of the continence mechanism (Fig. 4.12).

Using three-dimensional imaging techniques, combined with immunohistochemical staining, complete reconstructions of the male and female urethra were completed. The bladder neck is oriented in an oblique angle with the ventral aspect of the bladder neck in a cranial position. The muscle layers of the trigone and the rest of the bladder

were different in morphology. Below the ureteral orifices, the trigonal muscle narrowed and then broadened and thickened dorsally to the bladder and proximal urethra. The outer longitudinal muscle layer of the ventral bladder wall continued in a ventrolateral direction at the bladder neck to envelope the ventral circular muscle fibers of the proximal urethra. The dorsal division did not extend to the proximal urethra. The inner proximal urethra muscle layer could be traced to the internal meatus, where the detrusor inner muscle begins. The inner muscle layer of the urethra continues to the distal urethra [9].

The external urethra sphincter begins in the bladder neck and continues to the distal urethra. Cranially, the external urethral sphincter starts as horseshoe-shaped, only covering the ventral and lateral faces of the proximal and midurethra. The external urethral sphincter at the distal portion remains horseshoe-shaped, yet has a longer extension that covers the distal vagina [9].

The rectovaginal muscle, external urinary sphincter muscle, levator ani muscles, and bulbospongiosis muscle all converged on the median fibrous

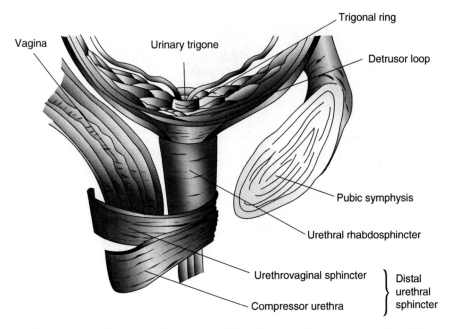

FIG. 4.12. Vaginal view of the pubourethral ligaments, rhabdosphincter, and compressor urethrae [2]

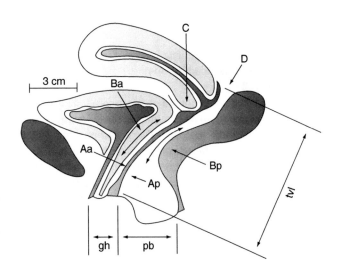

FIG. 4.13. POP classification of prolapse

raphe. The origins of Denonvilliers' fascia have been debated since the first description in 1836. Currently, taking into account the embryological origins, Denonvilliers' fascia is a condensation of the peritoneal cul-de-sac, resulting in a single layer. Denonvilliers' fascia then fuses with the posterior vaginal wall [11]. The illustration outlines the international pelvic organ prolapse; note that at

point D, there is a fusion of the Denonvilliers' fascia and the peritoneum (Fig. 4.13). Perineal body relaxation characteristically is associated with an increase in the diameter of the vaginal opening.

The female pelvis can be divided into two triangles by drawing a line between the ischial tuberosities. The line passes directly through the perineal body (Fig. 4.14).

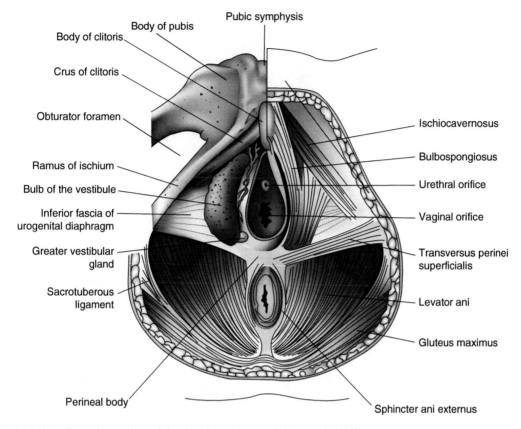

Body of clitoris

Crus of clitoris

Obturator foramen

Ramus of ischium

Bulb of the vestibule

Inferior fascia of
urogenital diaphragm

Greater vestibular
gland

Sacrotuberous
ligament

Perineal body

Body of pubis

Pubic symphysis

Ischiocavernosus

Bulbospongiosus

Urethral orifice

Vaginal orifice

Transversus perinei
superficialis

Levator ani

Gluteus maximus

Sphincter ani externus

Fɪɢ. 4.14. Anterior and posterior pelvic triangles with superficial muscles [12]

Vaginal Anatomy

Vagina

The vaginal wall is 2–3 mm thick and consists of an inner mucous coat, an outer fibrous sheath, and a muscular layer in between. The muscular coat is made of smooth muscle cell bundles, arranged in a spiral system, which allows for distention with tearing [4]. The vaginal depth and axis are maintained, as described by DeLancey in his three-tiered system (Fig. 4.10). The rectovaginal fascia attaches to the posterior vaginal wall, contributing to the overall support system of the vaginal vault [13]. (Fig. 4.15).

Tissue Planes of the Pelvis

The connective tissue planes of the pelvis allow for independent function of the uterus, bladder, and rectum. These connective tissue planes create potential spaces to allow for dissection during urologic and gynecologic procedures and also impede the spread of infection among adjacent organs/spaces. The septa dividing these areas envelope neurovascular and lymphatic structures supplying each organ (Fig. 4.16).

Vesicovaginal Space

The vesicovaginal space traverses the area posterior to the adventia of the bladder and anterior to the vagina. The lateral borders consist of the bladder septa containing the ureter and efferent veins, which attaches laterally inferiorly at the lateral portion of the bladder and extends up to the lateral portion of the cardinal ligaments. The vesicovaginal space fuses closed between the adventia of the bladder and uterus, forming the vesicovaginal septum, which progresses as the vesicocervical space.

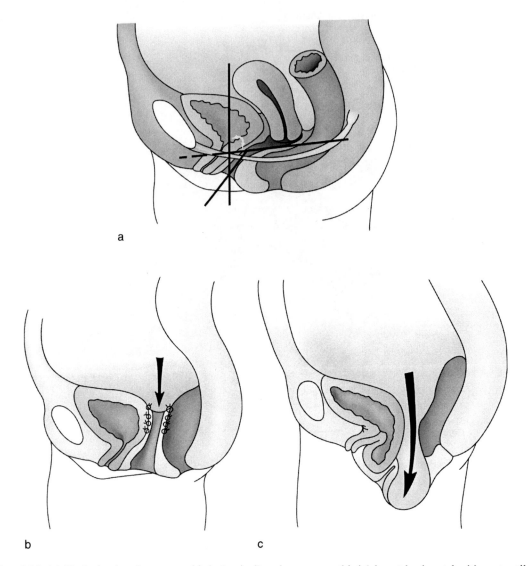

a

b   c

FIG. 4.15. (a) Vaginal axis – lower two thirds (vesical) and upper one third (almost horizontal with poster tilt). (b) Loss of axis post hysterectomy. (c) Apical and anterior compartment prolapse secondary to loss of axis

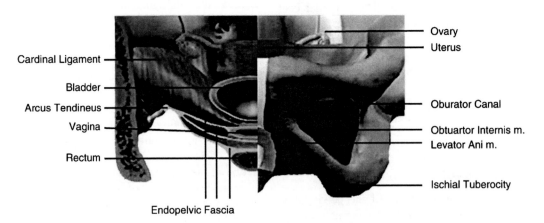

Cardinal Ligament

Bladder

Arcus Tendineus

Vagina

Rectum

Endopelvic Fascia

Ovary

Uterus

Oburator Canal

Obtuartor Internis m.
Levator Ani m.

Ischial Tuberocity

FIG. 4.16. Superficial and deep pelvis (anterior view) with potential dissecting planes

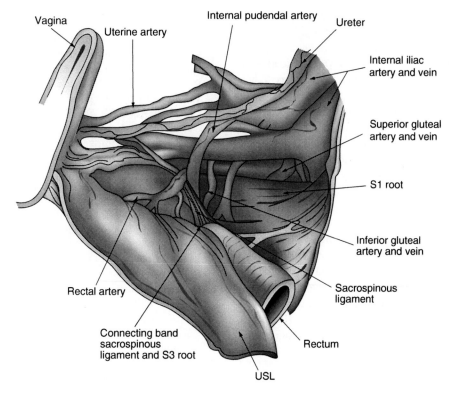

FIG. 4.17. Neurovascular anatomy of the pelvis (lateral review) [15]

Space of Retzius (Retropubic Space)

The prevesical space of Retzius extends from the posterior aspect of the pubis, anteriorly to the bladder, and then extends cephalad between the medial umbilical ligaments. It offers the space to approach the endopelvic fascia and arcus tendineus for suprapubic approach in continence procedures, as well as the space that needles traverse.

Paravesical Space

The paravesical spaces, which are preformed fat-filled spaces, are bilaterally bound, superiorly by the lateral umbilical ligaments and medially by the bladder separating the space. This lies superior to the cardinal ligaments. The lateral boundary consists of the fascia from the levator ani muscles and the obturator internus. The so-called paravaginal tear at the endopelvic fascia and its attachment to the arcus tendineus are described as a cause of lateral cystocele and urethral hypermobility.

Pararectal Space

The pararectal space is inferior to the cardinal ligaments, extends from the anteriolateral boundaries of the sacrum, and spans the area to the lateral borders of the rectum and the levator ani muscles. Superiorly, the rectum is contained within a single circular pararectal space, which is a confluence of the two inferior pararectal spaces.

Rectovaginal Space

The superior portion of the rectovaginal space is bound by the rectouterine pouch (Douglas) and inferiorly by the perineal body. The pelvic floor muscle (levator ani) inserts on the perineal body. The detachment of the endopelvic prerectal fascia from the perineal body results in a rectocele.

Pelvic organ prolapse is divided into three major categories (anterior, middle, and posterior). Anterior vaginal wall prolapse consists of two subtypes: lateral and central or posterior cystoceles. The lateral cystocele is associated with a hypermobility of the bladder neck, which includes the urethra. This condition results from the attenuation of the lateral supports (pubourethral and endopelvic fascia). In contrast to the central variant (bladder), this is secondary to laxity of the vesicopelvic fascia.

Vaginal vault prolapse is secondary to the loss of support from the sacrouterine and cardinal ligaments. Also, midline defects included enteroceles, which are most commonly associated with a laxity between the vagina and the rectum, and the length of the posterior vaginal wall is preserved [13]. There is a 75% incidence of enteroceles associated with vault eversion [14].

Posterior compartmental prolapse (rectocele) can be secondary to attenuation of the distal posterior wall, perineal membrane, and perineal body. The rectum has numerous attachments contributing to its overall support, including the Waldeyer's fascia, perineal body (anterior), ATFP (laterally), and rectovaginal fascial attachment to uterosacral ligaments (superior) [13].

Neurovascular Anatomy

The neurovascular anatomy of the pelvis is complex due to the venous and neural plexus widely spread through the entire pelvis. Presacral, retrotrigonal, and pararectal nerve dissection leads to functional impairment and violation of the prevesical spaces, resulting in significant bleeding. The arterial anatomy is more predictable with branches of the internal iliac supply of the pelvic organ. Vascular grafts for labia majora (Martius flap) can be anteriorly or posteriorly based.

The location of the neurovascular bundle, 1–2 cm medial to the ischial spine over the sacrospinalis ligament, is well recognized. Similarly, venous plexus in presacral space can be a cause of significant bleeding in the repair (Fig. 4.17).

References

1. Whiteside J, Walters M. Anatomy of the obturator region: Relations to a trans-obturator sling. Int Urogynecol J 2004;15:223–226.
2. Plzak L, Staskin D. Genuine stress incontinence: Theories of etiology and surgical correction. Urol Clin North Am 2002; 29:527–535.
3. Gosling J, Dixon J, Crichely H, Thompson S. A comparative study of the human external sphincter and periurethral levator ani muscles. Br J Urol 1981; 53(1):35–41.
4. Klutke C, Siegel C. Functional female pelvic anatomy. Urol Clin North Am 1995; 22(3):487–498.
5. DeCaro R, Aragona F, Herms A, Guidolin D. Morphometric analysis of the fibroadipose tissue of the female pelvis. J Urol 1998;160:707–713.
6. Safir MH, Gousse AE, Rovner ES, . 4-Defect repair of grade 4 cystocele. J Urol 1999; 161:587–594.
7. DeLancey J. Anatomy and biomechanics of genital prolapse. Clin Obstet Gynecol 1993; 36(4):897–909.
8. DeLancey JOL. Anatomic aspects of vaginal eversion after hysterectomy. Am J Obstet Gynecol 1992; 166:1717–1728.
9. Yucel S, Baskin L. An anatomical description of the male and female urethral sphincter complex. J Urol 2004;171:1890–1897.
10. Delancy J. Structural aspects of urethrovesical junction in the female. Neurourol Urodyn 1988; 7:509.
11. Cesoedes RD. The treatment of posterior compartment vaginal defects. Atlas Urol Clin 2004;12:233–241.
12. From Williams PL, Warwick R. Gray's anatomy, 35th British ed. Philadelphia, WB Saunders, 1973:1364.
13. Zhu H, Kluthke JJ, Lutke CG. MR imaging findings with female prolapse. Atlas Urol Clin 2003;11:101–112.
14 Nichols DH, Randall CL. Vaginal surgery, 4th ed. Baltimore, Williams and Wilkins.
15. Chesson RR, Shobeiri SA. Uterosacral suspension of the vaginal vault. Atlas Urol Clin 2003; 11:113–127.

Chapter 5
Pelvic Floor Prolapse: Cause and Effect

Matthew A. Barker and Mickey M. Karram

Introduction

Pelvic floor prolapse or pelvic organ prolapse (POP) (Fig. 5.1) is a common but poorly understood condition affecting millions of women worldwide. In the United States, the lifetime risk of undergoing surgery for POP or urinary incontinence is estimated to be 11%, and nearly 30% of these patients require another operation for recurrence [1]. The Women's Health Initiative (WHI) data revealed that approximately 40% of women had some form of POP [2]. This difference in rates of prolapse between surgical patients and patients being seen for routine gynecologic examinations reflects the often asymptomatic presentation of prolapse [3]. Understanding the progression of this disease may allow clinicians to apply more appropriate treatment to patients depending on the etiology of their prolapse and their symptoms. Despite the prevalence of POP, little is known regarding the mechanism for development and natural history of the disease. Much of this stems from the lack of a clear and standardized definition for POP, which limits our ability to study its etiologies. A conference on terminology assembled by the National Institutes of Health (NIH) recently focused on developing clear definitions for POP to foster more epidemiological research into the disease [4]. These studies are forthcoming, but with a 45% increase over 30 years in demand for services related to pelvic floor dysfunction, our understanding of its development will become important in meeting the treatment needs of the future [5]. Successful treatment will require the identification and management of risk factors that could potentially be involved in the development of POP.

In order to recognize risk factors for POP, a thorough understanding of pelvic anatomy is needed. As the female pelvis evolved from quadruped ambulation to bipedalism, supportive structures adapted to support pelvic viscera and enable parturition (see Chapter 4, Three-Dimensional surgical anatomy). Activities and events that are shaped by a bipedal lifestyle can contribute to failures in the supportive structure of the pelvis that can lead to POP. Maintaining or rehabilitating levator muscle bulk and strength may be the key to preventing many cases of pelvic organ prolapse [6]. Just as humans evolve, so too do the signs and symptoms of POP. Research into the evolution of POP should focus on the anatomical disruptions predisposed to by specific risk factors and physical insults to the female pelvis. It is not uncommon for urinary incontinence, fecal incontinence, and POP to coexist because of their anatomical relationships and common risk factors (Fig. 5.2). In this chapter we will focus specifically on the cause and effect of pelvic organ prolapse.

Causes

There are many postulated risk factors for POP, including genetics, race, pregnancy, vaginal childbirth, prior surgery, neuropathy, obesity, smoking, chronically increased intra-abdominal pressure, certain recreational or occupational activities, aging, and menopause. In reality, the etiology most likely is multifactorial and reflects a combination of some if not all of these risk factors [3]. Individuals will develop POP based on the combination of these risk factors. Bump and Norton described a useful

approach to understanding the development of POP by considering the risk factors as predisposing, inciting, promoting, and decompensating events [7] (Table 5.1).

Predisposing Events

Predisposing factors such as race and genetics may increase an individual's risk for developing POP. Unfortunately, many of the studies looking at the etiology of POP included predominately Caucasians. Data from the WHI showed African-Americans had a lower rate of POP compared to Caucasians, whereas Hispanics had a higher risk of developing uterine and anterior wall prolapse [2]. These differences may be related to differences in the bony pelvis and muscle mass or it may reflect a paucity of data regarding racial differences with pelvic floor dysfunction. Many ethnic and racial studies have small sample sizes that limit us from

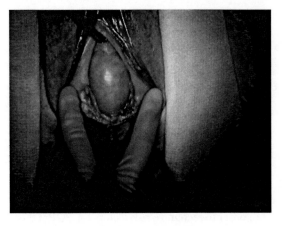

FIG. 5.1. Picture of pelvic organ prolapse

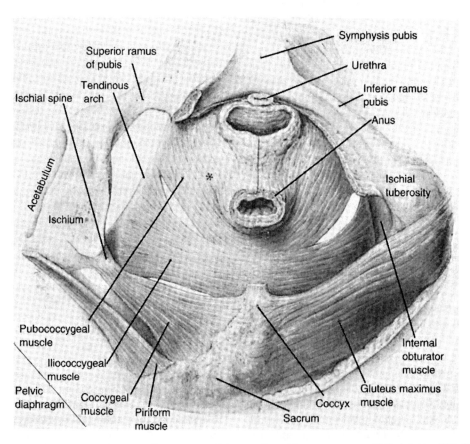

FIG. 5.2. Anatomy of the pelvic floor. (From: Anson BJ. *An atlas of human anatomy*. Philadelphia: WB Saunders, 1950, with permission.)

TABLE 5.1. Potential risk factors for pelvic organ prolapse.

Predispose	Incite	Promote	Decompensate
Genetics	Pregnancy	Obesity	Aging
Race	Delivery	Smoking	Menopause
	Pelvic surgery	Pulmonary disease	Myopathy
	Myopathy	Constipation	Neuropathy
	Neuropathy	Heavy lifting	Debilitation

drawing any statistically meaningful inferences. These studies may actually harm certain racial demographics by minimizing the need to assess certain ethnic groups or by providing inappropriate therapy [8]. Studies are limited and data often are contradictory in regard to racial differences in the incidence of pelvic organ prolapse, and it is impossible to draw any firm conclusions [9]. Further population-based studies are needed to decipher whether racial differences exist for POP so that appropriate care and counseling can be given.

Although no study exists that identifies individuals who are destined to develop POP, there are certain risk factors that may predispose women to POP. Just as race is inherited, so too are other familial traits such as the shape of bony pelvis. There have been studies showing that women are at greater risk for developing prolapse if their mothers or sisters reported the condition [10–13]. This association among relatives may have to do with similar collagen make up. Defective connective tissue such as that associated with joint hypermobility and diseases like Ehlers–Danlos syndrome may contribute to POP through defects in the underlining collagen of the pelvic floor [14]. The connective tissue that supports and suspends the pelvic organs can become structurally or biochemically defective, leading to POP. Women undergoing surgery for POP have a decrease in fibroblasts and an increase in abnormal collagen [15]. Other studies reaffirmed this imbalance of collagen, meaning that there was an increase in type III collagen, which is weaker and its overabundance may lead to POP [16]. It yet has to be determined whether this change in collagen is related to age, hypoestrogenic states, or remodeling secondary to an already present POP.

Just as breakdown in support can occur and lead to POP, pelvic neuropathies can cause similar effects. The resting tone of the levator ani helps support the pelvic floor and prevent prolapse;

any disruption to this innervation can predispose a women to POP. Occult spina bifida has been correlated with the development of POP, and 80% of newborn females and nulliparous women with spina bifida have uterine prolapse [17, 18]. Other conditions that affect the spinal cord pathway and pelvic nerve roots result in flaccid paralysis of the pelvic floor muscles and POP [19]. It is the loss of support, whether structural, biochemical, or denervation to pelvic tissues, that predisposes women to POP. This concept of loss of support at many levels is important when looking at other insults to the pelvic floor and its effects.

Inciting Events

The factors that may incite POP are related to events that lead to damage to the pelvic floor. This may include vaginal birth, nerve and muscle damage, and pelvic surgery. Parity is a risk factor often associated with POP and increasing parity is associated with advancing prolapse [20]. In data from the WHI the first birth doubled the risk of uterine prolapse as well as anterior and posterior wall prolapse; each additional birth increased the risk by 10–21% [2]. The Oxford Family Planning Study showed that women with two deliveries were 8.4 times more likely to have surgery for prolapse compared to nulliparous women (Fig. 5.3) [21]. Even though vaginal delivery is associated with POP, other obstetric risk factors exist that may contribute to POP. Operative deliveries, prolonged second stage, macrosomia, episiotomies, epidurals, and oxytocin have been implicated in causing prolapse [3].

The labor and delivery process may cause direct injury to the nerves and muscles and possible tissue disruption, all of which can cause pelvic floor dysfunction. Increased pressure on the pelvic floor may stretch and tear maternal tissues during delivery. Forceps and episiotomies are risk factors for

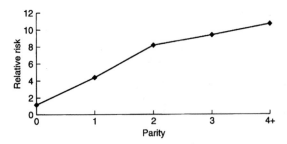

FIG. 5.3. Adjusted effects of parity on inpatient admission rates for genital prolapse. (From Mant J, Painter R, Vesse M. Epidemiology of genital prolapse: observations from the Oxford Family Planning Association Study. *Br J Obstet Gynaecol* 1997;104:579, with permission.)

pelvic floor dysfunction. Many argue for elective cesarean sections to prevent these injures to the pelvic floor [22–24]. Because there is no evidence that elective episiotomy and operative vaginal delivery are beneficial and the potential harm is great, some feel that the routine use of these procedures should be avoided [3]. Data relating vaginal delivery to the development of POP are confusing because most pelvic floor dysfunction occurs long after the vaginal birth, and most women who experience childbirth do not develop POP [7]. In a recent cross-sectional study comparing women who had undergone one or more vaginal deliveries compared to women who had only cesarean sections, the vaginal delivery cohort showed a significantly greater risk of developing symptomatic POP, after adjusting for age, parity, and obesity [25]. This study suggests that it is the labor process more so than the pregnancy that contributes to pelvic floor dysfunction. Yet, other studies exist that contradict these findings, and the problem that still persists is that pregnancy is a risk factor in itself; further data are needed to evaluate which has the greatest impact on pelvic floor dysfunction [20, 21].

The debate is ongoing about elective cesarean sections, but it seems reasonable to offer women with preexisting pelvic floor dysfunction or prior injury an elective cesarean section to prevent further worsening of their disease. Recently, the NIH held a conference on cesarean delivery and it was concluded that more research was needed before promoting elective operative deliveries [26]. What is interesting about the consensus group is that it still left open the possibility for planned cesarean deliveries, but thought it should be made on an individual

basis. This is exactly how we should approach women with risk factors for POP: individualize their care based on risk stratification and orient their treatment to their specific risk factors or causes of their POP. Ideally, physician's efforts should be aimed at identifying which women are at risk and which risk factors in the birthing process can be modified.

In addition to childbirth, pelvic surgery is an identifiable inciting factor for pelvic floor dysfunction. During radical pelvic surgery muscles and supportive tissues often are transected, predisposing women to POP. Hysterectomy alone is thought to double the risk of severe POP and prior surgery for pelvic organ prolapse is a risk factor for recurrence as well [27]. In the Oxford Family Planning Study, the incidence of surgery for POP was higher in women with a prior hysterectomy for reasons other than prolapse and substantially higher in women who had a hysterectomy for prolapse [21]. This may reflect surgical techniques that have resulted in high failure rates for surgical correction of POP or the disruption to the pelvic muscles, nerves, and tissues that occur during surgery. One study looked at the risk of developing POP after vaginal hysterectomy and found that a prophylactic McCall-type culdoplasty at the time of vaginal hysterectomy may prevent the development of posterior wall prolapse [28]. There is potential to modify our surgical techniques in order to improve clinical outcomes, decrease recurrence rates, and counsel patients who may be at risk for later POP development.

Promoting Events

The area that holds the greatest benefit to preventing the development of POP is modifying the behaviors and activities that are known risk factors for POP. We have discussed risk factors that predispose and incite POP, but there are many factors that promote the development of POP. Risk factors such as obesity, smoking, chronic coughing, constipation, and heavy lifting can be modified to prevent the cause-and-effect relationship we see with them and the development of POP.

Obesity is one of the few modifiable risk factors for POP identified so far [2, 21]. Data from the WHI showed that body mass index greater that 30 kg m^{-2} conferred a 40–75% increased risk of POP [2]. The data revealed that "apple" body-shaped women had a 17% increase of anterior and posterior vaginal wall prolapse. This supports the theory that chronic increases in intra-abdominal pressure lead to POP. There are limited data on the results of weight reduction and resolution of pelvic floor disorders. The prevalence of urinary and anal incontinence in the obese population is high, and weight loss may be able to reverse some of these symptoms [29]. The effects of increased weight and intra-abdominal pressure on the pelvic floor cause a mixture of pelvic floor dysfunction, with POP being a symptom of this. There is potential to possibly reverse urinary and defecatory symptoms with weight loss, and further data are needed to evaluate the potential to reverse the symptoms of POP.

The theory behind the development of POP from chronically increased intra-abdominal pressure is supported by many associations. Obesity, chronic constipation, chronic coughing and repetitive heavy lifting have been associated with the development of POP. The chronic straining associated with constipation is thought to lead to progressive pelvic neuropathy and dysfunction due to stretching of the pudendal nerve [30]. Women with a history of constipation and straining during bowel movements before the onset of pelvic floor dysfunction had an increased risk of developing both POP and urinary incontinence compared to women who did not have pelvic floor dysfunction [31]. Similar repetitive forceful straining also can occur with coughing usually associated with cigarette smoking and chronic obstructive pulmonary disease (COPD).

The data around smoking as a cause of POP are mixed, and one study suggests it may be protective [1, 2, 10, 20, 21, 32]. Interestingly, data analyzing COPD and its association with POP failed to show a correlation [1, 24]. Studies looking at urinary incontinence revealed an increase in stress urinary incontinence with smokers [33]. It was thought that smokers' more chronic and stronger coughing contributed to their incontinence. Again, POP is intuitively thought to be influenced by a similar mechanism, but data showing an association with COPD are lacking.

Activities that increase intra-abdominal pressure such as repetitive manual lifting are associated with POP. Nursing assistants who were exposed to repetitive heavy lifting were at increased risk of undergoing surgery for POP [34]. In a clinic-based study of Nepalese women with POP, their POP was associated with heavy lifting especially during the postpartum period [35]. Another report implicated the stress of airborne training in female paratroopers as a risk factor for the development of POP and urinary incontinence [36]. A survey of Olympic athletes in high-impact sporting events did not have any greater risk for the development of urinary incontinence years later compared with athletes competing in low-impact events [37]. This study did not look at prolapse and there is limited data showing an association of high impact forces on the pelvic floor and the development of POP.

A clear cause-and-effect relationship with increased intra-abdominal pressure and the development of POP has yet to be validated with large prospective studies. This is an area where research is clearly needed and could possibly help identify women at risk and possibly contribute to the prevention of POP. It also could potentially decrease the risk of POP recurrence, which is as high as 30% following pelvic surgery [1]. In a study looking at certain activities and intra-abdominal pressure measurements, there were wide variations in pressures generated, and many of the activities surgeons recommend patients avoid after surgery did not generate pressures greater than simply getting out of a chair [38]. A better understanding of the mechanisms that abdominal forces play on the pelvic floor is needed to help guide our understanding of the causes of POP and help us educate our patients better in terms of avoiding these promoting factors.

Decompensating Events

The normal pelvic floor anatomy of the female evolved to withstand the shift in abdominal forces from the anterior abdominal wall to the pelvis, stress from childbirth, and permit urinary and fecal evacuation. It often is affected by the direct strain these changes place on it, but it also is susceptible to factors extrinsic to the pelvic floor. Age, estrogen status, and comorbid diseases contribute to the development of POP, but studies are limited that show a direct relationship of these individual factors on the pelvic floor.

Advancing age is probably the greatest risk factor for POP. Prior studies have evaluated age as a risk factor for POP; utilizing multiple logistic regression analysis, the menopausal status becomes nonsignificant and age more than estrogen levels places a woman at risk for prolapse [2, 10, 20, 24]. Estrogen receptors are found throughout the vagina, but little is known about the potential independent effects of menopause or estrogen status on

POP. Dermatologic studies have shown that estrogen increases total skin collagen content and vaginal estrogen is routinely recommended to correct POP [39]. One study looking at selective estrogen receptor modulator (SERM) for osteoporosis was stopped before completion secondary to adverse affects including increased urinary incontinence and twofold increase in progression of prolapse [40]. In contrast to this study there is one case-controlled study showing a decreased risk of POP in postmenopausal women using hormone replacement therapy (HRT) for greater than 5 years [41]. It is not clear if HRT is truly protective, but other than in a SERM study HRT does not appear to have a negative effect on POP. The common use of topical vaginal estrogen cream in postmenopausal women with POP hopefully will generate future studies that examine estrogen status as an independent risk factor for prolapse.

Age and postmenopausal status are associated with many other medical illnesses. Medical diseases that lead to microvasculature damage and peripheral neuropathies potentially can cause POP. In one large study of the etiologies of POP the presence of any chronic illness was not associated with POP, but in another study hypertension was a risk factor [20, 24]. Large epidemiological studies evaluating women with POP are needed to examine and assess the impact diseases like diabetes, hypertension, and other chronic illnesses have on the pelvic floor.

Effects

The grouping of risk factors established by Bump and Norton enable clinicians to organize their thoughts about the development and progression of POP, but it does not enable them to predict who will be symptomatic from their POP or what type of pelvic floor dysfunction they will suffer [7]. The risk factors that lead to causes of POP usually manifest as symptoms perceived by an individual. The suggested definition of POP by the NIH conference to standardize the terminology of pelvic floor disorders relied on physical findings alone to define POP, but in clinical practice it is the patient's symptoms that lead them to seek treatment; there are limited data regarding the significance of asymptomatic POP [4]. The effects that POP have on individuals vary in severity in terms of the impact on their quality of life. Symptoms that individuals with POP traditionally describe can be broken down into anatomic, functional, or sexual symptoms. Because of the anatomical relationships of the urinary, reproductive, and digestive systems, much overlap often exists in symptoms associated with POP. These symptoms include vaginal bulging, pelvic pressure, voiding dysfunction, defecatory dysfunction, and sexual dysfunction (Table 5.2). Our understanding of the relationship between prolapse and pelvic floor symptoms have improved with the implementation of validated self-administered questionnaires that enable researchers to assess the impact different symptoms have on individuals and which correlate with POP [42].

Anatomic Symptoms

The failure of normal pelvic floor support leads to symptoms of POP. The protusion of the cervix or herniations of vaginal tissue through the vaginal introitus cause symptoms which patients describe as a "bulge," protrusion, pelvic or low back pain, or just pressure. The levator ani muscles and connective tissue attachments to the pelvic viscera provide the normal support to pelvic organs and their surrounding tissue (Fig. 5.4). The levator ani muscles have a normally contracted basal tone that

TABLE 5.2. Symptoms of pelvic floor prolapse.

Anatomic	Functional (urinary)	Functional (bowel)	Sexual
Sense "bulge"	Incontinence (stress and/or urge)	Incontinence (fecal/flatal)	Dyspareunia
Visualize "bulge"	Frequency and urgency	Urgency	Interference of POP during intercourse
Pressure/fullness	Incomplete bladder emptying	Incomplete rectal emptying	
	Hesitancy	Straining	
	Splinting to void	Splinting to defecate	

keeps the urogenital hiatus closed, but also can contract reflexively in response to certain actions that increase intra-abdominal pressure [43]. If there is damage or weakening of the levator ani muscles, the connective tissue around the pelvic organs will provide support until the load becomes too great [43]. The genital hiatus then will open with the loss of levator ani contraction and failure of the connective tissue allows for the pelvic organs and/or tissues to prolapse [43]. It is this failure of the normal anatomy caused by previously described risk factors that leads to the development of POP.

The varying complaints that patients report have led clinicians to investigate whether the extent of prolapse correlates with symptoms. In one study, the symptoms of POP increased when the leading edge of the prolapse was beyond the hymenal remnants [44]. The concept that symptoms worsen with stage of POP is important, but it does not explain why patients with similar degrees of POP present with different and multiple symptoms. Ellerkmann et al. found a correlation between patients being able to visualize a bulge and worsening stage of POP, but symptoms did not necessarily correlate with compartment-specific defects [45]. Also, they did not show a strong correlation between the stage of POP and other symptoms related to urinary and defecatory dysfunction. Other studies have confirmed that the typical symptom that is anatomically associated with POP is a "bulging" sensation and that other symptoms do not correlate with the severity of POP [46, 47]. The inability to correlate stage of prolapse with voiding and defecatory symptoms with stage of POP may imply that a different mechanism may be involved in the development of functional complaints in women with POP.

Functional Symptoms

The loss of normal urinary and bowel function in an individual can be very debilitating to an individual's quality of life. POP often is associated with different complaints that relate to the urinary and bowel function controlled by the pelvic floor. Individuals with POP often complain of urinary stress incontinence, urgency and or frequency, hesitancy, incomplete emptying, and splinting (digitally reducing prolapse) to fully evacuate urine. The bowel symptoms in individuals with POP consist of straining to defecate, incontinence of flatus and stool, incomplete rectal emptying, and splinting to complete defecation. All these symptoms can impact an individual's life in a negative way. It is important to question regarding these symptoms in anyone with any stage of POP because symptoms do not always correlate with stage of POP and these symptoms can be debilitating and need to be addressed [45–47].

The typical urinary symptoms that develop in women with POP are variable. Stress incontinence

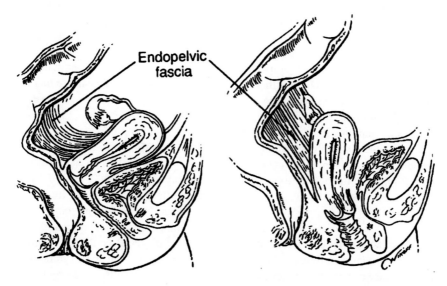

Endopelvic fascia

FIG. 5.4. Levator ani muscle and connective tissue supportive function of the pelvic floor. (From DeLancey JOL. Anatomy and biomechanics of genital prolapse. *Clin Obstet Gynecol* 1993;36:906, with permission.)

often is encountered in women with a hypermobile urethra, often seen in patients with anterior vaginal wall prolapse [42]. The symptom of stress incontinence can resolve as a prolapse worsens or even develop into obstructive urinary symptoms depending on the stage of the prolapse [45, 46, 48]. Often women with POP beyond the hymen have less stress incontinence symptoms, but have to splint (digitally reduce the prolapse) in order to urinate [46]. The reason patients with advanced stage prolapse are often continent of urine is because the urethra is kinked and urinary retention develops as the anterior vaginal wall prolapse worsens [42]. This becomes important in the evaluation of women considering both conservative management with a pessary or surgical correction because each can unmask occult stress urinary incontinence.

Symptoms of defecatory dysfunction are just as variable as that of urinary incontinence in women with POP. The defecatory symptom that seems to correlate most greatly with POP of the posterior compartment is the need to splint the vagina or perineum to defecate [42, 45, 46]. Unfortunately, the exam and extent of prolapse do not always correlate with symptoms, and factors involved in defecactory dysfunction usually benefit from an extensive workup looking at other causes than just POP [49]. Because symptoms of POP such as constipation and straining may contribute to POP, it is difficult to elicit whether the symptoms are the cause or effect or POP [30, 31, 42]. Other defecatory symptoms may have different etiologies, but are present in association with POP. Fecal incontinence is seen in 7–31% of women with POP [50–51]. Fecal incontinence typically is associated with rectal prolapse rather than POP, but the two disorders share similar risk factors including neuropathic and muscular injury to the pelvic floor [7, 42, 51]. Variation in symptoms may be related to the degree of insult to the pelvic floor, which may explain why people with more symptoms may have a greater degree of injury to the pelvic floor.

Sexual Symptoms

Female sexual dysfunction is characterized by problems with sexual desire, arousal, orgasm, or dyspareunia that cause personal distress [52]. Women with POP and urinary incontinence traditionally have been considered to have similar rates

of sexual activity to those of aged-matched individuals without POP and urinary incontinence [53]. Age more than POP and incontinence seems to contribute to sexual dysfunction. As POP increases in stage, women report more interference with sexual activity, but data are mixed on whether this limits their sexual activity or negatively affects their sexual satisfaction [45, 53, 54]. In another study looking at pelvic floor dysfunction and sexual function, POP did not reveal an association with sexual complaints, but this study did not use questionnaires designed for women with pelvic floor disorders [55]. Our understanding of the effects of POP rely on our ability to adequately study and measure these effects. In a study looking at patients presenting to a urogynecology office, only 10% of patients who were not sexually active reported that their POP was contributing to sexual dysfunction [56]. Clearly the overlap of disorders and symptoms in women with pelvic floor dysfunction contributes to their sexual function and further studies using validated measuring techniques are needed to further understand the effects of POP on sexual function.

Sexual dysfunction also includes pain symptoms, which are often frequent complaints in individuals with POP. Patients with POP often attribute their back pain or pelvic pain to their prolapse. Heit et al. examined women with POP and found no association between low back pain or pelvic pain [57]. Similar results were found in another study that did not show any pain association with severity of POP [44]. Just as sexual dysfunction is influenced by other factors, so too are pain symptoms. Individuals caring for women with POP who have pain symptoms should evaluate this further instead of just equating it with their other POP symptoms.

Conclusions

Pelvic organ prolapse is caused by multiple factors that lead to variable effects on the pelvic floor. There is as yet no large epidemiological study evaluating the natural history of women with asymptomatic POP or the type and frequency of symptoms in women with symptomatic POP [4]. Much of the difficulty in designing a large study lies in the fact that multiple factors are involved in the development of this condition and there is a lack of a standard definition. The future of understanding the etiology of POP will rest in our ability to design studies to look at individual factors that contribute to POP. Ideally, a model needs to be created to test these factors in controlled environments so that their individual effects on the pelvic floor can be studied. Recently computer- generated models have been developed based on radiological imaging and muscle morphology to study pelvic anatomy and the effect of vaginal birth on the pelvic floor muscles [58–60]. This advancement in the comprehension of pelvic anatomy and use of technology will lead to the development of a validated model to study the causes and effects of POP. Further understanding of the etiology and natural history of POP will enable clinicians to intervene and prevent disease progression in patients with recognized risk factors.

References

1. Olsen AL, Smith VJ, Bergstrom JO, et al. Epidemiology of surgically managed pelvic organ prolapse and urinary incontinence. Obstet Gynecol 1997;89:501–506.
2. Hendrix SL, Clark A, Nygaard I, et al. Pelvic organ prolapse in the Women's Health Initiative: Gravity and gravidity. Am J Obstet Gynecol 2002;186:1160–1166.
3. Schaffer JI, Wai CY, Boreham MK. Etiology of pelvic organ prolapse. Clin Obstet Gynecol 2005;48:639–647.
4. Weber AM, Abrams P, Brubaker L, et al. The standardization of terminology for researchers in female pelvic floor disorders. Int Urogynecol J 2001;12:178–186.
5. Luber KM, Boreo S, Choe JY. The demographics of pelvic floor disorders current observations and future projections. Am J Obstet Gynecol 2001;184:1496–1503.
6. Schimpf M, Tulikangas P. Evolution of the female pelvis and relationships to pelvic organ prolapse. Int Urogynecol J 2005;16:315–320.
7. Bump RC, Norton PA. Epidemiology and natural history of pelvic floor dysfunction. Obstet Gynecol Clin North Am 1998;25:723–746.
8. Mallett VT, Bump RC. The epidemiology of female pelvic floor dysfunction. Curr Opin Obstet Gynecol 1994;6:308–312.
9. Kim S, Harvey MA, Johnston S. A review of the epidemiology and pathophysiology of pelvic floor dysfunction: Do racial differences matter? J Obstet Gynaecol Can 2005;27:251–259.
10. Chiaffarino F, Chatenoud L, Dindelli M, et al. Reproductive factors, family history, occupation and risk of urogenital prolapse. Eur J Obstet Gynecol Reprod Biol 1999;82:63–67.
11. Buchsbaum G, Kerr L, Guzick D. Pelvic relaxation in nulliparous postmenopausal women and their parous sisters. Neurourol Urodyn 2003;22:508–509.
12. Buchbaum GM, Duecy EE, Kerr LA, et al. Pelvic organ prolapse in mulliparous women and their parous sisters. Obstet Gynecol 2006;108:1388–1393.
13. Jack GS, Nikolova G, Vilain E, et al. Familial transmission of genitovaginal prolapse. Int Urogynecol J Pelvic Floor Dysfunct 2005;17:498–501.
14. Norton P, Baker J, Sharp HC, et al. Genitourinary prolapse and joint hypermobiity in women. Obstet Gynecol 1995;85:225–228.
15. Makinen J, Soderstrom KO, Kiilhoma P, et al. Histological changes in the vaginal connective tissue of patients with and without uterine prolapse. Arch Gynecol 1986;239:17–20.
16. Norton P, Boyd C, Deak S. Abnormal collagen ratios in women with genitourinary prolapse. Neurourol Urodyn 1992;11:2–4.
17. Fidas A, MacDonald HL, Elton RA, et al. Prevalence of spina bifida occulta in patients with functional disorders of the lower urinary tract and its relation to urodynamic and neurophysiologic measurements. BMJ 1989;298:357–359.
18. Findley P. Prolapse of the uterus in nulliparous women. Am J Obstet Dis Women 1917;75:12.
19. DeMola JRL, Carpenter SE. Management of genital prolapse in neonates and young women. Obstet Gynecol Surv 1996;51:253–260.
20. Swift S, Woddman P, O'Boyle A, et al. Pelvic organ support study (POSST): The distribution, clinical definition and epidemiology of pelvic organ support defects. Am J Obstet Gynecol 2005;192:795–806.
21. Mant J, Painter R, Vessey M. Epidemiology of genital prolapse: Observations from the Oxford Family Planning Association study. Br J Obstet Gynaecol 1997;104:579–585.
22. Klein MC, Gauthier RJ, Robbins JM, et al. Relationship of episiotomy to perineal trauma and morbidity, sexual function, and pelvic floor relaxation. Am J Obstet Gynecol 1994;171:591–598.
23. Sultan AH, Kamm MA, Hudson CH, et al. Anal-sphincter disruption during vaginal delivery. N Engl J Med 1993;329:1905–1911.
24. Sultan AH, Kamm MA, Hudson CH, et al. Third degree obstetric anal sphincter tears: Risk factors and outcome of primary repair. BMJ 1994;308:887–891.
25. Lukacz ES, Lawrence JM, Contreras R, et al. Parity, mode of delivery, and pelvic floor disorders. Obstet Gynecol 2006;107:1253–1260.
26. National Institutes of Health state-of-the-science conference statement: Cesarean delivery on maternal

request March 27–29, 2006. Obstet Gynecol 2006;107:1386-1397.

27. Swift SE, Pound T, Dias JE. Case-control study of the etiology of severe pelvic organ prolapse. Int Urogynecol J 2001;12:187–192.

28. Cruikshank SH, Kovak SR. Randomized comparison of three surgical methods used at the time of vaginal hysterectomy to prevent posterior enterocele. Am J Obstet Gynecol 1999;180:859–865.

29. Richter HE, Burgio KL, Clements RH, et al. Urinary and anal incontinence in morbidly obese women considering weight loss surgery. Obstet Gynecol 2005;106:1272–1277.

30. Lubowski DZ, Swash M, Nichols RJ, et al. Increases in pudendal nerve terminal motor latency with defecation straining. Br J Surg 1988;75:1095–1097.

31. Spence-Jones C, Kamm MA, Henry MM, et al. Bowel dysfunction: A pathogenic factor in uterovaginal prolapse and urinary stress incontinence. Br J Obstet Gynaecol 1994;101:147–152.

32. Samuelsson EU, Victor FTA, Tibblin G, et al. Signs of genital prolapse in a Swedish population of women 20–59 years of age and possible related factors. Am J Obstet Gynecol 1999;180:299–305.

33. Bump RC, McClish DK. Cigarette smoking and urinary incontinence in women. Am J Obstet Gynecol 1992;167:1213–1218.

34. Jorgensen S, Hein HO, Gyntelberg F. Heavy lifting at work and risk of genital prolapse and herniated lumbar disk is assistant nurses. Occup Med 1994;44:47–49.

35. Bonetti TR, Erpelding A, Pathak LR. Listening to "felt needs": Investigating genital prolapse in western Nepal. Reprod Health Matters 2004;12:166–175.

36. Davis GD, Goodman M. Stress urinary incontinence in nulliparous female soldiers in airborne infantry training. J Pelvic Surg 1996;2:68–71.

37. Nygaard IE. Does prolonged high-impact activity cause urinary incontinence? A retrospective cohort study of female Olympians. Obstet Gynecol 1997;90:718–722.

38. Weir LF, Nygaard IE, Wilken J, et al. Postoperative activity restrictions: Any evidence? Obstet Gynecol 2006;107:305–309.

39. Brincat M, Versi E, Moniz CF, et al. Skin collagen changes in postmenopausal women receiving different regimens of estrogen therapy. Obstet Gynecol 1987;70:123–127.

40. Goldstein SR, Nanavati N. Adverse events that are associated with selective estrogen receptor modulator levormeloxifene in an aborted phase III osteoporosis study treatment study. Am J Obstet Gynecol 2002;187:521–527.

41. Moalli PA, Ivy SJ, Meyn LA, et al. Risk factors associated with pelvic floor disorders in women undergoing surgical repair. Obstet Gynecol 2003;101:869–874.

42. Barber MD. Symptoms and outcome measures of pelvic organ prolapse. Clin Obstet Gynecol 2005;48:648–661.

43. DeLancey JOL. Anatomy and biomechanics of genital prolapse. Clin Obstet Gynecol 1993;36:897–909.

44. Swift SE, Tate SB, Nicholas J. Correlation of symptoms with degree of pelvic organ support in a general population of women: What is pelvic organ prolapse? Am J Obstet Gynecol 2003;189:372–377.

45. Ellerkmann MR, Cundiff GW, Melick CF, et al. Correlation of symptoms with location and severity of pelvic organ prolapse. Am J Obstet Gynecol 2001;185:1332–1337.

46. Burrows LJ, Meyn LA, Walters MD, et al. Pelvic symptoms in women with pelvic organ prolapse. Obstet Gynecol 2004;104:982–988.

47. Ghetti C, Gregory WT, Edwards SR, et al. Pelvic organ descent and symptoms of pelvic floor disorders. Am J Obstet Gynecol 2005;193:53–57.

48. Romanzi LJ, Chaikin DC, Blaivas JG. The effect of genital prolapse on voiding. J Urol 1999;161:581–586.

49. Cundiff GW, Fenner D. Evaluation and treatment of women with rectocele: Focus on associated defecatory and sexual dysfunction. Obstet Gynecol 2004;104:1403–1421.

50. Jackson SL, Weber AM, Hull TL, et al. Fecal incontinence in women with urinary incontinence and pelvic organ prolapse. Obstet Gynecol 1997;89:423–427.

51. Nichols CM, Gill EJ, Nguyen T, et al. Anal sphincter injury in women with pelvic floor disorders. Obstet Gynecol 2004;104:690–696.

52. Basson R, Berman J, Burnett A, et al. Report of the international consensus development conference on female sexual dysfunction: Definitions and classifications. J Urol 2000:183:888–893.

53. Barber MD, Visco AG, Wyman JF, et al. Sexual function in women with urinary incontinence and pelvic organ prolapse. Obstet Gynecol 2002;1999:281–289.

54. Weber AM, Walters MD, Schover LR, et al. Sexual function in women with uterovaginal prolapse and urinary incontinence. Obstet Gynecol 1995;85:483–487.

55. Handa VL, Harvey L, Cundiff GW, et al. Sexual dysfunction among women with urinary incontinence and pelvic organ prolapse. Am J Obstet Gynecol 2004;191:751–756.

56. Pauls RN, Segal JL, Silva WA, et al. Sexual function in patients presenting to a urogynecology practice. Int Urogynecol J Pelvic Floor Dysfucnt 2006;17:576–580.

57. Heit M, Culligan P, Rosenquist C, et al. Is pelvic organ prolapse a cause of pelvic or low back pain? Obstet Gynecol 2002;99:23–28.
58. Hoyte L, Schierlitz L, Zou K, et al. Two- and 3-dimensional MRI comparison of levator ani structure, volume, and integrity in women with stress incontinence and prolapse. Am J Obstet Gynecol 2001;185:11–29.
59. Janda S, va der Helm FCT, deBlok SB. Measuring morphological parameters of the pelvic floor for finite element modeling purposes. J Biomech 2003;36:749–757.
60. Lien KC, Mooney B, DeLancey JOL, et al. Levator ani muscle stretch induced by simulated vaginal birth. Obstet Gynecol 2004;103:31–40.

Chapter 6
Hormonal Influences on Continence

Dudley Robinson and Linda Cardozo

Introduction

The female genital and lower urinary tract share a common embryological origin, arising from the urogenital sinus (Fig. 6.1). Both are sensitive to the effects of female sex steroid hormones. Estrogen is known to have an important role in the function of the lower urinary tract throughout adult life with estrogen and progesterone receptors demonstrated in the vagina, urethra, bladder, and pelvic floor musculature [1–4]. This is supported by the fact that estrogen deficiency occurring following the menopause is known to cause atrophic changes within the urogenital tract [5] and is associated with urinary symptoms such as frequency, urgency, nocturia, incontinence, and recurrent infection. These also may coexist with symptoms of vaginal atrophy such as dyspareunia, itching, burning, and dryness.

This chapter will review the role of estrogens in lower urinary tract function and dysfunction as well as the role of estrogen replacement therapy in the management of urogenital atrophy.

Estrogen Receptors and Hormonal Factors

The effects of the steroid hormone 17β-estradiol are mediated by ligand-activated transcription factors known as estrogen receptors. These share common features with both androgen and progesterone receptors and can be divided into several functional domains [6]. The classic estrogen receptor (ERα)

was first discovered by Elwood Jensen in 1958 and cloned from uterine tissue in 1986 [7], although it was not until 1996 that the second estrogen receptor (ERβ) was identified [8]. The precise role of the two different receptors remains to be elucidated, although ERα appears to play a major role in the regulation of reproduction while ERβ has a more minor role [9].

Estrogen receptors have been demonstrated throughout the female lower urinary tract and are expressed in the squamous epithelium of the proximal and distal urethra, vagina, and trigone of the bladder [3, 10], although not in the dome of the bladder, reflecting its different embryological origin. Pubococcygeus and the musculature of the pelvic floor also have been shown to be estrogen sensitive [11, 12], although estrogen receptors have not yet been identified in the levator ani muscles [13].

The distribution of estrogen receptors throughout the urogenital tract also has been studied with both α and β receptors being found in the vaginal walls and uterosacral ligaments of premenopausal women, although the latter were absent in the vaginal walls of postmenopausal women [14]. In addition, α receptors are localized in the urethral sphincter and when sensitized by estrogens are thought to help maintain muscular tone [15].

In addition to estrogen receptors both androgen and progesterone receptors are expressed in the lower urinary tract, although their role is less clear. Progesterone receptors are expressed inconsistently, having been reported in the bladder, trigone, and vagina. Their presence may be dependent on

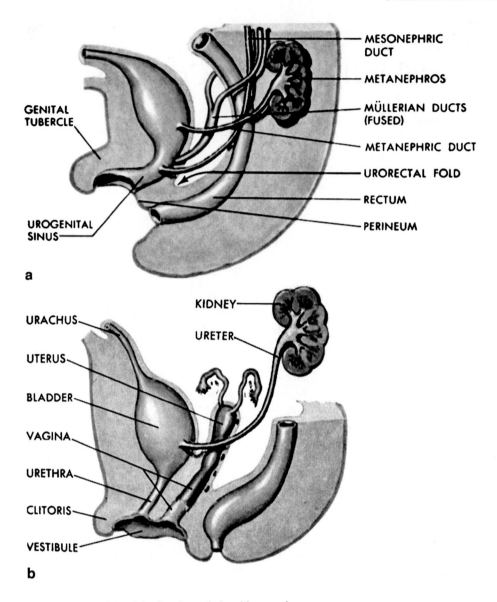

FIG. 6.1. Embryological origin of the female genital and lower urinary tract

estrogen status [5]. While androgen receptors are present in both the bladder and urethra, their role has not yet been defined [16]. Interestingly, estrogen receptors also have been identified in mast cells in women with interstitial cystitis [17, 18] and in the male lower urinary tract [19].

The incidence of both estrogen and progesterone expression has been examined throughout the lower urinary tract in 90 women undergoing gynecologic surgery; 33 were premenopausal, 26 postmenopausal without hormone replacement therapy, and 31 postmenopausal and taking hormone replacement

therapy [20]. Biopsies were taken from the bladder dome, trigone, proximal urethra, distal urethra, vagina, and vesicovaginal fascia adjacent to the bladder neck. Estrogen receptors were found to be consistently expressed in the squamous epithelia, although they were absent in the urothelial tissues of the lower urinary tract of all women, irrespective of estrogen status. Progesterone receptor expression, however, showed more variability, being mostly subepithelial, and it was significantly lower in postmenopausal women not taking estrogen replacement therapy.

Hormonal Influences on Lower Urinary Tract Symptoms

In order to maintain continence the urethral pressure must remain higher than the intravesical pressure at all times except during micturition [21]. Estrogens play an important role in the continence mechanism with bladder and urethral function becoming less efficient with age [22]. Elderly women have been found to have a reduced flow rate, increased urinary residuals, higher filling pressures, reduced bladder capacity, and lower maximum voiding pressures [23]. Estrogens may affect continence by increasing urethral resistance, raising the sensory threshold of the bladder, or by increasing α adrenoreceptor sensitivity in the urethral smooth muscle [24, 25]. In addition, exogenous estrogens have been shown to increase the number of intermediate and superficial cells in the vagina of postmenopausal women [26]. These changes also have been demonstrated in the bladder and urethra [27].

More recently a prospective observational study has been performed to assess cell proliferation rates throughout the tissues of the lower urinary tract [28]. Fifty-nine women were studied of whom 23 were premenopausal, 20 were postmenopausal and not taking hormone replacement therapy, and 20 were postmenopausal and taking hormone replacement therapy. Biopsies were taken from the bladder dome, trigone, proximal urethra, distal urethra, vagina, and vesicovaginal fascia adjacent to the bladder neck. The squamous epithelium of estrogen-replete women was shown to exhibit greater levels of cellular proliferation than in those women who were estrogen deficient.

Cyclical variations in the levels of both estrogen and progesterone during the menstrual cycle have been shown to lead to changes in urodynamic variables and lower urinary tract symptoms with 37% of women noticing a deterioration in symptoms prior to menstruation [29]. Measurement of the urethral pressure profile in nulliparous premenopausal women shows there is an increase in functional urethral length midcycle and early in the luteal phase corresponding to an increase in plasma estradiol [30]. Furthermore, progestogens have been associated with an increase in irritative bladder symptoms [31, 32] and urinary incontinence in those women taking combined hormone replacement therapy [33]. The incidence of detrusor overactivity in the luteal phase of the menstrual cycle may be associated with raised plasma progesterone following ovulation and progesterone has been shown to antagonize the inhibitory effect of estradiol on rat detrusor contractions [34]. This may help to explain the increased prevalence of detrusor overactivity found in pregnancy [35].

The role of estrogen therapy in the management of women with fecal incontinence also has been investigated in a prospective observational study using symptom questionnaires and anorectal physiological testing before and after 6 months of estrogen replacement therapy. At follow up 25% of women were asypmtomatic and a further 65% were improved in terms of flatus control, urgency, and fecal staining. In addition, anal resting pressures and voluntary squeeze increments were significantly increased following estrogen therapy, although there were no changes in pudendal nerve terminal latency. The authors conclude that estrogen replacement therapy may have a beneficial effect, although larger studies are needed to confirm these findings [36].

Hormonal Influences on Urinary Tract Infection

Urinary tract infection also is a common cause of urinary symptoms in women of all ages. This is a particular problem in the elderly, with a reported incidence of 20% in the community and over 50% in institutionalized patients [37, 38]. Pathophysiological changes such as impairment of bladder emptying, poor perineal hygiene, and both fecal and urinary incontinence partly may account for the high prevalence observed. In addition, changes in the vaginal flora due to estrogen depletion lead to colonization with gram-negative bacilli, which in addition to causing local irritive symptoms also act as uropathogens. These microbiological changes may be reversed with estrogen replacement following the menopause, offering a rationale for treatment and prophylaxis.

Hormonal Influences on Lower Urinary Tract Function

Neurological Control

Sex hormones are known to influence the central neurological control of micturition, although their exact role in the micturition pathway has yet to be elucidated. Estrogen receptors have been demonstrated in the cerebral cortex, limbic system, hippocampus, and cerebellum [39, 40], while androgen receptors have been demonstrated in the pontine micturition center and the preoptic area of the hypothalamus [41].

Bladder Function

Estrogen receptors, although absent in the transitional epithelium at the dome of the bladder, are present in the areas of the trigone which have undergone squamous metaplasia [10]. Estrogen is known to have a direct effect on detrusor function through modifications in muscarinic receptors [42, 43] and by inhibition of movement of extracellular calcium ions into muscle cells [44]. Consequently, estradiol has been shown to reduce the amplitude and frequency of spontaneous rhythmic detrusor contractions [45] and there also is evidence that it may increase the sensory threshold of the bladder in some women [46].

Urethra

Estrogen receptors have been demonstrated in the squamous epithelium of both the proximal and distal urethra [10] and estrogen has been shown to improve the maturation index of urethral squamous epithelium [47]. It has been suggested that estrogen increases urethral closure pressure and improves pressure transmission to the proximal urethra, promoting continence [48–51]. Additionally, estrogens have been shown to cause vasodilatation in the systemic and cerebral circulation, and these changes also are seen in the urethra [52–54].

The vascular pulsations seen on urethral pressure profilometry secondary to blood flow in the urethral submucosa and urethral sphincter have been shown to increase in size following estrogen administration [55], while the effect is lost following estrogen withdrawal at the menopause. The urethral vascular bed is thought to account for around a third of the urethral closure pressure and estrogen replacement therapy in postmenopausal women with stress incontinence has been shown to increase the number of periurethral vessels [56].

Collagen

Estrogens are known to have an effect on collagen synthesis and they have been shown to have a direct effect on collagen metabolism in the lower genital tract [57]. Changes found in women with urogenital atrophy may represent an alteration in systemic collagenase activity [58] and urodynamic stress incontinence, and urogenital prolapse has been associated with a reduction in both vaginal and periurethral collagen [59–61]. Furthermore, there is a reduction in skin collagen content following the menopause [62] with rectus muscle fascia being shown to become less elastic with increasing age, resulting in a lower energy requirement to cause irreversible damage [63]. Changes in collagen content also have been identified, the hydroxyproline content in connective tissue from women with stress incontinence being 40% lower than in continent controls [64].

Lower Urinary Tract Symptoms

Urinary Incontinence

The prevalence of urinary incontinence is known to increase with age, affecting 15–35% of community-dwelling women over the age of 60 years [65] and other studies reporting a prevalence of 49% in women over 65 years [66]. In addition, rates of 50% have been reported in elderly nursing home residents [67]. A recent cross-sectional population prevalence survey of 146 women aged 15–97 years found that 46% experienced symptoms of pelvic floor dysfunction defined as stress or urge incontinence, flatus, or fecal incontinence, symptomatic prolapse, or previous pelvic floor surgery [68].

Little work has been done to examine the incidence of urinary incontinence, although a study in New Zealand of women over the age of 65 years found 10% of the originally continent developed urinary incontinence in the 3-year study period [69].

Epidemiological studies have implicated estrogen deficiency in the etiology of lower urinary tract symptoms, with 70% of women relating the onset of urinary incontinence to their final menstrual period [5]. Lower urinary tract symptoms have been shown to be common in postmenopausal women attending a menopause clinic, with 20% complaining of severe urgency and almost 50% complaining of stress incontinence [70]. Urge incontinence in particular is more prevalent following the menopause and the prevalence would appear to rise with increasing years of estrogen deficiency [71]. There is, however, conflicting evidence regarding the role of estrogen withdrawal at the time of the menopause. Some studies have shown a peak incidence in perimenopausal women [72, 73], while other evidence suggests that many women develop incontinence at least 10 years prior to the cessation of menstruation, with significantly more premenopausal women than postmenopausal women being affected [74].

Urogenital Atrophy

Urogenital atrophy is a manifestation of estrogen withdrawal following the menopause and symptoms may appear for the first time more than 10 years after the last menstrual period [75]. In addition, increasing life expectancy has led to an increasingly elderly population and it is now common for women to spend a third of their lives in the estrogen-deficient postmenopausal state [76], with the average age of the menopause being 50 years [77].

Postmenopausal women comprise 15% of the population in industrialized countries, with a predicted growth rate of 1.5% over the next 20 years. Overall, in the developed world 8% of the total population have been estimated to have urogenital symptoms [78]; this represents 200 million women in the United States alone.

It has been estimated that 10–40% of all postmenopausal women are symptomatic [79], although only 25% are thought to seek medical help (Table 6.1). In addition, two out of three women report vaginal symptoms associated with urogenital atrophy by the age of 75 years [80]. However, the prevalence of symptomatic urogenital atrophy is difficult to estimate, since many women accept the changes as being an inevitable consequence of the ageing process, and thus do not seek help; this leads to considerable underreporting (Table 6.2).

A study assessing the prevalence of urogenital symptoms in 2,157 Dutch women recently has been reported [81]. Overall, 27% of women complained of vaginal dryness, soreness, and dyspareunia, while the prevalence of urinary symptoms such as leakage and recurrent infections was 36%. When considering severity, almost 50% reported moderate to severe discomfort, although only a third had received medical intervention. Interestingly, women who previously had had a hysterectomy reported moderate to severe complaints more often than those who had not.

The prevalence of urogenital atrophy and urogenital prolapse also has been examined in a population of 285 women attending a menopause clinic [82]. Overall, 51% of women were found to have anterior vaginal wall prolapse, 27% posterior vaginal prolapse, and 20% apical prolapse. In addition, 34% of women were noted to have urogenital atrophy and 40% complained of dyspareunia. While urogenital atrophy and symptoms of dyspareunia were related to menopausal age, the prevalence of prolapse showed no association.

However, while urogenital atrophy is an inevitable consequence of the menopause, women may not always be symptomatic. A recent study of 69 women attending a gynecology clinic were asked to fill out a symptom questionnaire prior to examination and vaginal cytology [83]. Urogenital symptoms were found to be relatively low and were poorly correlated with age and physical examination findings, although not with vaginal cytological maturation index (Fig. 6.2). Women who were taking estrogen replacement therapy had higher symptom scores and physical examination scores.

In order to clinically grade and quantify the changes associated with urogenital atrophy a scoring system has been developed based on a five-point scale [84] (Table 6.3). From this evidence it would appear that urogenital atrophy is a universal consequence of the menopause, although often elderly women may be minimally symptomatic. Hence, treatment should not be the only indication for replacement therapy.

TABLE 6.1. Symptoms of urogenital atrophy.

Vaginal dryness
Dyspareunia
Vaginal burning
Pruritis
Urinary symptoms: urgency, frequency, nocturia, dysuria, recurrent infection
Prolapse

TABLE 6.2. Signs of urogenital atrophy.

Pallor/inflammation
Petechiae
Epithelial or mucosal thinning
Decreased elasticity
Urogenital prolapse

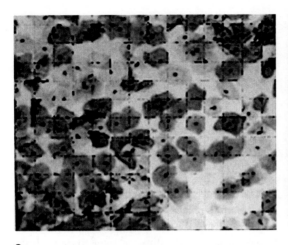
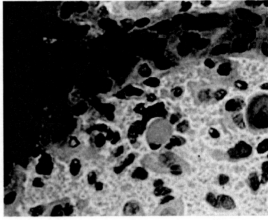

a   b

FIG. 6.2. Vaginal cytology in (**a**) a healthy premenopausal woman and (**b**) following the menopause in a woman with symptomatic vaginal atrophy

TABLE 6.3. The vaginal health index.

Overall elasticity
Fluid secretion (type and consistency)
pH
Epithelial integrity
Moisture

Management of Lower Urinary Dysfunction

Estrogens in the Management of Incontinence

Estrogen preparations have been used for many years in the treatment of urinary incontinence [85, 86], although their precise role remains controversial. Many of the studies performed have been uncontrolled observational series examining the use of a wide range of different preparations, doses, and routes of administration. The inconsistent use of progestogens to provide endometrial protection is a further confounding factor making interpretation of the results difficult.

In order to clarify the situation a meta-analysis from the Hormones and Urogenital Therapy (HUT) Committee has been reported [87]. Of 166 articles identified that were published in English between 1969 and 1992, only six were controlled trials and 17 were uncontrolled series. Meta-analysis found an overall significant effect of estrogen therapy on subjective improvement in all subjects and for subjects with urodynamic stress incontinence alone. Subjective improvement rates with estrogen therapy in randomized controlled trials ranged from 64 to 75%, although placebo groups also reported an improvement of 10–56%. In uncontrolled series subjective improvement rates were 8–89%, with subjects with urodynamic stress incontinence showing improvement of 3–73%. However, when assessing objective fluid loss there was no significant effect. Maximum urethral closure pressure was found to increase significantly with estrogen therapy, although this outcome was influenced by a single study showing a large effect [88] (Table 6.4).

A further meta-analysis performed in Italy has analyzed the results of randomized controlled clinical trials on the efficacy of local and systemic estrogen treatment in postmenopausal women with urinary incontinence [89]. A search of the literature (1965–1996) revealed 72 articles of which only four were considered to meet the meta-analysis criteria. There was a statistically significant difference in subjective outcome between estrogen and placebo, although there was no such difference in objective or urodynamic outcome. The authors conclude that this difference could be relevant, although the studies may have lacked objective sensitivity to detect this.

TABLE 6.4. Summary of randomized controlled trials assessing the use of estrogens in the management of urinary incontinence.

Study	Year	Type of incontinence	Estrogen	Route
Henalla et al. [88]	1989	Stress incontinence	Conjugated estrogen	Vaginal
Hilton et al. [103]	1990	Stress incontinence	Conjugated estrogen	Vaginal
Beisland et al. [102]	1984	Stress incontinence	Estriol	Vaginal
Judge [138]	1969	Mixed incontinence	Quinestradol	Oral
Kinn and Lindskog [25]	1988	Stress incontinence	Estriol	Oral
Samsioe et al. [106]	1985	Mixed incontinence	Estriol	Oral
Walter et al. [98]	1978	Urge incontinence	Estradiol and estriol	Oral
Walter et al. [139]	1990	Stress incontinence	Estriol	Oral
Wilson et al. [97]	1987	Stress incontinence	Piperazine estrone sulfate	Oral

The most recent meta-analysis of the effect of estrogen therapy on the lower urinary tract has been performed by the Cochrane group [90]. Overall, 28 trials were identified, including 2,926 women. In the 15 trials comparing estrogen to placebo there was a higher subjective impression of improvement rate in those women taking estrogen, and this was the case for all types of incontinence (RR for cure 1.61; 95% CI 1.04–2.49). Equally, when subjective cure and improvement were taken together there was a statistically higher cure and improvement rate for both urge (57% vs. 28%) and stress (43% vs. 27%) incontinence. In those women with urge incontinence the chance of improvement was 25% higher than in women with stress incontinence; overall, about 50% of women treated with estrogen were cured or improved compared to 25% on placebo. The authors conclude that estrogens can improve or cure incontinence and that the effect may be most useful in women complaining of urge incontinence.

Systemic HRT and Urinary Incontinence

Several large-scale systemic HRT studies recently have been reported that have led to greater controversy regarding the role of oral estrogens on the lower urinary tract. The role of estrogen replacement therapy in the prevention of ischemic heart disease has been assessed in a 4-year randomized trial: the Heart and Estrogen/progestin Replacement Study (HERS) [91], involving 2,763 postmenopausal women younger than 80 years with intact uteri and ischemic heart disease. In the study, 55% of women reported at least one episode of urinary incontinence each week and were randomly assigned to oral conjugated estrogen plus medroxyprogesterone acetate (MPA) or placebo daily. Incontinence improved in 26% of women assigned to placebo compared to 21% receiving HRT, while 27% of the placebo group complained of worsening symptoms compared with 39% in the HRT group ($P = 0.001$). The incidence of incontinent episodes per week increased an average of 0.7 in the HRT group and decreased by 0.1 in the placebo group ($P < 0.001$). Overall, combined hormone replacement therapy was associated with worsening stress and urge urinary incontinence, although there was no significant difference in daytime frequency, nocturia, or number of urinary tract infections.

These findings also have been confirmed in the Nurse's Health Study, which followed 39,436 postmenopausal women aged 50–75 years over a 4-year period. The risk of incontinence was found to be elevated in those women taking HRT compared to those who had never taken HRT. There was an increased risk in women taking oral estrogen (RR 1.54; 95% CI 1.44–1.65), transdermal estrogen (RR 1.68; 95% CI 1.41–2.00), oral estrogen and progesterone (RR 1.34; 95% CI 1.24–1.34), and transdermal estrogen and progesterone (RR 1.46; CI 1.16–1.84). In addition, while there was a small risk that remained after the cessation of HRT (RR 1.14; 95% CI 1.06–1.23), by 10 years the risk was identical (RR 1.02; 95% 0.91–1.41) and was identical to those women who had never taken HRT [92].

In addition, the effects of oral estrogens and progestogens on the lower urinary tract have been assessed in 32 female nursing home residents [93] with an average age of 88 years. Subjects were randomized to oral estrogen and progesterone or placebo for 6 months. At follow-up there was no difference between severity of incontinence, prevalence of bacteriuria, or the results of vaginal cultures, although there was an improvement in atrophic vaginitis in the placebo group.

The most recent paper to be reported by the Women's Health Initiative (WHI) writing group also studied the effect of estrogens, with and without progestogens, on urinary incontinence [94]. This paper represents another subanalysis of the data, although it should be remembered that the study was not designed to assess urinary incontinence, and thus may lack the appropriate power to do so conclusively.

In this study 27,347 postmenopausal women aged 50–79 years were assessed in a multicenter, double-blind, placebo-controlled trial. Of these, 23,296 were known to complain of lower urinary tract symptoms at baseline and at 1-year follow-up. Women were randomized based on hysterectomy status to active treatment or placebo in either the estrogen and progestogen or estrogen-only trials. The estrogen was conjugated equine estrogen (CEE), while the progestogen was MPA. The main outcome measure was the incidence of urinary incontinence at 1 year among women who were continent at baseline and the severity of urinary incontinence at 1 year in those who were incontinent at baseline.

Overall, HRT was found to increase the incidence of all types of urinary incontinence at 1 year in those women continent at baseline. The risk was highest for stress incontinence [CEE + MPA; RR 1.87 (1.61–2.18); CEE alone; RR 2.15 (1.77–2.62)] followed by mixed incontinence [CEE + MPA; RR 1.49 (1.10–2.01); CEE alone; RR 1.79 (1.26–2.53)]. However, the effect on urge urinary incontinence was not uniform – [CEE + MPA; RR 1.15 (0.99–1.34); CEE alone; RR 1.32 (1.10–1.58)].

When considering those women who were symptomatic at baseline, urinary frequency was found to increase in both arms [CEE + MPA; RR 1.38 (1.28–1.49); CEE alone; RR 1.47 (1.35–1.61)] and the incidence of urinary incontinence was seen to increase at 1 year [CEE + MPA; RR 1.20 (1.06–1.36); CEE alone; RR 1.59 (1.39–1.82)]. In addition, while no formal quality of life (QoL) assessment was reported, women receiving HRT were more likely to report that urinary incontinence limited their daily activities and bothered and disturbed them.

These results, while supportive of the previously reported HERS study and Nurse Health study, would certainly seem to contradict much of the previous work assessing the use of estrogens in the management of lower urinary tract symptoms. There are several possible explanations why these findings may differ.

First, this trial was not designed specifically to assess urinary symptoms and the questionnaires used may have lacked the sensitivity to correctly identify incontinent women. The question, "Have you ever leaked even a very small amount of urine involuntarily and you couldn't control it," may have overestimated the actual prevalence of urinary incontinence in this population, and this is supported by the findings that over 45% of 60 to 69-year-old women in the study were found to be incontinent.

In addition to a possible overestimation of the population the relatively large age range of this trial (50–79 years) and considerable comorbidities of participants may not accurately reflect the current clinical use of HRT. Since the majority of women receive hormone replacement for symptomatic relief in the perimenopausal period, it may be more appropriate to stratify the results with respect to age, as this may more accurately reflect current clinical practice.

Furthermore, the treatment regimens themselves also may not be representative of current clinical practice, and certainly in Europe there has been a move away from the use of CEEs to favor the use of estradiol. It also is important to remember that this trial has only examined the use of oral systemic replacement therapy, while local topical estrogens have been shown to be effective in the management of troublesome lower urinary tract symptoms and have minimal systemic effect.

Neither menopausal symptoms nor urinary incontinence are life-threatening conditions, although both have a significant effect on QoL. The current evidence from all trials suggests that estrogen replacement therapy may have a minor role in lower urinary tract dysfunction and the findings of the WHI studies should not prevent its use in women who complain of troublesome menopausal symptoms after appropriate counseling and discussion.

Estrogens in the Management of Stress Incontinence

In addition to the studies included in the HUT meta-analysis, several authors also have investigated the role of estrogen therapy in the management of urodynamic stress incontinence only. Oral estrogens have been reported to increase the maximum urethral pressures and lead to symptomatic improvement in 65–70% of women [95, 96], although other work has not confirmed this [97, 98]. More recently, two placebo-controlled studies have been performed examining the use of oral estrogens in the treatment of urodynamic stress incontinence in postmenopausal women. Neither CEEs and medroxyprogesterone [99], or unopposed estradiol valerate [100] showed a significant difference in either subjective or objective outcomes. Furthermore, a review of 8 controlled and 14 uncontrolled prospective trials concluded that estrogen therapy was not an efficacious treatment for stress incontinence but may be useful for symptoms of urgency and frequency [101].

From the available evidence estrogen does not appear to be an effective treatment for stress incontinence, although it may have a synergistic role in combination therapy. Two placebo-controlled studies have examined the use of oral and vaginal estrogens with the α-adrenergic agonist, phenylpropanolamine, used separately and in combination. Both studies found that combination therapy was superior to either drug given alone, although while there was subjective improvement in all groups [102], there was only objective improvement in the combination therapy group [103]. This may offer an alternative conservative treatment for women who have mild urodynamic stress incontinence, although because of its pressor effects phenylpropanolamine now has been withdrawn in the United States [104].

A recently reported meta-analysis has helped determine the role of estrogen replacement in women with stress incontinence [105]. Of the papers reviewed, 14 were nonrandomized studies, 6 were randomized trials (of which 4 were placebo controlled), and 2 were meta-analyses. Interestingly, there was only a symptomatic or clinical improvement noted in the nonrandomized studies, while there was no such effect noted in the randomized trials. The authors concluded that currently the evidence would not support the use of estrogen replacement alone in the management of stress incontinence.

Estrogens in the Management of Urge Incontinence

Estrogens have been used in the treatment of urinary urgency and urge incontinence for many years, although there have been few controlled trials to confirm their efficacy. A double-blind, placebo-controlled crossover study using oral estriol in 34 postmenopausal women produced subjective improvement in 8 women with mixed incontinence and 12 with urge incontinence [106]. However, a double-blind, multicenter study of the use of estriol (3 mg d^{-1}) in postmenopausal women complaining of urgency has failed to confirm these findings [107], showing both subjective and objective improvement but not significantly better than placebo. Estriol is a naturally occurring weak estrogen that has little effect on the endometrium and does not prevent osteoporosis, although it has been used in the treatment of urogenital atrophy. Consequently, it is possible that the dosage or route of administration in this study was not appropriate in the treatment of urinary symptoms and higher systemic levels may be required.

The use of sustained-release 17β-estradiol vaginal tablets (Vagifem, Novo Nordisk) also has been examined in postmenopausal women with urgency and urge incontinence or a urodynamic diagnosis of sensory urgency or detrusor overactivity. These vaginal tablets have been shown to be well absorbed from the vagina and to induce maturation of the vaginal epithelium within 14 days [108]. However, following a 6-month course of treatment the only significant difference between active and placebo groups was an improvement in the symptom of urgency in those women with a urodynamic diagnosis of sensory urgency [109]. A further double-blind, randomized, placebo-controlled trial of vaginal 17β-estradiol vaginal tablets has shown lower urinary tract symptoms of frequency, urgency, and urge and stress incontinence to be significantly improved, although there was no objective urodynamic assessment performed [110]. In both of these studies the subjective improvement in symptoms may simply represent local estrogenic effects reversing urogenital atrophy rather than a direct effect on bladder function.

More recently a randomized, parallel group, controlled trial has been reported comparing the estradiol-releasing vaginal ring (Estring, Pharmacia, Uppsala, Sweden) with estriol vaginal pessaries in the treatment of postmenopausal women with bothersome lower urinary tract symptoms [111]. Low-dose vaginally administered estradiol and estriol were found to be equally efficacious in alleviating lower urinary tract symptoms of urge incontinence (58% vs. 58%), stress incontinence (53% vs. 59%), and nocturia (51% vs. 54%), although the vaginal ring was found to have greater patient acceptability.

To try and clarify the role of estrogen therapy in the management of women with urge incontinence a meta-analysis of the use of estrogen in women with symptoms of "overactive bladder" has been reported by the HUT Committee [112]. In a review of ten randomized placebo-controlled trials estrogen was found to be superior to placebo when considering symptoms of urge incontinence, frequency, and nocturia, although vaginal estrogen administration was found to be superior for symptoms of urgency. In those taking estrogens there also was a significant increase in first sensation and bladder capacity compared to placebo.

Estrogens in the Management of Recurrent Urinary Tract Infection

Estrogen therapy has been shown to increase vaginal pH and reverse the microbiological changes that occur in the vagina following the menopause [113]. Initial small uncontrolled studies using oral or vaginal estrogens in the treatment of recurrent urinary tract infection appeared to give promising results [114, 115], although unfortunately this has not been supported by larger randomized trials. Several studies have been performed examining the use of oral and vaginal estrogens, although these have had mixed results (Table 6.5).

Kjaergaard and colleagues [116] compared vaginal estriol tablets with placebo in 21 postmenopausal women over a 5-month period and found no significant difference between the two groups. However, a subsequent randomized, double-blind, placebo-controlled study assessing the use of estriol vaginal cream in 93 postmenopausal women during an 8-month period did reveal a significant effect [117].

Kirkengen randomized 40 postmenopausal women to receive either placebo or oral estriol and found that although initially both groups had a significantly decreased incidence of recurrent infections, after 12 weeks estriol was shown to be significantly more effective [118]. These findings, however, were not confirmed subsequently in a trial of 72 women postmenopausal women with recurrent urinary tract infections randomized to oral estriol or placebo. Following a 6-month treatment period and a further 6-month follow-up estriol was found to be no more effective than placebo [119].

The role of vaginal estriol cream also has been assessed in 93 postmenopausal women with a history of recurrent urinary tract infections in a randomized double-blind, placebo-controlled trial [120]. Overall the incidence of urinary tract infection in the estriol group was lower than the placebo group (0.5 vs. 5.9 episodes per patient year; $P < 0.001$) and more of the women in the estriol group remained infection free. In addition, lactobacilli were absent in all vaginal cultures before treatment and reappeared after 1 month in 61% of estriol-treated women but in none of the placebo group ($P < 0.001$), and the rate of vaginal colonization with Enterobacteriaceae fell from 67 to 31% in the treatment group compared to 67 to –63% in the placebo arm.

More recently a randomized, open, parallel-group study assessing the use of an estradiol-releasing silicone vaginal ring (Estring; Pharmacia, Uppsala, Sweden) in postmenopausal women with recurrent infections has been performed that showed the cumulative likelihood of remaining infection free was 45% in the active group and 20% in the placebo group [121]. Estring also was shown to decrease the number of recurrences per year and to prolong the interval between infection episodes.

Estrogens in the Management of Urogenital Atrophy

Symptoms of urogenital atrophy do not occur until the levels of endogenous estrogen are lower than that required to promote endometrial proliferation [122]. Consequently, it is possible to use a low dose of estrogen replacement therapy in order to alleviate urogenital symptoms while avoiding the risk of endometrial proliferation and removing the necessity of providing endometrial protection with progestogens [123].

TABLE 6.5. Summary of randomized controlled trials assessing the use of estrogens in the management of recurrent lower urinary tract.

Study	Study group	Type of estrogen	Route of delivery	Duration of therapy	Results
Kjaergaard et al. 1990 [116]	21 postmenopausal women with recurrent cystitis *10 active group 11 placebo*	Estradiol	Vaginal tablets	5 months	Number of positive cultures not statistically different between the two groups
Kirkengen et al. 1992 [118]	40 postmenopausal women with recurrent UTIs *20 active group 20 placebo*	Estriol	Oral	12 weeks	Both estriol and placebo significantly reduced the incidence of UTI's ($p < 0.05$) After 12 weeks estriol was significantly more effective than placebo ($p < 0.05$)
Raz and Stamm 1993 [120]	93 postmenopausal women with recurrent UTIs *50 active group 43 placebo*	Estriol	Vaginal cream	8 months	Significant reduction in the incidence of UTI's in the group given estriol compared to placebo ($p < 0.001$)
Cardozo et al. 1998 [119]	72 postmenopausal women with recurrent UTIs *36 active group 36 placebo*	Estriol	Oral	6 month treatment period with a further 6 months follow-up	Reduction in urinary symptoms and incidence of UTI's in both groups. Estriol no better than placebo
Eriksen 1999 [120]	108 women with recurrent UTIs *53 active group 55 no treatment*	Estradiol	Estring	36 weeks for the active group 36 weeks or until first recurrence for the controls	Cumulative likelihood of remaining free of infection was 45% in active group and 20% in control group ($p = 0.008$)

Vaginal Estrogens

The dose of estradiol commonly used in systemic estrogen replacement is usually 25–100 μg, although studies investigating the use of estrogens in the management of urogenital symptoms have shown that 8–10 μg of vaginal estradiol is effective [124]. Thus only 10–30% of the dose used to treat vasomotor symptoms may be effective in the management of urogenital symptoms. Since 10–25% of women receiving systemic hormone replacement therapy still experience the symptoms of urogenital atrophy [125], low-dose local preparations may have an additional beneficial effect (Table 6.6).

The addition of local vaginal estrogen replacement as an adjunct to systemic therapy has been assessed in a randomized, double-blind, placebo-controlled study of 27 women with menopausal symptoms and atrophic vaginitis [126]. In addition to systemic therapy with transdermal 17β-estradiol and oral MPA, women were randomized to adjuvant 0.5-mg vaginal estriol or placebo. When considering the results overall there were no differences between the two groups in terms of symptoms or cytological changes, although those women taking additional vaginal estrogens exhibited a shorter latency period for urinary symptoms. While this small short-term study would not appear to support the use of adjuvant vaginal estrogen replacement, this may be explained by the fact that estriol is a relatively weak estrogen, and thus the dose may have been too low.

The efficacy and safety of vaginally administered low-dose 25-μg 17β-estradiol (Vagifem, NovoNordisk) has been reported in a multicenter double-blind, placebo-controlled study in 1,612 women [127]. Patients were randomized to 25- μg estradiol or placebo once daily for 2 weeks and twice weekly thereafter. Overall there was a significant improvement in symptoms of urogenital atrophy in the treatment arm compared to placebo (85.5% vs. 41.4%) and also an improvement in cystometric capacity, first desire to void, and strong desire to void on urodynamic testing. Reassuringly there appeared to be no effect on serum estrogen levels and there were no cases of endometrial proliferation.

These findings are supported by a 12-week observational study assessing the safety and efficacy of low-dose, 25-μg 17β-estradiol (Vagifem, NovoNordisk) in 91 symptomatic postmenopausal women [128]. Overall there was a significant improvement in the symptoms of vaginal dryness, vaginal itching, and dyspareunia. When considering safety, despite a significant increase in serum estradiol in relation to baseline ($P < 0.001$) and decrease in FSH levels (47.4–45.5 mIU ml^{-1}; $P < 0.003$), these levels remained within the normal range for postmenopausal women.

Two studies also have assessed the efficacy of using ultra-low-dose vaginal estrogens. The first was a single-blind, single-arm study to determine the effects of de-escalating doses of vaginal estrogens on symptoms of urogenital atrophy, vaginal pH, and vaginal and urethral cytology [129]. Overall, 10-μg vaginal estradiol was found to have an 82% clinical response in symptoms as well as causing a statistical improvement in vaginal cytology, urethral cytology, and vaginal pH. The endometrium remained atrophic and serum estradiol remained within the normal postmenopausal range. The second study evaluated the effects of 25- and 10-μg 17β-estradiol in 58 symptomatic postmenopausal women in a double-blind, randomized, parallel-group study [130]. After 12 weeks of therapy the area under the curve, maximal, and average over 24 hr, estradiol concentration was higher in the 25-μg arm (563 pg hr ml^{-1}, 49 and 23 pg ml^{-1}) than the 10-μg (264 pg hr ml^{-1}, 22 and 11 pg ml^{-1}). Overall, 74% in the 25-μg group and 96% in the 10-μg group had low systemic absorption of estradiol (<500 pg ml^{-1}), absorption patterns remained consistent, and there was no evidence of accumulation. These two studies thus would suggest that ultra-low-dose vaginal estradiol may be safe and efficacious in the treatment of urogenital symptoms in postmenopausal women.

Vaginal estradiol also has been compared to vaginal CEEs in the management of urogenital atrophy. A multicenter, open-label, randomized, parallel-group study compared 25-μg 17β-estradiol with 1.25 mg CEE vaginal cream in 159 menopausal

TABLE 6.6. Vaginal estrogen preparations.

Type of estrogen	Mode of administration
Estriol	Cream: *Ovestin*
	Pessary: *Orthogynest*
Estradiol	Tablets: *Vagifem*
	Ring: *Estring*
Conjugated	Cream: *Premarin*

women over 24 weeks [131]. While both treatment regimens provided relief of the symptoms associated with atrophic vaginitis, increases in serum estradiol and suppression of follicle-stimulating hormone (FSH) were found to be significantly higher in those women using CEEs compared to vaginal estradiol tablets ($P < 0.001$). In addition, fewer patients who were using the vaginal tablets experienced endometrial proliferation or hyperplasia. In terms of satisfaction, significantly more women favored vaginal tablets and they also were associated with lower rates of withdrawal (10% vs. 32%). These findings have been confirmed by a further study of 53 women randomized to 25 μg estradiol or 1 gm conjugated estrogen cream for 12 weeks [132]. Both groups showed improvement in urogenital symptoms, vaginal health index, and vaginal cytology after 4 weeks of therapy, although the vaginal cream was found to be superior in terms of vaginal dryness and dyspareunia.

The use of the continuous low-dose estradiol-releasing silicone vaginal ring (Estring; Pfizer) releasing estradiol 5–10 μg/24 h also has been investigated in postmenopausal women with symptomatic urogenital atrophy [112]. There was a significant effect on symptoms of vaginal dryness, pruritis vulvae, dyspareunia, and urinary urgency with improvement being reported in over 90% of women in an uncontrolled study, while the maturation of vaginal epithelium also was significantly improved. The patient acceptability was high, and while the maturation of vaginal epithelium (Fig. 6.3) was significantly improved, there was no effect on endometrial proliferation.

These findings were supported by a 1-year multicenter study of Estring in postmenopausal women with urogenital atrophy, which found subjective and objective improvement in 90% of patients up to 1 year. However, there was a 20% withdrawal rate with 7% of women reporting vaginal irritation – two having vaginal ulceration and three complaining of vaginal bleeding – although there were no cases of endometrial proliferation [133]. Long-term safety has been confirmed by a 10-year review of the use of the estradiol ring delivery system, which has found its safety, efficacy, and acceptability to be comparable to other forms of vaginal administration [134]. A comparative study of safety and efficacy of Estring with CEE vaginal cream in 194 postmenopausal women

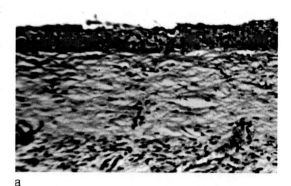

a

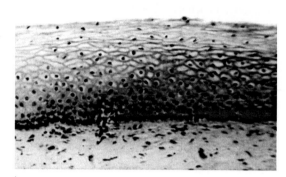

b

Fig. 6.3. Topical vaginal estrogen replacement increases the number of intermediate and superficial cells in the vaginal mucosa; (**a**) prior to treatment and (**b**) following treatment

complaining of urogenital atrophy found no significant difference in vaginal dryness, dyspareunia, and resolution of atrophic signs between the two treatment groups. Furthermore, there was a similar improvement in the vaginal mucosal maturation index and a reduction in pH in both groups with the vaginal ring being found to be preferable to the cream [135].

In order to clarify the situation a review of estrogen therapy in the management of urogenital atrophy has been performed by the HUT Committee [136]. Ten randomized trials and 54 uncontrolled series were examined from 1969 to 1995 assessing 24 different treatment regimens. Meta-analysis of ten placebo-controlled trials confirmed the significant effect of estrogens in the management of urogenital atrophy.

The route of administration was assessed and oral, vaginal, and parenteral (transcutaneous patches and subcutaneous implants) were compared. Overall, the vaginal route of administration was found to correlate with better symptom relief, greater improvement in cytological findings, and higher serum estradiol levels.

With regard to the type of estrogen preparation estradiol was found to be most effective in reducing patient symptoms, although conjugated estrogens produced the most cytological change and the greatest increase in serum levels of estradiol and estrone.

Finally, the effect of different dosages was examined. Low-dose vaginal estradiol was found to be the most efficacious according to symptom relief, although oral estriol also was effective. Estriol had no effect on the serum levels of estradiol or estrone, while vaginal estriol had minimal effect. Vaginal estradiol was found to have a small effect on serum estrogen, although not as great as systemic preparations. In conclusion it would appear that estrogen is efficacious in the treatment of urogenital atrophy and low-dose vaginal preparations are as effective as systemic therapy.

A more recent meta-analysis of the use of estrogens in the management of urogenital atrophy has been reported by the Cochrane group [137]. Overall, 16 trials with 2,129 women were included in the meta-analysis. When comparing the efficacy of estrogen-containing preparations there were significant differences favoring creams, tablets, and the estradiol ring compared to placebo and nonhormonal gel. Fourteen trials assessed safety; four examined endometrial hyperplasia, four endometrial stimulation, and six adverse effects. One trial found a significant increase in adverse effects (uterine bleeding, breast pain, and perineal pain) associated with CEE cream compared to estradiol tablets (1 RCT; OR 0.18, 95% CI: 0.07–0.50). In addition, two studies showed significant endometrial stimulation with CEE cream compared to the estradiol ring (OR 0.29; 95% CI: 0.11–0.78). While not significant, there was a 2% incidence of simple hyperplasia in the estradiol ring group compared to CEE cream and a 4% incidence of endometrial hyperplasia (one simple, one complex) in the conjugated estrogen cream group compared to the estradiol vaginal tablets. Acceptability was assessed in nine studies, and overall found a significant preference for the estradiol-releasing ring.

Conclusions

Estrogens are known to have an important physiological effect on the female lower genital tract throughout adult life, leading to symptomatic, histological, and functional changes. Urogenital atrophy is the manifestation of estrogen withdrawal following the menopause, presenting with vaginal and/or urinary symptoms. The use of estrogen replacement therapy has been examined in the management of lower urinary tract symptoms as well as in the treatment of urogenital atrophy, although only recently has it been subjected to randomized placebo-controlled trials and meta-analysis.

Estrogen therapy alone has been shown to have little effect in the management of urodynamic stress incontinence. At present there are no data regarding the synergistic use of estrogens and duloxetine, a combined serotonin and noradrenaline reuptake inhibitor, and the only drug to be licensed for the treatment of stress urinary incontinence.

When considering the irritive symptoms of urinary urgency, frequency, and urge incontinence estrogen therapy may be of benefit, although this may simply represent reversal of urogenital atrophy rather than a direct effect on the lower urinary tract. The role of systemic estrogen replacement therapy in the management of women with recurrent lower urinary tract infection remains to be determined, although there is now good evidence that vaginal administration may be efficacious. While low-dose vaginal estrogens have been shown to be have an important role in the treatment of urogenital atrophy in postmenopausal women and would appear to be as effective as systemic preparations, at present the role of adjuvant vaginal estrogen remains uncertain.

References

1. Cardozo LD. Role of oestrogens in the treatment of female urinary incontinence. J Am Geriatr Soc 1990; 38: 326–328.
2. Iosif S, Batra S, Ek A, Astedt B. Oestrogens receptors in the human female lower urinary tract. Am J Obstet Gynaecol 1981; 141: 817–820.
3. Batra SC, Fossil CS. Female urethra, a target for oestrogen action. J Urol 1983; 129: 418–420.

4. Batra SC, Iosif LS. Progesterone receptors in the female urinary tract. J Urol 1987; 138: 130–134.

5. Iosif C, Bekassy Z. Prevalence of genitourinary symptoms in the late menopause. Acta Obstet Gynaecol Scan 1984; 63: 257–260.

6 Beato M, Herrich P, Schutz G. Steroid hormone receptors: Many actors in search of a plot. Cell 1995; 83: 851–857.

7. Green S, Walter P, Kumar V, et al. Human oestrogen receptor cDNA: Sequence, expression and homology to v-erbA. Nature 1986; 320: 134–139.

8. Kuiper G, Enmark E, Pelto-Huikko M, et al. Cloning of a novel oestrogen receptor expressed in rat prostate and ovary. Proc Natl Acad Sci USA 1996; 93: 5925–5930.

9. Warner M, Nilsson S, Gustafsson JA. The oestrogen receptor family. Curr Opin Obstet Gynecol 1999; 11: 249–254.

10. Blakeman PJ, Hilton P, Bulmer JN. Mapping oestrogen and progesterone receptors throughout the female lower urinary tract. Neurourol Urodyn 1996; 15: 324–325.

11. Ingelman-Sundberg A, Rosen J, Gustafsson SA. Cytosol oestrogen receptors in urogenital tissues in stress incontinent women. Acta Obstet Gynecol Scand 1981; 60: 585–586.

12. Smith P. Oestrogens and the urogenital tract. Acta Obstet Gynaecol Scand 1993; 72(Suppl): 1–26.

13. Bernstein IT. The pelvic floor muscles: Muscle thickness in healthy and urinary-incontinent women measured by perineal ultasonography with reference to the effect of pelvic floor training. Oestrogen receptor studies. Neurourol Urodyn 1997; 16(4): 237–275.

14. Chen GD, Oliver RH, Leung BS, et al. Oestrogen receptor α and β expression in the vaginal walls and uterosacral ligaments of premenopausal and postmenopausal women. Fertil Steril 1999; 71(6): 1099–1102.

15. Screiter F, Fuchs P, Stockamp K. Oestrogenic sensitivity of α receptors in the urethral musculature. Urol Int 1976; 31: 13–19.

16. Blakeman PJ, Hilton P, Bulmer JN. Androgen receptors in the female lower urinary tract. Int Urogynaecol J 1997; 8: S54.

17. Pang X, Cotreau-Bibbo MM, Sant GR, Theoharides TC. Bladder mast cell expression of high affinity oestrogen receptors in receptors in patients with interstitial cystitis. Br J Urol 1995; 75: 154–161.

18. Letourneau R, Pang X, Sant GR, Theoharides TC. Intragranular activation of bladder mast cells and their association with nerve processes in interstitial cystitis. Br J Urol 1996; 77: 41–54.

19. Bodker A, Balsev E, Juul BR, et al. Oestrogen receptors in the human male bladder, prostatic urethra and prostate. Scan J Urol Nephrol 1995; 29: 161–165.

20. Blakeman PJ, Hilton P, Bulmer JN. Oestrogen and progesterone receptor expression in the female lower urinary tract, with reference to oestrogen status. BJU Int 2000; 86: 32–38.

21. Abrams P, Blaivas JG, Stanton SL, et al. The standardisation of terminology of lower urinary tract dysfunction. Br J Obstet Gynaecol 1990; 97: 1–16.

22. Rud T, Anderson KE, Asmussen M, et al. Factors maintaining the urethral pressure in women. Invest Urol 1980; 17: 343–347.

23. Malone-Lee J. Urodynamic measurement and urinary incontinence in the elderly. In: Brocklehurst JC, ed. Managing and measuring incontinence. Proceedings of the Geriatric Workshop on Incontinence, July 1988 (Geriatric Medicine).

24. Versi E, Cardozo LD. Oestrogens and lower urinary tract function. In: Studd JWW, Whitehead MI, eds. The menopause. Oxford: Blackwell Scientific Publications, 1988:76–84.

25. Kinn AC, Lindskog M. Oestrogens and phenylpropanolamine in combination for stress incontinence. Urology1988; 32: 273–280.

26. Smith PJB. The effect of oestrogens on bladder function in the female. In: Campbell S, ed. The management of the menopause and postmenopausal years. Carnforth: MTP 1976:291–298.

27. Samsioe G, Jansson I, Mellstrom, D, Svandborg A. Occurrence, nature and treatment of urinary incontinence in a 70 year old female population. Maturitas 1985; 7: 335–342.

28. Blakeman PJ, Hilton P, Bulmer JN. Cellular proliferation in the female lower urinary tract with reference to oestrogen status. Br J Obstet Gynaecol 2001; 8: 813–816

29. Hextall A, Bidmead J, Cardozo L, Hooper R. Hormonal influences on the human female lower urinary tract: A prospective evaluation of the effects of the menstrual cycle on symptomatology and the results of urodynamic investigation. Neurourol Urodyn 1999; 18(4): 282–283.

30. Van Geelen JM, Doesburg WH, Thomas CMG. Urodynamic studies in the normal menstrual cycle: The relationship between hormonal changes during the menstrual cycle and the urethral pressure profile. Am J Obstet Gynaecol 1981; 141: 384–392.

31. Burton G, Cardozo LD, Abdalla H, et al. The hormonal effects on the lower urinary tract in 282 women with premature ovarian failure. Neurourol Urodyn 1992; 10: 318–319.

32. Cutner A, Burton G, Cardozo LD, et al. Does progesterone cause an irritable bladder? Int Urogynaecol J 1993; 4: 259–261.

33. Benness C, Gangar K, Cardozo LD, Cutner A. Do progestogens exacerbate urinary incontinence in women on HRT? Neurourol Urodyn 1991; 10: 316–318.

34. Elliot RA, Castleden CM. Effect of progestogens and oestrogens on the contractile response of rat detrusor muscle to electrical field stimulation. Clin Sci 1994; 87: 342.

35. Cutner A. The urinary tract in pregnancy. MD Thesis, 1993, University of London.

36. Donnelly V, O'Connell PR, O'Herlihy C. The influence of hormonal replacement on faecal incontinence in post menopausal women. Br J Obstet Gynaecol 1997; 104: 311–315.

37. Sandford JP. Urinary tract symptoms and infection. Annu Rev Med 1975; 26: 485–505.

38. Boscia JA, Kaye D. Asymptomatic bacteria in the elderly. Infect Dis Clin North Am 1987; 1: 893–903.

39. Maggi A, Perez J. Role of female gonadal hormones in the CNS. Life Sci 1985; 37: 893–906.

40. Smith SS, Berg G, Hammar M, eds. The modern management of the menopause. Hormones, mood and neurobiology – a summary. Carnforth, UK: Parthenon Publishing;1993: 204.

41. Blok EFM, Holstege G. Androgen receptor immunoreactive neurones in the hypothalamic preoptic area project to the pontine micturition centre in the male cat. Neurourol Urodyn 1998; 17(4): 404–405.

42. Shapiro E. Effect of oestrogens on the weight and muscarinic receptor density of the rabbit bladder and urethra. J Urol 1986; 135: 1084–1087.

43. Batra S, Anderson KE. Oestrogen induced changes in muscarinic receptor density and contractile responses in the female rat urinary bladder. Acta Physiol Scand 1989; 137: 135–141.

44. Elliott RA, Castleden CM, Miodrag A, Kirwan P. The direct effects of diethylstilboestrol and nifedipine on the contractile responses of isolated human and rat detrusor muscles. Eur J Clin Pharmacol 1992; 43: 149–155.

45. Shenfield OZ, Blackmore PF, Morgan CW, et al. Rapid effects of oestriol and progesterone on tone and spontaneous rhythmic contractions of the rabbit bladder. Neurourol Urodyn 1998; 17(4): 408–409.

46. Fantl JA, Wyman JF, Anderson RL, et al. Post menopausal urinary incontinence: Comparison between non-oestrogen and oestrogen supplemented women. Obstet Gynaecol 1988; 71: 823–828.

47. Bergman A, Karram MM, Bhatia NN. Changes in urethral cytology following oestrogen administration. Gynaecol Obstet Invest 1990; 29: 211–213.

48. Rud T. The effects of oestrogens and gestogens on the urethral pressure profile in urinary continent and stress incontinent women. Acta Obstet Gynaecol Scand 1980; 59: 365–270.

49. Hilton P, Stanton SL. The use of intravaginal oestrogen cream in genuine stress incontinence. Br J Obstet Gynaecol 1983; 90: 940–944.

50. Bhatia NN, Bergman A, Karram MM, et al. Effects of oestrogen on urethral function in women with urinary incontinence. Am J Obstet Gynaecol 1989; 160: 176–180.

51. Karram MM, Yeko TR, Sauer MV, et al. Urodynamic changes following hormone replacement therapy in women with premature ovarian failure. Obstet Gynaecol 1989; 74: 208–211.

52. Ganger KF, Vyas S, Whitehead RW, et al. Pulsitility index in the internal carotid artery in relation to transdermal oestradiol and time since the menopause. Lancet 1991; 338: 839–842.

53. Jackson S, Vyas S. A double blind, placebo controlled study of postmenopausal oestrogen replacement therapy and carotid artery pulsatility index. Br J Obstet Gynaecol 1998; 105(4): 408–412.

54. Penotti M, Farina M, Sironi L, et al. Long term effects of postmenopausal hormone replacement therapy on pulsatility index of the internal carotid and middle cerebral arteries. Menopause J North Am Menopause Soc 1997; 4(2): 101–104.

55. Versi E, Cardozo LD. Urethral instability: Diagnosis based on variations in the maximum urethral pressure in normal climateric women. Neurourol Urodyn 1986; 5: 535–541.

56. Girao MJ, Jarmy-Di Bella ZI, Sartori MG, et al. Doppler velocimetry parameters of periurethral vessels in postmenopausal incontinent women receiving oestrogen replacement. Int Urogynaecol 2001; 12: 241–246.

57. Falconer C, Ekman-Ordeberg G, Ulmsten U, et al. Changes in paraurethral connective tissue at menopause are counteracted by oestrogen. Mauturitas 1996; 24: 197–204.

58. Kushner L, Chen Y, Desautel M, et al. Collagenase activity is elevated in conditioned media from fibroblasts of women with pelvic floor weakening. Int Urogynaecol 1999; 10(S1): 34.

59. Jackson S, Avery N, Shepherd A, et al. The effect of oestradiol on vaginal collagen in postmenopausal women with stress urinary incontinence. Neurourol Urodyn 1996; 15: 327–328.

60. James M, Avery N, Jackson S, et al. The pathophysiological changes of vaginal skin tissue in women with stress urinary incontinence: A controlled trial. Int Urogynaecol 1999; 10(S1): 35.

61. James M, Avery N, Jackson S, et al. The biochemical profile of vaginal tissue in women with genitourinary prolapse: A controlled trial. Neurourol Urodyn 1999; 18(4): 284–285.

62. Brincat M, Moniz CF, Studd JWW. Long term effects of the menopause and sex hormones on

skin thickness. Br J Obstet Gynaecol 1985; 92: 256–259.

63. Landon CR, Smith ARB, Crofts CE, Trowbridge EA. Biochemical properties of connective tissue in women with stress incontinence of urine. Neurourol Urodyn1989; 8: 369–370.

64. Ulmsten U, Ekman G, Giertz G. Different biochemical composition of connective tissue in continent and stress incontinent women. Acta Obstet Gynaecol Scand 1987; 66: 455.

65. Diokno AC, Brook BM, Brown MB. Prevalence of urinary incontinence and other urological symptoms in the non-institutionalised elderly. J Urol 1986; 136: 1022.

66. Yarnell J, Voyle G, Richards C, Stephenson T. The prevalence and severity of urinary incontinence in women. J Epidemiol Commun Health 1981; 35: 71–74.

67. Ouslander JG. Urinary incontinence in nursing homes. JAGS 1990; 38: 289–291.

68. MacLennan AH, Taylor AW, Wilson AW, Wilson D. The prevalence of pelvic floor disorders and their relationship to gender, age, parity, and mode of delivery. Br J Obstet Gynaecol 2000; 107: 1460–1470.

69. Kok AL, Voorhorst FJ, Burger CW, et al. Urinary and faecal incontinence in community residing elderly women. Age Ageing 1992; 21: 211.

70. Cardozo LD, Tapp A, Versi E, eds. The lower urinary tract in peri- and postmenopausal women. In: The urogenital deficiency syndrome. Bagsverd, Denmark: Novo Industri AS, 1987: 10–17.

71. Kondo A, Kato K, Saito M, et al. Prevalence of hand washing incontinence in females in comparison with stress and urge incontinence. Neurourol Urodyn 1990; 9: 330–331.

72. Thomas TM, Plymat KR, Blannin J, et al. Prevalence of urinary incontinence. Br Med J 1980; 281: 1243–1245.

73. Jolleys JV. Reported prevalence of urinary incontinence in a general practice. Br Med J 1988; 296: 1300–1302.

74. Burgio KL, Matthews KA, Engel B. Prevalence, incidence and correlates of urinary incontinence in healthy, middle aged women. J Urol 1991; 146: 1255–1259.

75. Iosif CS. Effects of protracted administration of oestriol on the lower genitourinary tract in postmenopausal women. Acta Obstet Gynaecol Scand 1992; 251: 115–120.

76. American National Institute of Health Population Figures. US Treasury Department. NIH, 1991.

77. Research on the menopause in the 1990's. Report or a WHO Scientific Group. In: WHO Technical Report Series 866 Geneva, Switzerland, 1994.

78. Barlow D, Samsioe G, van Geelan H. Prevalence of urinary problems in European countries. Maturitas 1997; 27: 239–248.

79. Greendale GA, Judd JL. The menopause: Health implications and clinical management. J Am Geriatr Soc 1993; 41: 426–436.

80. Samsioe G, Jansson I, Mellstrom D, Svanborg A. The occurrence, nature and treatment of urinary incontinence in a 70 year old population. Mauturitas 1985; 7: 335–343.

81. Van Geelen JM, Van de Weijer PH, Arnolds HT. Urogenital symptoms and resulting discomfort in non-institutionalised Dutch women aged 50–75 years. Int Urogynecol J Pelvic Floor Dysfunct 2000; 11(1): 9–14

82. Versi E, Harvey MA, Cardozo L, et al. Urogenital prolapse and atrophy at menopause: A prevalence study. Int Urogynaecol J Pelvic Dysfunct 2001; 12(2): 107–110

83. Davila GW, Karapanagiotou I, Woodhouse S, et al. Are women with urogenital atrophy symptomatic? Obstet Gynaecol 2001; 97(4 Suppl 1): S48.

84. Bachman GA. Urogenital aging: An old problem newly recognised. Maturitas 1995; 22: S1–S5.

85. Salmon UL, Walter RI, Gast SH. The use of oestrogen in the treatment of dysuria and incontinence in postmenopausal women. Am J Obstet Gynaecol 1941; 14: 23–31.

86. Youngblood VH, Tomlin EM, Davis JB. Senile urethritis in women. J Urol 1957; 78: 150–152.

87. Fantl JA, Cardozo LD, McClish DK, the Hormones and Urogenital Therapy Committee. Oestrogen therapy in the management of incontinence in postmenopausal women: A meta-analysis. First report of the Hormones and Urogenital Therapy Committee. Obstet Gynaecol 1994; 83: 12–18.

88. Henalla SM, Hutchins CJ, Robinson P, Macivar J. Nonoperative methods in the treatment of female genuine stress incontinence of urine. Br J Obstet Gynaecol 1989; 9: 222–225.

89. Zullo MA, Oliva C, Falconi G, et al. Efficacy of oestrogen therapy in urinary incontinence. A meta-analytic study. Minerva Gynecol 1998; 50(5): 199–205.

90. Moehrer B, Hextall A, Jackson S. Oestrogens for urinary incontinence in women. Cochrane Database Syst Rev 2003; (2): CD001405.

91. Grady D, Brown JS, Vittinghoff E, et al. Postmenopausal hormones and incontinence: The Heart and Estrogen/Progestin Replacement Study. Obstet Gynaecol 2001; 97: 116–120.

92. Grodstein F, Lifford K, Resnick NM, Curhan GC. Postmenopausal hormone therapy and risk of developing urinary incontinence. Obstet Gynaecol 2004; 103: 254–260.

93. Ouslander JG, Greendale GA, Uman G, et al. Effects of oral oestrogen and progestin on the lower urinary tract among female nursing home residents. Am Geriatr Soc 2001; 49(6): 803–807.

94. Hendrix SL, Cochrane BR, Nygaard IE, et al. Effects of estrogen with and without progestin on urinary incontinence. JAMA 2005; 293(8): 935–948.

95. Caine M, Raz S. The role of female hormones in stress incontinence. In: Proceedings of the 16th Congress of the International Society of Urology, Amsterdam, The Netherlands.

96. Rud T. The effects of oestrogens and gestogens on the urethral pressure profile in urinary continent and stress incontinent women. Acta Obstet Gynaecol Scand 1980; 59: 265–270.

97. Wilson PD, Faragher B, Butler B, et al. Treatment with oral piperazine oestrone sulphate for genuine stress incontinence in postmenopausal women. Br J Obstet Gynaecol 1987; 94: 568–574.

98. Walter S, Wolf H, Barlebo H, Jansen H. Urinary incontinence in postmenopausal women treated with oestrogens: A double-blind clinical trial. J Urol 1978; 33: 135–143.

99. Fantl JA, Bump RC, Robinson D, et al. Efficacy of oestrogen supplementation in the treatment of urinary incontinence. Obstet Gynaecol 1996; 88: 745–749.

100. Jackson S, Shepherd A, Brookes S, Abrams P. The effect of oestrogen supplementation on post-menopausal urinary stress incontinence: A double-blind, placebo controlled trial. Br J Obstet Gynaecol 1999; 106: 711–718.

101. Sultana CJ, Walters MD. Oestrogen and urinary incontinence in women. Maturitas 1995; 20: 129–138.

102. Beisland HO, Fossberg E, Moer A, et al. Urethral insufficiency in post-menopausal females: Treatment with phenylpropanolamine and oestriol separately and in combination. Urol Int 1984; 39: 211–216.

103. Hilton P, Tweddel AL, Mayne C. Oral and intravaginal oestrogens alone and in combination with alpha adrenergic stimulation in genuine stress incontinence. Int Urogynecol J 1990; 12: 80–86.

104. Horwitz RI, Brass LM, Kernan WN, Viscoli CM. Phenylpropanolamine and risk of hemorrhagic stroke: Final report of the Hemorrhagic Stroke Project, May 10, 2000.

105. Ahmed Al-Badr, Ross S, Soroka D, Drutz HP. What is the available evidence for hormone replacement therapy in women with stress urinary incontinence? J Obstet Gynaecol Can 2003; 25(7): 567–574.

106. Samsicoe G, Jansson I, Mellstrom D, Svanberg A. Urinary incontinence in 75 year old women. Effects of oestriol. Acta Obstet Gynaecol Scand 1985; 93: 57.

107. Cardozo LD, Rekers H, Tapp A, et al. Oestriol in the treatment of postmenopausal urgency: A multicentre study. Maturitas 1993; 18: 47–53.

108. Nilsson K, Heimer G. Low dose oestradiol in the treatment of urogenital oestrogen defiiciency – A pharmacokinetic and pharmacodynamic study. Maturitas 1992; 15: 121–127.

109. Benness C, Wise BG, Cutner A, Cardozo LD. Does low dose vaginal oestradiol improve frequency and urgency in postmenopausal women. Int Urogynaecol J 1992; 3(2): 281.

110. Eriksen PS, Rasmussen H. Low dose 17β-oestradiol vaginal tablets in the treatment of atrophic vaginitis: A double-blind placebo controlled study. Eur J Obstet Gynaecol Reprod Biol 1992; 44: 137–144.

111. Lose G, Englev E. Oestradiol-releasing vaginal ring versus oestriol vaginal pessaries in the treatment of bothersome lower urinary tract symptoms. Br J Obstet Gynaecol 2000; 107: 1029–1034.

112. Cardozo L, Lose G, McClish D, Versi E. Estrogen treatment for symptoms of an overactive bladder, results of a meta-analysis. Int J Urogynaecol 2001; 12(3): V.

113. Brandberg A, Mellstrom D, Samsioe G. Low dose oral oestriol treatment in elderly women with urogenital infections. Acta Obstet Gynaecol Scand 1987; 140: 33–38.

114. Parsons CL, Schmidt JD. Control of recurrent urinary tract infections in postmenopausal women. J Urol 1982; 128: 1224–1226.

115. Privette M, Cade R, Peterson J, et al. Prevention of recurrent urinary tract infections in postmenopausal women. Nephron 1988; 50: 24–27.

116. Kjaergaard B, Walter S, Knudsen A, et al. Treatment with low dose vaginal oestradiol in postmenopausal women. A double blind controlled trial. Ugeskr Laeger 1990; 152: 658–659.

117. Raz R, Stamm WE. A controlled trial of intravaginal oestriol in postmenopausal women with recurrent urinary tract infections. New Engl J Med 1993; 329: 753–756.

118. Kirkengen AL, Anderson P, Gjersoe E, et al. Oestriol in the prophylactic treatment of recurrent urinary tract infections in postmenopausal women. Scand J Prim Health Care 1992; 10: 142.

119. Cardozo LD, Benness C, Abbott D. Low dose oestrogen prophylaxis for recurrent urinary tract infections in elderly women. Br J Obstet Gynaecol 1998; 105: 403–407.

120. Raz R, Stamm WE. A controlled trial of intravaginal oestriol in postmenopausal women with recurrent urinary tract infections. New Engl. J Med 1993; 329: 753–756.

121. Eriksen B. A randomised, open, parallel-group study on the prevetitive effect of an oestradiol-releasing vaginal ring (Estring) on recurrent urinary tract infections in postmenopausal women. Am J Obstet Gynaecol 1999; 180: 1072–1079.

122. Samicoe G. Urogenital ageing – A hidden problem. Am J Obstet Gynaecol 1998; 178(5): S245–S249.

123. Mettler L, Olsen PG. Long term treatment of atrophic vaginitis with low dose oestradiol vaginal tablets. Maturitas 1991; 14: 23–31.

124. Smith P, Heimer G, Lindskog, Ulmsten U. Oestradiol releasing vaginal ring for treatment of postmenopausal urogenital atrophy. Maturitas 1993; 16: 145–154.

125. Smith RJN, Studd JWW. Recent advances in hormone replacement therapy. Br J Hosp Med 1993; 49: 799–809.

126. Palacios S, Castelo-Branco C, Cancelo MJ, Vazquez F. Low dose vaginally administered oestrogens may enhance local benefits of systemic therapy in the treatment of urogenital atrophy in postmenopausal women on hormone replacement therapy. Maturitas 2005; 50: 98–104.

127. Simunic V, Banovic I, Ciglar S, et al. Local oestrogen treatment in patients with urogenital symptoms. Int J Gynaecol Obstet 2003; 82: 187–197.

128. Akrivis Ch, Varras M, Thodos A, et al. Action of 25 mcg 17β oestradiol vaginal tablets in the treatment of vaginal atrophy in Greek postmenopausal women; clinical study. Clin Exp Obstet Gynaecol 2003; 30: 229–234.

129. Santen RJ, Pinkerton JV, Conaway M, et al. Treatment of urogenital atrophy with low dose oestradiol: Preliminary results. Menopause 2002; 9: 179–187.

130. Notelovitz M, Funk S, Nanavati N, Mazzeo M. Oestradiol absorption from vaginal tablets in postmenopausal women. Obstet Gynaecol 2002; 99: 556–562.

131. Rioux JE, Devlin C, Gelfend MM, et al. 17β Oestradiol vaginal tablet versus conjugated equine oestrogen vaginal cream to relieve menopausal atrophic vaginitis. Menopause 2000; 7: 156–161.

132. Manonai J, Theppisai U, Suthutvoravut S, et al. The effect of oestradiol vaginal tablet and conjugated oestrogen cream on urogenital symptoms in postmenopausal women: A comparative study. J Obstet Gynaecol Res 2001; 27: 255–260.

133. Henriksson L, Stjernquist M, Boquist L, et al. A one-year multicentre study of efficacy and safety of a continuous, low dose, oestradiol-releasing vaginal ring (Estring) in postmenopausal women with symptoms and signs of urogenital aging. Am J Obstet Gynaecol 1996; 174: 85–92.

134. Bachmann G. Oestradiol-releasing vaginal ring delivery system for urogenital atrophy. Experience over the last decade. J Reprod Med 1998; 43: 991–998.

135. Ayton RA, Darling GM, Murkies AL, et al. A comparative study of safety and efficacy of low dose oestradiol released from a vaginal ring compared with conjugated equine oestrogen vaginal cream in the treatment of postmenopausal vaginal atrophy. Br J Obstet Gynaecol 1996; 103: 351–358.

136. Cardozo LD, Bachmann G, McClish D, et al. Meta-analysis of oestrogen therapy in the management of urogenital atrophy in postmenopausal women: Second report of the Hormones and Urogenital Therapy Committee. Obstet Gynaecol 1998; 92: 722–727.

137. Suckling J, Lethaby A, Kennedy R. Local oestrogen for vaginal atrophy in postmenopausal women. Cochrane Database Syst Rev 2003; (4): CD001500.

138. Judge TG. The use of quinestradol in elderly incontinent women: A preliminary report. Gerontol Clin 1969; 11: 159–164.

139. Walter S, Kjaergaard B, Lose G, et al. Stress urinary incontinence in postmenopausal women treated with oral oestrogen (oestriol) and an α-adrenoceptor stimulating agent (phenylpropanolamine): A randomised double-blind placebo-controlled study. Int. Urogynaecol. J. 1990; 1: 74–79.

Part III
Management of Stress Urinary Incontinence

Chapter 7
Pelvic Floor Rehabilitation

Kari Bø

Introduction

In 1948, Kegel [1] was the first to report pelvic floor muscle training (PFMT) to be effective in treatment of female urinary incontinence. In spite of his reports of cure rates of >84%, surgery soon became the first choice of treatment, and not until the 1980s was there renewed interest for conservative treatment. This new interest for conservative treatment may have developed because of higher awareness among women on incontinence and health and fitness activities, cost of surgery, and morbidity, complications, and relapses reported after surgical procedures.

Today several consensus statements based on systematic reviews have recommended conservative treatment and especially PFMT as the first choice of treatment for stress urinary incontinence (SUI) [2–5]. However, many physicians seem to be skeptical about PFMT. This skepticism may be based on inadequate knowledge of exercise science and physical therapy, and beliefs that there is insufficient evidence for the effectiveness of PFMT, that evidence for long-term effects is lacking or poor, and that women are not motivated to regularly perform PFMT. In this chapter the focus will be to report evidence-based knowledge on the above-mentioned points related to PFMT for SUI.

Methods

This review is limited to the effect of physical therapy on patients with a history of or urodynamic SUI. Only outcomes from randomized controlled trials (RCT) are included. Computerized search on the PubMed, studies, data, and conclusions from the two latest International Consultations on Incontinence (ICI) [2, 5], and the Cochrane Library of systematic reviews [3, 4] have been used as background sources. This overview will comprise rehabilitation with PFMT with or without biofeedback or cones in addition to the use of electrical stimulation.

Is PFMT Effective in Treatment of Female SUI?

The gold standard research design to evaluate the effect of an intervention (surgery, pharmaceutical, training) is RCT. However, there are high- and low-quality RCTs. High methodology quality is judged on concealment of treatment allocation, blinding of assessors, sufficient sample size (based on power calculation if possible), use of reproducible and valid outcome measurements, and handling of dropouts and low adherence (intention to treat analysis).

Equally important, but less written about in textbooks of statistics and research methodology, is the quality of the intervention, e.g., surgery in the hands of well-experienced surgeons or research-based and high-quality conducted PFMT. A lot of ineffective or even harmful treatments can be put into a RCT of high-methodology quality. Herbert and Bø [6] found that by adding studies with high sample size but low training dosage and nonsupervised training to smaller studies with adequate training dosage in a meta-analysis, the effect size may change dramatically in disfavor of high-quality smaller studies.

For PFMT studies there is an additional problem. Several research groups have shown that >30% of women are not able to voluntarily contract the pelvic floor muscles at their first consultation even after thorough individual instruction [7–10]. Hay-Smith et al. [3] reported that only in 15 of 43 RCTs on the effect of PFMT for SUI, urge and mixed incontinence, ability to contract was checked before training started. A common mistake is to strain instead of squeeze and lift. If women are straining instead of performing a correct contraction, the training may harm and not improve pelvic floor muscles (PFM) function.

The numerous reports by Kegel with >80% cure rate comprised uncontrolled studies with the inclusion of a variety of incontinence types and no measurement of urinary leakage before and after treatment. However, since then, several RCTs have demonstrated that PFMT is more effective than no treatment to treat SUI [11–15]. In addition, a number of RCTs have compared PFMT alone with either the use of vaginal resistance devices, biofeedback, or vaginal cones [4]. Only one study did not show any significant effect of PFMT on urinary leakage [3]. Interestingly, in this study there was no check of the women's ability to contract, adherence to the training protocol was poor, and the placebo group contracted gluteal muscles and external rotators of the hips; activities that may give co-contractions of the PFM[16, 17].

Improvement Rates

As for surgery [18] and pharmacology studies [19], a combination of cure and improvement measures often is reported. To date there is no consensus on what outcome measure to choose as the gold standard for cure [urodynamic diagnosis, no leakage episodes, ≤2 g of leakage on pad test (tests with standardized bladder volume, 1, 24, and 48 h?), women's report, etc.] [20]. Subjective cure/improvement rates of PFMT including studies of both SUI and mixed incontinence reported in RCTs varies between 56 and 70% [3, 21].

Cure Rates

It often is reported that PFMT is more commonly associated with improvement of symptoms rather than a total cure. However, in several RCTs cure has been reported. In a study by Bø et al. [22] cure rate was defined as conversion of negative to positive closure pressure during cough and a cure rate of 60% was found. This corresponded with the number of women reporting to be continent or almost continent. In newer RCTs short-term cure rates of 44–70% defined as <2 g of leakage on different pad tests has been found after PFMT [11, 13, 14, 23–26]. The highest cure rate from PFMT alone was shown in a single-blind RCT where the female subjects had thorough individual instruction by a trained physical therapist (PT), combined training with biofeedback, and close follow-up once and every second week. The training period lasted 6 months. Adherence was high and dropout was low [25]. The third ICI meeting concludes that PFMT should be offered as first-line therapy to all women with stress, urge, or mixed urinary incontinence [5].

The Most Effective PFMT Program

Because of use of different outcome measures and instruments to measure PFM function and strength, it is impossible to combine results among studies and it is difficult to conclude which training regimen is the more effective. Also the exercise dosage (type of exercise, frequency, duration, and intensity) varies significantly between studies [3, 5].

Several research groups have found that either more intensive training, more frequent training, or supervised training is more effective than lower dosage of training [22, 23, 27, 28]. Bø et al. combined individual assessment and teaching of correct contraction with strength training in groups in a 6-month training program [11, 22]. The women were randomized to either an (1) intensive training program consisting of seven individual sessions with a PT, combined with 45 min weekly PFMT classes, and three sets of 8–12 contractions per day at home or (2) the same program without the weekly intensive exercise classes (Figs. 7.1 and 7.2). The results showed a much better improvement in both muscle strength and urinary leakage in the intensive exercise group. Sixty percent reported to be continent/almost continent in the intensive exercise group compared to 17% in the less intensive group. A significant reduction of urinary leakage, measured by pad test with standardized bladder volume, was demonstrated only in the intensive exercise group.

This study demonstrated that a huge difference in outcome can be expected according to the intensity and follow-up of the training program and very little effect can be expected after training

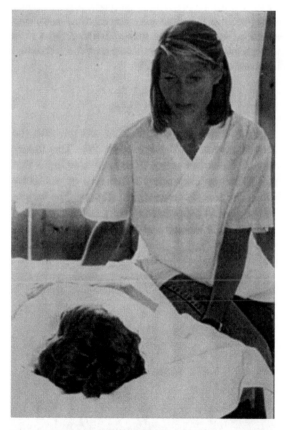

FIG. 7.1. Individual assessment of ability to contract the pelvic floor muscles correctly is necessary to assure effective training. Vaginal palpation is used to give direct feedback to the patient about muscle performance

without close follow-up. It is worth noting that the significantly less effective group in this study had seven visits with a skilled PT and that adherence to the home-training program was high. Nevertheless, the effect was only 17%. There is a dose–response issue in all sorts of training regimens [29]. Hence, one reason for disappointing effects shown in some clinical practices or research studies may be due to insufficient training stimulus and low dosage [30]. Furthermore, if low-dosage programs are chosen as one arm in a RCT comparing PFMT with other methods, PFMT is bound to be less effective. The third ICI recommends that clinicians should provide the most intensively supervised PFMT program possible within service constraints [5].

PFMT with Biofeedback

Biofeedback has been defined as "a group of experimental procedures where an external sensor is used to give an indication on bodily processes, usually in the purpose of changing the measured quality" [31]. Biofeedback equipment has been developed within the area of psychology, mainly for measurement of sweating, heart rate, and blood pressure during different forms of stress. Kegel [1] always based his training protocol on thorough instruction of correct contraction using vaginal palpation and clinical observation. He combined PFMT with use of vaginal squeeze pressure measurement as biofeedback during exercise. Today, a variety of biofeedback apparatuses are commonly used in clinical practice to assist with PFMT.

In urology or urogynecology textbooks the term "biofeedback" often is used to classify a method different from PFMT. However, biofeedback is not a treatment by itself. It is an adjunct to training, measuring the response from a single PFM contraction. For PFMT, both vaginal and anal surface electromyograms (EMG) and urethral and vaginal squeeze pressure measurements have been used to help make the patients more aware of muscle function and to enhance and motivate patients' effort during training [3].

Since Kegel first presented his results, several RCTs have shown that PFMT without biofeedback is more effective than no treatment for SUI [3, 5]. In women with stress or mixed incontinence, all but one of RCTs have failed to show any additional effects of adding biofeedback to the training protocol.

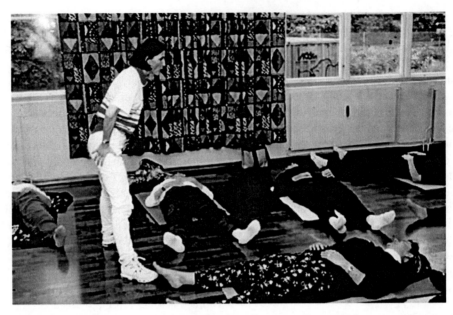

FIG. 7.2. After individual instruction and assurance of ability to contract the pelvic floor muscles correctly, regular strength training of the muscles can be done in groups. This may be more fun, motivating, and less time-consuming for both the patients and the physical therapists. In between the pelvic floor muscle strength training, focus is on other muscle groups such as the abdominals, back, arm, and thigh muscles. The program also comprises relaxation and breathing exercise and practice on correct lifting techniques and ergonomics [11, 22]

In the study of Glavind et al. [23] a positive effect was demonstrated. However, this study was confounded by a difference in training frequency, and the effect might be due to double-training dosage, the use of biofeedback, or both. Hence, the results of the above-mentioned study support the studies that conclude there is a dose–response issue in PFMT [22, 27, 28].

Since PFMT is effective without biofeedback, a large sample size may be needed to show any beneficial effect of adding biofeedback to an effective training protocol. In most of the published studies the sample sizes are small, and type II error may have been the reason for negative findings. However, in the two largest RCTs published, no additional effects were demonstrated [3, 25].

Many women may not like to undress, lock the room, and insert a vaginal or rectal device in order to exercise [32]. On the other hand, some women find it motivating to use biofeedback to control and enhance the strength of the contractions when training. Any factor that may stimulate high adherence and intensive training should be recommended to enhance the effect of a training program. Hence, there is a place for biofeedback in PFMT.

PFMT with Vaginal Cones

Vaginal cones are weights that are put into the vagina above the levator plate [4]. The theory behind the use of cones in strength training is that the PFM are contracted reflexively or voluntary when the cone is perceived to slip out. The weight of the cone is supposed to give a training stimulus and make the women contract harder with progressive weight (Fig. 7.3). It has been concluded that

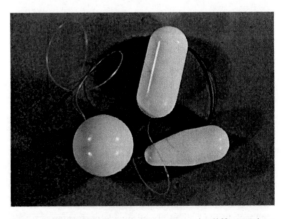

FIG. 7.3. Vaginal weighted cones comes in different sizes and shapes

training with vaginal cones is more effective than no treatment [4]. Several RCTs have been found comparing PFMT with and without vaginal cones for SUI [11, 33–36]. Bø et al. [11] found that PFMT was significantly more effective than training with cones both to improve muscle strength and to reduce urinary leakage. In the three other studies there was no difference between PFMT with and without cones [33–35]. Cammu and Van Nylen [34] reported very low compliance, and therefore did not recommend use of cones. Bø et al. [11] reported that women in the cones group reported great motivational problems and Laycock et al. [35] had a total dropout rate in their study of 33%.

The use of cones can be questioned from an exercise science perspective. Holding the cone for as long as 15–20 min as recommended might cause decreased blood supply, decreased oxygen consumption, muscle fatigue and pain, and recruit contraction of other muscles instead of the PFM. In addition, many women report that they dislike using cones [34]. On the other hand, the cones may add benefit to the training protocol if used in a different way. Arvonen et al. [36] used "vaginal balls" and followed general strength training principles with dynamic contractions. They found that training with the balls was significantly more effective in reducing urinary leakage than regular PFMT.

Electrical Stimulation

The aim of electrical stimulation for SUI is to strengthen the PFM mirroring voluntary contractions. Several consensus reports have concluded that strength training is more effective than electrical stimulation to increase muscle strength for other skeletal muscles [37, 38]. In most physical therapy practices, electrical stimulation has been used for partially paralyzed muscles and to stimulate to activity when the patients were not able to contract. As soon as the patient can contract voluntarily, most PTs would stop using electrical stimulation and continue with regular muscle training. Surprisingly, in the area of PFM rehabilitation, there has been a great interest especially among gynecologists and general practitioners to treat urinary incontinence with electrical stimulation alone. In one of the first studies in this area, Eriksen et al. [39] used long-term stimulation (8 h a day, usually during sleep, with 10 Hz) and showed significant improvement in urodynamic parameters

and urinary leakage. However, the study design was uncontrolled and unblinded.

Today there are several RCTs on the effect of electrical stimulation on female SUI [5]. A number of different currents, apparatus, and stimulation regimens have been used. For SUI, short-term stimulation applying 35–50 Hz has been used in most of the studies. Electrical stimulation was compared with sham or untreated control in six studies for SUI. Henalla et al. [14], Sand et al. [40], and Yamanishi et al. [41] found a significant effect compared to control or sham stimulation, while Luber and Wolde Tsadik [42], Brubaker et al. [43], and Bø et al. [11] did not find significant effect. It has been concluded that more studies are needed to clarify whether electrical stimulation is effective in treatment of female SUI [5].

PFMT or Electrical Stimulation?

Hennalla et al. [14] and Bø et al. [11] found that PFMT was significantly better than electrical stimulation to treat SUI. Laycock and Jerwood [44] and Hahn et al. [45] found no difference, and Smith [46] found that electrical stimulation was significantly better. In addition, several research groups have found no effect of adding electrical stimulation to PFMT [28, 47, 48]. Many of these studies are flawed by small numbers of subjects, and future RCTs with better methodological quality should be repeated [5]. However, electrical stimulation has shown to have side effects [40] and to be less tolerable to women than PFMT [11]. In addition, Bø and Talseth [49] found that voluntary PFM contraction increases urethral pressure significantly more than electrical stimulation.

Adverse Effects of PFM Rehabilitation Methods

Few, if any, adverse effects have been found after PFMT [5]. The only reported adverse effect is from Lagro-Jansson [50] where one woman reported pain with exercise and three had an uncomfortable feeling during the exercises. In other studies no side effects have been found [11].

Reported adverse effects after electrical stimulation have been pain, discomfort, vaginal irritations or infections, urinary tract infections, and diarrhea [11, 40, 51]. In a Norwegian study of 3,100 women who had used electrical stimulation 51% reported one or more side effect [51]. The most common side effects were soreness/local irritation (26%), pain (20%), and psychological distress. Most of the cases were mild. Reported adverse effects of cones have been abdominal pain, vaginities, and bleeding [11].

Two Concepts of How and Why PFMT May Work in Treatment of SUI

There are two main concepts of explaining how PFMT may work for SUI [21]:

1. *Use of conscious cocontraction of the PFM with increase in abdominal pressure.* Precontractions before increases in intra-abdominal pressures have been part of PFMT in many physical therapy practices for years [52]. Miller et al. [15] showed that teaching women how to contract and encourage them to contract before coughing significantly reduced urinary leakage within a week. They named the precontraction "the Knack," and there is evidence that the conscious contraction can clamp the urethra [21]. However, Bump et al. [10] showed that only 49% of women were able to contract the PFM in a way that effectively closed the urethra, and we do not know the amount of strength necessary to close the urethra.
2. *Strength training.* Kegel [1] described his training program as a tightening up of the pelvic floor. Strength training of the pelvic floor aims to build up a permanently better structural support for the bladder and urethra by lifting the anatomical location of the pelvic floor to a higher position, hypertrophying the muscle fibers, increasing stiffness in the muscles and connective tissue, and closing the levator hiatus. A strong structural support (stiff pelvic floor) may prevent descent of the bladder neck and urethra and close the urethra during abrupt increase in intra-abdominal pressure. There is some evidence in the literature showing such morphological changes after PFMT, put so far only from noncontrolled trials [21].

The theoretical rationale will decide how the therapist teaches PFMT. The literature shows that only one research group has used the Knack only, and very few researchers report the use of a combination of strength training and the Knack. Most of the protocols describe regular strength training only. In continent subjects, the PFM contraction is an automatic response without conscious voluntary contraction before activity. In addition, conscious precontractions are only possible before single bouts of physical exertion (for instance, coughing and sneezing). Nobody can run or dance over a longer period of time and contract the PFM voluntarily all the time. Therefore, the main goal of PFMT is to build the muscles to improve stiffness of the pelvic floor to avoid the occurrence of descent. The following recommendations on effective training to increase strength and muscle volume is given by the American College of Sport Sciences (ACSM) [53]:

1. Initial training: 8–12 repetition maximum (RM) (close to maximum effort) 2–3 times a week.
2. Intermediate to advanced training: 1–12 RM in a periodized fashion with heavy loading 4–5 times a week.

Typically higher intensity (close to maximum contraction) is recommended for maximizing hypertrophy [53]. However, the authors state that the recommendations should be viewed in the context of the individual's target goals, physical capacity, and training status. Hence, optimally PFMT should be based on a thorough evaluation of the function of the PFM (Fig. 7.4.). In all RCTs on PFMT to treat SUI the women have been encouraged to do everyday exercise.

Long-Term Effects of PFMT

Long-term effects of any exercise program cannot be expected if the persons stop exercising. Several studies have reported long-term effects of PFMT [3]. However, usually women in the nontreatment or less effective intervention groups have gone on to receive treatment after cessation of the study period. Follow-up data therefore usually are reported for either all women or for only the group with best effects. As for surgery [54], there are only a few long-term studies that include clinical examination [55–57]. Klarskov et al. [55] assessed only a few of the women originally participating in the study. Lagro-Janssen et al. [56] evaluated 88 out of 110 women with stress, urge, or mixed incontinence 5 years after cessation of training, and found that 67% remained satisfied with the

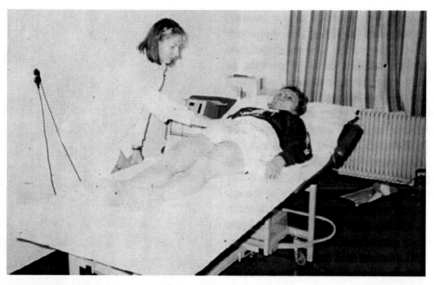

FIG. 7.4. Measurement of pelvic floor muscle function is important when teaching pelvic floor muscle training. There are different apparatuses available commercially. Ideally, all apparatuses should be tested for responsiveness, reliability, and validity before use. The picture shows Camtech squeezemeter (Camtech AS, Sandvika, Norway)

condition. Only 7of 110 had been treated with surgery. Moreover, satisfaction was closely related to adherence to training and type of incontinence, with mixed incontinent women being more likely to lose the effect. SUI women had the best long-term effect, but only 39% of them were exercising daily or "when needed."

Cammu et al. [58] sent postal questionnaires and evaluated medical files of 52 women who had participated in an individual course of PFMT for urodynamic SUI. Eighty-seven percent were suitable for analysis. Thirty-three percent had had surgery after 10 years. However, only 8% had undergone surgery in the group originally being successful after training, whereas 62% had undergone surgery in the group initially dissatisfied with training. Successful results were maintained after 10 years in two thirds of the patients originally classified as successful.

In a 5-year follow-up, Bø and Talseth [57] found that urinary leakage was significantly increased after cessation of organized training. Three of 23 had been treated with surgery. Two of these women who had not been cured after the initial training, were satisfied with their surgery, and had no leakage on pad test. The third women had been cured after initial PFMT. However, after 1 year she stopped training because of personal problems

connected to the death of her husband. Her incontinence problems returned and she had surgery 2 years before the 5-year follow-up. She was not satisfied with the outcome after surgery and had visible leakage on cough test and 17 g of leakage on the pad test. Fifty-six percent of the women had a positive closure pressure during cough and 70% had no visible leakage during cough at 5-year follow-up. Seventy percent of the patients were still satisfied with the results and did not want other treatment options. However, following up the same patients with questionnaires 15 years after cessation of organized training, the short-term significant effect of intensive training was no longer present [59]. Fifty percent from both groups had interval surgery for SUI; however, more women in the less intensive training group had surgery within the first 5 years after ending the training program. At 15 years follow-up there were no differences in reported frequency or amount of leakage between nonoperated and operated women, but women who had surgery reported significantly more severe leakage and to be more bothered by urinary incontinence during daily activities than those who did not have surgery.

The general recommendations for maintaining muscle strength are one set of 8–12 contractions twice a week [60]. The intensity of the contraction seems to be more important than frequency of training. So far, no studies have evaluated how many contractions subjects have to perform to maintain PFM strength after cessation of organized training. In the study of Bø and Talseth [57] PFM strength was maintained 5 years after cessation of organized training, with 70% exercising more than once a week. However, number and intensity of exercises varied considerably among successful women [61]. One series of 8–12 contractions easily could be taught in aerobic dance classes or recommended as part of women's general strength training programs. On the other hand, we do not know how a voluntary precontraction before increase in intra-abdominal pressure will maintain or increase muscle strength. In the study of Cammu et al. [58] the long-term effect of PFMT appeared to be attributed to the precontraction before sudden increases in intra-abdominal pressure and not so much to regular strength training. Unfortunately, muscle strength was not measured in their study.

PFMT in Prevention of SUI

Only a few RCTs have been found to prevent urinary incontinence and in some of the studies women with symptoms or diagnoses of SUI, urge, and mixed incontinence have been included. As far as this author has ascertained there are no primary prevention studies in the general population using PFMT for nonsymptomatic women to avoid the occurrence of SUI sometime in the future [5]. The focus of most of the prevention studies has been to evaluate the effect of PFMT during pregnancy and after childbirth. Four RCTs have been found that assess the effect of PFMT during pregnancy (Fig. 7.5). Sampselle et al. [62] found significantly less incontinence symptoms in the PFMT group at 6 weeks and 6 months postpartum. However, the effect was no longer present at 12 months postpartum. Huges et al. [63] did not find any effect of only one session of physical therapy to prevent urinary leakage during pregnancy. On the other hand, Reilly et al. [64] found a significant reduction in the prevalence of urinary leakage in a group of primigravida women with bladder neck mobility, and Mørkved et al. [65] found significant reduction in the prevalence of urinary leakage after

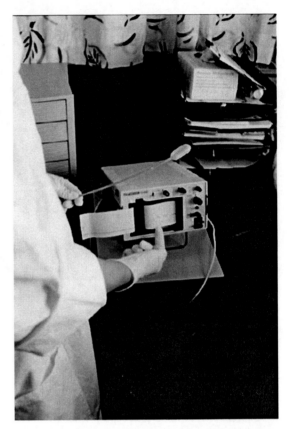

Fig. 7.5. Since randomized controlled trials have demonstrated effects on reducing and preventing urinary incontinence during pregnancy and after childbirth, strength training of the pelvic floor muscles should start antenatally. Much important general information about health issues during pregnancy and after childbirth can be discussed in the class

18 weeks of supervised group training combined with home exercise.

Three RCTs and one matched controlled trial have been found that evaluate the effect of postpartum PFMT. Sleep and Grant [66] did not find any effect of midwives counseling postpartum women to perform PFMT. However, Mørkved and Bø [67], Meyer et al. [68], and Chiarelli and Cochburn [69] found significant reduction of urinary incontinence in favor of PFMT. In the matched controlled trial of Mørkved and Bø [67] a 50% reduction in prevalence was found in the training group. Hence, there is evidence from high-quality RCTs to recommend PFMT both antenatally and postpartum.

Motivation

Some women may find the exercises difficult to conduct on a regular basis [70]. However, when analyzing results of RCTs, adherence to the exercise program is generally high and dropout rate is low [3, 5]. In a few studies low adherence and high dropout rates have been reported [35, 71]. The PTs knowledge about behavioral sciences such as pedagogy and health psychology and their ability to explain and motivate patients may be a crucial factor to enhance adherence and minimize dropouts from training. In some studies such strategies have been followed, and high adherence has been achieved [70, 72]. In other studies specific strategies have not been reported, but much emphasis has been put on creating a positive, enjoyable, and supportive training environment. Group training after thorough individual instruction may be a good concept if led by a skilled and motivating therapist [11, 22]. PFMT concepts with 0 dropouts [73] and adherence >90% [11] are possible. In a study by Alewijnse [70] most women followed the adviceto train four to six times a week 1 year after cessation of the training program. The following factors predicted adherence with 50%: positive intention to adhere, high short-term adherence levels, positive self-efficacy expectations, and frequent weekly episodes of leakage before and after initial therapy. Patients do not comply with treatment for a wide variety of reasons: long-lasting and time-consuming treatments, requirement of lifestyle changes, poor client/patient interaction, cultural and health beliefs, poor social support, inconvenience, lack of time, motivational problems, and travel time to clinics have been listed as important factors [74].

In a Japanize study, Sugaya et al. [75] used a computerized pocket-size device that emits a sound three times a day to remind the person to perform PFMT. To stop the sound the person needed to push a button, and by pushing the button for each contraction, adherence was registered. Forty-six women were randomly assigned to either instruction to contract the PFM following a pamphlet or the same pamphlet together with the sound device and instruction in how to use the device. Interestingly, the results showed a significant improvement in daily incontinence episodes and pad test only in the device group. Forty-eight percent were satisfied in the device group compared to 15% in the control group.

In most countries patients receive physical therapy on physicians' referrals only. This means that the motivation of the general practitioner, gynecologist, or urologist for PFMT and conservative treatment is extremely important. If these professions are not updated on the effect of PFMT, do not know any trained PTs in their area, or think PFMT is boring and a big demand, the patients may not even be introduced to the option of training. PFMT can be put forward either as a "boring demanding task you need to do the rest of your life" or it can be introduced as a method that is "easy, at a low cost and with no side effects. It may take less than 10 min per day to build up strength if it is conducted correctly (three sets of 8–12 contractions a day), and it takes even less to maintain it." The number of PTs specializing in women's health and pelvic floor issues vary among countries. In order to recruit more PTs into the area, it may be important to advocate for a mandatory curriculum on pelvic floor dysfunction and treatment at undergraduate education level, add courses on postgraduate level, and stimulate urologists to participate in the teaching of PTs.

Is PFMT Effective only for the Young and Those with Minor Leakage?

Several researchers have looked into factors affecting outcome of PFMT on urinary incontinence [5]. No single factor has been shown to predict outcome, and it has been concluded that many factors traditionally supposed to affect outcomes such as age and severity of incontinence may be less crucial than previously thought. Factors that appear to be most associated with positive outcome are thorough teaching of correct contraction, motivation, adherence with the intervention, and intensity of the program [5].

Conclusion

RCT and systematic reviews have shown that PFMT with or without biofeedback or cones has proved to be effective in the treatment of female SUI. There is increasing evidence that PFMT can prevent urinary incontinence when performed antenatally and postpartum. Compared to surgery PFMT has no known side effects and is relatively inexpensive, and women should be motivated to intensively perform PFMT as first-line treatment. However, more than 30% do not contract correctly at their first consultation, and thorough individual instruction is needed. Manual techniques and electrical stimulation may be used to teach how to contract. Three sets of 8–12 close to maximum contractions every day or every second day is recommended based on general strength training theory and results of high-quality RCTs. In addition, the women should learn to precontract before increase in intra-abdominal pressure.

Most women need motivation and encouragement to perform regular strength training. This can be achieved in individual training sessions or in specifically designed PFMT classes. When sufficient function has been achieved, PFM strength has to be maintained by ongoing training but with lower frequency. More research is needed to find out how much exercise is needed to improve and maintain optimal PFM function and whether the effect is attributed to a conscious precontraction, the building up of a firm structural support giving automatic cocontractions, or a combination. There is a need for better collaboration between physicians and PTs to organize a better health service for SUI patients and for planning of future high-quality clinical trials.

References

1. Kegel AH. Progressive resistance exercise in the functional restoration of the perineal muscles. Am J Obstet Gynecol 1948; 56:238–249.
2. Wilson PD, Bø KH-SJ, Nygaard I, et-al. Conservative treatment in women. In: Abrams P, Cardozo L, Khoury S, Wein A, eds. Incontinence. Plymouth: Plymbridge, Health Publication, 2002: 571–624.
3. Hay-Smith E, Bø K, Berghmans L, et al. Pelvic floor muscle training for urinary incontinence in women (Cochrane review).[3] . Oxford, UK: The Cochrane Library, 2001.
4. Herbison P, Plevnik S, Mantle J. Weighted vaginal cones for urinary incontinence. Oxford, UK: The Cochrane Library, 2000; 1–24.
5. Wilson PD, Berghmans B, Hagen S, et al. Adult conservative management. In: Abrams P, Cardozo L, Khoury S, Wein A, eds. Incontinence, Vol 2, Management. Paris: Health Publications 2005: 855–964
6. Herbert RD, Bø K. Analysis of quality of interventions in systematic reviews. BMJ 2005; 331:507–509.
7. Kegel AH. Stress incontinence and genital relaxation. Ciba Clin Symp 1952; 2:35–51.
8. Benvenuti F, Caputo GM, Bandinelli S, et al. Reeducative treatment of female genuine stress incontinence. Am J Phys Med 1987; 66(4):155–168.
9. Bø K, Larsen S, Oseid S, et al. Knowledge about and ability to correct pelvic floor muscle exercises in women with urinary stress incontinence. Neurourol Urodyn 1988; 7(3):261–262.
10. Bump R, Hurt WG, Fantl JA, et al. Assessment of Kegel exercise performance after brief verbal instruction. Am J Obstet Gynecol 1991; 165:322–329.
11. Bø K, Talseth T, Holme I. Single blind, randomised controlled trial of pelvic floor exercises, electrical stimulation, vaginal cones, and no treatment in management of genuine stress incontinence in women. BMJ 1999; 318:487–493.
12. Lagro-Janssen TLM, Debruyne FMJ, Smits AJA, et al. Controlled trial of pelvic exercises in the treatment of urinary stress incontinence in general practice. Br J Gen Pract 1991; 41:445–449.
13. Henalla S, Millar D, Wallace K. Surgical versus conservative management for post-menopausal genuine stress incontinence of urine. Neurourol Urodyn 1990; 9(4):436–437.
14. Henalla SM, Hutchins CJ, Robinson P, et al. Non-operative methods in the treatment of female genuine stress incontinence of urine. J Obstet Gynaecol 1989; 9:222–225.
15. Miller JM, Ashton-Miller JA, DeLancey J. A pelvic muscle precontraction can reduce cough-related urine loss in selected women with mild SUI. J Am Geriatr Soc 1998; 46:870–874.
16. Bø K, Kvarstein B, Hagen R, et al. Pelvic floor muscle exercise for the treatment of female stress urinary incontinence: II. Validity of vaginal pressure measurements of pelvic floor muscle strength and the necessity of supplementary methods for control of correct contraction. Neurourol Urodyn 1990; 9:479–487.
17. Peschers U, Gingelmaier A, Jundt K, et al. Evaluation of pelvic floor muscle strength using four different techniques. Int Urogynecol J 2001; 12:27–30.
18. Smith T, Daneshgari F, Dmochowski R, et al. Surgical treatment of incontinence in women. In: Abrams P, Cardozo L, Khoury S, Wein A, eds. Incontinence. Plymouth, UK: Plymbridge Distributors, 2002: 823–863.
19. Andersson K, Appell R, Awad S, et al. Pharmacological treatment of urinary incontinence. In: Abrams P, Cardozo L, Khoury S, Wein A, eds. Incontinence. Plymouth: Plymbridge Distributors, 2002: 479–511.
20. Blaivas JG, Appell RA, Fantl JA, et al. Standards of efficacy for evaluation of treatment outcomes in

urinary incontinence: Recommendations of the urodynamic society. Neurourol Urodyn 1997; 16(145):147.

21. Bø K. Pelvic floor muscle training is effective in treatment of female stress urinary incontinence, but how does it work? Int Urogynecol J 2004; 15:76–84.

22. Bø K, Hagen RH, Kvarstein B, et al. Pelvic floor muscle exercise for the treatment of female stress urinary incontinence: III. Effects of two different degrees of pelvic floor muscle exercise. Neurourol Urodyn 1990; 9:489–502.

23. Glavind K, Laursen B, Jaquet A. Efficacy of biofeedback in the treatment of urinary stress incontinence. Int Urogyn J 1998; 9:151–153.

24. Wong K, Fung B, Fung, et al. Pelvic floor exercises in the treatment of stress urinary incontinence in Hong Kong chinese women. Papers to be read by title, ICS 27th annual Meeting, Yokohama, Japan, 1997: 62–63.

25. Mørkved S, Bø K, Fjørtoft T. Is there any additional effect of adding biofeedback to pelvic floor muscle training? A single-blind randomized controlled trial. Obstet Gynecol 2002; 100 (4):730–739.

26. Dumoulin C, Lemieux M, Bourbonnais D, et al. Physiotherapy for persistent postnatal stress urinary incontinence: A randomized controlled trial. Obstet Gynecol 2004; 104:504–510.

27. Wilson PD, Samarrai TAL, Deakin M, et al. An objective assessment of physiotherapy for female genuine stress incontinence. Br J Obstet Gynaecol 1987; 94:575–582.

28. Goode PS, Burgio KL, Locher JL, et al. Effect of behavioral training with or without pelvic floor electrical stimulation on stress incontinence in women. JAMA 2003; 290(3):345–352.

29. Bouchard C, Shephard RJ, Stephens T. Physical activity, fitness, and health. International procedings and consensus statement. 1st ed. Champaign: Human Kinetics Publishers, 1994.

30. Bø K. Pelvic floor muscle exercise for the treatment of stress urinary incontinence. An exercise physiology perspective. Int Urogynecol J 1995; 6:282–291.

31. Schwartz G, Beatty J. Biofeedback: Theory and research. New York: Academic Press, 1977.

32. Prashar S, Simons A, Bryant C, et al. Attitudes to vaginal touching and device placement in women with urinary incontinence. Int Urogynecol J 2000; 11:4–8.

33. Pieber D, Zivkovic F, Tamussino K. Beckenbodengymnastik allein oder mit Vaginalkonen bei pramenopausalen Frauen mit milder und massiger Stressharninkontinenz. Gynecol Geburtshilfliche Rundsch 1994; 34:32–33.

34. Cammu H, Van Nylen M. Pelvic floor exercises versus vaginal weight cones in genuine stress incontinence. Eur J Obstet Gynecol Reprod Biol 1998; 77:89–93.

35. Laycock J, Brown J, Cusack C, et al. Pelvic floor reeducation for stress incontinence: Comparing three methods. Br J Commun Nurs 2001; 6(5):230–237.

36. Arvonen T, Fianu-Jonasson A, Tyni-Lenne R. Effectiveness of two conservative modes of physical therapy in women with urinary stress incontinence. Neurourol Urodyn 2001; 20:591–599.

37. Dudley GA, Harris RT. Use of electrical stimulation in strength and power training. In: Komi PV, ed. Strength and power in sport. Oxford: Blackwell Scientific Publications, 1992: 329–337.

38. Vuori I, Wilmore JH. Physical activity, fitness, and health: Status and determinants. In: Bouchard C, Shephard RJ, Stephens T, eds. Physical activity, fitness and health. Consensus statement. Champaign: Human Kinetics Publishers, 1993: 33–40.

39. Eriksen B, Eik-Nes SH. Long-term electrostimulation of the pelvic floor: Primary therapy in female stress incontinence? Urol Int 1989; 44:90–95.

40. Sand PK, Richardson DR, Staskin SE, et al. Pelvic floor stimulation in the treatment of genuine stress incontinence: A multicenter placebo-controlled trial. Am J Obstet Gynecol 1995; 173:72–79.

41. Yamanishi T, Yasuda K, Sakakibara R. Pelvic floor electrical stimulation in the treatment of stress incontinence: An investigational study and a placebo controlled double-blind trial. J Urol 1997; 158:2127–2131.

42. Luber KM, Wolde-Tsadik G. Efficacy of functional electrical stimulation in treating genuine stress incontinence: A randomized clinical trial. Neurourol Urodyn 1997; 16:543–551.

43. Brubaker L, Benson JT, Bent A, et al. Transvaginal electrical stimulation for female urinary incontinence. Am J Obstet Gynecol 1997; 177:536–540.

44. Laycock J, Jerwood D. Does pre-modulated interferential therapy cure genuine stress incontinence? Physiotherapy 1996; 79 (8):553–560.

45. Hahn I, Sommar S, Fall M. A comparative study of pelvic floor training and electrical stimulation for treatment of genuine female stress urinary incontinence. Neurourol Urodyn 1991; 10:545–554.

46. Smith JJ. Intravaginal stimulation randomized trial. J Urol 1996; 155:127–130.

47. Knight S, Laycock J, Naylor D. Evaluation of neuromuscular electrical stimulation in the treatment of genuine stress incontinence. Physiotherapy 1998; 84(2):61–71.

48. Bidmead J, Mantle J, Cardozo L, et al. Home electrical stimulation in addition to pelvic floor exercises. A useful adjunct or expensive distraction? Neurourol Urodyn 2002; 21(4):372–373

49. Bo K, Talseth T. Change in urethral pressure during voluntary pelvic floor muscle contraction and vaginal electrical stimulation. Int Urogyn J 1997; 8:3–7.

50. Lagro-Janssen A, Debruyne F, Smiths A, et al. The effects of treatment of urinary incontinence in general practice. Fam Pract 1992; 9(3):284–289.

51. Indrekvam S, Hunskaar S. Side-effects, feasability, and adherence to treatment during home-managed electrical stimulation for urinary incontinence: A Norwegian national cohort of 3198 women. Neurourol Urodyn 2002; 21:546–552.

52. Mantle J. Physiotherapy for incontinence. In: Cardozo L, Staskin D, eds. Textbook of female urology and urogynecology. London: Isis Medical Media, 2001: 351–358.

53. Kraemer J, Adams, K, Cafarelli E, et al. Progression models in resistance training for healthy adults. American College of Sport Medicine. Position Stand. Med Sci Sports Exerc 2002; 34(2):364–380.

54. Black NA, Downs SH. The effectiveness of surgery for stress incontinence in women: A systematic review. Br J Urol 1996; 78(497):510.

55. Klarskov P, Nielsen KK, Kromann-Andersen B, Maegaard E. Long-term results of pelvic floor training for female genuine stress incontinence. Int Urogynecol J 1991; 2:132–135.

56. Lagro-Janssen T, van Weel C. Long-term effect of treatment of female incontinence in general practice. Br J Gen Pract 1998; 48:1735–1738.

57. Bø K, Talseth T. Long term effect of pelvic floor muscle exercise five years after cessation of organized training. Obstet Gynecol 1996; 87 (2):261–265.

58. Cammu H, Van Nylen M, Amy J. A ten-year follow-up after Kegel pelvic floor muscle exercises for genuine stress incontinence. BJU Int 2000; 85:655–658.

59. Bø K, Kvarstein B, Nygaard I. Lower urinary tract symptoms and pelvic floor muscle exercise adherence after 15 years. Obstet Gynecol 2005, 105:999–1005.

60. Pollock ML, Gaesser GA, Butcher JD, et al. The recommeneded quantity and quality of exercise for developing and maintaining cardiorespiratory and muscular fitness, and flexibility in healthy adults. Med Sci Sports Exerc 1998; 30(6):975–991.

61. Bø K. Adherence to pelvic floor muscle exercise and long term effect on stress urinary incontinence. A five year follow up. Scand J Med Sci Sports 1995; 5:36–39.

62. Sampselle CM, Miller JM, Mims BL, et al. Effect of pelvic muscle exercise on transient incontinence during pregnancy and after birth. Obstet Gynecol 1998; 91(3):406–412.

63. Hughes P, Jackson S, Smith P, et al. Can antenatal pelvic floor exercises prevent postnatal incontinence. Neurourol Urodyn 2001; 20(4):447–448.

64. Reilly E, Freeman R, Waterfield M, et al. Prevention of postpartum stress incontinence in primigravidae with increased bladder neck mobility: A randomised controlled trial of antenatal pelvic floor exercises. BJOG 2002; 109:68–76.

65. Mørkved S, Bø K, Schei B, et al. Pelvic floor muscle training during pregnancy to prevent urinary incontinence: A single blind randomized controlled trial. Obstet Gynecol 2003; 101:313–319.

66. Sleep J, Grant A. Pelvic floor exercises in postnatal care. Midwifery 1987; 3:158–164.

67. Mørkved S, Bø K. The effect of postpartum pelvic floor muscle exercise in the prevention and treatment of urinary incontinence. Int Urogynecol J 1997; 8:217–222.

68. Meyer S, Hohlfield P, Achtari C, et al. Pelvic floor education after vaginal delivery. Obstet Gynecol 2001; 97:673–677.

69. Chiarelli P, Cockburn J. Promoting urinary continence in women after delivery: Randomised controlled tiral. BMJ 2002; (324):1241–1246.

70. Alewijnse D. Urinary incontinence in women. Long term outcome of pelvic floor muscle exercise therapy. Maastricht Health Research Institute for Prevention and Care/Department of Health Education and Health Promotion. Doctoral thesis, 2002.

71. Ramsey IN, Thou M. A randomized, double blind, placebo controlled trial of pelvic floor exercise in the treatment of genuine stress incontinence. Neurourol Urodyn 1990; 9(4):398–399.

72. Chiarelli P, Cockburn J. Promoting urinary continence in women after delivery: Randomised controlled trial. BMJ 2002, (324):1241.

73. Berghmans LCM, Frederiks CMA, deBie RA, et al. Efficacy of biofeedback, when included with pelvic floor muscle exercise treatment, for genuine stress incontinence. Neurourol Urodyn 1997; 15:37–52.

74. Paddison K. Complying with pelvic floor exercises: A literature review. Nurs Stand 2002; 16(39):33–38.

75. Sugaya K, Owan T, Hatano T, et al. 2003 Device to promote pelvic floor muscle training for stress incontinence. Int J Urol 10:416–422.

Chapter 8
Pharmacotherapy of Stress Urinary Incontinence

David Castro-Diaz and Sergio Fumero

Introduction

Stress urinary incontinence (SUI) is a very common condition that affects an average of 49% (24–75%) of incontinent women between 18 and 90 years of age [1]. SUI incontinence is much less common in men than in women by a 1:2 ratio, ranging from 2 to 39% with advancing age [2].

Although it is not a life-threatening condition, SUI may produce a considerable impact on female quality of life. Treatment of SUI is indicated if it begins to affect the sufferer's quality of life and if the symptom cannot be properly managed by an increase of voluntary micturition or reduction of physical activity. Possible therapies range from absorbent pads and pelvic floor muscles training (PFMT) to several drugs, devices, and surgical procedures. Various drugs, including estrogens, α-adrenoceptor agonists, β-adrenoceptor agonists, and tricyclic antidepressants have been used off label. With the advent of new targets and drugs with a different mechanism of action, pharmacological treatment of SUI is currently regaining interest.

There are several factors involved in the pathogenesis of SUI including the urethral support, the bladder neck function, and the function of the muscles of the urethra and pelvic floor [3]. As women with SUI have lower resting urethral pressures than age-matched continent women [4, 5], it appears likely that there is a reduced urethral closure pressure in most women with SUI. Consequently, it seems logical to increase urethral pressure in order to improve continence. Urethral closure is

the result of several contributing factors, including tone of urethral smooth and striated muscle and passive properties of the vasculature of urethral lamina propria. Although the relative contribution of each of these factors to intraurethral pressure is not fully understood, there is ample pharmacological evidence that a substantial part of urethral tone is mediated through stimulation of a-adrenoceptors in the urethral smooth muscle by release of norepinephrine. Lack of estrogens, mainly in elderly women, may be another contributing factor promoting a lack of mucosal function [6].

Pharmacotherapies for SUI aim to increase intraurethral closure forces by increasing tone in the urethral smooth and striated muscles. Several drugs may contribute to achievement of this goal, but limited efficacy or side effects often have limited their clinical use.

Hormonal Therapy

In postmenopausal women, hormone replacement therapy (HRT) is thought to increase the urethral closure pressure, to raise the sensory threshold of the bladder and urethra, and to increase the number of epithelial cells lining the bladder and urethra [7]. It also has been observed that estrogens increase the response to α-adrenoceptor agonists by increasing the number of α-adrenoceptors in an animal model [8, 9]. A symptomatic or clinical improvement has been observed in nonrandomized studies, but the actual role of HRT in the management of

SUI has not been established. There is a lack of well-designed, randomized placebo-controlled trials documenting a benefit of HRT therapy among women with SUI. In a recent analysis of 28 clinical trials including 2,926 women with SUI or urge urinary incontinence (UUI) using varying combination of estrogens, dosages, duration of treatments, and length of follow-up, little benefit of estrogens for SUI was found [10].

In the 4-year follow-up of the Heart and Estrogen/Progestin Replacement Study, 1,525 postmenopausal women were randomized to either daily oral estrogen plus progestogen therapy or placebo. Overall, daily doses of oral estrogen plus progestogen therapy were associated with worsening urinary incontinence. The authors suggested that the beneficial effect of estrogen-only is negated by the addition of progestogens to the regimen [11]. In addition, there is new evidence suggesting that long-term estrogen/progestogen increases the risk of stroke, heart attack, and ovarian cancer, making this therapeutic modality much less attractive [12]. At the International Consultation on Incontinence it was agreed to recommend estrogens as an optional therapy (grade of recommendation: C) as there was no evidence of good quality that showed a benefit for the treatment of SUI [6]. A recent multicenter double-blind, placebo-controlled, randomized clinical trial of menopausal hormone therapy, which included 27,347 women, showed that the use of estrogens alone or in combination with progestin was associated with an increased risk for urinary incontinence among continent women and worsening of characteristics of urinary incontinence among symptomatic women. The authors concluded that estrogens alone or in combination with progestin should not be prescribed for the prevention or relief of urinary incontinence [13]. In spite of their known effects on urethral pressure in the animal model and those trophic effects on the urethral epithelium, estrogens play little, if any, role in the treatment of SUI. Estrogen therapy may be more effective in improving irritative symptoms of urinary urgency, frequency, and urgency incontinence.

α-Adrenoceptor Agonists

α-Adrenoceptor agonists have been widely used for SUI treatment because they effectively increase bladder outlet resistance during bladder filling in animal models [14]. They have been found to be effective for SUI in both open-label and controlled clinical trials [15–17]. These drugs also have been used in combination with estrogens and conservative therapies such as pelvic floor exercises and electrical stimulation; nevertheless, there is a lack of long-term, randomized controlled clinical trials [18]. Phenylpropanolamine was withdrawn from the US market by the FDA because of the risk of hemorrhagic stroke in women [19]. Furthermore, α-adrenoceptor agonists lack exclusive selectivity for urethral α-adrenoceptors and may cause elevated blood pressure, sleep disturbances, nausea, dry mouth, headache, tremor, palpitations, and exacerbation of abnormal cardiac rhythms [20].

Midodrine is another a-adrenoceptor agonist prescribed mainly for orthostatic hypotension, which has been used for the treatment of SUI in some countries. However, in a randomized, double-blind, placebo-controlled multicenter study in 80 women with SUI, midodrine did not significantly improve urodynamic measures [21]. Methoxamine is a similar α-adrenoceptor agonist that was studied in a placebo-controlled crossover trial. No significant increases in maximum urethral pressure compared with placebo were observed. Furthermore, all patients experienced systemic adverse effects, including piloerection, headache, and cold extremities. The investigators suggested that the clinical usefulness of direct, peripherally acting selective α_1-adrenoceptor agonists in the treatment of SUI may be limited by adverse effects [22].

Ro 115–1240 is a new selective $\alpha_{1A/1L}$-adrenoceptor partial antagonist known to produce a maximal increase in urethral tension at doses that had no effect on blood pressure [23]. In a randomized, crossover study in women with SUI, Ro 115–1240 was associated with a significantly lower mean weekly number of SUI episodes than placebo (8.4 vs. 6.0: $P = 0.0079$), a 28% relative improvement over placebo. There also was a significantly lower mean number of pads used and wet pads changed/week with Ro 115–240 than with placebo ($P = 0.0055$ and 0.0066, respectively). Treatment-emergent adverse events were transient and mild to moderate in intensity. There were no cardiovascular effects or clinically significant changes in electrocardiograms or laboratory tests [24]. However, another phase II trial did not achieve the same level as seen in the earlier study; furthermore, studies on the rat showed some carcinogenic effects. For these reasons the manufacturing company decided to discontinue the development of this compound [25].

β-Adrenoceptor Antagonists

The theoretical basis for the use of β-adrenoceptor antagonists in the treatment of SUI is that blockade of urethral β-adrenoceptors may enhance the effects of norepinephrine on urethral β-adrenoceptors. Although it has been suggested that propranolol might promote some improvement in patients with SUI [26], there are no randomized controlled trials demonstrating such effect. In addition, although it has been suggested that the use of these compounds might be an alternative to a-adrenoceptor agonists in hypertensive patients with SUI, these agents have major potential cardiac and pulmonary side effects that limit their utility [6].

β-Adrenoceptor Agonists

β-Adrenoceptor agonists are indicated as bronchodilators in the treatment of asthma. It has been suggested that β_2-adrenoceptor agonists, such as clenbuterol, which initially was developed as a bronchodilator, may increase the contractility of the urethral striated sphincter by releasing acetylcholine at the neuromuscular junction [27]. In a placebo-controlled, double-blind trial, clenbuterol produced clinically significant improvement and an increase in mean maximal urethral closure pressure in 165 women with SUI [28]. Seventy-three percent of women in the clenbuterol arm showed significant improvement versus 55% of significant improvement in the placebo arm. In a 12-week randomized trial, clenbuterol was compared with pelvic floor exercises and a combination of both in 61 female patients with SUI [27]. The frequency of SUI episodes, the volume of each leakage, and the patient's own impression were the outcome variables. Clenbuterol alone improved incontinence in 76.9% of patients, pelvic floor exercises in 52.6%, and the combination of both therapies improved incontinence in 89.5% of patients. Adverse effects of clenbuterol included tremors, tachycardia, and headache. In spite of these promising results, to date, there have no been good studies documenting the effects of clenbuterol as a potential treatment for SUI. Consequently, there is a need of well-designed, randomized placebo-controlled trials in order to study the actual applicability of these agents for the treatment of SUI (level of evidence 2, grade of recommendation C) [6].

Tricyclic Antidepressants

Tricyclic antidepressants (TCA) are indicated for depressive disorders and have been reported to produce beneficial effects in patients with urinary incontinence. Imipramine is the main tricyclic antidepressant that has been used in the treatment of urinary incontinence, mainly in nocturnal enuresis in children but also in patients with SUI [29]. The mechanism of action is not fully understood. If adequately dosed, all TCA inhibit the reuptake of norepinephrine and serotonin into nerve endings. Moreover, some TCA such as imipramine have a marked anticholinergic action. At the urethral level, the effects on amine uptake can be expected to enhance the contractile effects of norepinephrine on smooth muscle, which also may influence the striated muscles in the urethra and pelvic floor by effects at the spinal cord level [20]. In an open-label study, Gilja et al. reported that imipramine produced subjective continence in 70% of patients and also increased the urethral closure pressure [30]. In a prospective study in 40 women with SUI, Lin et al. found that imipramine improved SUI in 60% of patients [31]. However, imipramine has not been studied in good-quality, randomized controlled clinical trials. Furthermore, imipramine has troublesome adverse effects including dry mouth, blurred vision, constipation, orthostatic hypotension, sedation, drowsiness, and heart rhythm abnormalities [32]. At the last International Consultation on Incontinence imipramine was considered to have level of evidence 3 (case-control studies, case series) and was granted a grade of recommendation D (evidence inadequate/conflicting) [6] (Table 8.1).

Serotonin and Norepinephrine Reuptake Inhibitors: Duloxetine

In the last decade, in vivo animal studies have demonstrated that serotonin and norepinephrine have a role in the neural control of the micturition

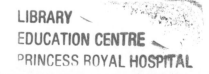

TABLE 8.1. Summary of characteristics and level of evidence of pharmacological agents prescribed off-label for stress urinary incontinence.

Pharmacological agents prescribed off-label for stress urinary incontinence
Hormone replacement therapy (HRT)
Thought to increase the urethral closure pressure
Thought to increase the response of α-adrenoreceptor agonists
Clinical improvement shown in nonrandomized studies
Lack of well-designed randomized studies showing efficacy
May increase the risk for urinary incontinence among symptomatic women
Level of evidence 2, grade of recommendation D
α-Adrenoceptor agonist
Found to be effective for SUI in both open-label and controlled clinical trials
Lack of long-term randomized controlled trials
Phenylpropanolamine withdrawn by the FDA because of risk of hemorrhagic stroke in women
Level of evidence 23, grade of recommendation C–D
β-Adrenoceptors agonists: Clenbuterol
Thought to increase urethral striated sphincter activity
Lack of well-designed randomized clinical trials
Level of evidence 2, grade of recommendation C
Tricyclic antidepressants
Mechanism of action not fully understood: marked systemic anticholinergic action and weak inhibition of reuptake of norepinephrine and serotonin at nerve ending
Physiologically/pharmacologically effective. Clinically widely used, but evidence from randomized studies is scarce
Know antiarrhythmic effect
Level of evidence 3, grade of recommendation D

cycle. Studies in the anesthetized cat model have demonstrated that serotonin 5-HT receptor agonists suppress parasympathetic activity and enhance sympathetic and somatic activity in the bladder. These effects promote urine storage by relaxing the bladder and increasing urethral resistance. Duloxetine hydrochloride is a balanced dual serotonin and norepinephrine reuptake inhibitor, which has affinity for binding to these neurotransmitters uptake sites. In an acetic acid-induced model of irritated bladder in the cat, duloxetine significantly increased bladder capacity and sphincteric muscle activity, presumably by acting at the central level via both motor and sensory afferent modulation [33]. These effects were not reproduced by a combination of two separate single reuptake inhibitors [34]. Duloxetine is believed to affect SUI by blocking the reuptake of serotonin and norepinephrine and causing accumulation of serotonin and norepinephrine at the synapses in Onuf's nucleus, an area in the sacral spinal cord that has a high density of 5-HT and norepinephrine receptors. Pudendal motor neurons located in Onuf's nucleus regulate the urethral striated muscle sphincter. Serotonin and norepinephrine stimulate these neurons, increasing the strength of urethral sphincter contractions [32–36] (Fig. 8.1). Phase I safety studies showed that duloxetine is well tolerated in healthy volunteers [18]. In a phase II dose-finding clinical trial conducted in 48 centers in the United States, duloxetine was associated with a significant reduction in SUI episodes. Five hundred thirty-three women aged 18–65 years, with at least four incontinence episodes per week, were randomized to 12 weeks of treatment with placebo or duloxetine at one of three doses (20, 40, or 80 mg/day). Duloxetine was associated with significant dose-dependent decreases in incontinence episode frequency (IEF). This decrease paralleled improvements in the Patient Global Impression of Improvement (PGI-I) scale and the Incontinence Quality of Life (I-QOL) questionnaire. The median IEF decrease with placebo was 41% compared with 54% for duloxetine 20 mg/day ($P = 0.06$), 59% for duloxetine 40 mg ($P = 0.002$), and 64% for duloxetine 80 mg/day ($P < 0.001$) [37]. Duloxetine was well tolerated and no adverse events were considered to be clinically severe. Discontinuation rates due to adverse events were 5% for placebo and 9, 12, and 15% for duloxetine 20, 40, and 80 mg/day, respectively ($P = 0.04$).

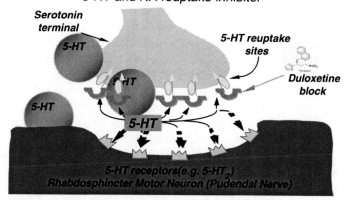

Duloxetine : a balanced dual
5-HT and NA reuptake inhibitor

Duloxetine is a balanced dual 5-HT and NA neuronal reuptake inhibitor
Duloxetine blocks the reuptake of 5-HT and NA and causes accumulation of 5-HT and NA
at the synapses in Onuf's nucleus. This facilitates pudendal nerve activity and increases
rhabdosphincter contraction during the storage phase of the micturition cycle

FIG. 8.1.

Nausea was the most common symptom that led to discontinuation. According to these data, duloxetine 80 mg/day (40 mg twice daily) was determined to be the optimum dose in women with SUI [38]. In a phase III clinical study conducted in North America, which included 683 women aged 22–84 years with a weekly IEF of at least 7, duloxetine was associated with a significant decrease in IEF (median decrease 50% vs. 27%, $P < 0.001$) and improvement in the I-QOL scores (+11 vs. + 6.8, $P < 0.001$). Improvements in IEF were associated with significant increases in voiding intervals compared with placebo. At the end of the study period 10.5% of duloxetine-treated patients and 5.9% of placebo-treated patients had no incontinence episodes ($P < 0.05$). In a subgroup of 436 patients with severe SUI a similar significant improvement in both IEF and I-QOL was observed. The PGI-I results showed that 62% of duloxetine-treated patients had a better bladder condition compared with 39.6% in the placebo group. Furthermore, the I-QOL showed significant improvements compared with placebo in the three domains of avoidance and limiting behavior, social embarrassment, and psychosocial impact [38]. The effects of duloxetine were confirmed in a simultaneous phase III, placebo-controlled trial conducted in several centers in Europe and Canada. Compared with placebo, duloxetine-treated patients showed a significant decrease in IEF (median decrease of 50% vs. 29%, $P = 0.002$) with comparable significant improvements in those subjects with more severe incontinence. A total of 52% of women taking duloxetine experienced a 50–100% reduction in IEF compared with 34% of women taking placebo ($P < 0.001$). A significant improvement in the I-QOL was observed as well (7.3 in duloxetine group vs. 4.3 in the placebo group) [39]. In another randomized, double-blind, placebo-controlled clinical trial conducted in several geographic regions including Argentina, Australia, Brazil, Finland, Poland, South Africa, and Spain, 458 incontinent women were assigned to duloxetine 40 mg twice daily (227) or placebo (231) for 12 weeks. A significantly greater median decrease in IEF was observed with duloxetine (54%) compared with placebo (40%), and comparable significant improvement in quality of life (I-QOL score increases of 10.3 vs. 6.4, $P = 0.007$). Improvements with duloxetine were associated with significantly greater increases in voiding intervals than with placebo (20.4 vs. 8.5 min, $P < 0.001$). In this study the placebo responses were higher than those reported in the North American and European phase III studies, which is thought to be related to a higher number of patients being naïve for incontinence management [40].

In a randomized clinical trial conducted in women awaiting surgery for SUI it was observed that at the conclusion of the study 20% of duloxetine-treated women were no longer interested in surgery compared with 0 of 45 placebo-treated women [41]. Most common (>5%) treatment-emergent adverse events observed in active treatment arms in clinical trials with duloxetine include nausea, fatigue, insomnia, dry mouth, constipation, dizziness. and headache, with nausea being the most common adverse event (23–28%) and the most common reason for discontinuation (5.7%) [37–41]. Nausea tended to be mild-to-moderate, transient (lasting 1 week to 1 month), and not progressive [38–40]. In a recent double-blind placebo-controlled study assessing the impact of duloxetine dose escalation on tolerability and efficacy in the treatment of SUI, it was found that starting duloxetine at 20 mg bid for 2 weeks before increasing to 40 mg bid significantly improved tolerability but did not impact duloxetine efficacy after all subjects had been on 40 mg bid for at least 2 weeks [42]. Consequently, dose escalation seems to be an appropriate way of reducing the risk of nausea in patients starting with duloxetine.

Duloxetine has not been associated with cardiovascular side effects in short-term clinical trials. Data from a long-term study in patients with depression indicate that after 1 year of use, duloxetine was not associated with sustained elevations in blood pressure and did not prolong corrected QT intervals. Duloxetine significantly increased heart rate around two beats per minute compared with placebo [43].

Duloxetine also has been studied in association with pelvic floor muscle exercises. In a randomized, controlled clinical trial of duloxetine alone, PFMT alone, combined treatment, and no active treatment of women with SUI, it was found that combination therapy of duloxetine and PFMT was more efficacious in reducing urinary incontinence episodes than either one alone. Combined therapy also showed an improvement of quality of life [44].

Duloxetine has been found to be useful in the treatment of women with symptoms of mixed urinary incontinence (MUI). A recent multicenter, multinational trial compared the efficacy and safety of duloxetine and placebo in women with symptoms of MUI. Overall, IEF decreases were significantly greater with duloxetine than placebo (mean change of 7.30 vs. 5.65 IEF/week, $P < 0.05$, median percent change 60 vs. 47%, $P < 0.001$). Significant benefits also were demonstrated with duloxetine compared with placebo for changes in

I-QOL, ICIQ-SF, score as well as for PGI-I ratings ($P = 0.001$) [45].

Duloxetine also has been studied in women with overactive bladder. In a recent double-blind, placebo-controlled study 306 women with symptoms of overactive bladder and evidence of absence of SUI were randomly assigned to placebo or duloxetine. Patients randomized to duloxetine demonstrated significant improvements compared with patients randomized to placebo for decreases in micturition and incontinence episodes and quality of life, indicating that this drug may be an alternative to antimuscarinics in the treatment of overactive bladder [46].

In healthy volunteers coadministration of duloxetine and tolterodine was well tolerated and demonstrated no significant safety findings in the studied population [47]. Age did not influence pharmacokinetics of elderly healthy volunteers [48].

The impact of demographic characteristics and comorbidities on efficacy of duloxetine has been studied recently using an integrated database including data from four large randomized controlled trials. Several subgroups were studied with regard to ethnicity, age, body mass index (BMI), chronic lung disease, hypoestrogenism, diabetes mellitus, and depression. It was observed that the reduction in IEF was minimal and not significantly different between duloxetine and placebo in women with chronic lung disease, while no differences with regard to the rest of the subgroups. Interestingly, the improvement in quality of life was higher in the subgroups of patients with higher BMI. With regard to age, reductions in IEF and increases in I-QOL were more pronounced in women younger than 65 years of age, suggesting that older women may be less likely to respond to treatment directed at the striated sphincter [49].

Duloxetine is licensed at 40 mg twice daily for the treatment of SUI in the European Union, Canada, and some South-American countries but not in the United States. However, duloxetine has been licensed for depression and for diabetic polyneuropathic pain in the European Union and in the United States. There have been some reports by the FDA of increased suicidal ideation in adults with depression who are taking antidepressants, but none has been reported in clinical trials on urinary incontinence. Communications with the US FDA's Division of Reproductive and Urologic Drug Products (DRUDP) led the sponsoring companies to conclude in January 2005 that DRUDP was not prepared to grant approval for duloxetine for the treatment of the SUI population based on the data package submitted. This led to the withdrawal of the New Drug Application in January 2005. The sponsoring companies believe that the current overall benefit/risk evaluation by DRUDP includes considerations regarding all three elements of the benefit/risk equation: (1) the perceived severity and impact of SUI as a medical condition, (2) the magnitude of the drug's benefit in the SUI patient population, and (3) the safety profile as it applies to the SUI patient population [50].

In any case, duloxetine, being the only proven medical therapy for SUI, is being used in many Europeans countries. According to very preliminary data, indications for its use are at present being extended to males with SUI [51], although definitive conclusions with regard to its use in males can be obtained only if formal evaluation is conducted with adequate placebo control and standardized follow-up [52] (Tables 8.2 and 8.3).

TABLE 8.2. Summarary of mechanism of action, indications, and level of evidence of duloxetine.

Serotonin and norepinephrine reuptake inhibitors: duloxetine
Duloxetine blocks the reuptake of serotonin and norepinephrine at the synapses in Onuf's nucleus, stimulating pudendal neurons increasing the strength of urethral sphincter contractions
Demonstrated efficacy in high quality double-blind placebo controlled trials. Level of evidence 1, grade of recommendation A
Nausea is the most common side effect. Tolerability can be improved with dose escalation starting with 20 mg 2 weeks before increasing to 40 mg bid
Duloxetine has proven efficacy in patients with symptoms of mixed urinary incontinence and overactive bladder
Not FDA approved in the United States

TABLE 8.3. Summarary of efficacy and safety issues of drugs used for stress urinary incontinence.

Class	Drug	Efficacy	Safety issues
Estrogen replacement	Estrogens/progestogens	Overall subjective improvement No significant objective effect	Breast and ovarian cancer Stroke, heart attack
β-Adrenoceptor agonists	Ephedrine, phenypropanolamine, phenylpropanolamine pseudoephedtrine, midodrine, methoxamine, norfenefrine	Stimulated urethral smooth muscle contraction; efficacy demonstrated in	Hypertension, sleep disturbances dry mouth, headache, tremor, palpitations, tachycardia
β-Adrenoceptor agonists	Clenbuterol	It is thought to increase contractility of urethral striated sphincter	Tremors
			Tachycardia Headache
β-Adrenoceptor antagonists	Propanolol	Thought to increase contractility of urethral smooth muscle; no controlled studies	Orthostatic hypotension
			Cardiac decompensation
Tricyclic antidepressants	Imipramine	No controlled studies	Anticholinergic symptoms Orthostatic hypotension Cardiac arrhythmia Weight gain
Serotonin and norepinephrine reuptake inhibitors	Duloxetine	Increased bladder capacity, decreased incontinence episodes, and improved quality of life	Nausea, dry mouth, insomnia, constipation, dizziness

Conclusion

Although the female lower urinary tract is under hormonal influences, hormonal therapy for SUI has not proved to be efficacious. α-Adrenergic agonists may increase urethral resistance by modifying urethral pressure, but there is not a current acceptable agent to be used for the treatment of SUI.

Duloxetine has proved to be efficacious in reducing the frequency of incontinence episodes. More than 50% of duloxetine-treated patients experience an improvement higher than 50%. Nausea is the most common side effect. Dose escalation seems to improve tolerability without any impact on efficacy. Combination of PFMT and duloxetine is more efficacious in reducing urinary incontinence episodes than either one alone.

References

1. Hunskaar S, Burgio K, Diokno, et al. Epidemiology and natural history of urinary incontinence. In Abrams P, Cardozo L, Khoury S, et al., eds. Incontinence. Plymouth, UK: Health Publication Ltd. 2002:165–201.

2. Hunskaar S, Burgio K, Clark A, et al. Epidemiology of urinary (UI) and faecal (FI) incontinence and pelvic organ prolapse. In: Abrams P, Cardozo L, Khoury S, Wein A eds. Incontinence, Vol. I: Basics and evaluation. Plymouth, UK: Health Publication Ltd. 2005: 255–312.

3. DeLancey JOL. The pathophysiology of stress urinary incontinence in women and its implications for surgical treatment. World J Urol 1997; 15(5):268–274.

4. Henriksson L, Anderson. K-E, Ulmsten U. The urethral pressure profiles in continent and stress incontinent women. Scand J Urol Nephrol 1979; 13(1):5–10.

5. Hilton P, Stanton SL. Urethral pressure measurement by microtransducer: The results in symptom-free women and in those with genuine stress incontinence. Br J Obstet Gynaecol 1983; 90(10):919–933.

6. Anderson KE, Appell R, Caardozo L, et al. Pharmacological treatment of urinary incontinence. In: Abrams P, Cardozo L, Khoury S, Wein A, eds. Incontinence: 3rd International Consultation on Incontinence. Plymouth, UK: Health publication Ltd. 2005: 809–854.

7. Versi E, Cardozo L. Estrogens and the lower urinary tract function. London: Blackwell Scientific, 1988.

8. Hodson BJ, Dumas S, Bolling DR, et al. Effect of estrogen on sensitivity of rabbit bladder and urethra to phenylephrine. Invest Urol 1978; 16 (1):67–69.

9. Larsson B, Andersson KJ, Batra S, et al. Effect of estradiol on norepinephrine-induced contraction, alpha adrenorecptor number and norepinephrine content in the female rabbit uretra. J Pharmacol Exp Ther 1984; 229:557–563.

10. Moehrer B, Hextall A, Jackson S. Oestrogens for urinary incontinence in women (Cochrane Review). In: The Cochrane Library, Issue 4. Chichester, UK: Wiley, 2003.

11. Grady D, Brown JS, Vittinghoff E, et al. Postmenopausal hormones and incontinence: The Heart and Estrogen/Progestin Replacement Study. Obstet Gynecol 2001; 97(1):116–120.

12. Al-Badr A. Ross A, Soroka D, et al. What is the available evidence for hormone replacement therapy in women stress urinary incontinence. J Obstet Gynecol Can 2003; 25(7):567–574.

13. Hendrix SL, Cochrane BB, Nygaard IE, et al. Effects of estrogen with and without progestin on urinary incontinence. JAMA 2005; 293(8):998–1001.

14. Brune ME, O'Neill AB, Gauvin DM, et al. Comparison of alpha 1-adrenoceptor agonists in canine urethral pressure profilometry and abdominal leak point pressure models. J Urol 2001; 166(4):1555–1559.

15. Diokno AC, Taub M. Ephedrine in treatment of urinary incontinence. Urology 1975; 5(5):624–625.

16. Collste L, Lindskog M. Phenylpropanolamine in treatment of female stress urinary incontinence: Double-blind placebo controlled study in 24 patients. Urology 1987; 30(4):398–403.

17. Siltberg H, Larsson G, Hallen B, et al. Validation of cough-induced leak point pressure measurement in the evaluation of pharmacological treatment of stress incontinence. Neurourol Urodyn 1999; 18(6):591–602.

18. Zinner NR, Koke SC, Viktrup L. Pharmacotherapy for stress urinary incontinence. Present and future options. Drugs 2004;64(14):1503–1516.

19. Fleming G. The FDA regulation and the risk of stroke. N Engl J Med 2000; 343(25):1886–1887.

20. Anderson KW, Appell R, Awad S, et al. Pharmacological treatment of urinary incontinence. In: Abrams P, Khoury S, Wein A eds. Incontinence. Plymouth, UK: Health Publications Ltd.2002: 418–511.

21. Weil EH, Eerdmans PH, Dijkman GA, et al. Randomized double-blind placebo-controlled multicenter evaluation of efficacy and dose finding of midodrine hydrochloride in women with mild to moderate stress urinary incontinence: A phase II study. Int Urogynecol J Pelvic Floor Dysfunct 1998; 9(3):145–150.

22. Radley SC, Chapple CR, Bryan NP, et al. Effect of methoxamine on maximum urethral pressure

in women with genuine stress incontinence: A placebo-controlled, double-blind crossover study. Neurourol Urodyn 2001; 20(1):43–52.

23. Blue DR. Pharmacological characteristics of Ro 115–1240, a selective a1A/1L-adrenoceptor partial agonist: A potential therapy for stress urinary incontinence. BJU Int 2003; 93:164–172.

24. Musselman DM, Ford APDW, Gennevois DJ, et al. A randomized crossover study to evaluate Ro 115–1240, a selective a1A/1L-adrenoceptor partial agonist in women with stress urinary incontinence. BJU Int. 2004; 93(1):78–83).

25. Script. World Pharmaceutical News. April 28th, 2004. No. 2947.

26. Kaisary AV. Beta adrenoceptor blockade in the treatment of female urinary stress incontinence. J Urol (Paris) 1984; 90(5):351–353.

27. Ishiko O, Ushiroyama T, Saji F, et al. Beta2-adrenergic agonists and pelvic floor exercises for female stress incontinence. Int J Gynaecol Obstet 2000; 71(1):39–44.

28. Yasuda K, Kawabe K, Takimoto Y, et al. A double-blind clinical trial of a beta2-adrenergic agonist in stress incontinence. Int Urogynecol J 1993; 4:146–151.

29. Hunsballe JM, Djurhuus JC. Clinical options for imipramine in the management of urinary incontinence. Urol Res 2001; 29(2):118–125.

30. Gilja I, Radej M, Kovacic M, et al. Conservative treatment of female stress incontinence with imipramine. J Urol 1984; 132(5):909–911.

31. Lin HH, Sheu BC, Lo MC, et al. Comparison of treatment outcomes for imipramine for female genuine stress incontinence. Br J Obstet Gynaecol 1999; 106(10):1089–1092.

32. Frazer A. Pharmacology of antidepressants. J Clin Psychopharmacol 1997; 17(Suppl 1):2s–18s.

33. Thor KB, Katofiasc MA. Effects of duloxetine, a combined serotonin and norepinephrine reuptake inhibitor, on central neural control of lower urinary tract function in the chloralose-anesthesized female cat. J Pharmacol Exp Ther 1995; 274:1014–1024.

34. Katofiasc MA, Nissen J, Audia JE, Thor KB. Comparison of the effects of serotonin selective, norpepinephrine selective, and dual serotonin and norpepinephrine reuptake inhibitors on lower urinary tract function in cats. Life Sci 2002; 71:1227–1236.

35. Bymaster FP, Dresfield-Ahmad LJ, Threlkeld PG, et al. Comparative affinity of duloxetine and venlafaxine for serotonin and norpepinephrine transporters in vitro and in vivo, human serotonin receptor subtypes, and other neuronal receptors. Neuropsychopharmacology 2001; 25(6):871–880.

36. Michel MC, Oelke M, Duloxetine in the treatment of stress urinary incontinence. Women's Health 2005; 1(3):345–358.

37. Norton PA, Zinner NR, Yalcin I, Bump RC. Duloxetine versus placebo in the treatment of stress urinary incontinence. Am J Obstet Gynecol 2002; 187(1):40–48.

38. Dmochowski RR, Miklos JR, Norton PA, et al. Duloxetine versus placebo for the treatment of non-American women with stress urinary incontinence. J Urol 2003; 170:1259–1263.

39. van Kerrebroeck, Abrams P, Lange R, et al. Duloxetine vs. placebo in the treatment of European and Canadian women with stress urinary incontinence. BJOG 2004; 11:249–257.

40. Millard RJ, Moore K, Rencken R, et al. for the Duloxetine Study Group. Duloxetine vs. placebo in the treatment of stress urinary incontinence: A four-continent randomized clinical trial. BJUI 2004; 93:3111–318.

41. Cardozo L, Drutz HP, Baygani SK, Bump RC. Pharmacological treatment of women awaiting surgery for stress urinary incontinence. Obstet Gynecol. 2004; 104(3):511–519.

42. Castro-Diaz D, Palma PC, Bouchard C, et al. Effect of dose escalation on the tolerability and efficacy of duloxetine in the treatment of women with stress urinary incontinence. Int Urogynecol J Pelvic Floor Disfunct 2007; 18:919–929.

43. Mallinckrodt C, Goldstein DJ, Detke MJ, et al. Duloxetine: A long term treatment for the emotional and physical symptoms of depression. Primary Care Companion J Clin Psych 2003:5:19–28.

44. Ghoniem GM, Van Leeuwen JS, Elser DM, et al. A randomized controlled trial of duloxetine alone, pelvic floor muscle training alone, combined treatment and no active treatment in women with stress urinary incontinence. J Urol 2005;173(5):1647–1653.

45. Bump RC, Bent AE, Gousse AE, et al. Duloxetine treatment of women with mixed urinary incontinence (MUI). (IUGA) [abstract No. 31]. Int Urogynecol J 2006; 17(Suppl 2):S57–S100.

46. Bump R, Steers W, Herschorn S, et al. Duloxetine compared with placebo for the treatment of women with symptoms of bladder overactivity. International Continence Society, 36th Annual Meeting. Abstract No. 127.

47. Hua TC, Pan A, Chan C, et al. Effect of duloxetine on tolterodine pharmacokinetics in healthy volunteers. BJ Clin Pharm 57(5):652.

48. Skinner MH, Kuan HY, Skerjanec A, et al. Effect of age on the pharmacokinetics of duloxetine in women. BJ Clin Pharm 2004; 57(1):54.

49. Viktrup L, Yalcin I. Duloxetine treatment of stress urinary incontinence in women: Effects of demographics, obesity, chronic lung disease, hypoestrogenism, diabetes mellitus and depression on efficacy. Eur J Obstet Gynecol Reprod Biol. 2007; 133:105–113.

50. Castro-Diaz D, Pascual MA. Pharmacotherapy for stress urinary incontinence. Curr Opin Urol 2005; 15(4):227–230.

51. Schlenker B, Gratzke C, Reich O, et al. Preliminary results of the off-label use of duloxetine for the treatment of stress incontinence after radical prostatectomy or cystectomy. Eur Urol 2006; 49:1075–1078.

52. Chapple CR. Duloxetine for male stress incontinence. Eur Urol 2006; 49:958–960.

Chapter 9
Radio Frequency Therapy for the Treatment of Female Stress Urinary Incontinence

Roger R. Dmochowski and Emily Cole

Introduction

The demographics of stress incontinence suggest that a significant percentage of the female population is affected by this condition and that the number of women who report discomfort due to stress incontinence is increasing [1–4]. Stress incontinence is associated with quality of life aberrations that, while often managed by changes in physical activity, lead to treatment-seeking behavior on the part of the sufferer in order to regain normal physical function. Cure of stress incontinence is the ultimate goal of any intervention aimed at this symptom; however, complete symptom resolution often is not attained with therapy. Yet, it is now becoming evident from evolving outcomes analysis research that symptom improvement, when attained after intervention, is viewed as a significant and positive aspect of intervention, even if absolute cure is not obtained [5]. When compared to the well-defined prevalence of stress incontinence, the actual number of surgical procedures (colposuspensions and slings) performed for this condition reveal a significant disparity in absolute numbers of women who actually undergo surgical intervention. This numeric difference implies that women may be reluctant to undergo operative interventions due to concerns about morbidity, recovery times, or other perceived risk/lifestyle issues [2, 6, 7].

Nonsurgical modalities, despite the associated noninvasive nature of these options, are plagued by durability and efficacy concerns [8, 9].

Radio frequency (RF) energy application to the endopelvic fascia has been proposed recently as an option for the treatment of women with less bothersome stress incontinence as a less invasive, initial surgical procedure. RF tissue remodeling has been used for other indications such as fecal incontinence [10] and gastroesophageal reflux disease [11] in which luminal contents pass through a poorly functional anatomic and/or physiological barrier. The goal of the RF energy procedure is to correct the laxity and elasticity of the fascial "hammock" that underlies the proximal urethra and bladder neck and which is thought to contribute to anatomic stress incontinence [12] by creating thermally induced tissue shrinkage and contraction [13]. Focal RF application produces heating of the endopelvic fascia, which denatures collagen fibers, resulting in acute contraction (shrinkage) of the target area and which then results in a chronic fibrotic response [14]. Within 4–6 weeks, collagen ingrowth and fibrosis further shrink and stabilize the endopelvic fascia. These dynamic tissue changes result in a decreased compliance to intra-abdominal pressure increases and produce stabilization of the position of the bladder neck [15]. The theory of RF effect subsequently will be reviewed in light of clinical experience.

Theory of Radio Frequency Tissue Interaction and Treatment of the Endopelvic Fascia for the Treatment of Stress Urinary Incontinence

Several factors are thought to contribute to the pathophysiology of stress urinary incontinence in women: (1) damage or loss of the intrinsic closure mechanism ("seal") of the proximal urethra; (2) loss of active and passive support of the urethra from tissue stretching and loss of stability; and (3) disruption of the neurological control of the pelvic floor and urethra [12, 16–18]. Loss of urethral support results in urethral hypermobility, which contributes to poor urethral compression during periods of increased abdominal pressure and produces urinary incontinence [19–21]. Endopelvic support defects may be compounded by urethral displacement, which results in the unequal distribution of intra-abdominal pressure changes, further compounding urinary loss due to unequal pressure transmission to the bladder and urethra.

It has been hypothesized that RF application to the collagen-rich endopelvic fascia would produce collagenous ultrastructural changes mimicking a "tightening" or contraction of the fascia, which then would stabilize the tissue during increased abdominal pressure events. The ultimate goal would approximate a resuspension of the proximal urethral mechanism. Based on surgical experiences from other specialties, this technology also was envisioned as being accomplished with minimally invasive techniques with minimal morbidity. Ideally, a method to perform this intervention without an incision would provide the optimal form of intervention delivery.

Thermally induced contraction of collagen is dependent on several unique characteristics of the collagen molecule. Collagen exists in vivo as a fibrillar structure that has a triple helix configuration. The helical configuration is maintained by cross-linking hydrogen bonds, which are unstable when subjected to heat. The fibrillar structure is maintained by thermally stable bonds, and therefore is more resistant to deformation when subjected to thermal stress. Thermal energy in the range of 60–80°C will cause unwinding of the helix, due to disruption of the intramolecular cross-links, yet the heat-stable fibrillar structure remains intact. The overall effect is shrinkage of the molecule along the longitudinal axis associated with distortion (swelling) of the individual fibrils [13].

RF energy has been used clinically to achieve tissue shrinkage via collagen denaturation for numerous indications including ophthalmologic, orthopedic, and dermatologic [13, 22–25]. RF energy is imparted to the tissue via direct application (contact) to the target area using electrodes. During this energy application, tissue heating ensues due in large part to tissue resistance to the flow of the RF energy. A three-dimensional thermal effect is created as heat spreads from areas of high to low temperature. Overall thermal effects vary according to the electrode configuration, the actual amount of RF energy delivered, and inherent tissue resistance that may be affected by intrinsic as well external factors (such as excess free fluid in the energy delivery area).

Several basic and clinical studies have substantiated the theoretic effect of RF energy-induced collagenous changes. While evaluating the use of monopolar RF energy to treat bovine joint capsular tissue in vivo, Hecht et al. noted that the application of RF energy produced acute tissue inflammatory reaction with associated degradation of collagen. Subsequently, new collagen developed over a 12-week period, which produced a remodeling of the articular capsular tissue. They noted that the primary treatment effect was collagen denaturation produced by the thermal application with attendant tissue shrinkage (loss of three-dimensional volume). These effects were noted to maximally occur at 60–80°C. Histological evaluation of the treated tissue demonstrated that the thermal effects were very localized to the specific area of energy application with little or no changes being seen beyond the area of thermal effect (7–10 mm). At 3 months posttreatment, further histological study showed fibroblast proliferation and capillary ingrowth producing complete tissue healing [13]. Other types of dense collagenous structures also have been studied to assess RF thermal effects. Fresh bovine heart tendons were mounted in a tension-free device, RF energy was imparted to the tissue, and tissue volume changes (degree of shrinkage) were measured as a function of time and temperature variables associated with thermal delivery [26]. Threshold values for time and temperature were noted to be required for maximal tissue shrinkage (volume loss) to occur. Interestingly, the optimal temperature to effect near-maximal shrinkage when applied for a minimum of 30 s was 70°C. Less effective shrinkage was noted to occur with temperatures below 70°C. This finding was found to be independent of the duration of energy delivery.

Given these reproducible effects, RF energy delivery was evaluated for potential salubrious effects in the treatment of stress incontinence in women. It was postulated that thermal energy application to the endopelvic fascia could produce a "resuspension" of the proximal urethra, decreasing hypermobility and reducing or curing urinary incontinence. Clinical studies were undertaken to assess this effect.

Technique

The first commercially available RF bladder neck suspension procedure was known as the SURx transvaginal system (SURx System, Cooper Surgical, Inc. Trumbull, CT). The device is composed of an applicator and a RF generator (see Fig. 9.1). The generator produces bipolar radio frequency, while monitoring tissue temperature and resistance. The sterile, single-use applicator is composed of a handle, with a triggering mechanism and a 270°-rotational tip with microbipolar electrodes and a saline drip at the distal end of the probe. Accurate monitoring of treatment tissue temperatures is performed by a thermistor that is located in the applicator tip between the electrodes.

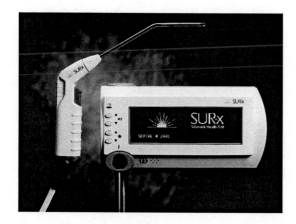

FIG. 9.1. External applicator and radiofrequency generator

The RF procedure may be performed either laparoscopically or transvaginally, with thermal energy being applied to the endopelvic fascia at least 1 cm lateral to the midurethra on each side of midline. RF energy produces a similar treatment effect when applied either to the superior or inferior surface of the endopelvic fascia depending on the surgical approach.

Patients considered to be candidates for the RF procedure as performed by the SURx system should be evaluated carefully prior to surgery with a history and physical (demonstrating proximal urethral hypermobility of greater than 30° associated with objective urinary incontinence associated with either Valsalva's effort or cough), voiding diary, and urodynamics when indicated. Transvaginal RF procedures may be performed in the ambulatory setting using either general or regional anesthesia. The thermal energy delivered by this procedure makes local anesthesia difficult, although the combination of sedation and local techniques may be feasible.

For the transvaginal approach, the patient is placed in the dorsal lithotomy position and the bladder is drained with a Foley catheter. The catheter is left in place and the balloon inflated for purposes of anatomic identification of the proximal urethra and bladder neck junction. A full thickness vaginal incision approximately 2–3 cm is created 1 cm lateral to the urethra at the level mid- and proximal urethra. Hydrodissection of the vaginal wall may be done prior to the incision using either 20 U vasopressin in 50 ml injectable saline or epinephrine at a 1:200,000 dilution in injectable saline to minimize mucosal bleeding. After the incision is performed, the vaginal mucosa is dissected away from the underlying endopelvic fascia laterally toward the ischium so as to expose a 1.5 cm × 2 cm area of the inferior aspect of the endopelvic fascia. The endopelvic fascia should not be disrupted during the dissection. Hemostasis is critical, as excess fluid (whether blood, serum, or remnant hydrodissection fluid) acts as a heat-dissipating interface and circumvents adequate thermal delivery to the underlying tissue.

After completion of the mucosal dissection, the applicator tip is placed in contact with the underlying endopelvic fascia avoiding excess pressure (the probe should simply touch the fascia). RF delivery parameters include: minimum of 70°C to the target tissue, a minimum of 30 s of application time, and an absence of excess fluid in the operative area. During RF application, a visual blanching of the fascia occurs which is associated with tissue volume loss (shrinkage). Tissue charring is to be avoided as this effect also dissipates thermal delivery. Power delivered by the RF system approximates 15 W with the bipolar probe. The RF probe is applied to the fascia with a slow, sweeping manner parallel to the urethra, making sure to remain 1 cm lateral to the urethra at all times. The entire exposed fascial surface should be treated with this technique. During thermal application, continuous monitoring of tissue temperature and tissue impedance is accomplished by the RF generator via the thermistor in the probe tip. When optimal resistance parameters are obtained, an aural tone is delivered by the generator indicating attainment of optimal parameters. The same technique then is accomplished on the contralateral side.

After the completion of RF application, the incisions are closed with delayed resorbable suture such a polydioxanone. A vaginal packing is placed for 2–4 h, after which packing and catheter are removed. Activity constraints include avoidance of intercourse for 6 weeks and lifting limitations of 5 pounds for a similar period.

The laparoscopic RF technique is similar. After insertion of laparoscopic ports (per surgeon preference for optimal visualization of the pelvis), dissection exposes the intrapelvic aspect of the endopelvic fascia. RF treatment is delivered to the superior aspect of the endopelvic fascia so as to remain 1 cm lateral to the urethra, which can be confirmed by ascertaining the location of the urethral catheter. Similar heat intensity and tissue impedance criteria are used for this approach.

Therapeutic Results

Two prospective FDA investigational device (IDE) approved clinical trials have been completed to demonstrate the therapeutic index of the RF procedure [27, 28]. A total of 214 patients with stress urinary incontinence were enrolled at 16 US study sites. Of this group, 94 (44%) were treated with a laparoscopic approach and an additional 120 (56%) underwent the transvaginal technique. Acute and chronic safety and clinical efficacy at 6-month follow-up was assessed in both treatment groups. All patients were primary incontinence patients (had received no prior surgical intervention for stress incontinence), without grade III or IV anterior vaginal wall prolapse or other vaginal support defects. Urodynamics were performed to exclude detrusor overactivity and to assess other vesical storage parameters. Prohibited medications included antidepressants, a-adrenergics, and anticholinergics. Per protocol, all women had had previous unsuccessful outcomes after at least 3 months of conservative, noninvasive pelvic floor therapies such as Kegel exercises or electrical stimulation. Parameters for efficacy included number of incontinence pads used and change in daily incontinence episodes. Additionally, Valsalva effort also was assessed for all patients with physical examination and urodynamics. Also, quality of life was assessed at baseline and at completion of follow-up.

Efficacy was defined as cured, improved, or failed. "Cure" was defined as a negative Valsalva on physical examination and "improved" was defined as decreased daily incontinence episodes or pad use. Results are shown in Table 9.1. No reported device-related events occurred during the study, specifically no injury to the urethra or bladder (no identified urinary tract fistulas) (Table 9.2). Post hoc assessment of study outcomes and delivered thermal parameters

TABLE 9.1. Clinical efficacy.

	Laparoscopic group			Transvaginal group		
	Baseline	1-year	Long-term	Baseline	1-year	Long-term
N	94	85	61	120	96	73
Neg Valsalva (%)	0	79	71	0	76	66
Pt QOL assessment (%)		88	79		74	73
Uses <1 pad per day or none (%)		85	60		72	58

TABLE 9.2. Summary of reported complications.

	Laparoscopic group	Transvaginal group
Bladder (%)	2	0
Cardiovascular (%)	0	0
Pulmonary (%)	0	0
Additional surgery (%)	0	0
Transfusion (%)	0	0
Retention > 4 weeks (%)	0	0
UT infection (%)	2	0
Sexual dysfunction (%)	0	0
Postop urgency (%)	1	1

TABLE 9.3. Self explanatory.

Adverse event	Sham arm ($n = 63$)	RF arm ($n = 110$)	P Value
Urinary retention	0%	0.9% (1)	1.0
Urinary tract infection	4.8% (3)	4.5% (5)	1.0
Hematuria	0%	0.9% (1)	1.0
Dysuria	1.6% (1)	9.1% (10)	0.06
Hesitancy	1.6% (1)	0%	0.4
Asymptomatic detrusor overactivity	6.3% (4)	1.8% (2)	0.2
Dry overactive bladder	3.2% (2)	7.3% (8)	0.3
Wet overactive bladder	9.5% (6)	10% (11)	1.0

From [30]

revealed two treatment parameters that significantly impacted efficacy: (1) early and persistent increases of impedance due to excessive fluid in the surgical field which causes energy dissipation and resultant superficial, insufficient treatment; and (2) lack of continuity of thermal delivery to the treatment area (intermittent energy applications resulting from multiple "on/off" cycles which produces inadequate thermal delivery to the targeted tissues).

Using these additional criteria, the original patient cohort was assessed using the same outcome criteria at longer follow-up. The average follow-up times were 38 ± 3.51 months in the laparoscopic group and 30 ± 3.29 months in the transvaginal group. Using an actuarial survival analysis of objective and subjective outcomes from the initial evaluation, results projected to 30 ± 3.3 months demonstrated relative stability [29].

Future Directions

Transurethral delivery of RF energy recently has been described. Appell et al. [30] have used a system introduced by Novasys (Novasys Medical, Inc., Newark, CA) that is composed of a 21-French transurethral RF microremodeling probe mated to an RF generator. This system is monopolar and uses a standard return electrode ("grounding pad"), which is placed on the patient and connected to the RF generator. The urethral mucosa is continuously irrigated to avoid injury from heat application, with a tubing line carrying sterile, room-temperature water routed through a pump on the RF generator to the probe.

The technique does not require cystoscopic visualization. The RF probe is placed into the bladder lumen and a retention balloon on the end of the probe is insufflated and then palpably anchored within the bladder outlet, identical to positioning a Foley catheter. Immediately below the retention balloon, four 23-gauge needle electrodes are located within the probe. After probe localization, the needles are simultaneously deployed, and the needle tips are deployed through the urethral mucosa into the submucosa. Four separate submucosal tissue targets are treated with the needles, microremodeling requiring 60 s of current delivery at each site. Subsequently, a series of rotational maneuvers between periods of RF delivery result in the four needles residing in nine different positions (a total of 9 min of RF delivery). The goal of treatment is microremodeling of 36 microscopic, submucosal, circumferential targets ranging from the proximal urethra to the bladder neck.

In the pilot study, 110 women were randomized to the RF treatment group and 63 patients to a sham treatment group (probe insertion only). Subjective outcomes included the rate of ≥ 10 point Incontinence Quality of Life (I-QOL) score improvement and magnitude of perceived improvement based on patient satisfaction with treatment. Objective outcomes assessed included the change in mean leak-point pressure (LPP), and the number of women with $\geq 25\%$ reduction in both incontinence episode frequency and pad weight during stress testing. Adverse events were noted for both groups.

The 12-month safety profile was identical between the two groups (Table 9.3). Of the women with moderate to severe stress incontinence, 74% experienced [3]10 point I-QOL score improvement at 12 months following RF remodeling versus

50% of women who underwent sham treatment (P = 0.03). Of the women with mild incontinence, 22% of women who received RF treatment reported improvement versus 35% of women who received sham treatment (P = 0.2). Changes in the LPP between the two groups were noted. Although a high degree of variability was noted [RF treatment group demonstrated an increase in mean LPP at 12 months (13.2 ± 39.2 cm H_2O)], women in the sham treatment group demonstrated a reduction in mean LPP at 12 months [−2.0 ± 33.8 cm H_2O (P = 0.02)].

Summary

RF-induced tissue responses are well-defined and reproducible [12, 13]. Immediate effects reflect a denaturation of collagen fibers, with resultant loss in collagen fibril integrity. After 1 week, generalized granulation response is seen with resolution of acute inflammatory infiltrate. At 3 weeks, fibrosis and initial collagen remodeling are predominant. At 6 weeks posttreatment, continued resolution of inflammatory components has occurred, with further progression of the expected fibrotic healing response [15]. The final histological result is replacement of the elastic fascia by fibrotic tissue. The overall structural result is shortening, stiffening, and thickening of the fascia, which results in increased support of the bladder neck and proximal urethra and a decrease in hypermobility of these structures. These reproducible RF thermal tissue effects have been used in dermatology, in orthopedics, and for treatment of varicose veins [28]. The contractile response to RF energy also has been applied to the treatment of tendinous and ligamentous attachments within joints to shorten and strengthen these structures [27].

Loss of integrity of the endopelvic fascia generally is thought to be caused by pregnancy and childbirth [31, 32]. However, fascial support defects also may occur in other women such as athletes and those possibly at risk due to familial propensity, resulting in stress incontinence [33]. Hypermobility of the proximal urethra and bladder neck now are felt to be contributory but not causative to the development of stress urinary incontinence. Hypermobility of these structures is considered to be resultant from increased elasticity of the surrounding fascial tissues. Clinical studies performed thus far indicate that the RF procedure offers a safe and effective modality to impart thermal energy to the endopelvic fascia, replacing elastic tissue with inelastic fibrotic scar. Stabilization of the proximal urethra and bladder neck, which recapitulates support of the suburethral tissue, results from these changes, producing improvement and in some cases cure of stress urinary incontinence.

Overall, efficacy results must be balanced against any adverse events or safety issues resulting from an intended intervention, and both these considerations must be taken in the context of patient expectations for therapy [31–33]. For women with mild to moderate incontinence, continued evaluation of new therapies is ongoing in an effort to best balance risks and benefits of these therapies as opposed to those associated with more invasive procedures. Such considerations as voiding dysfunction after surgery requiring short- or long-term urethral catheterization, restrictions on future pregnancy that are inherent to sling and suspension procedures, and concerns regarding the use of biomaterials and possible adverse events resulting from these materials including erosion and poor tissue healing can impact patient preference for intervention. Given these issues, new therapies that potentially may decrease adverse events yet maintain relatively significant degrees of efficacy as compared to more invasive procedures are intriguing.

The RF approach does not rely on the use of implanted materials for structural support, thereby eliminating the concerns of voiding dysfunction resulting from sling placement and the potential for foreign material erosion. The minimal invasiveness of the procedure resulting from either the small incision and dissection used in the SURx technique or the probe insertion used in the Novasys procedure provides a therapeutic option for stress incontinence without the potential for injury to the lower urinary tract, bowel, and major vessels.

Inherent weaknesses exist, however, regarding the evidence extant for RF interventions for stress urinary incontinence. Longer-term follow-up analysis is necessary to determine the ultimate efficacy of RF interventions, as is the necessity for more uniform outcomes reporting using both objective and subjective criteria. Whether or not these procedures will be generally adopted also will depend on the overall comparative therapeutic index for RF therapy as compared to midurethral sling or bulking interventions. Ideally, RF thermal delivery could be carried out under local anesthesia as an ambulatory intervention. The SURx device is not as amenable to this technique, but possible further device evolution may allow this consideration. The Novasys system is much more applicable to the ambulatory, minimal anesthesia setting and further data may indeed support its use under these circumstances.

References

1. Hannestad YS, Rortveit G, Sandvik H, et al. A community based epidemiological survey of female urinary incontinence: The Norwegian EPINCONT study. J Clin Epidemiol, 53:1150–1157, 2000.
2. Luber KM. The definition, prevalence, and rick factors for stress urinary incontinence. Rev Urol, 6(Suppl 3):S3–S9, 2004.
3. Luber KM, Boero S, Choe JY. The demographics of pelvic floor disorders: Current observations and future projections. Am J Obstet Gynecol, 184:1496–1501, 2001.
4. Hampel C, Weinhold N, Eggersmann C, et al. Definition of overactive bladder and epidemiology of urinary incontinence. Urology, 50(Suppl 6A):4–14, 1997.
5. Elkadry EA, Kenton KS, Fitzgerald MP, et al. Patient selected goals: A new perspective on surgical outcome. Am J Obstet Gynecol, 189:1551–1558, 2003.
6. Kinchen KS, Burgio K, Diokno AC, et al. Factors associated with women's decisions to seek treatment for urinary incontinence. J Women's Health, 12:687–698, 2003.
7. Norton PA, MacDonald LD, Sedgwick PM, et al. Distress and delay associated with urinary incontinence, frequency, and urgency in women. BMJ, 297:1187–1189, 1988.
8. Cammu H, Van Nylen M, Amy JJ. A 10-year follow-up after Kegel pelvic floor muscle exercises for genuine stress incontinence. BJU Int, 85:655–658., 2000.
9. Goode PS, Burgio KL, Locher JL, et al. Effect of behavioral training with or without pelvic floor electrical stimulation on stress incontinence in women: A randomized controlled trial. JAMA, 290:345–352, 2003.
10. Takahashi T, Garcia-Osogobio S, Valdovinos MA, et al. Extended two-year results of radio-frequency energy delivery for the treatment of fecal incontinence (the Secca Procedure). Dis Colon Rectum, 46:711–715, 2003.
11. Fanelli RD, Gersin KS, Bakhsh A. The Stretta procedure: Effective endoluminal therapy for GERD. Surg Technol Int, 11:129–134, 2003.
12. DeLancey JO. Structural support of the urethra as it relates to stress urinary incontinence: The hammock hypothesis. Am J Obstet Gynecol, 170:1713–1720, 1994.
13. Hecht P, Hayashi K, Lu Y, et al. Monopolar radiofrequency energy effects on joint capsular tissue: Potential treatment for joint instability. An in-vivo mechanical, morphological, and biochemical study using an ovine model. Am J Sports Med, 27:761–771, 1999.
14. Galen DL. Histologic results of a new treatment for stress urinary incontinence without implantable materials. Obstet Gynecol, 95:530–533, 2000.
15. Fulmer BR, Sakamoto K, Turk TM, et al. Acute and long-term outcomes of RF BNS. J Urol, 167:141–144, 2002.
16. Smith A, Hosker GL, Warrell DW. The role of partial denervation of the pelvic floor in the aetiology of genito-urinary prolapse and stress incontinence of urine. A neurophysical study. Br J Obstet Gynaecol, 96:24–28, 1989.
17. Allen R, Hosker GL, Smith AR, et al. Pelvic floor damage and childbirth: A neurophysiologic study. Br J Obstet Gyaecol, 97:770–779, 1990.
18. Keane DP, Sims TJ, Abrams P, et al. Analysis of collagen status in premenopausal nulliparous women with genuine stress incontinence. Br J Obstet Gynaecol, 104:994–998, 1997.
19. Norton P. Pelvic floor disorders: The role of fascia and ligaments. Clin Obstet Gynecol, 36:929–939, 1993.
20. Aronson M, Bates SM, Jacoby AF, et al. Periurethral and paravaginal anatomy: An endovaginal magnetic resonance imaging study. Am J Obstet Gynecol, 173:1702–1710, 1995.
21. Richardson, A. Cystocele. Paravaginal repair. In: Female pelvic floor disorders. Benson J, ed. New York: Norton Medical Books, 1992: 280.
22. Osmond C, Hecht P, Hayashi K, et al. Comparative effects of laser and radio frequency energy on joint capsule. Clin Orthoped, 286:299, 2000.
23. Hecht P, Hayashi K, Cooley AJ, et al. The thermal effect of monopolar radio frequency energy on the properties of joint capsule. An in-vivo histologic study using a sheep model. Am J Sports Med, 26:808, 1998.
24. Lopez MJ, Hayashi K, Fanton GS, et al. The effect of radio frequency energy on the ultrastructure

of joint capsular collagen. Arthroscopy, 14:495, 1998.

25. Allain JC, Le Lous M, Cohen S, et al. Isometric tensions developed during the hydrothermal swelling of rat skin. Connect Tissue Res, 7:127–132, 1980.

26. Chen SS, Wright NT, Humphrey JD. J Biomech Eng, 119:372–378, 1997.

28. Ross J, Galen D, Abbott K, et al. A prospective multisite study of radiofrequency biopolar energy for treatment of genuine stress incontinence. J Am Assoc Gynecol Laparosc, 9:493–499,2002.

29. Dmochowski RR, Ross JW, Levy BS, et al. Three-year cure and improvement rates of a transvaginal radio frequency procedure for genuine stress incontinence. Unpublished data, 2005.

30. Appell RA, Juma S, Wells WG, et al. Transurethral radiofrequency energy collagen micro-remodeling for the treatment of female stress urinary incontinence. Neurourol Urodyn, 25(4):331–336, 2006.

31. Tincello DG, Alfirevic Z. Important clinical outcomes in urogynecology: Views of patients, nurses and medical staff. Int Urogynecol J Pelvic Floor Dysfunct, 13:96–98, 2002.

32. Hullfish KL, Bovbjerg VE, Gibson J, et al. Patient-centered goals for pelvic floor dysfunction surgery: What is success, and is it achieved? Am J Obstet Gynecol, 187:88–92, 2002.

33. Robinson D, Anders K, Cardozo L, et al. What women want – their interpretation of the concept of cure. Neurourol Urodyn, 21:429–430, 2002.

Chapter 10
Surgery for Stress Urinary Incontinence: Historical Review

Matthew P. Rutman and Jerry G. Blaivas*

Why a historical survey of surgery for stress incontinence? There are several reasons. First, there is much to learn from the mistakes of the past. In the words of Miguel de Santayana, "Those who fail to heed the lessons of history are doomed to repeat it." There was a time, for example, when surgeons were taught that to be effective, slings needed to be tied tightly enough to compress the urethra. That resulted in some disastrous complications and we do not do that any more. Second, as pointed out by Issac Newton, the accumulated experience of those who have gone before forms the substrate on which we formulate the innovations of the future. Relating to his own work, he said, "If I have seen further, it is by standing on the shoulders of giants." Relating to stress incontinence, the history of proposed pathophysiology and classification serves as a cogent example of this concept.

In Hinman's textbook of urology, published in 1935, fewer than 2 of 1,111 pages were devoted to incontinence. It was classified as (1) true incontinence, (2) false incontinence, (3) paradoxical (overflow) incontinence, and (4) essential incontinence. True incontinence was defined as "constant urinary leakage....resulting from a permanent dysfunction of the urinary reservoir or its sphincteral apparatus." No real distinction was made between the two. In 1961, Green proposed the first formal classification system for stress incontinence based on the radiographic appearance of the bladder neck and urethra during increases in abdominal pressure. He described two types. In type 1 SUI there was loss of the posterior urethrovesical angle,

whereas in type 2 there was in addition a rotational descent of the urethra [1]. This remained the only classification until 1980, when McGuire defined type 3 SUI [later termed intrinsic sphincter deficiency (ISD)], as a low urethral closure pressure associated with an open vesical neck at rest [2]. McGuire's classification was based on his own astute clinical observations. He noticed that there was an unusually high failure rate among women who underwent retropubic urethropexy after prior unsuccessful anti-incontinence surgery. He sought to find the reason why using newly refined urodynamic techniques. He found that those who had what he termed type 3 stress incontinence were the ones with the high failure rates, and he subsequently found that those patients fared better after autologous fascial sling surgery instead of urethropexy.

Until that time urodynamic studies were not used very often for women with stress incontinence; rather, they were reserved mostly for patients with neurogenic bladder. McGuire's contribution in utilizing urodynamics in women cannot be overstated. Using videourodynamic techniques, Blaivas and Olson (1988) further refined this Green/McGuire classification by adding type 0 stress incontinence [3]. Type 0 SUI was defined as a woman who complains of stress incontinence, but is not incontinent during the urodynamic study, yet has the substrate for type 2 stress incontinence (rotational descent of the urethra and opening of the vesical neck and proximal urethra). They further observed that some patients with apparent hypermobility, the bladder neck and proximal urethra were not hypermobile at all; rather, they were scarred (from previous surgery) in a low-lying position. They called this type 2B SUI. The implications for surgical treatment of type 2B SUI is that a urethrolysis was necessary at the time of sling procedure.

Thereafter, the Green/McGuire/Blaivas classification of SUI became an important clinical tool for helping to determine which anti-incontinence procedure to choose in an effort to minimize surgical failures [2, 3]. Subsequently, it has been documented over and over that sling procedures have good efficacy in treating type 3 SUI, whereas, retropubic urethropexy and transvaginal suspension do not fare as well. This fact, and the decreased morbidity associated with vaginal approaches, has led to widespread use of sling procedures as a first-line option to treat SUI.

The Green/McGuire/Blaivas classification is still widely utilized today, but as urodynamic techniques became more sophisticated and more widely used in clinical research, it became apparent that deficient anatomy was only part of the pathophysiology of sphincteric incontinence. Until McGuire's reported observation in 1980, it was thought that urethral hypermobility was the only cause of sphincteric incontinence and that surgical treatment should be aimed at restoring the proximal urethra to its normal "high retropubic position [1, 4].

Based on these observations, during the decade of the 1990s, it became fashionable to classify sphincteric incontinence into two distinct categories: urethral hypermobility and intrinsic sphincter deficiency based on the leak point pressure [5, 6]. The need for this classification was fortified when in the United States Medicare regulations required that in order to receive payment for periurethral injection of collagen, the leak point pressure must be less than 60 cm H_2O, i.e., intrinsic sphincter deficiency. At the time it was widely believed that women with urethral hypermobility should be treated with bladder neck suspensions and those with ISD should undergo a sling procedure. However, further studies revealed that these two conditions can (and often do) coexist in the same patient and that the expected inverse relationship between leak point pressure and urethral hypermobility does not exist [7, 8]. Accordingly, we (the authors) no longer classify SUI according to any

of these schemas; rather, we simply characterize it by the leak point pressure (a measure of sphincter strength) and the degree of urethral hypermobility (Q-tip angle).

Of course, the linchpin of all of these classifications systems is the underlying pathophysiology. For most of the twentieth century, until the innovative work of Petros and Ulmsten, it was widely believed that the bladder neck is the primary mechanism of continence [9, 10]. Reinforced by a number of basic science and clinical studies, it was postulated that increased abdominal pressure normally is transmitted equally to both bladder and urethra. When the proximal urethra descends too far, increases in abdominal pressure become unequally transmitted, and when vesical pressure exceeds urethral pressure, stress urinary incontinence ensues [11–15].

However, further studies unexpectedly showed that many women with significant urethral hypermobility remain continent, suggesting that urethral hypermobility is not the sole cause [16]. In fact, in McGuire's original description of type 3 SUI, he noted that it denoted an intrinsic malfunction of the urethral sphincter independent of urethral mobility. Further, as early as 1981, Constantinou demonstrated that pressure changes during stress are highest in the midurethra in continent woman and that this is lost in women with stress incontinence [12]. Subsequently, Petros and Ulmsten proposed that the midurethra, supported anteriorly by the pubourethral ligaments, is the primary continence mechanism, and from their worked emerged the midurethral sling procedures surgical procedures that have become the current rage [9, 10, 12, 17–21].

Petros and Ulmsten further expounded on the pathophysiology of incontinence with their "integral theory." The integral theory posits that stress and urge incontinence have a common etiology [9]. It states that support of the anterior vaginal wall is provided by three separate, but synergistic mechanisms: (1) the anterior pubococcygeus muscle lifts the anterior vaginal wall to compress the urethra, (2) the bladder neck is closed by traction of the underlying vaginal wall in a backward and downward fashion, and, (3) the pelvic floor musculature, under voluntary control, draws the hammock upward, closing the bladder neck. Overall laxity of the anterior vaginal wall causes a dissipation of all of these forces, resulting in stress incontinence. They further suggested that laxity of the anterior vaginal wall causes activation of stretch receptors in the bladder neck and proximal urethra, which can trigger an inappropriate micturition reflex, resulting in detrusor overactivity. Based on this theoretical work, they devised an operation: the tension-free vaginal tape (TVT) placed at the midurethra rather than the bladder neck. Subsequently, this and other midurethral operations have been shown to be successful in treating stress incontinence, at least in the short term [22–26].

In the 1990s a group of investigators at Johns Hopkins, using fast scan MRI and real-time perineal ultrasound, proposed that another mechanism causing SUI is unequal movement of the anterior and posterior walls of the bladder neck and proximal urethra during stress; the urethral lumen is literally pulled open as the posterior wall moves away from the anterior wall [27, 28]. According to this theory, it is the relative strength of the anterior and posterior urethral attachments that determine continence. If both are equally strong (or weak), the urethral walls will either not move at all or will move equally and continence will be maintained. If the anterior attachments are stronger than the posterior ones when there is sufficient force to cause movement, the posterior wall will be pulled open and incontinence will ensue. These investigators also demonstrated that the common denominator in SUI is opening of the bladder neck (funneling), not urethral hypermobility.

In 1995, John DeLancey proposed the hammock theory of urethral support [29]. He postulated that continence is maintained when the urethra is compressed against the hammocklike musculofascial structures on which the bladder and urethra rest. In this model, it is not the degree of urethral mobility, but the weakness of the supporting layers that cause sphincteric incontinence.

Upon first reflection, the preceding discussion might appear to be one of semantics, just splitting hairs. In fact, though, it is the understanding of pathophysiology and the mechanisms by which treatments affect pathophysiology that provides the requisite knowledge base for innovation. Based on this understanding (or misunderstanding), the surgical treatment of SUI has evolved from compression of the urethra to restoring the bladder neck to a high retropubic position to preventing descent to

creating a backboard against which the urethra can be compressed. Additionally, the focus of attention has turned from the bladder neck to the midurethra. In fact some of the most popular procedures for the treatment of stress incontinence do not change the position of the urethra or even correct hypermobility [30–32]. Just as the current treatments have evolved from those of the past, future treatments will evolve from those of the present. Exploring the century-long history of retropubic suspensions and slings provides a critical background and comprehension of where we are currently and hopefully what the future has in store for the treatment of SUI.

Surgical Procedures for SUI

The surgical treatment of SUI has evolved along three different lines: retropubic suspensions, transvaginal placations, and pubovaginal slings. The latest iteration of the former is the laparoscopic and robotic Burch colposuspension and transvaginal bladder neck suspension and the latter is the midurethral sling. The latest, of course, is not necessarily the best!

Transvaginal Plication

In 1914, Kelly first reported plication of the "lateral tissues" of the bladder neck under the urethra in "women without manifest injury to the bladder" [33]. His initial report revealed an 80% short-term success rate in 20 patients. Kennedy, nearly a quarter of a century later, described his modification to the Kelly procedure to include dissection of the urethra from the vaginal wall with plication of the injured sphincter muscle at the urethrovesical junction. The procedure became commonly known as the Kelly-Kennedy plication [34]. Although both of these procedures had relatively poor long-term success rates, they remained very popular because of their simplicity, lack of significant complications, and the ease with which they could be performed at the time of prolapse surgery [35]. The Ball–Burch procedure used a combined approach, performing a transabdominal Burch procedure with transvaginal imbrication of the urethra. Compared with the Burch or Kelly plication alone, the Ball–Burch procedure had improved continence rates in women with SUI and low urethral pressures [36, 37]. However, in a meta-analysis of the English language literature, Leach et al. concluded that the overall success rate of the Kelly–Kennedy procedure was only about 60% compared to over 85% for slings and retropubic operations [35].

Retropubic Suspensions

The retropubic suspensions or urethropexy procedures use existing tissues to reinforce, reposition, and stabilize the bladder neck into a high retropubic position. This procedure was first described in the United States by George White in 1909, as part of a retropubic paravaginal repair done for a cystocele repair [38]. The abdominal paravaginal repair was later popularized by Richardson in the early 1980s [39]. The paravaginal repair reattaches the endopelvic fascia that has pulled away form its attachment to the arcus tendinous fascia pelvis. It was reported to result in the cure of SUI; however, there was a paucity of literature demonstrating good efficacy. A recent prospective evaluation comparing the paravaginal defect repair to the Burch procedure showed a much higher failure rate in those undergoing the former [40]. At the present time, most surgeons who perform paravaginal repair combine it with a Marshall–Marchetti–Krantz (MMK) or a Burch colposuspension in order to treat SUI [41].

The original MMK procedure was first reported in 1949 [42]. The rationale for the MMK was based on observations made in men who presented with urinary retention after abdominoperineal (AP) resection of the rectum: "...Most of the patients... had mobility and marked sagging of the vesical base and outlet...lack of elevation and fixation...In some cases firm upward pressure on the perineum with a fist or harness would provide temporary elevation and fixation and these patients could thereby void satisfactorily." The first MMK was actually performed on a man who developed urinary retention after AP resection: "Two transurethral resections resulted in total incontinence even though the external urethral sphincter had not been damaged. Perineal pressure would provide good control. Simple suprapubic suspension of the vesical outlet by suturing to the pubis immediately and completely corrected his urinary control which has remained normal for a period of 46 months. By

analogy, the knowledge gained from the study of these rectal cases was applied to the problem of the common stress incontinence of females." The first operation on a woman was performed on June 8, 1944.

In the original description of the MMK procedure, two sutures were placed on either side of the periurethral tissues and anchored to the periosteum of the pubic symphysis. The operation resulted in "a simple elevation and immobilization of the vesical neck and urethra by suturing them to the pubis and rectus muscles" [43]. In a large review of 56 articles, the overall complication rate was 21.1% with a 5% wound complication rate and a 2.5% incidence of osteitis pubis [44]. In some instances, osteitis pubis resulted in severe and prolonged pubic pain with significant discomfort and disability [45]. Subsequently, to avoid these problems, sutures were placed in the cartilage of the symphysis.

In a further modification, Burch, in 1958, described the operation that now bears his name. Three sutures of 2–0 chromic were placed bilaterally, attaching the periurethral tissue directly to the ileopectineal ligament of Cooper [46]. Tanagho reported his modification of the original Burch procedure in 1976 at the Western Section of the American Urological Association meeting [47]. His adjustments included placement of more lateral sutures and emphasizing the avoidance of excess tension between Cooper's ligament and the anterior vaginal wall. Tanagho was the first to suggest the concept of avoiding overelevation of the vaginal wall during urethropexy surgery in an effort to limit prolonged voiding dysfunction. The retropubic urethropexy remains an important part of the choices available to the surgeon and the Burch colposuspension is its gold standard. Cure rates have been reported to range from 69 to 93.7% in long-term (10–15 year) follow-up [48–50].

Laparoscopic Retropubic Urethropexy

Laparoscopic approaches to retropubic urethropexy were introduced to address the morbidity associated with open procedures, but the overall success rate has been disappointing. It was first described in 1991, using a transperitoneal approach [51]. Currently, most laparoscopic urethropexy surgery uses an extraperitoneal approach mimicking the open procedure. Both Burch and MMK procedures have been reported using laparoscopic techniques, but reported cure rates have been lower than the open technique (80% vs. 96% at minimum 1-year follow-up) [52]. Techniques for suture placement have varied from instrument suturing (duplicating the open procedure) to stapling and tacking devices that attach mesh to Cooper's ligament. Recent publications have revealed an increase in the use of laparoscopy and robotic-assisted laparoscopy for vaginal prolapse surgery, which may lead to an increase in the number of concomitant laparoscopic urethropexies. Theoretically, performing the procedure laparoscopically in an identical manner to the open approach should reveal equivalent outcomes with potentially less morbidity, but theory is far from practice.

Transvaginal Needle Suspensions

Transvaginal needle suspension procedures evolved in an effort to provide a simpler and less morbid treatment option, yet preserve the excellent results of retropubic urethropexy. The initial goal of these operations was to elevate the bladder neck and proximal urethra in that high retropubic position with the use of nonabsorbable suture. Armand Pereyra introduced the first transvaginal needle suspension in 1959, because of his observational failures with the MMK procedure. The Peyera operation used a ligature carrier to suspend the "pericervical" fascia from the rectus fascia with stainless steel sutures [53]. He later modified the procedure to include chromic suture material for helical passes through the pubourethral endopelvic fascia. Further multiple modifications were developed under the generic name of "modified Pereyra procedures." In 1973, Thomas Stamey further modified the procedure by passing the suture through a polyester buttress (Dacron pledgets) that was placed superficial to the endopelvic fascia in an attempt to prevent the observed high rate of suture pull-through with the modified Pereyra procedure. He also recommended performing cystoscopy to identify the position of the bladder neck and aid in placing the sutures in a more accurate

manner and to recognize inadvertent passage of the suture through the bladder or urethra [54]. Stamey devised a single-holed ligature carrier (Stamey needle) that was the forerunner of the instruments used to pass sutures from the abdomen to the vagina. The Stamey procedure, as it was known, became very popular and remained so until the mid 1980s when it was supplanted by a further modification reported by Shlomo Raz. In 1981, Raz further modified the modified Pereyra by including the vaginal wall (beneath the epithelium) and the pubocervical fascia (which he later called the urethropelvic ligament) within the helical suture [55]. Raz reported a greater than 90% success rate, but this was not reproducible by other surgeons. In 1987, Ruben Gittes and Kevin Loughlin reported yet another modification, which they called the "incisionless suspension." They passed the helical sutures through the vaginal wall without any incision and used stab puncture wounds suprapubically with blind passage of a needle ligature passer [56]. This operation also gained some popularity for a while and became known as the Gittes procedure.

All these operations were reported to have excellent short-term results (without, of course, any meaningful or validated outcome measures), but longer follow-up revealed a high rate of recurrent incontinence attributed to pull through of the sutures from their vaginal attachments. Further, many complications went unreported (suture granulomas, erosions, ureteral injuries). Transvaginal needle suspensions were evaluated by the American Urological Association Female Stress Urinary Incontinence Clinical Guidelines Panel and their recommendation for these procedures was "low" or "marginal" due to low long-term cure rates [35], and these operations fell into disfavor. The lessons learned from all these operations, though, paved the way for the next generation of operations: anterior vaginal wall suspensions, vaginal wall slings, and bone anchor suspensions. All these operations were intended to improve on the rate of suture pull-through by incorporating stronger fixation points in the repair.

In 1989, Raz described the "four-corner suspension," a transvaginal needle suspension operation that repaired anterior vaginal wall prolapse in addition to its anti-incontinence mechanism. He accomplished this by placing a second set of sutures at the cystocele base. The four sutures were transferred suprapubically by a ligature carrier and secured to the anterior rectus fascia. He reported subjective cure rates of 94 and 98% for incontinence and cystocele, respectively. Longer-term follow-up revealed significant cystocele recurrences [57]. Using a rabbit model, Bruskewitz and colleagues compared different anchoring materials and suture pull-through rates, reporting that loops of suture and greater cross-sectional area of the anchor would lead to lower pull-through rates and higher success rates [58]. Based on that research, Leach and Zimmern modified the Raz procedure by obtaining a broader anterior vaginal wall anchor to decrease the rate of suture tissue pull-through. They referred to this procedure as the "anterior vaginal wall suspension" [59]. This procedure is still advocated by some due to its technical ease, low morbidity, and reproducibility, particularly in patients with a small to moderate cystocele and urethral hypermobility, but in our judgment has the same high failure rate accorded the other procedures.

Pubovaginal Sling

The pubovaginal sling originally was described nearly a century ago. Urologists and gynecologists used the sling procedure in an attempt to replace the sphincter mechanism due to anatomic sphincter defects. It has undergone numerous modifications and advances, and what once was an operation considered only for severe and refractory SUI, it has now become the most commonly performed and efficacious procedure for treating SUI. While the autologous rectus fascial sling remains the gold standard for treating SUI, synthetic midurethral slings are gaining momentum and are the most commonly performed operations in the industrialized world today.

In 1907, Von Giordano described the first rudimentary pubovaginal sling, where via an abdominal approach he wrapped a gracilis muscle graft around the urethra [60]. Three years later, Goebell performed a sling constructed from pyrimidalis muscle, tunneling the muscle flaps through the retropubic space and suturing them together under the bladder neck [61]. In 1914, Frangenheim modified Goebell's technique, incorporating the overlying rectus fascia in the flap to allow for a longer sling [62]. Three years later, Stoeckl further modified the technique by adding a combined abdominal and vaginal approach to plicate the bladder neck [63]. This later became known as the Goebell–Frangenheim–Stoeckel technique and was the first to use a combined abdominal–vaginal approach. In 1923, Thompson sutured rectus muscle and fascia around the urethra [64]. Martius, in 1929, described the interposition of bulbocavernosus muscle and the labial fat pad between the vaginal wall and urethra [65]. While novel in concept and important historically, each of these procedures caused urethral compression and obstruction, resulting in high rates of urethral sloughing, fistula occurrence, and recurrent cystitis.

In 1933, Price became the first to report using autologous fascia lata, which he passed beneath the urethra from an antegrade approach. The ends of the fascia then were secured to the rectus muscle [66]. In 1942, Aldridge, in a single case report, described the use of rectus fascia as a fascial sling placed through the retropubic space under the urethra. He detached strips of rectus fascia and external oblique aponeurosis laterally, leaving them attached medially. He was the first to suggest that the sling resulted in urethral compression during times of increased intra-abdominal pressure. Aldridge also identified the periurethral fascia and described the bloodless plane that permitted entry into the space of Retzius (retropubic space) [67]. The anatomic drawings of surgical technique that accompanied the original paper are superb and probably contributed greatly to its short-term popularity [68]. There were, however, several significant limitations to the Aldridge sling: (1) the attached medial edges of rectus fascia limited the mobility of the sling, (2) the sling length was not always long enough to pass under the urethra, and (3) there was no method to avoiding excess tension under the bladder neck and proximal urethra, resulting in outlet obstruction. As a result of these drawbacks, several modifications were made to Aldridge's operation over the ensuing decades in an attempt to improve mobility, increase sling length, and avoid excess tension. Despite these changes, multiple complications (fistulas, urethral slough, obstruction, infections, and sepsis) and poor outcomes limited the use of sling surgery for SUI.

McGuire, in 1978, ushered in the modern era of sling surgery when he described a modified technique using autologous rectus fascia for women with the entity that he first described: type 3 SUI [69]. The operation was performed with a combined vaginal and abdominal approach. A strip of rectus fascia, 1 × 12 cm in length, was isolated leaving it attached laterally on one side. The other end of the fascial strip was passed through the rectus muscle and positioned under the urethra before reattaching it to the other side of the rectus fascia. In his initial series of 52 women with type 3 SUI, the success rate was 80% with 2.3 year mean follow-up. The obvious problem with this technique was the fact that there was no way to adjust the tension as long as one end of the sling was left attached. To remedy this, Blaivas reported a modification that utilized a free graft of rectus fascia whose tension could be adjusted [70].

A major paradigm shift for the surgical treatment of SUI occurred when Blaivas reported on the use of autologous rectus fascial sling for all type of SUI, not just for those with type 3 SUI or ISD. At the time, this was a major development because it was commonly thought that such slings should be reserved for those with severe incontinence, since the operation was believed to be difficult to master and plagued by complications. Subsequently, numerous reports have documented the safety, efficacy, and long-term durability of the autologous fascia pubovaginal sling with medium-term cure rates of 73–93% [71–74]. The complication rate is relatively low, with risks of prolonged retention of less than 5%, and de novo urgency incontinence around 3% [75]. The risk of urethral erosion with autologous fascia is miniscule. This resurrected sling surgery and paved the way for the current era of slings as a first-line option for women with or without urethral hypermobility. It remains the gold standard to which all sling procedures using new materials and anchoring techniques are compared.

Materials

Multiple materials have been utilized in pubovaginal sling surgery. These can be subdivided into autologous, allograft, xenograft, and synthetic sling materials.

1. Autologous fascia. Two sources of autlogous fascia have been used for slings: rectus abdominis and fascia lata. Autologous fascia lata sling surgery initially was described by Price in 1933 [66]. After McGuire's work reinvigorated the pubovaginal sling, rectus fascia became the most commonly used source, but many authors reported the use of fascia lata to avoid the morbidity of the abdominal incision employed for harvesting of the rectus fascia. Fascia lata is obtained from the iliotibial tract, with skin incisions located between the greater trochanter and the lateral epicondyle of the femur. Advantages of harvested fascia lata included the quality and length of available fascia, and the increased tensile strength of nonscarred tissue. Disadvantages included the additional time associated with harvesting and patient repositioning, as well as pain and cosmetic deformity at the incision site. Autologous fascia (rectus or fascia lata) remains the gold standard material for pubovaginal sling surgery. Significant complications with autologous fascia are rare and are limited mostly to urinary retention and de novo detrusor overactivity, likely the result of the sling tension and not the material itself.

2. Allograft. Allograft tissues are those harvested from human donors, typically cadavers, and transplanted into human recipients. Use of these tissues in pubovaginal sling surgery avoids the incision and time associated with harvesting of autologous fascia, resulting in shorter operating room time and quicker convalescence. In addition, it avoids the potential infection and erosion complications seen with the use of synthetic materials. Allograft materials used in sling surgery include lyophilized dura mater, fascia lata, and acellular dermis. European urologists have used lyophilized dura mater for many years. It has been used in bladder augmentations, vesicovaginal fistula repair, urethroplasty, and surgery for Peyronie's disease [76–79]. Several reports of dura in sling surgery have shown 89–92% cure rates with short- and intermediate-term follow-up [80, 81]. Cadaveric fascia lata (CFL) was first reported in incontinence surgery by Handa et al. in 1996 [82]. Prior to this it was used in orthopedic and ophthalmologic surgery for 15 years. The allograft tissue is obtained from a tissue bank and the process is regulated by the American Association of Tissue Banks. Although a thorough sterilization process is employed, the major safety issue concerning

the use of cadaveric allografts remains possible disease transmission, including human immunodeficiency virus (HIV) and Creutzfeldt–Jakob disease (CJD) as well as other prion diseases. All cadaveric tissues undergo serological screening for HIV and hepatitis B, but false-negative results are possible. The risk of HIV transmission is estimated to between 1 in 1,667,600 and 1 in 8 million, and the risk of CJD around 1 in 3.5 million [83–85]. There have been no reports of disease transmission with an allograft sling, but there have been reports of bacterial contamination including several cases of fatal transmission of clostridial infections in orthopedic surgery [86, 87]. DNA has been detected in solvent-dehydrated and freeze-dried CFL, as well as acellular dermis [88, 89]. Only one case of HIV transmission has been reported, occurring in 1985 in a woman receiving a bone allograft transplant [90]. One case of CJD was reported in a nonurological procedure where a patient received a cadaveric dura graft 12 years earlier [91]. No cases of CJD have been reported with the use of CFL. However, there have been reports of fatal CJD with allograft dura and we recommend that it no longer be used [92, 93].

CFL is processed by one of several techniques: solvent dehydration and gamma irradiation (Tutoplast®), freeze drying (FasLata®), and fresh frozen. Rehydration after processing is required for 15–30 min. Various processing techniques and early reported allograft failures have brought significant debate to the tensile strength of CFL. Chaikin et al. reported the first failure of a CFL sling in 1998, in a patient whose SUI recurred 3 days postoperatively. At reoperation, the edges of the graft had frayed and sutures had pulled through [94]. Sutaria et al. found no difference in tensile strengths of freeze-dried CFL, solvent-dehydrated CFL, and acellular cadaveric dermis [95]. Lemer et al. reported freeze-dried CFL had decreased tensile strength and tissue consistency [96]. The early reports on CFL sling demonstrated cure rates of 62.6–98% and were similar to those cure rates reported with autologous fascia [85, 97–99]. Fitzgerald et al. published their results on 35 women who underwent a pubovaginal sling with freeze-dried and irradiated CFL [100]. Eight of the 35 patients (23%) failed both sub-

jectively and objectively within 6 months, of whom 7 had been initially cured. On reexploration, the fascia had diminished to remnants or could not be identified. Similar findings were reported by Carbone and Raz at UCLA [101]. Frederick and Leach recently reported durable cystocele repair results, but noted a decrease in continence rates with the use of cadaveric tissues [102]. More recently, several acellular dermal allografts have been marketed for use in sling surgery, including Repliform®, Dermal Allograft®, and Alloderm®. Dermal allografts are strong, have similar mechanical properties to autologous tissues in vitro, and integrate well into tissue. In addition, it rehydrates in 5to 10 min, whereas CFL takes 15–30 min of hydration prior to implantation.

3. Xenografts. Xenografts are derived from nonhuman animal tissue. Zenoderm® was the first xenograft used in pubovaginal sling surgery. It is derived from porcine corium, treated with proteolytic enzymes to remove the noncollagenous material, and immersed in glutaraldehyde to cros-link the collagen molecules and reduce antigenicity. Cure rates of 78–90% have been reported, although there were several reports of significant wound infection rates [103–105]. Porcine corium also has been marketed under the brand names Pelvicol? and DermMatrix?. In contrast to Zenoderm®, these are cross-linked by diisocyanate and they avoid the graft mineralization that may occur with glutaraldehyde. Barrington et al. reported an 85% cure rate in 40 patients who underwent sling surgery with Pelvicol? with 12-month mean follow-up [106]. Stratasis®, a graft derived from porcine small intestinal submucosa (SIS), has been marketed recently for use in vaginal sling surgery. Rutner reported a 94% continence rate in 115 women who underwent a sling procedure, with infrapubic bone screws and SIS, with 36-month follow-up [107]. Bovine pericardium also has been marketed in several preparations for sling surgery. Using UroPatch? and infrapubic bone screws, Pelosi reported a 95% cure rate in 22 patients with 20-month mean follow-up [108].

4. Synthetic sling materials. Autologous fascia remains the gold-standard of materials, but few would deny that synthetic materials have stronger biomechanical properties. It is hypothesized that

the superior biomechanical properties will result in greater long-term efficacy and durability. The perfect synthetic material should have great tensile strength, be noncarcinogenic, inexpensive, nonallergenic, nonimmunogenic, and user-friendly. Synthetic slings vary in many ways including pore size, composition, and flexibility. They can be absorbable or permanent. Interstices, or interstitial pores, located in multifilament mesh, are much smaller than standard pores. This can prevent macrophage and immune influx yet allow bacteria free entry. The small pore size also can retard the fibrocollagenous ingrowth and inhibit sling scaffolding into neighboring tissues. Synthetic slings carry no risk of disease transmission aside from the theoretic potential of contamination with pathogens which has not been reported.

Synthetic materials were first used for slings in the 1950s in select patients (supposedly) devoid of usable fascia. In 1951, Bracht reported using nylon for sling construction [109]. The following year, Anselmino described Perlon as a sling material [110]. In 1961, Zoedler reported using nylon strips for a suburethral sling [111]. In 1962, Williams and TeLinde described the use of a 5-mm-wide piece of Mersilene (Dacron) ribbon, a permanent multi-filament synthetic, for sling surgery [112]. These synthetic procedures were all prone to obstruction at the bladder neck, potentially resulting in urinary retention, suprapubic abscess formation, and ure-thral fistula. In 1968, in an effort to decrease complications, Moir utilized a wider piece of Mersilene in a modified Aldridge sling, which was called the "gauze hammock operation" [113]. He felt the Aldridge sling and prior Mersilene surgeries resulted in complications due to the narrow size of the sling itself. His gauze hammock operation consisted of a 30 cm-long piece of Mersilene which had a center portion 2.5 cm in width placed under the bladder neck. The two ends of the synthetic were then secured to the rectus fascia. He reported an 81% cured or improved rate in 71 patients with up to 5-year follow-up. Nichols reported similar success in 1973 [114]. Both Moir and Nichols reported their success rates using physician assessment, not patient self-assessment.

In 1970, Morgan reported the use of a Marlex mesh for the treatment of recurrent stress urinary incontinence [115]. Marlex is a stiff polypropylene, permanent monofilament mesh with large pores and is devoid of interstices. Morgan described using a 2 cm strip of polypropylene mesh that he anchored to Cooper's ligament using a two-team combined abdominal and vaginal approach. His initial results revealed a 100% success rate. Longer follow-up, published 15 years later, revealed this number was closer to 80%. However, there were significant complication rates, as with prior types of sling surgery, including 6% rates of both urethral erosion and chronic retention, and a 5% rate of postoperative frequency and urgency [116].

Many other synthetic materials have been described in the last two decades. Stanton reported the first use of a sling made from Silastic, a material made from layers of silicone reinforced with Dacron. It is a permanent multifilament mesh with submicron pore size. This was theorized to be advantageous due to the sheath that surrounds the sling. In case of complications necessitating sling removal, it was thought that the sheath would make it easier to identify and remove the sling, while still preserving continence. Long-term data revealed a 71% cure rate at 5 years, but again there were high complication rates, particularly sinus formation and rejection [117], and subsequently the use of Silastic was abandoned.

In 1988, Horbach described using Gore-tex as a synthetic sling material [118]. Gore-tex is an expanded polytetrafluoroethylene, which is nonabsorbable and inert, and was theorized to incorporate with less foreign body reaction than other synthetic materials. It is a permanent multifilament with small pores. Initial short-term results were promising, but longer follow-up dropped the cure rate from 86 to 61% [119]. In addition, women with Gore-tex slings demonstrated wound infections, rejection, and erosion rates of 30–35%. Norris and Staskin later described the Gore-tex patch sling, reducing the amount of Gore-tex sling material to decrease infection rates. Despite success rates of 88–90%, 5–7% of patients had prolonged urinary retention and 4% had vaginal erosions [120–122]. Eventually, because of the high erosion rate, Gore-tex slings were taken off the market. The ProtoGen sling, a woven mesh of nonabsorbable polyester impregnated with bovine collagen matrix, gained great popularity and was widely used before it was recalled from the US market in 1999 due to complications including intractable pain and erosion rates as high as 55% [123]; it, too, was taken off the market.

The latest iteration of the synthetic sling is a polypropylene nonabsorbable monofilament mesh with large pores. It is more flexible and contains larger pores than Marlex mesh and lacks small interstices. It is widely considered to be the best synthetic material for sling surgery and the material of choice in the majority of the new generation "midurethal" slings.

Midurethral Slings

Midurethral slings were the brainchild of Peter Petros and Ulm Ulmsten based on their pioneering, innovative, and decades-long research into the physiology and pathophysiology of stress incontinence [9, 10]. Until their work, virtually all operations for SUI focused on the bladder neck. In 1994, Petros and Ulmsten were the first to report a procedure where polypropylene mesh was placed under the midurethra with the intention of being tension-free [124–127]. After several modifications, this later became known as the tension-free vaginal tape technique (TVT) [18]. In this technique, a wide, sharp trocar was passed from the vagina to the abdomen. Although largely unreported, within the first decade of its use, there were about 15–20 deaths worldwide using this technique due to perforation of iliac vessels and bowel. In addition, there were innumerable, also underreported major complications including nonfatal vessel and bowel injuries; urethral and vaginal erosions; vesicovaginal, urethrovaginal, and colovescial fistulas; and even ureteral injuries. These are listed in the MAUDE database, which reports adverse events involving medical devices. The data consist of voluntary reports since June 1993, user facility reports since 1991, distributor reports since 1993, and manufacturer reports since August 1996.

Fueled by industry, a large number of minor modifications of the TVT were introduced under the mantra of "midurethral sling kits." What these kits all have in common is that they are composed of disposable, onetime use trocars and sling materials and sutures, although they are expensive [18–20, 22, 25, 128–130]. All these procedures, including the TVT, usually can be completed in

less than 30 min. They can be done in the outpatient setting with local anesthesia in suitable patients. They all pass a synthetic material beneath the midurethra with the intention of creating a tension-free sling. Each employs a small anterior vaginal wall incision(s) with minimal or no dissection of the urethra. Trocars or needle passers are passed in an antegrade or retrograde fashion and the mesh is secured by design of the material to anchor in the soft tissue. All rely on blind passage of trocars and pose a risk of bladder perforation, nerve and vascular injury, bowel injury, and even death as discussed above.

One midurethral sling, though, is different from the others, and in our judgment safer: the distal urethral polypropylene sling devised by Raz [128]. This operation requires no disposable instruments (so it is not expensive), and because the endopelvic fascia (urethropelvic ligament of Raz) is perforated under direct vision, the chances of serious injury is negligible in the hands of experienced surgeons.

Because of the known complications of blind needle passage through the retropubic space and in order to obtain a more anatomically correct course for the sling, the transobturator technique was developed. It was introduced by Delorme who described placement of a sling material through a vaginal incision passed out through the obturator foramen near the medial thigh. He described an outside to inside passage of a hooked needle [19]. De Leval later described an inside-out transobturator urethral sling using TVT tape [129]. This was hypothesized to decrease potential injury to the urethra, bladder, and vagina. To date, almost all of the midurethral slings have demonstrated acceptable short-term results and the TVT has shown 4-year efficacy as good as the autologous rectus fascial sling [23, 25, 26].

Alternative Fixation Techniques

Although the composition of the sling is an important consideration, the point of fixation is important as well. In 1949, the MMK procedure was the first to rely on pubic bone fixation anchoring the periurethral tissues to the pubic symphysis. Burch described anchoring to Cooper's ligament. With the introduction of transvaginal needle suspensions, the rectus fascia became the most popular fixation

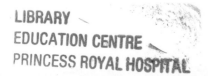

point. In 1998, Leach described his bony anchor fixation technique, where he manually attached his suspension sutures to the pubic bone [131]. He reported no cases of osteitis pubis or osteomyelitis in this series. Several transvaginal bony anchoring systems have been introduced since that rely on an infrapubic or transvaginal approach. They drill small screws with preattached suture directly into the bone. The sutures then can be passed through autologous, allogenic, or synthetic material resulting in a sling secured at the pubic bone. There is only limited long-term data assessing their use in sling surgery.

Sphincter Prosthesis

The artificial urinary sphincter (AUS) was the brainchild of F. Brantley Scott who also developed the inflatable penile prosthesis [132, 133]. Brantley, as he was known, intended the sphincter prosthesis to become a primary operation for SUI, and in fact, he implanted many prostheses in woman. Although the sphincter prosthesis is the mainstay of treatment for SUI in men, it never became the operation in women that Scott intended it to be, despite the reports of excellent efficacy by Pierre Costa [134, 135]. Its use in women is largely reserved for patients with severe and refractory incontinence with low leak point pressures who have failed other surgeries. The prosthesis is composed of three components: a sphincter cuff that is implanted around the bladder neck, a fluid reservoir implanted in the retropubic space or behind the rectus muscle, and a control pump component implanted in the subcutaneous tissue of the labia majora. The original prosthesis was plagued with mechanical problems, primarily tubing kinks and leaks, but these have been largely eliminated by using reinforced tubing and sutureless connectors [136, 137].

As originally described by Scott, the operation was performed entirely through a retropubic approach. This proved to be a particularly challenging operation from a technical standpoint, mostly because of the difficulty creating a plane between the anterior vaginal wall and proximal urethra. To this end, Scott devised a special instrument that more or less blindly cut behind the bladder neck, resulting in the almost inevitable complications of urethral damage, erosion, or fistula. These compli-

cations went largely unreported, but contributed to the lack of enthusiasm among other surgeons. In an attempt to improve on these complications, armed with the surgical skills learned from transvaginal urethropexies and slings, Appel reported using a transvaginal approach for implanting the sphincter cuff. This, too, though met with little enthusiasm.

Those who advocate the AUS over a suburethral sling cite the ability to provide circumferential compression around the entire urethra. The cure rates are greater than 90% in some series [135]. However, there remains a high revision rate that approaches from 20 to 90% at 10 years [138]. Additionally, there is a risk of erosion of the pump or cuff. Nevertheless, the AUS remains a viable treatment option in the rare patient with SUI who has failed prior intervention. It also can be used in patients with impaired detrusor contractility preferentially over a suburethral sling to lessen the chances of postoperative urinary retention.

Almost a century has passed since the initial sling procedure was described for stress incontinence. New techniques and new materials have come and gone and there are still many questions to be answered. Integral to the future of incontinence surgery is an understanding of the past. The lessons we have learned can help answer questions and guide research efforts in the future.

References

1. Green TH, Jr. Development of a plan for the diagnosis and treatment of urinary stress incontinence. Am J Obstet Gynecol 1962; 83:632–648.
2. McGuire EJ, et al. The value of urodynamic testing in stress urinary incontinence. J Urol 1980; 124(2):256–258.
3. Blaivas JG, Olsson CA. Stress incontinence: Classification and surgical approach. J Urol 1988; 139(4):727–731.
4. Hodgkinson CP. Relationships of the female urethra and bladder in urinary stress incontinence. Am J Obstet Gynecol 1953; 65(3):560–573.
5. McGuire EJ et al. Clinical assessment of ur ethral sphincter function. J Urol 1993; 150(5 Pt 1):1452–1454.
6. Horbach NS, Ostergard DR. Predicting intrinsic urethral sphincter dysfunction in women with stress urinary incontinence. Obstet Gynecol 1994; 84(2):188–192.
7. Nitti VW, Combs AJ. Correlation of Valsalva leak point pressure with subjective degree of stress

urinary incontinence in women. J Urol 1996; 155(1):281–285.

8. Fleischmann N et al. Sphincteric urinary incontinence: Relationship of vesical leak point pressure, urethral mobility and severity of incontinence. J Urol 2003; 169(3):999–1002.

9. Petros PE, Ulmsten UI. An integral theory of female urinary incontinence. Experimental and clinical considerations. Acta Obstet Gynecol Scand Suppl 1990; 153:7–31.

10. Petros PP, Ulmsten U. An anatomical classification – a new paradigm for management of female lower urinary tract dysfunction. Eur J Obstet Gynecol Reprod Biol 1998; 80(1):87–94.

11. McGuire EJ, Herlihy E. The influence of urethral position on urinary continence. Invest Urol 1977; 15(3):205–207.

12. Constantinou, CE, Govan DE. Contribution and timing of transmitted and generated pressure components in the female urethra. Prog Clin Biol Res 1981; 78:113–20.

13. Constantinou CE. Resting and stress urethral pressures as a clinical guide to the mechanism of continence. Clin Obstet Gynaecol 1985; 12(2):343–356.

14. Bump RC, Fantl JA, Hurt WG. Dynamic urethral pressure profilometry pressure transmission ratio determinations after continence surgery: Understanding the mechanism of success, failure, and complications. Obstet Gynecol 1988; 72(6):870–874.

15. Westby M, AsmussenM, Ulmsten U. Location of maximum intraurethral pressure related to urogenital diaphragm in the female subject as studied by simultaneous urethrocystometry and voiding urethrocystography. Am J Obstet Gynecol 1982; 144(4):408–412.

16. Versi E et al. Internal urinary sphincter in maintenance of female continence. Br Med J (Clin Res Ed) 1986; 292(6514):166–167.

17. Rodriguez LV, BermanJ, Raz S. Polypropylene sling for treatment of stress urinary incontinence: An alternative to tension-free vaginal tape. Tech Urol 2001; 7(2):87–89.

18. Ulmsten U et al., An ambulatory surgical procedure under local anesthesia for treatment of female urinary incontinence. Int Urogynecol J Pelvic Floor Dysfunct 1996; 7(2):81–85; discussion 85–86.

19. Delorme E. [Transobturator urethral suspension: Mini-invasive procedure in the treatment of stress urinary incontinence in women]. Prog Urol 2001; 11(6):1306–1313.

20. Tash, J, Staskin DR. Artificial graft slings at the midurethra: Physiology of continence. Curr Urol Rep 2003; 4(5):367–370.

21. de Leval J. Novel surgical technique for the treatment of female stress urinary incontinence: Transobturator vaginal tape inside-out. Eur Urol 2003; 44(6):724–730.

22. Ulmsten U, et al. A multicenter study of tension-free vaginal tape (TVT) for surgical treatment of stress urinary incontinence. Int Urogynecol J Pelvic Floor Dysfunct 1998; 9(4):210–213.

23. Nilsson CG, et al. Long-term results of the tension-free vaginal tape (TVT) procedure for surgical treatment of female stress urinary incontinence. Int Urogynecol J Pelvic Floor Dysfunct 2001; 12(Suppl 2):S5–8.

24. Olsson I, Kroon U. A three-year postoperative evaluation of tension-free vaginal tape. Gynecol Obstet Invest 1999; 48(4):267–269.

25. Rezapour M, Ulmsten U. Tension-free vaginal tape (TVT) in women with recurrent stress urinary incontinence—a long-term follow up. Int Urogynecol J Pelvic Floor Dysfunct 2001;; 12(Suppl 2):S9–11.

26. Nilsson CG. Falconer C, Rezapour M. Seven-year follow-up of the tension-free vaginal tape procedure for treatment of urinary incontinence. Obstet Gynecol 2004; 104(6):1259–1262.

27. Yang A et al. Pelvic floor descent in women: Dynamic evaluation with fast MR imaging and cinematic display. Radiology 1991; 179(1):25–33.

28. Mostwin JL et al. Radiography, sonography, and magnetic resonance imaging for stress incontinence. Contributions, uses, and limitations. Urol Clin North Am 1995; 22(3):539–549.

29. DeLancey JO. Structural support of the urethra as it relates to stress urinary incontinence: The hammock hypothesis. Am J Obstet Gynecol 1994; 170(6):1713–1720; discussion 1720–1723.

30. Lo TS et al. Ultrasonographic and urodynamic evaluation after tension free vagina tape procedure (TVT). Acta Obstet Gynecol Scand 2001; 80(1):65–70.

31. Sarlos D, Kuronen M, Schaer GN. How does tension-free vaginal tape correct stress incontinence? Investigation by perineal ultrasound. Int Urogynecol J Pelvic Floor Dysfunct 2003; 14(6):395–398.

32. Minaglia S et al. Effect of transobturator tape procedure on proximal urethral mobility. Urology 2005; 65(1):55–59.

33. Kelly HA. Dunn W. Urinary incontinence in women without manifest injury to the bladder. Surg Gynecol Obstet 1914; 18:444–450.

34. Kennedy WT. Incontinence of urine in the female: The urethral sphincter mechanism, damage of function, and restoration of control. Am J Obstet Gynecol 1937; 34:576.

35. Leach GE et al. Female stress urinary incontinence clinical guidelines panel summary report on surgical

management of female stress urinary incontinence. The American Urological Association. J Urol 1997; 158(3 Pt 1):875–880.

36. Bergman A, , Koonings PP, Ballard CA. The Ball–Burch procedure for stress incontinence with low urethral pressure. J Reprod Med 1991; 36(2):137–140.

37. Elia G, Bergman A. Genuine stress urinary incontinence with low urethral pressure. Five-year follow-up after the Ball–Burch procedure. J Reprod Med 1995; 40(7):503–506.

38. White GR. A radical cure by suturing lateral sulci of vagina to white line of pelvic fascia. JAMA 1909; 21:1707–1708.

39. Richardson AC. Edmonds PB, Williams NL. Treatment of stress urinary incontinence due to paravaginal fascial defect. Obstet Gynecol 1981; 57(3):357–362.

40. Colombo M et al. A randomized comparison of Burch colposuspension and abdominal paravaginal defect repair for female stress urinary incontinence. Am J Obstet Gynecol 1996; 175(1):78–84.

41. Bruce RG, El-Galley RE, Galloway NT. Paravaginal defect repair in the treatment of female stress urinary incontinence and cystocele. Urology 1999; 54(4):647–651.

42. Marshall VF, Krantz KE The correction of stress incontinence by simple urethrovesical suspension. Surg Gynecol Obstet 1949; 88:509.

43. Marshall VF, Marchetti AA, Krantz KE. The correction of stress incontinence by simple vesicourethral suspension. J Urol 2002; 168(4 Pt 1):1326–1331.

44. Mainprize TC, Drutz HP. The Marshall–Marchetti–Krantz procedure: A critical review. Obstet Gynecol Surv 1988; 43(12):724–729.

45. O'Leary JA. Osteitis pubis following vesicourethral suspension. Obstet Gynecol 1964; 24:73–77.

46. Burch J. Urethrovesical fixation to Cooper's ligament for correction of stress incontinence, cystocele, and prolapse. Am J Obstet Gynecol 1961; 81:281.

47. Tanagho EA. Colpocystourethropexy: The way we do it. J Urol 1976; 116(6):751–753.

48. Herbertsson G, Iosif CS. Surgical results and urodynamic studies 10 years after retropubic colpourethrocystopexy. Acta Obstet Gynecol Scand 1993; 72(4):298–301.

49. Langer R, et al., Long-term (10–15 years) follow-up after Burch colposuspension for urinary stress incontinence. Int Urogynecol J Pelvic Floor Dysfunct 2001; 12(5):323–326; discussion 326–327.

50. Alcalay M, Monga A, Stanton SL. Burch colposuspension: A 10–20 year follow up. Br J Obstet Gynaecol 1995; 102(9):740—745.

51. Vancaillie TG, Schuessler W. Laparoscopic bladder neck suspension. J Laparoendosc Surg 1991; 1(3):169–173.

52. Su TH et al. Prospective comparison of laparoscopic and traditional colposuspensions in the treatment of genuine stress incontinence. Acta Obstet Gynecol Scand 1997; 76(6):576–582.

53. Pereyra AJ. A simplified surgical procedure for the correction of stress incontinence in women. West J Obstet Gynecol 1959; 67:223–226.

54. Stamey TA. Cystoscopic suspension of the vesical neck for urinary incontinence. Surg Gynecol Obstet 1973; 136:547–554.

55. Raz S. Modified bladder neck suspension for female stress incontinence. Urology 1981; 17(1):82–85.

56. Gittes RF, Loughlin KR. No-incision pubovaginal suspension for stress incontinence. J Urol 1987; 138(3):568–570.

57. Raz S, Klutke CG, Golomb J. Four-corner bladder and urethral suspension for moderate cystocele. J Urol 1989; 142(3):712–715.

58. Bruskewitz RC et al. Bladder neck suspension material investigated in a rabbit model. J Urol 1989; 142(5):1361–1363.

59. Zimmern PE, Leach G, Sirls L. Four-corner bladder neck suspension. In: Atlas of the urological clinics of North America, Leach, GE editor, W.B. Saunders: Philadelphia, 1994:29–36.

60. Ridley J. The Goebel–Stockel sling operation. In: TeLinde's operative gynecology, Thompson J, Mattingly RF editors, . Lippincott: Philadelphia, 1985.

61. Goebel R. Zur operativen besteitigung der angerborenen incontinenz vesicae. Zeitscher Gynakol 1910; 2:187–191.

62. Frangenheim P. Zu operativen behandlung der inkontinenz der mannlichen harnohre. Ver Dtsch Ges 1914; 43:149–154.

63. Stoeckel W. Uber die verwendung der museuli pyramidalis bei der operitaven behandlung der incontinentia urinae. Zentralbl Gynakol 1917; 41:11–19.

64. Thompson R. A case of epispadias associated with complete incontinence treated by rectus transplantation. Br J Dis Child 1923; 20:146–151.

65. Martius H. Sphnicter-und Harnrohrnplastik aus dem Musculus Bulbocavernosus. Chirurg 1929; 1:769.

66. Price P. Plastic operations for incontinence of urine and feces. Arch Surg 1933; 26:1043–1048.

67. Aldridge A. Transplantation of fascia for relief of urinary stress incontinence. Am J Obstet Gynecol 1942; 44:398–411.

68. McLaren HC. Late results from sling operations. J Obstet Gynaecol Br Commonw 1968; 75(1):10–13.

69. McGuire EJ, Lytton B. Pubovaginal sling procedure for stress incontinence. J Urol 1978; 119(1):82–84.

70. Blaivas JG, Jacobs BZ. Pubovaginal fascial sling for the treatment of complicated stress urinary incontinence. J Urol 1991; 145(6):1214–1218.

71. Morgan TO, Jr, Westney OL, McGuire EJ. Pubovaginal sling: 4-Year outcome analysis and quality of life assessment. J Urol 2000; 163(6):1845–1848.

72. Chaikin DC, Rosenthal J, Blaivas JG. Pubovaginal fascial sling for all types of stress urinary incontinence: Long-term analysis. J Urol 1998; 160(4):1312–1316.

73. Mason RC, Roach M. Modified pubovaginal sling for treatment of intrinsic sphincteric deficiency. J Urol 1996; 156(6):1991–1994.

74. McGuire EJ et al. Experience with pubovaginal slings for urinary incontinence at the University of Michigan. J Urol 1987; 138(3):525–526.

75. Cross CA, Cespedes RD, McGuire EJ. Our experience with pubovaginal slings in patients with stress urinary incontinence. J Urol 1998; 159(4):1195–1198.

76. Romero Perez P et al. [Partial parietal cystectomy and cystoplasty using a lyophilized human dura mater patch as an alternative in palliative surgery for bladder cancer]. Arch Esp Urol 1990; 43(8):867–875.

77. Ramos C et al. [Vesicovaginal fistulas: Correction using lyophilized dura mater]. Actas Urol Esp 1991; 15(2):143–147.

78. Sampaio JS et al. Surgical correction of severe Peyronie's disease without plaque excision. Eur Urol 1992; 22(2):130–133.

79. Villavicencio Mavrich H et al. Experience with lyophilized human dura mater for urethral strictures. J Urol 1998; 160(4):1310–1311.

80. Enzelsberger H, Helmer H, Schatten C. Comparison of Burch and lyodura sling procedures for repair of unsuccessful incontinence surgery. Obstet Gynecol 1996; 88(2):251–256.

81. Rottenberg RD et al. Urodynamic and clinical assessment of the Lyodura sling operation for urinary stress incontinence. Br J Obstet Gynaecol 1985.;92(8):829–834.

82. Handa VL et al. Banked human fascia lata for the suburethral sling procedure: A preliminary report. Obstet Gynecol 1996; 88(6):1045–1049.

83. Buck BE, Malinin TI. Human bone and tissue allografts. Preparation and safety. Clin Orthop Relat Res 1994; 303:8–17.

84. Buck BE, Malinin TI, Brown MD. Bone transplantation and human immunodeficiency virus. An estimate of risk of acquired immunodeficiency syndrome (AIDS). Clin Orthop Relat Res 1989; 240:129–136.

85. Amundsen CL et al. Outcome in 104 pubovaginal slings using freeze-dried allograft fascia lata from a single tissue bank. Urology 2000; 56(6 Suppl 1):2–8.

86. Malinin TI et al. Incidence of clostridial contamination in donors' musculoskeletal tissue. J Bone Joint Surg Br 2003; 85(7):1051–1054.

87. Kainer MA et al. Clostridium infections associated with musculoskeletal-tissue allografts. N Engl J Med 2004; 350(25):2564–2571.

88. Hathaway JK, Choe, JM. Intact genetic material is present in commercially processed cadaver allografts used for pubovaginal slings. J Urol 2002; 168(3):1040–1043.

89. Choe JM, Bell T. Genetic material is present in cadaveric dermis and cadaveric fascia lata. J Urol 2001; 166(1):122–124.

90. Simonds RJ et al. Transmission of human immunodeficiency virus type 1 from a seronegative organ and tissue donor. N Engl J Med 1992; 326(11): 726–732.

91. Liscic RM et al. Creutzfeldt–Jakob disease in a patient with a lyophilized dura mater graft. Acta Med Croatica 1999; 53(2):93–96.

92. Miyashita K et al. Creutzfeldt–Jakob disease in a patient with a cadaveric dural graft. Neurology 1991; 41(6):940–941.

93. Fushimi M et al. PLEDs in Creutzfeldt–Jakob disease following a cadaveric dural graft. Clin Neurophysiol 2002; 113(7):1030–1035.

94. Chaikin DC, Blaivas JG. Weakened cadaveric fascial sling: An unexpected cause of failure. J Urol 1998; 160(6 Pt 1):2151.

95. Pa S Sutaria. Tensile strength of cadaveric fascia lata allograft is not affected by current methods of tissue preparation. 1998; J Urol 161:(4) Abstract 1194.

96. Lemer ML. Chaikin DC, Blaivas JG. Tissue strength analysis of autologous and cadaveric allografts for the pubovaginal sling. Neurourol Urodyn 1999; 18(5):497–503.

97. Wright EJ et al. Pubovaginal sling using cadaveric allograft fascia for the treatment of intrinsic sphincter deficiency. J Urol 1998; 160(3 Pt 1): 759–762.

98. Brown SL, Govier FE. Cadaveric versus autologous fascia lata for the pubovaginal sling: Surgical outcome and patient satisfaction. J Urol 2000; 164(5):1633–1637.

99. Kobashi KC, Mee SL, Leach GE. A new technique for cystocele repair and transvaginal sling: The cadaveric prolapse repair and sling (CAPS). Urology 2000; 56(6 Suppl 1):9–14.

100. Fitzgerald MP, Mollenhauer J, Brubaker L. Failure of allograft suburethral slings. BJU Int 1999; 84(7):785–788.

101. Carbone JM et al. Pubovaginal sling using cadaveric fascia and bone anchors: Disappointing early results. J Urol 2001; 165(5):1605–1611.

102. Frederick RW, Leach GE. Cadaveric prolapse repair with sling: Intermediate outcomes with 6 months to 5 years of follow-up. J Urol 2005; 173(4):1229–1233.

103. Jarvis GJ, Fowlie A. Clinical and urodynamic assessment of the porcine dermis bladder sling in the treatment of genuine stress incontinence. Br J Obstet Gynaecol 1985; 92(11):1189–1191.

104. Hilton P. A clinical and urodynamic study comparing the Stamey bladder neck suspension and suburethral sling procedures in the treatment of genuine stress incontinence. Br J Obstet Gynaecol 1989; 96(2):213–220.

105. Iosif CS. Porcine corium sling in the treatment of urinary stress incontinence. Arch Gynecol 1987; 240(3):131–136.

106. Barrington JW et al. The use of porcine dermal implant in a minimally invasive pubovaginal sling procedure for genuine stress incontinence. BJU Int 2002; 90(3):224–227.

107. Rutner AB, Levine SR, Schmaelzle JF. Processed porcine small intestine submucosa as a graft material for pubovaginal slings: Durability and results. Urology 2003; 62(5):805–809.

108. Pelosi MA II, Pelosi MA III, Pelekanos M. The YAMA UroPatch sling for treatment of female stress urinary incontinence: A pilot study. J Laparoendosc Adv Surg Tech A 2002; 12(1):27–33.

109. Bracht, [Simplified operation for incontinence.]. Arch Gynakol, 1951; 180: 163–164.

110. Hohenfellner R, Petrie E. Sling procedure in surgery. In: Surgery of female incontinence, Stanton, STE editor, . Springer:: Berlin, 1986: 105–113.

111. Zoedler D. Zur operativen Behandlung der weiblichen Stress inkontinenz. Z Urol 1961; 54:355.

112. Williams TJ, Telinde RW. The sling operation for urinary incontinence using mersilene ribbon. Obstet Gynecol 1962; 19:241–245.

113. Moir JC. The gauze-hammock operation. (A modified Aldridge sling procedure). J Obstet Gynaecol Br Commonw 1968; 75(1):1–9.

114. Nichols DH. The Mersilene mesh gauze-hammock for severe urinary stress incontinence. Obstet Gynecol 1973; 41(1):88–93.

115. Morgan JE. A sling operation, using Marlex polypropylene mesh, for treatment of recurrent stress incontinence. Am J Obstet Gynecol 1970; 106(3):369–377.

116. Morgan JE, Farrow G.A, Stewart FE. The Marlex sling operation for the treatment of recurrent stress urinary incontinence: A 16-year review. Am J Obstet Gynecol 1985; 151(2):224–226.

117. Stanton SL, Brindley GS, Holmes DM. Silastic sling for urethral sphincter incompetence in women. Br J Obstet Gynaecol 1985; 92(7):747–750.

118. Horbach NS et al. A suburethral sling procedure with polytetrafluoroethylene for the treatment of genuine stress incontinence in patients with low urethral closure pressure. Obstet Gynecol 1988; 71(4):648–652.

119. Weinberger MW, Ostergard DR. Long-term clinical and urodynamic evaluation of the polytetrafluoroethylene suburethral sling for treatment of genuine stress incontinence. Obstet Gynecol 1995; 86(1):92–96.

120. Choe JM, Staskin DR. Gore-Tex patch sling: 7 years later. Urology 1999; 54(4):641–646.

121. Norris JP, Breslin DS, Staskin DR. Use of synthetic material in sling surgery: A minimally invasive approach. J Endourol 1996; 10(3):227–230.

122. Staskin DR, Choe JM, Breslin DS. The Gore-tex sling procedure for female sphincteric incontinence: Indications, technique, and results. World J Urol 1997; 15(5):295–299.

123. Kobashi KC et al. Erosion of woven polyester pubovaginal sling. J Urol 1999; 162(6):2070–2072.

124. Ulmsten U, Johnson P, Petros P. Intravaginal slingplasty. Zentralbl Gynakol 1994; 116(7):398–404.

125. Ulmsten U, Petros P. Intravaginal slingplasty (IVS): An ambulatory surgical procedure for treatment of female urinary incontinence. Scand J Urol Nephrol 1995; 29(1):75–82.

126. Petros PP. The intravaginal slingplasty operation, a minimally invasive technique for cure of urinary incontinence in the female. Aust N Z J Obstet Gynaecol 1996; 36(4):453–461.

127. Petros PE. New ambulatory surgical methods using an anatomical classification of urinary dysfunction improve stress, urge and abnormal emptying. Int Urogynecol J Pelvic Floor Dysfunct 1997; 8(5):270–277.

128. Rodriguez LV, Raz S. Polypropylene sling for the treatment of stress urinary incontinence. Urology 2001; 58(5):783–785.

129. Deval B et al. A French multicenter clinical trial of SPARC for stress urinary incontinence. Eur Urol 2003; 44(2):254–258; discussion 258–259.

130. Dargent D et al. Insertion of a sub-urethral sling through the obturating membrane for treatment of female urinary incontinence. Gynecol Obstet Fertil 2002; 30(7–8):576–582.

131. Leach GE. Bone fixation technique for transvaginal needle suspension. Urology 1988; 31(5):388–390.

132. Scott FB, Bradley WE, Timm GW. Treatment of urinary incontinence by an implantable prosthetic urinary sphincter. J Urol 1974; 112(1):75–80.

133. Scott FB, Bradley WE, Timm GW. Management of erectile impotence. Use of implantable inflatable prosthesis. Urology 1973; 2(1):80–82.

134. Costa P et al. The artificial urinary sphincter AMS 800: Our experience in women with or without uterine prolapse. Acta Urol Belg 1995; 63(2):45–46.

135. Costa P et al. The use of an artificial urinary sphincter in women with type III incontinence and a negative Marshall test. J Urol 2001; 165(4):1172–1176.

136. Leo ME, Barrett DM. Success of the narrow-backed cuff design of the AMS800 artificial urinary sphincter: Analysis of 144 patients. J Urol 1993; 150(5 Pt 1): 1412–1414.

137. Light JK, Reynolds JC. Impact of the new cuff design on reliability of the AS800 artificial urinary sphincter. J Urol 1992; 147(3):609–611.

138. Wang Y, HR. Artificial sphincter: Transvaginal approach In: Female urology, Raz S editor, W.B. Saunders: Philadelphia, 1996.

Chapter 11
Surgery for Stress Urinary Incontinence: Open Approaches

Meidee Goh and Ananias C. Diokno

Open Retropubic Suspensions

Marshall–Marchetti–Krantz Procedure

Historical Perspective

The abdominal approach for repair in incontinence is premised on recreating the elevation of the bladder neck. In 1949, Marshall et al. reported on their experiences with 50 patients [1]. They had observed that patients with urinary retention following rectal resection were not helped by transurethral resection of the vesical neck; however, if the perineum were elevated, patients then could void. Based on these findings, they proposed a technique to elevate the bladder neck and the anterior bladder wall out of the pelvis. In their series, 82% of patients had excellent results.

The initial description of the Marshall–Marchetti–Krantz (MMK) procedure by Marshall et al. [1] in 1949 called for three pairs of figure-eight periurethral sutures placed through the lateral urethral wall on either side of midline. The stitches then are sutured to the appropriate location into the periosteum of the symphysis pubis. Number 1 chromic catgut was the suture recommended by Marshall and his colleagues. Additionally, three stitches were placed in the musculature of the lower and lateral portions of the bladder. These then were placed into the posterior portion of the rectus muscle. The goal of the second set of sutures was to pull the bladder anteriorly into the space of Retsius. A penrose drain was placed prior to closure.

Later, Marchetti [2] provided an update of his results and a modification of the original proce-dure. He found that elevation and fixation of the bladder neck to the posterior surface of the perios-teum to be critical for success. The procedure was modified to avoid placing stitches through the wall of the urethra. This reduced the incidence of hema-turia and risk of urethral injury. He recommended a "stout bite of the vaginal wall" in a periurethral location. In addition, he stopped placing a drain in seven of his patients.

Operative Technique

Over the years, modifications include foregoing the sutures placed in the anterior bladder wall, the total number of sutures placed, and the type of suture. The basic procedure starts with placing the patient in a low lithotomy position or frog-legged supine on the operating table. The abdomen and vagina should be prepped and a catheter placed to depend-ent drainage. A lower midline or Pfannenstiel inci-sion can be made. The rectus muscle then is split in the midline and the space of Retsius cleared over-lying the urethra and the bladder neck. In patients with previous repair, Webster and Guralnick advo-cate a formal urethrolysis in order to fully mobilize the bladder neck [3].

The surgeon's nondominant hand should be placed in the vagina to assist elevation of the paravaginal tissues adjacent to the bladder neck and urethra. Absorbable (0-chromic) suture or permanent suture (0-Prolene, Ethicon, Somerville, NJ) should be placed first at the bladder neck in a periurethral loca-tion through the anterior vaginal wall (Fig. 11.1). The stitch should be placed approximately 2–3 mm

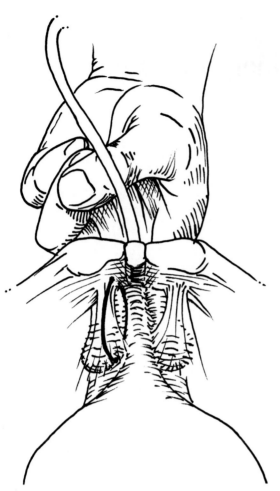

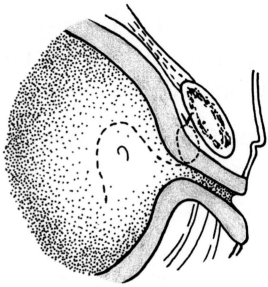

FIG. 11.2. Sagittal section showing support of the bladder neck and urethra following the tying of the sutures to the fibrocartilage of the symphysis pubis. Overelevation of the urethra should be avoided to prevent kinking of the urethra

FIG. 11.1. The first suture is placed in the periurethral tissue at the bladder neck and secured to the periosteum of the symphysis pubis. Elevation of the anterior vaginal wall with the hand may be helpful to determine the appropriate depth for suture placement

away from the urethra in the midline. One or two additional sutures can be placed more distally on either side of midline. Each of these sutures would then be placed into the fibrocartilage of the symphysis pubis (Fig. 11.2). Following tying these sutures, the bladder and urethra then be can inspected cystoscopically to ensure that there is no injury to the urethra or ureters [4]. Care should be taken to recognize and treat any bladder injury during this dissection. Instillation of the bladder with indigo carmine or methylene blue could facilitate identification of an injury. If significant venous bleeding occurs, a figure-eight suture to control the bleeding may be necessary.

Outcomes A meta-analysis by Mainprinze and colleagues showed a wide range of success from 29 to 100% [5]. In their review of 56 articles, they found that some authors worried that failure occurred secondary to use of an absorbable suture and they tried other suture material such as linen, silk, Mersilene (Ethicon, Somerville, NJ), and Tevdek (Teleflex Medical, Research Triangle Park, NC) suture. One surgeon tried placing talc in the wound in an attempt to facilitate scar formation. The overall success rate was 86.1%; however, 11.4% of the patients did not have long-term data to complete analysis. Furthermore, the success rate decreases over time. At 15 years, the overall success rate had decreased to 75% [6].

Clemens et al. [7] noted a more substantial loss in efficacy over time. Using Kaplan–Meier analysis, they estimated the 10- and 15-year cure rates to be 59 and 41%, respectively. The most rapid loss of continence occurred within the first 5 postoperative years. Their initial cure rate was lower at 57%. Czalpicki and colleagues reported on similar decreases in the cure rate over time. They found a reduction of success from 81% at 6 months to a low of 28% at 10 years. Mean duration of continence was approximately 6½ years [8].

In their review of 680 patients, Park and Miller [9] found that the MMK provided a cure in 86% of their 680 patients regardless of suture type (absorbable vs. nonabsorbable). Others have reported success rates from 83 to 100% [10, 11].

Quadri and colleagues studied 30 women randomized to MMK or Burch and found 100% continence in the MMK group and 66% continence in the Burch group. They believed that the use of videourethroscopy during the MMK procedure allowed better control of the tensioning of the sutures, thus leading to their high success rate. Nonetheless, they noted a delay of recovery of spontaneous voiding in some patients. Their average time to spontaneous voiding was 20.5 days (range of 13.4 days) [11].

Successful outcomes also may depend on patient selection. Bladder instability, prolapse, and recurrence of incontinence following a previous surgery could contribute to a poor outcome. Milani et al. reported that surgery was successful in 83% of those with stable bladders but only 38% in those with unstable bladders [12]. Arnold et al. reported similar findings in 1973 [13].

Complications

With the MMK procedure, the complications of concern include osteitis pubis, postoperative urinary retention, and de novo bladder urgency/overactivity. Studies report overall complication rates ranging from 11.4 to 21% [5, 10].

The most worrisome complication is osteitis pubis, which presents as discomfort over the pubis. Coughing and ambulation may worsen the discomfort. Radiographic studies are not always conclusive for osteitis pubis. The reported incidence of osteitis pubis ranged from 3.2 to 10%, with symptoms occurring within 1–8 weeks following surgery [10, 14, 15]. The recommended treatment includes rest, nonsteroidal anti-inflammatory agents, and systemic steroid treatment.

Postoperative urinary retention can be divided into short-term and long-term urinary retention. In Parnell's series [10], 27% of patients had short-term urinary retention with an average duration of retention of 12.2 days. Only 2 of the 158 patients (1.4%) had long-term urinary retention. Carr and Webster reported that approximately 12% of patients undergoing MMK develop chronic urinary retention [16]. The majority of patients notice the symptoms immediately postoperatively. Resolution of the retention was achieved in 86% of patients who underwent a retropubic urethrolysis and 73% of patients who underwent a transvaginal urethrolysis.

Other complications noted in the review by Mainprize and Drutz [5] include direct injuries to the urinary tract: bladder tears (0.7%), urethral obstruction (0.5%), and sutures in either the bladder or urethra (0.1%). Prolonged retention occurred in 3.6%, retroperitoneal hematoma in 0.3%, and fistulae in 0.3%. They reported an overall surgical complication rate of 21%.

Burch Colposuspension

Historical Perspective

In 1961, John C. Burch reported on a modification of the MMK procedure [17]. He had encountered difficulty performing the MMK when the sutures in the periosteum would not hold. He had first tried securing the sutures to the arcus tendineus fascia pelvis with the goal of also treating an anterior and posterior cystocele. Over time he found that this was a poor site to anchor sutures, and he then settled on using Cooper's ligament. He recommended the placement of three sutures of No. 2 chromic catgut to be placed in the paravaginal tissues at the bladder neck and then secured to the appropriate location in the ligament. He reported 100% continence in his first 53 patients.

He then reported on a larger series of 143 patients with 93% continence [18]. Critics complained that this high continence rate might have been secondary to the fact that most patients had the Burch as their first incontinence operation. His preference for chromic catgut remained. He believed the catgut was less likely to be problematic if the bladder was entered and that it would not form a fistula tract if placed through and through in the vagina. Thus, the Burch procedures performed today are based on his initial work.

Operative Technique

The patient can be placed in low lithotomy position with Allen Yellofin® stirrups (Allen Medical Systems, Inc., Acton, MA) or in a frog-legged position on the operating table. Administration of prophylactic antibiotic and use of sequential compression devices to prevent deep venous thrombosis are advised. The abdomen, vagina, and perineum should be prepped. A foley catheter should be placed in a sterile fashion to allow identification of the bladder neck and drain the bladder.

The retropubic space then is reached through a low midline or Pfannesteil incision. The anterior bladder wall and urethra should be freed of overlying fat in order to facilitate identification of the bladder neck junction. Care should be taken during this dissection, as this area is extremely vascular.

Fingers placed in the vagina allow the elevation of the lateral vaginal fornix. Two pairs of sutures of a No. 1 or 0 nonabsorbable monofilament sutures should be placed on the endopelvic fascia and vaginal wall lateral to the bladder neck and proximal urethra (Fig. 11.3). The distal sutures should be placed first at the level proximal urethra, followed by one or two pairs of sutures placed more proximally at the bladder neck. If bleeding occurs during placement of these sutures, additional figure-eight sutures may be necessary. Under most circumstances, hemostasis is accomplished once the sutures are tied to Cooper's ligament.

The sutures then are attached to Cooper's ligament in the position directly above the suture (Fig. 11.4). With all sutures secured to Cooper's

ligament, the sutures are tied to elevate the paraurethral tissue. There should be no compression of the urethra against the pubic bone. A suture bridge between the ligament and the vaginal wall may be present. Once the sutures are tied, cystoscopy with administration of indigo carmine can be performed to rule out ureteral and vesical neck injury.

Prior to closure, a penrose drain or closed suction drain may be placed lateral to the sutures, although this is not required [19]. The authors have not used any drains in the last 15 years and have not had an adverse event. If a drain is used, the drain then can be removed on the first to third day following surgery. A voiding trial can be performed on the first postoperative day, although the average time to voiding reported by McLennan and colleagues was 6.7 days [20]. In our experience, 85% of patients undergoing the Burch procedure have a successful voiding trial during the first 1 or 2 days postprocedure.

Outcomes

Initial success rates for the Burch procedure reported in studies range from 75–90% [21–23]. Long-term outcomes reported by Nithara and colleagues are less positive [24]. Continence in 60 patients was evaluated over a mean period of 6.9 years. Sixty-nine percent of the patients remained continent at long-term follow-up. Galloway [25] also reported deterioration of continence over time. While 84% of patients in his study were dry immediately following surgery, only 44% were dry at mean follow-up of 4.5 years. Furthermore, Galloway showed individuals who had previous incontinence surgery had a lower success rate (63%).

In contrast, Feyereisl and colleagues [23] noted that success was not diminished by previous surgical procedures for incontinence. They found that

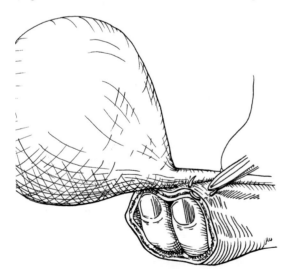

FIG. 11.3. Burch sutures should be placed lateral to the bladder in the area of the vaginal fornix. Locating the vaginal fornix can be facilitated by elevation of the anterior vaginal wall

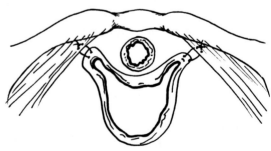

FIG. 11.4. Burch sutures elevate and support the urethra

continence was maintained in 81.6% of the women 5–10 years after a Burch procedure. In a Cochrane Library database review of 33 trials by Lapitan and colleagues [26], the overall cure rate of those studies ranged from 68.9 to 88%. They found a slight decrease in the success rate to 70% at 5 years. Alcalay et al. demonstrated that the decline in the cure rate stabilized at 69% at 10–12 years [22].

Sand and colleagues [27] suggested patients with a low preoperative urethral closure pressure (UCP) were more likely to fail. They found the failure rate to be 54% in those with a UCP less than 20 cm of H_2O, while those with a UCP greater than 20 cm of H_2O had a lower failure rate of 18%. Earlier work by McGuire [28] and Hilton and Stanton [29] had suggested that patients who have failed multiple anti-incontinence procedures in the past are likely to have lower urethra closure pressures. Koonings et al. [30] also found a lower cure rate in those with low urethral pressure versus those with normal urethral pressures (50% vs. 77%).

The number of sutures may affect outcome. In a study by Ladwig et al. [31], the Burch procedure was modified to allow use of only one pair of sutures in 86% of 374 patients. Subjective cure rates ranged from 39.7 to 50%, depending on the severity of the incontinence. Results of this study suggest that placement of additional sutures may affect long-term outcomes. However, approximately 30% of the patients in Ladwig's study had at least one previous failed anti-incontinence procedure.

Complications

Postoperative complications of the Burch procedure include voiding dysfunction, de novo urge, and pelvic organ prolapse, in particular enteroceles. The duration of catheterization can range from 1 to 12 days. Kjølhede and Ryden reported that 8.8% of Burch procedure patients had an in-dwelling catheter longer than 2 weeks [32]. In the study with Nitihara et al. 90% of their patients were able to void 5 days following surgery [24], while mean time to resumption of voiding following a Burch procedure was 6.5 days in a study by Quadri et al. [11].

In one long-term study, a 16% incidence of de novo urge resulted in patient dissatisfaction with surgery despite the correction of the anatomy [24]. Other studies estimate the incidence of de novo urgency at 6–27% [33, 34]. Gleason et al. [35] reported the development of urgency in 50% of patients; however, their procedure had been modified to include a cystotomy to aid determination of suture tension. Anticholinergics were helpful but were given judiciously in order to avoid development of urinary retention.

In his series of 143 cases, Burch reported the development of a postoperative enterocele in 7.6% of cases [18]. Galloway reported enterocele formation in 2 of 50 (4%) patients and uterine prolapse in 2 of 50 (4%) patients [25]. Others report an incidence of enterocele formation at between 2 and 27% [4].

Laparoscopic Retropubic Suspensions

Laparoscopic retropubic urethropexies were introduced by Vancaillie and Schuessler [36] as a minimally invasive option for management of stress urinary incontinence. Many variations of the technique have been tried including use of staples and mesh, staples and suture, gasless laparoscopy, and different numbers of sutures.

Most of the laparoscopic studies have reported success in the range of 69–100%, with decreases in length of stay, intra-operative blood loss, less de novo urgency, and postoperative voiding dysfunction [37]. However, in most of the studies the mean operative time was increased in comparison to the open technique.

Liu et al. [38] published a study of 132 patients that demonstrated a 97% cure rate and a 10% complication rate (follow-up ranged from 3 to 27 months). The complications experienced included four bladder injuries and one uretheral obstruction. In the beginning of his series, Liu had performed the laparoscopic Burch procedure with one suture per side, but he eventually switched to two sutures per side [39]. He had concerns as to whether one set of sutures was sufficient in the long term.

Moehrer et al. [40] performed a meta-analysis of four randomized clinical trials in the Cochrane Incontinence Review Group's database and demonstrated no difference in outcomes between open and laparoscopic Burch procedure. Subjective perception of cure was equivalent between the laparoscopic and open Burch groups. When the success rate was evaluated on the basis of urodynamic testing, the cure rate was lower in the laparoscopic Burch group.

Although operating time was longer, the laparoscopic Burch procedure patients experienced less postoperative pain, shorter length of stay in the hospital, and time to return to normal function was shortened [40]. However, the complication rate with the laparoscopic procedure was found be higher and was related to surgeon experience. The major intraoperative and short-term complications included bladder and bowel injury in 0–25% [37]. The most common injury was bladder perforation and the incidence decreased with increasing experience. Two cases of foreign body erosions have been reported following the use of tacks and mesh to assist the laparoscopic procedure [41].

While initial results for the laparoscopic procedure have been good, few studies have reported on long-term follow-up. At the 3 years following initial surgery, the percentage of cured patients ranged from 40 to 60% [42]. McDougall and colleagues showed even further deterioration in success at 4 years to 30% [43]. In contrast, a study by Ross did not demonstrate deterioration in efficacy at 5 years [44].

Pubovaginal Sling

Historical Perspective

Von Giordano introduced the first urethral sling by wrapping a gracilis muscle graft around the urethra in 1907 [45]. The first true pubovaginal sling was performed in 1910, when Goebell rotated the pyramidalis muscle beneath the urethra and joined them in the midline [46]. Aldridge further modified the technique by suturing two strips of fascia beneath the urethra [47].

In 1978, McGuire and Lytton popularized the modern autologous fascial sling with the use of rectus fascia [48]. Since then, there have been many adaptations to the sling, including changing the type of sling material (Table 11.1), as well as the use of bone anchors to secure the sling in position.

Operative Technique

Prior to the procedure, patients can be taught intermittent self-catherization. However, if they are physically unable to catherize themselves, a suprapubic tube can be placed at the time of surgery in order to facilitate checking their postvoid residuals following surgery. Perioperative antibiot-

TABLE 11.1. Pubovaginal sling material options.

Material	Source
Autologous	Rectus fascia, fascia lata, vaginal wall
Allogenic	Cadaveric fascia lata, cadaveric dermis
Xenografts	Porcine dermis, porcine intestinal submucosa
Synthetics	Polyester, Gore-tex, silicone, polypropylene, polytetrafluoroethylene

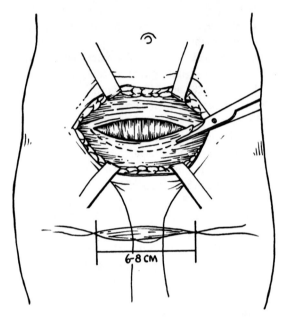

FIG. 11.5. The rectus fascial strip measuring 6–8 cm can be harvested from the lower leaf of the rectus fascia

ics and prophylaxis for deep venous thrombosis should be utilized. The patient should be placed in the lithotomy position and a foley catheter placed to drain the bladder.

A combined abdominal and vaginal approach can be used. A low transverse midline incision can be made and dissection carried down to the rectus fascia. The rectus fascia then is cut transversely and freed inferiorly from the attachments to the muscle below in a cephalad and caudad manner. A strip of rectus fascia measuring 1.5 cm in width by 6–8 cm in length can be harvested (Fig. 11.5) [49]. Additional lengths of fascia have been utilized. Blaivas [50] advocates the use of a full-length rectus fascia sling (15 cm), while others have used much shorter "patch" slings [51, 52]. The ends of the sling then are prepared for transfer with placement

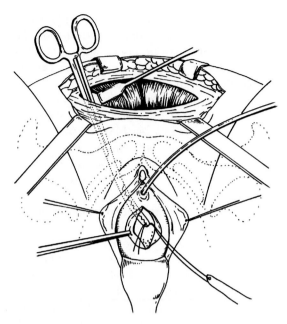

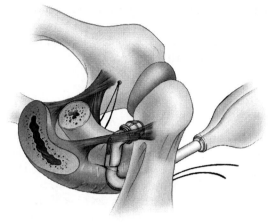

FIG. 11.7. In-Fast™ Ultra Sling System anchoring system for placement of cadaveric transvaginal sling. The bone anchors are placed into the pubic bone. Image courtesy of American Medical System, Minnetonka, MN

FIG. 11.6. The Crawford clamp is passed from the abdominal incision through the endopelvic fascia to the vaginal incision below

of a 0-Vicryl suture (Ethicon, Somerville, NJ) in a helical fashion.

A midline incision should be made in the anterior vaginal wall at the level of the bladder neck. Hydrodissection of the anterior vaginal wall can be done to facilitate the dissection. The dissection of the anterior vaginal wall is completed laterally on both sides up to the level of the endopelvic fascia. Using a sharp and blunt dissection, a Crawford clamp is passed from the abdominal incision below the rectus fascia to the tunnel in the anterior vaginal wall (Fig. 11.6). Cystoscopy with a 70° lens then should be performed to check for bladder perforation once both clamps have been passed. Typically, the injury occurs at the 1 o'clock and 11 o'clock position within the bladder. If an injury has occurred, the clamp should be removed and repassed. The foley catheter should be left in place for a longer period if perforation should occur. A larger injury may require formal closure.

If both clamps are in position, the sling sutures then can be grasped and pulled upward to the abdominal incision from the vaginal incision. The sling can be secured in position at the bladder neck using 2–0 Vicryl (Ethicon, Somerville, NJ) suture. Care should be taken to ensure that both ends of the sling pass through the endopelvic fascia [53]. The sling sutures then should be passed under the

lower leaf of the rectus fascia. The rectus fascia then should be closed before tying the sutures in the midline over the fascia. The sutures should be tied with enough to tension to stabilize the urethra but still allow easy passage of two fingers under the suture.

Wright and colleagues [54] recommend checking sling tension by placing a cystoscope in the urethra. The sling should be tied such that 30° rotational descent of the scope is still possible. Govier et al. [55] recommend easy placement of one finger under the sling suture. The urethra should be able to move approximately 1 cm with traction on the foley. Ghoniem [56] advocates adjusting the sling using the Q-tip method.

The abdominal and vaginal incisions are then closed. A vaginal pack can be left in place and the catheter allowed to dependently drain. A voiding trial can be performed the following day as long as the patient is ambulatory.

Alternatively, the procedure can be performed through a vaginal approach alone using the cadaveric transvaginal sling (CaTS) technique popularized by Kobashi and Leach [45]. This alternative technique allows placement of the sling with only a vaginal incision. An inverted U-shaped incision is made in the anterior vaginal wall from the distal urethra to the bladder neck. The pubic bone is then exposed lateral to the urethra and the inferior surface of the bone cleared of tissue. Bone anchors are then placed transvaginally into the under surface of the pubic bone (Fig. 11.7). The 0-Prolene sutures (Ethicon, Somerville, NJ) then are passed through the ends of a prepared cadaveric strip of fascia (2 × 7 cm). The sling should be tied with a right angle between the urethra and the sling. The urethral incision then is closed and a vaginal pack placed.

Outcomes

Autologous Slings

In McGuire and Lytton's paper, 80% of the 52 patients were cured and 20 of 29 (67%) patients had their detrussor instability resolved [57]. This was updated further by Morgan et al., who reviewed their 4-year experience with 247 women [58]. Overall continence rate was 88% at a mean follow-up of 51 months. Patients with type 2 (abdominal leak point pressure greater than 90 cm H_2O and urethral mobility greater than 2 cm) stress incontinence had a higher success rate (91%) than patients with type 3 (abdominal leak point pressure less than 90 cm H_2O) stress urinary incontinence (84%). In the 88 patients with at least 5 years of follow-up, 85% were still continent. Eighty-one of the 109 (74%) patients with preoperative urge incontinence had resolution of their urge symptoms.

Chaikin et al. reported excellent long-term results as well [50]. One year following surgery, 94% of their patients were cured of their stress urinary incontinence, and at 10 years, 95% of their patients remained continent. Most of the failures were secondary to persistent urge symptoms. De novo urge incontinence occurred in 3%. The patients who had persistent stress incontinence despite surgical treatment were found to have a fixed pipe-stem urethra.

Others have seen similar results with 94 to 97% of patients cured of their stress urinary incontinence and urgency resolved in two thirds of patients with OAB [59, 60]. De novo urgency rates were reported at 2–12%.

Allograft/Synthetic Material

Cure rates for stress urinary incontinence in studies using cadaveric allograft are comparable to autograft. In a study by Wright et al. [61], 92 patients were followed for 11.5 months. Fifty-nine patients received allograft fascia lata and 33% received autograft. The success rate was 93% for the autograft group and 93% for the allograft group. Mean duration of suprapubic tube placement was equivalent: 12 days for the autograft and 11 days for the allograft. Flynn and Yap [62] presented additional data to support the equivalence of cadaveric fascia lata to autograft fascia at 2-year follow-up. Seventy-one percent of the allograft group was cured, while 77% of the autograft group was cured. The majority of failures presented at 2 to 3 years following initial surgery. Brown and Govier [63] reported similar outcomes for 104 patients who underwent pub-ovaginal slings with cadaveric fascia lata versus autologous fascia lata. Eighty-five percent of the cadaveric fascia group was cured of stress incontinence, while 90% of the autologous fascia group was cured.

Other groups have cautioned against the use of allograft material due to issues of durability. Fitzgerald and colleagues [64] reported on 7 of 35 patients who autolyzed their sling within 6 months of surgery. Carbone et al. [65] raised similar concerns about the longevity of allograft material. In their study of 154 patients who underwent pubovaginal sling with cadaveric fascia lata and bone anchors, 40% of the patients developed recurrent stress urinary incontinence. Most of these failures occurred within the first 10 months postprocedure.

Cure rates for synthetic slings range from 77 to 90%, with mean follow-up duration of 4–8 years [66]. Erosions into the vagina and into the urethra remain concerns with using synthetic materials [67].

Complications

The pubovaginal sling has not been popular despite the high success rate. This may be due to the higher risk of complications in comparison to other alternatives for management of stress urinary incontinence. Most of the issues arise from tensioning the sling too tightly, which is more likely to occur with a new practitioner of the technique. Possible problems that could arise include retention, de novo urge incontinence, and erosion, particularly with the use of synthetic slings [50].

Postoperative urinary retention is the most common complication following placement of pubovaginal slings. The retention is likely to resolve within the first month postoperatively; however, if retention has not resolved during this period, it is unlikely to do so. The risk for retention ranges from 0 to 17% [49].

Morgan and colleagues [58] reported that 94% of their patients experienced transient urinary retention. Mean duration of catherization was 8.4 days. Within 1 month of their operation, 92% of the patients had returned to normal voiding. Five patients had voiding difficulty secondary to urethral hypersuspension, which resolved following urethrolysis. No sling erosions were reported.

Zaragosa [60] reported that 60% of his patients developed transient urinary retention. All patients who developed urinary retention subsequently were able to void within 10 days. Chaikin et al. [50] reported permanent urinary retention in four patients in a series of 251. Two of the four had concomitant prolapse repairs.

Rates of de novo urge have ranged from 5 to 11% [50, 60, 68]. A trial of anticholinergics, either single or combination, can be attempted. If urgency is persistent, outlet obstruction secondary to the sling should be ruled out. However, if the urgency has been present for a long duration, the symptoms are unlikely to resolve even with treatment of the obstruction. In a refractory situation, a trial of sacral neuromodulation can be attempted.

There have been many synthetic materials on the market: polypropylene, nylon, silicone, polyglactin, and polytetrafluoroethylene. The American Urological Association guidelines in 1997 reported 0.007% vaginal or urethral erosions with autologous fascial slings and 0.027% erosion rate with synthetic slings [67]. The erosion rates (vagina and urethra) are highest for silicone, polytetrafluroethylene, and polyester; these rates range from 11 to 55% [69–71]. The bovine collagen-impregnated woven polyester mesh sling ProtoGen™ (Boston Scientific, Natick, MA) subsequently was taken off the market in 1999 due to its high erosion rate. The erosions typically occurred within the first year of placement, but they can occur up to 7 years following initial surgery. Average time to erosion was 7.3 months [72, 73]. Many erosions presented as recurrent urinary tract infections, obstructive voiding symptoms, vaginal pain or pressure, suprapubic pain, and recurrent stress urinary incontinence. Factors that may increase the risk of urethral erosion include poor vascularity secondary to estrogen deficiency or previous radiation treatment, excessive tension at time of surgery, traumatic catherization, and forceful urethral dilation [74]. A transvaginal approach can be utilized

to remove the eroded sling. If the sling eroded into the urethra, synthetic material should be removed as completely as possible, followed by debridment of the urethral edges and closure in multiple layers. A Martius labial fat pad graft can be placed to bolster the repair. Both Kobashi et al. and Amundsen et al. recommend delayed sling placement to manage recurrent SUI [75, 76].

Artificial Urinary Sphincters

Historical Perspective

The first artificial urinary sphincter (AS-721) was placed in 1973 by Scott and colleagues [77]. The device (Fig. 11.8, see also Chap. 29) had four components: a fluid reservoir, an inflatable cuff, an inflation pump, and a deflation pump. In order to

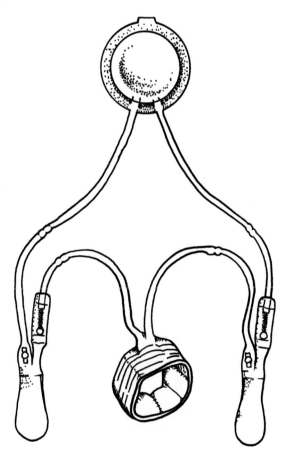

FIG. 11.8. First artificial urinary sphincter (AS-721) had four components: reservoir, reinflation pump, cuff, and deflation pump (clockwise from the top)

void, patients would squeeze the deflation pump on the left side. The fluid then would run back into the reservoir. When they were done voiding, the right-sided inflation pump then was squeezed to return fluid back to the cuff from the reservoir. There was a valve in the system that would regulate the pressure in the cuff. Failures of the device tended to occur at this valve [78]. The subsequent modifications of the device revolved around replacing the valve with a pressure balloon and changing the cuff material to an all-silicone elastomer [79].

The AMS-800 (Fig. 11.9) was introduced in 1982, with three components: a cuff, a pressure-regulating balloon, and a pump. The pump consists of a valve, a refill-delay resistor, and a deactivation button. The refill-delay resistor enables the cuff to refill automatically in approximately 2 min, allowing the patient adequate time to finish voiding. After 1987, the narrow backing cuff was introduced to allow more even distribution of pressure across the urethra, increasing the durability of the device.

While popular in men with postprostatectomy stress urinary incontinence, the use of artificial urinary sphincters (AUS) in women has not been as popular. This may be due in part to the technical challenge related to the scarring created by

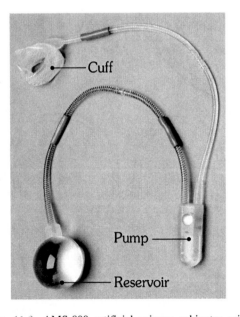

FIG. 11.9. AMS-800 artificial urinary sphincter with cuff, pressure-regulating balloon reservoir, and pump. The pump contains a refill-delay resistor, which allows automatic refilling of the cuff

previous attempts at anti-incontinence procedures and the availability of sling options with less risk. However, the AUS still should be considered for a woman with stress incontinence who has failed sling surgery.

Operative Technique

The patient should receive preoperative broad-spectrum antibiotics, such as ampicillin/vancomycin and gentamicin. The patient should be positioned in low lithotomy or frog-legged position to allow access to the vagina and urethra. The abdomen, perineum, and vagina should be prepped and draped in a sterile fashion.

In women, the cuff of sphincter is placed at the bladder neck. Two approaches are possible: abdominal and transvaginal [80, 81]. In either approach, the artificial sphincter is left deactivated at the end of the case. The artificial sphincter is activated 6 weeks following surgery.

In the retropubic approach, a Pfannensteil incision is made and a plane is developed in the space of Retsius to expose the bladder neck. The dissection is often difficult in the midline if the patient has undergone previous incontinence surgery. In this situation, the dissection can begin in the lateral perivesical space where there is less scar tissue and continued medially until the adhesions in the midline are taken down sharply. A modified right-angle clamp is placed in the urethrovaginal septum to separate the bladder neck and urethra from the vagina (Fig. 11.10). A hand in the vagina during this dissection can be helpful. If there is difficulty in identifying the vesicourethrovaginal junction, a midline cystotomy can be made [82]. A 2-cm area should be cleared at the bladder neck to allow placement of the cuff. Once the cuff is placed, the cuff tubing then is advanced through the rectus muscle and anterior rectus fascia to a location close to the internal inguinal ring. The pump then is placed in a subcutaneous pocket in the labia. The reservoir then is placed in the prevesical space, underneath the rectus fascia (Fig. 11.11). All connections then are made.

Alternatively, Hadley [83] and Appell [81] suggest that approaching cuff placement around the bladder neck transvaginally may be technically easier. An inverted U-shaped incision should be made in the anterior vaginal wall. Dissections then should be continued laterally to the endopelvic

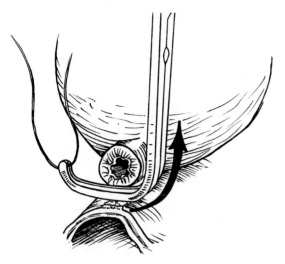

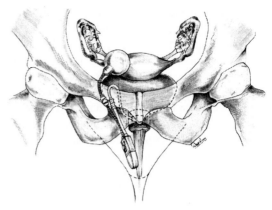

FIG. 11.11. The reservoir for the AMS 800 is placed under rectus fascia. The pump is placed in the labium majora

FIG. 11.10. Placement of a modified right-angle clamp to facilitate dissection of the posterior wall of the urethra from the anterior vaginal wall. Placement of a nondominant hand in the vagina also could assist dissection in this plane

fascia on both sides of the urethra. The endopelvic fascia is penetrated laterally and the retropubic space entered. The anterior wall of the urethra then is mobilized sharply off of the posterior aspect of the pubic bone. Following completion of this dissection, the bladder neck is sized and the appropriate cuff placed. A limited Pfannenstiel incision then is made to place the reservoir under the rectus fascia. The tubing from the cuff then is passed from the vaginal incision to the abdominal incision using a tonsil clamp. The subcutaneous tunnel to the labia from the abdominal incision then is made to place the pump. All the tubing is connected. The incisions are all closed and a vaginal pack with estrogen cream can be placed.

Outcomes

Appell [81] reported that in his 34 patients undergoing the transvaginal technique 91% of his patients were dry when the device was originally placed. The remaining three patients were dry after revisions for mechanical issues. Others report an 81–92% continence rate [84, 85]. Petero and Diokno [86] reported 84% satisfactory continence rate with their long-term review of 55 women who had received artificial sphincters. Thirty-five (64%) of the women were completely dry. Interestingly, nine of the women were dry without activation of the device. With a mean follow-up of 8.1 years, 56% of the women

eventually required revisions. The revisions were mechanical in approximately half the cases. The remaining revisions were secondary to nonmechanical failure (cuff erosion, loose/tight cuff, infection, pain, reservoir migration, insufficient pressure in reservoir) and iatrogenic issues (prolonged catherization leading to erosions).

Webster and colleagues [87] also published their long-term data on 25 women with artificial sphincters. Ninety-two percent had marked improved of their incontinence with use of no pads. Four (17%) of the patients have had an average of two revisions in 7–8 years following initial placement of AUS. They had noticed that none of the revisions had occurred after 1983, when a modification had been made to the design of the cuff.

In terms of pregnancy with AUS, Fishman and Scott [88] reported that delivery can occur safely even if the cuff is not deactivated. They published a series of seven women who underwent five vaginal deliveries and four cesarean sections. All the devices were functioning postpartum. Toh and Diokno recommend deactivation of the artificial urinary sphincter in order to minimize the risk for cuff erosion following labor [89].

Summary

Open retropubic suspensions (MMK and Burch) have excellent outcomes both short and long term. The MMK does have a higher incidence of voiding dysfunction in comparison to the Burch procedure. Both techniques require experience in tensioning the sutures to avoid producing an overcorrection of the urethral position and subsequent voiding dysfunction. Both techniques may be less successful in the situation of low UCPs (<20 cm H_2O). In this situation, pubovaginal slings may be more versatile. Pubovaginal slings can be used to manage both hypermobility and intrinsic sphincter deficiency.

For the patient with the fixed pipe-stem urethra, AUS may be most helpful. Of all four open surgical procedures for stress incontinence, artificial sphincters require the most experience to place in women. Most of the women presenting for AUS placement have failed several anti-incontinence procedures, making periurethral dissection for cuff placement challenging.

Both the introduction of tension-free vaginal tape (TVT) in 1996 by Ulmsten and the transobturator tape (TO) in 2003 by De Lorme have dramatically changed the treatment of stress incontinence. Both procedures are minimally invasive and adjustable. The ability to loosen the sling within the first postoperative week and to quickly resolve retention has reduced dramatically the morbidity of incontinence surgery. As more data become available regarding the long-term efficacy of TVT and TO, the role of the open procedures in the management of stress urinary incontinence will continue to evolve.

References

1. Marshall V, Marchetti, A, Krantz K. The correction of stress incontinence by simple vesicourethral suspension. Surg Gynec Obstet 1949; 88:509–518.
2. Marchetti A. The female bladder and urethra before and after correction for stress incontinence. Am J Obstet Gynec 1949; 58:1145–1154.
3. Webster G, Guralnick M. Retropubic suspension surgery for female incontinence. In: Walsh PC, Retik AB, Vaughn ED, et al., eds. Campbell's urology, 8th edition. Philadelphia: Saunders 2002:1140–1150.
4. Alcalay M, Stanton J. Retropubic suspensions. In: Stanton S, Zimmern P, eds. Female pelvic reconstructive surgery. London: Springer, 2003:83–107.
5. Mainprize TC, Drutz HP. The Marshall–Marchetti–Krantz procedure: A critical review. Obstet Gynecol Surg 1988; 43:724–729.
6. McDuffie RW, Litin RB, Blundon KE. Urethrovesical suspension(Marshall–Marchetti–Krantz):Experience with 204 cases. Am J Surg 1981; 141: 297–298.
7. Clemens JQ, Stern JA, Bushman WA, et al. Long-term results of the stamey bladder neck suspension:

8. Czaplicki M, Dobroński P, Torz C, et al. Long-term subjective results of Marshall–Marchetti–Krantz procedure. Eur Urol 1998; 34:118–123.
9. Park GS, Miller EJ. Surgical treatment of stress urinary incontinence: A comparison of the Kelly plication, Marshall–Marchetti–Krantz, and Pereyra procedure. Obstet Gynecol 1998; 71:575–579.
10. Parnell JP, Marshall Vh, Vaughan, ED. Primary management of urinary stress incontinence by the Marshall–Marchetti–Krantz vesicourethropexy. J Urol 1982; 127:679–682.
11. Quadri G, Magatti, F, Belloni C, Barisani D, Natale N.Marshall–Marchetti–Krantz urethropexy and Burch colposuspension for stress urinary incontinence in women with low pressure and hypermobility of the urethra: Early results of a prospective randomized clinical trial. Am J Obstet Gynecol 1999; 181:12–18.
12. Milani R, Scalambrino S, Quadri G, Algeri M, Marchesin R. Marshall–Marchetti–Krantz procedure and Burch colposuspension in the surgical treatment of female urinary incontinence. Br J Obstet Gynecol 1985; 92:1050–1053.
13. Arnold EP, Webster JR, Loose H, Brown AD, et al. Urodynamics of female incontinence: Factors influencing the results of surgery. Am J Obstet Gynecol 1973; 117:805–813.
14. Zorzos I, Paterson PJ. Quality of life after a Marshall–Marchetti–Krantz procedure for stress urinary incontinence. J Urol 1996; 155:259–262.
15. Lee RA, Symmonds RE, Goldstein RA. Surgical complications and results of modified Marshall–Marchetti–Krantz procedure for urinary incontinence. Obstet Gynecol 1979; 53:447–450.
16. Carr LK, Webster GD. Voiding dysfunction following incontinence surgery: Diagnosis and treatment with retropubic or vaginal urethrolysis. J Urol 1197; 157:821–823.
17. Burch JC. Urethrovaginal fixation to Cooper's ligament for correction of stress incontinence, cystocele and prolapse. Am J Obstet Gynecol 1961; 81:281–290.
18. Burch JC. Cooper's ligament urethrovesical suspension for stress incontinence. Am J Obstet Gynecol 1968; 764–774.
19. Tanagho EM. Colpocystourethropexy: The way we do it. J Urol 1976; 116:751–753.
20. McLennan MT, Bent AE. Fascia lata suburethral sling vs. Burch retropubic urethropexy: A comparison of morbidity. J Reprod Med 1998; 43:488–494.
21. Columbo M, Scalambrino S, Maggioni A, et al. Burch colposuspension versus modified Marshall–

Marchetti–Krantz urethropexy for primary genuine stress urinary incontinence: A prospective, randomized trial. Am J Obstet Gynecol 171:1573–1579.

22. Alcalay M, Monga A, Stanton SL. Burch colposuspension: A 10–20 year follow up. Br J Obstet Gynaecol 1995; 102:740–745.

23. Feyereisl J, Dreher E, Haenggi W, et al. Long-term results after Burch colposuspension. Am J Obstet Gynecol 1994; 171:647–652.

24. Nitahara KS, Aboseif S, Tanagho EA. Long-term results of coplocystourethropexy for persistent or recurrent stress incontinence. J Urol 1999; 162: 138–141.

25. Galloway NTM, Davies N, Stephenson TP. The complications of colposuspension. Br J Urol 1987; 60–122–124.

26. Lapitan MC, Cody DJ, Grant AM.Open retropubic suspension for urinary incontinence in women. Cochrane Database Syst Rev 2003; 1:CD002912.

27. Sand PK, Bowen LW, Panganiban R, et al. The low pressure urethra as a factor in failed retropubic urethropexy. Obstet Gynecol 1987; 69:399–402.

28. McGuire EJ. Urodynamic findings in patients after failure of stress incontinence operations. Prog Clin Biol Res 1981; 78:351–360.

29. Hilton P, Stanton SL. Urethral pressure measurement by microtransducer: The results in symptom-free women and in those with genuine stress incontinence. Br J Obstet Gynaecol 1983; 90: 919–933.

30. Koonings PP, Bergman A, Ballard CA. Low urethral pressure and stress urinary incontinence in women: Risk factor for failed retropubic surgical procedures. Urology 1990; 36:245–248.

31. Ladwig D, Milkjkovic-Petrovic L, Hewson AD. Simplified colposuspension: A 15-year follow-up. Aust N Z J Obstet Gynaecol 2004; 44:39–45.

32. Kjølde P, Ryden G. Prognostic factors and long-term results of the Burch colposuspension: A retrospective study. Acta Obstet Gynecol Scand 1994; 73:642–647.

33. Langer R, Ron-El R, Newman M, et al. Detrusor instability following colposuspension for urinary stress incontinence. Br J Obstet Gynecol 1988; 95:607–610.

34. Lose G, Jorgensen L, Mortensen SO, et al. Voiding difficulties after colposuspension. Obstet Gynecol 1987; 69:33–38.

35. Gleason DM, Reilly RJ, Pierce JA. Vesical neck suspension under vision with cystotomy enhances treatment of female incontinence. J Urol 1976; 115:555–557

36. Vancaillie TG, Schuessler W. Laparoscopic bladder neck suspension. J Laparoendosc Surg 1:169–173.

37. Paraiso MF, Walters MD. Laparoscopic surgery for stress urinary incontinence and pelvic organ prolapse. Clin Obstet Gynecol 2005; 48:724–736.

38. Liu CY. Laparoscopic treatment of genuine urinary stress incontinence. Clin Obstet Gynecol 1994; 8:789–798.

39. Lui CY. Laparoscopic retropubic colposuspension (Burch procedure): A review of 58 cases. J Reprod Med 1993; 38:526–530.

40. Moehrer B, Carey M, Wilson D. Laparoscopic colposuspension: A systematic review. Br J Obstet Gynaecol 2003; 110:230–235.

41. Kenton K, Fitzgerald MP, Brubaker L. Multiple foreign body erosions after laparoscopic colposuspension with mesh. Am J Obstet Gynecol 2002; 157:252–253.

42. Winfield HN. Laparoscopic bladder neck suspensions. In: Stanton Sl, Zimmern PE, eds.Female pelvic reconstructive surgery. London: Springer, 2003: 101–107.

43. McDougall EM, Heidorn CA, Portis AJ, et al. Laparoscopic bladder neck suspension fails the test of time. J Urol 1999; 162:2078–2081.

44. Ross J. Laparoscopy or open Burch colposuspension. Curr Opin Obstet Gynecol 1998; 10:405–409.

45. Kobashi KC, Leach GE. Fascial slings. In: Stanton Sl, Zimmern PE, eds. Female pelvic reconstructive surgery. London: Springer, 2003:93–101.

46. Wilson TS, Lemack GE, Zimmern PE. Management of intrinsic sphincteric deficiency in women. J Urol 2003; 169:1662–1669.

47. Aldridge AH. Transplantation of fascia for relief of urinary stress incontinence. Am J Obstet Gynecol 1942; 44:398–411.

48. McGuire EJ, Lytton B. Pubovaginal sling procedure for stress incontinence. J Urol 1978; 119:82–84.

49. McGuireEJ, Clemens JQ. Pubovaginal slings. In: Walsh PC, Retik AB, Vaughn ED, et-al., eds. Campbell's urology, 8th edn. Philadelphia: Saunders 2002:1140–1150.

50. Chaikin DC, Rosenthal J, Blaivas JG. Pubovaginal fascial sling for all types of stress urinary incontinence: Long-term analysis. J Urol 1998; 167:1312–1316.

51. Chopra A, Raz S, Stothers L. Technique of rectangular fascial slings. In: Raz S, editor. Female urology. New York: Springer, 1995:392–394.

52. Karram MM, Bhatia NN. Patch procedure: Modified transvaginal fascia lata sling for recurrent or severe stress urinary incontinence. Obstet Gynecol 1990; 75:461–463.

53. McGuireEJ, Clemens JQ. Pubovaginal slings. In: Walsh PC, Retie AB, Vaughn ED, et al., eds. Campbell's urology, 8th edn. Philadelphia: Saunders 2002:1140–1150.

54. Wright EJ, Iselin CE, Carr LK, et al. Pubovaginal sling using cadaveric allograft fascia for the treatment of intrinsic sphincter deficiency. J Urol 1998; 160:759–762.

55. Govier Fe, Gibbons RP, Correa RJ, et al. Pubovaginal slings using fascia lata for the treatment of intrinsic sphincter deficiency. J Urol 1997; 157:117–121.

56. Ghoniem GM. Modified rectus fascia suburethral sling. Tech Urol 1996; 2:16–21.

57. McGuire EJ, Lytton B. Pubovaginal sling procedure for stress incontinence. J Urol 1978; 119:82–84.

58. Morgan TO, Westney OL, McGuire EJ. Pubovaginal sling: 4-year outcome analysis and quality of life assessment. J Urol 2000; 163:1845–1848.

59. Fulford SC, Flynn R, Barrington J, et al. An assessment of the surgical outcome of urodynamic effects of the pubovaginal sling for stress incontinence and the associated urge symptoms. 1999; 1:135–137.

60. Zaragosa MR. Expanded indications for the pubovaginal sling: treatment of type 2 or 3 stress urinary incontinence. J Urol 1996; 156:1620–1622.

61. Wright JE, Iseling CE, Carr LK, et al. Vaginal sling using cadaveric allograft fascia for the treatment of intrinsic sphincter deficiency. J Urol 1998; 759–762.

62. Flynn BJ, Yap WT. Pubovaginal sling using allograft fascia late versus autograft fascia for all types of stress urinary incontinence: 2-year minimum follow-up. J Urol 2002; 167:608–612.

63. Brown S, Govier F. Cadaveric versus autologous fascia lata for the pubovaginal sling: Surgical outcome and patient satisfaction. J Urol 2000; 164:1633–1637.

64. Fitzgerald MP, Mollenhauer J, Brubaker. Failure of allograft suburethral slings. BJU Int 1999; 84:785–788.

65. Carbone JM, Kavaler E, Hu JC, Raz, S. Pubovaginal sling using cadaveric fascia and bone anchors: Disappointing early results. J Urol 2001; 165:1605–1611.

66. Choe JM, Ogan K, Battino BS. Antimicrobial mesh versus vaginal wall sling: A comparative outcomes analysis. J Urol 2000; 163:1829–1834.

67. Leach GE, Dmochowski RR, Appell RA, et al. Female stress urinary incontinence clinical guidelines panel summary report on surgical management of female stress urinary incontinence. J Urol 1997; 158:875–880.

68. Carr LK, Walsh PJ, Abraham VE, et al. Favorable outcome of pubovaginal slings for geriatric women with stress incontinence. J Urol 1997; 157:125–128.

69. Chin YK, Stanton SL. A follow-up of silastic sling for genuine stress urinary incontinence. Br J Obstet Gynaecol 1195; 102:143–147.

70. Leach GE, Kobashi KC, Mee SL, et al. Erosion of women's polyester synthetic sling ("ProtoGen") pubovaginal sling. J Urol 1999; 161:106, abstract 400

71. Bent AE, Ostergard DR, Zwick-Zaffuto M. Tissue reaction to expanded polytetrafluoroethylene suburethral sling for urinary incontinence: Clinical and histological study. Am J Obstet Gynecol 1993; 169:1198–2004.

72. Ahmed MM, Hai MA, Ibrahim SA, et al. Outcomes following polypropylene mesh pubovaginal slings for stress urinary incontinence. J Urol Suppl 1999; 162:2070, abstract 397.

73. Kobashi KC, Dmochowski R, Mee SL, et al. Erosion of woven polyester pubovaginal sling. J Urol 1999; 162:2070–2072.

74. Amundsen CL, Flynn BJ, Webster GD. Urethral erosions after synthetic and nonsynthetic pubovaginal slings: Difference in management and continence outcome. J Urol 2003; 170:134–137.

75. Amundsen CL, Flynn BJ, Webster GD. Urethral erosions after synthetic and nonsynthetic pubovaginal slings: Difference in management and continence outcome. J Urol 2003; 170:134–137

76. Kobashi KC, Dmochowski R, Mee SL, et al. Erosion of woven polyester pubovaginal sling. J Urol 1999; 162:2070–2072.

77. Scott FB, Bradley WE, Timm GW. Treatment of urinary incontinence by an implantable prosthetic sphincter. J Urol 1974; 112:75–80, discussion 1130.

78. Seigel SW. History of the prosthetic treatment of urinary incontinence. Urol Clin North Am 1989; 16:99–104.

79. Scott BF. The artificial urinary sphincter: Experience in adults. Urol Clin North Am 1989; 16:105–117.

80. Abbassian A. A new operation for the insertion of the artificial urinary sphincter. J Urol 1988; 140:512–513.

81. Appell RA. Techniques and results in the implantation of the artificial urinary sphincter in women with type III stress urinary incontinence by vaginal approach. Neurourol Urodyn 1988; 7:613–619.

82. Salisz JA, Diokno AC. The management of injuries to the urethra, bladder or vagina encountered during difficult placement of the artificial urinary sphincter in the female patient. J Urol 1992:1528–1530.

83. Hadley HR. Insertion of artificial urinary sphincter in women. In: Vasavada SP, Appell RA, Sand PK, et al., eds. Female urology, urogynecology, and voiding dysfunction. New York: Marcel Decker, 2005:319–328.

84. Thomas H, Venn SN, Mundy AR. Outcome of the artificial sphincter in female patients. J Urol 2002; 167:1720–1722.

85. Light JK, Scott FB. Management of urinary incontinence in women with the artificial urinary sphincter. J Urol 1985; 134:476–478.
86. Petero VG, Diokno A. Comparison of the long-term outcomes between incontinent men and women treated with artificial urinary sphincter. J Urol 2006; 175:604–609.
87. Webster GD, Perez LM, Khoury JM, Timmons SL. Management of type III stress urinary incontinence using artificial urinary sphincter. Urology 1992; 36:499–503.
88. Fishman IJ, Scott FB. Pregnancy in patients with the artificial urinary sphincter. J Urol 1993; 150 (2 pt 1):340–341.
89. Khailee T, Diokno AC. Management of intrinsic sphincter deficiency in adolescent females with normal bladder emptying function. J Urol 2002; 168:1150–1153.

Chapter 12
Surgery for Stress Urinary Incontinence: Minimally Invasive Procedures

Eric A. Hurtado and Rodney A. Appell

Introduction

The idea of increasing urethral resistance by an injectable agent was first reported in 1938. Twenty women had either sodium morrhuate or cod-liver oil injected into the anterior vaginal wall to provoke an inflammatory response, resulting in scar formation and contracture of tissue around the urethra. Seventeen patients reported being cured or improved, but pulmonary infarction and cardiopulmonary arrest were reported [1]. In 1955, the first injections into the urethra were reported by Quackels. Two patients were treated successfully without complications [2]. In 1963, Sachse used Dondren, a sclerosing agent, to treat 7 women and 24 men. Four women and 12 men were reported as cured but several patients experienced pulmonary embolism [3]. These first bulking agents were far from ideal. Such an ideal agent would be nonimmunogenic, hypoallergenic, biocompatible, and nonmigratory, and would heal with minimal fibrosis and retain its bulking effect over a long period of time [4].

Mechanism

Injectable agents work by forming a "seal" through restoring mucosal coaptation (see Fig. 12.1). They have several advantages over surgical procedures in treating stress urinary incontinence (SUI). Compared to surgical procedures that create a functional obstruction, injectable agents restore continence by increasing urethral resistance at rest. With bulking agents, the urethra maintains its ability to funnel and open, keeping urethral resistance low during micturition. This spares a resultant increase in detrusor pressure (P_{det}), which could lead to overactive bladder symptoms and/or upper tract damage. In comparison, surgical procedures may result in increased resistance at rest and during micturition by not allowing the urethra the same physiological movement. Most bulking agents are placed at the level of the bladder neck within the smooth muscle in the area of the continence mechanism (see Fig. 12.2). Since the placement is within the urethra, "intraurethral" is more accurate than the commonly used terms "periurethral" or "submucosal."

Criteria for Selection

Ideal patients for intraurethral bulking have SUI due to intrinsic sphincter deficiency (ISD) and a normal contractile bladder. Clues such as leaking a large amount of urine with cough or sneeze, significant leakage on exertion, leakage while supine, bed-wetting, or leakage with the sensation of urinary urgency may suggest ISD. On physical examination, the patient should have a well-supported, fixed urethra. This can be determined by placing a cotton swab through the urethra with the tip just past the urethrovesical junction. If the angle is greater than 30° from the horizontal or change in angle is greater than 30° when the patient

149

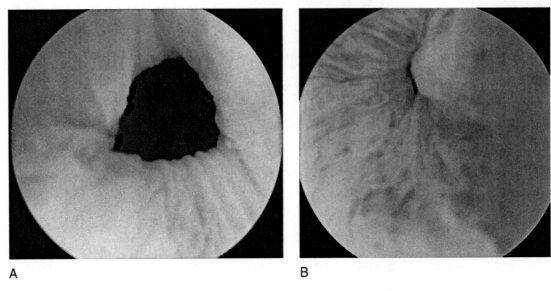

A   B

Fig. 12.1. (a) Bladder neck prior to injection. (b) Bladder neck after injection

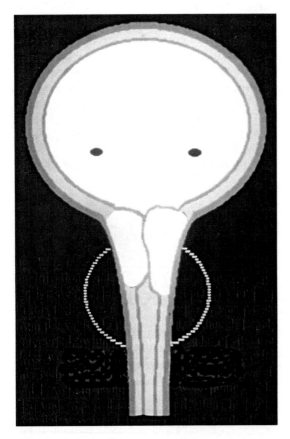

Fig. 12.2. Illustration of coaptation at continence mechanism

bears down or coughs, the patient is said to have a hypermobile rather than fixed urethra [5, 6].

The use of intraurethral bulking agents in women with urethral hypermobility, type II incontinence, is an area of controversy. A comparison between pubovaginal slings and intraurethral collagen injections was performed by Kreder et al. In their study, they compared success rates in patients with ISD alone or mixed with urethral hypermobility. In the mixed group, those receiving a pubovaginal sling faired better with a cure rate of 81% versus 25% in the collagen group [7]. However, the collagen group received only a single injection, whereas it has been demonstrated that many patients require between two and three injection sessions to affect their continence [8]. In another study, despite more injections and amount of material injected in the group with urethral hypermobility, both those with and without hypermobility had equal success [9]. In a later study by Herschorn and Radomski, no statistically significant difference was found between those with and without urethral hypermobility. Over time, 72% remained dry at 1 year, 57% at 2 years, and 45% at 3 years with no significant difference between the type of incontinence and time to failure [10]. Others have documented similar findings in patients with urethral hypermobility or type II incontinence [11–14].

Urodynamics should be performed to rule out other causes of urinary incontinence such as detrusor overactivity. Urethral function can be assessed by measuring the abdominal leak point pressure (ALPP), which is the amount of abdominal pressure (P_{abd}) necessary to overcome the bladder's continence mechanism. The definition of ISD by ALPP has varied from a low ALPP (65 cm H_2O) to an ALPP less than 100 cm H_2O. An absolute value for ALPP suggesting ISD has become unimportant due to limitations in urodynamic testing as well as different values used by different clinicians. With videourodynamics, radiographic evidence of an open bladder neck and proximal urethra without detrusor contraction during the storage phase of the bladder is believed to imply ISD.

As more is understood about the continence mechanism, it appears that most women with SUI have some component of ISD, since there are numerous women with urethral hypermobility who do not leak with significant intra-abdominal pressures. Women who do have a fixed, nonmobile urethra, however, are more likely to have a greater degree of ISD [15]. Exclusion criteria for intraurethral bulking would include urinary incontinence due to abnormal detrusor contractions, active urinary tract infection, or allergy to the material used as a bulking agent.

Key Concept

- Ideal patients for intraurethral bulking have SUI due to ISD and a normal contractile bladder
- Most women with SUI have some component of ISD

Injection Techniques

When performing intraurethral bulking, precise placement of the bulking material into the wall of the proximal urethra near the bladder neck in the area of the continence mechanism is of the utmost importance. The plane of delivery, tissue quality at the injection site, and cause of incontinence are all important factors in successful therapy. If material is delivered too distally, the treatment is likely to fail and may cause irritative voiding symptoms. Prior to injection, patients are placed in lithotomy position and prepped in standard sterile fashion.

A local anesthetic in the form of 20% benzocaine ointment or cream may be applied to the vestibule covering the urethra and a topical 2% lidocaine jelly may be applied to urethra. Two to four milliliters of 1% lidocaine are then injected periurethrally at the 3 and 9 o'clock positions.

Key Concept

- Precise placement of the bulking material into the wall of the proximal urethra near the bladder neck in the area of the continence mechanism is of the utmost importance.

Transurethral Injection

There are several approaches that may be taken when performing injections of bulking agents. It may be performed by placing a needle through a cystourethroscope and injecting suburothelially, also known as a "transurethral injection" [16]. A 0-, 12-, or 30-degree lens is best for providing a good view of the urethra as well as the injection needle. Once the cystourethroscope is placed into the urethra and passed into the bladder, the bladder usually is drained as the patient's bladder may become distended toward the end of the procedure. The endoscope then is backed to the midurethra at which time the needle is deployed at the 4 o'clock position. The needle then is inserted submucosally into the urethral muscle beyond the midurethra and advanced to the proximal urethra near the bladder neck. Once the desired positioning is achieved, the bulking agent is slowly delivered to allow it to spread underneath the urethral mucosa. Once the mucosa on that side has expanded to the midline, the needle is slowly withdrawn while injecting. Attention is then turned to the 8 o'clock position where the technique is repeated. After completion of both sides, a fair amount of coaptation should be noted.

In order to create an easier, more reliable transurethral delivery, a new device has been created called the "implacer" (Q-Med AB, Uppsala, Sweden). This device consists of four preloaded syringes with bulking material covered by an outer sleeve that is placed into the urethra. Once the syringes are advanced, the needles enter the submucosa at the midurethra in four distinct areas. The location of the midurethra is measured by a

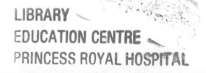

urethral catheter. The only recommended anesthesia consists of intraurethral lidocaine and a periurethral block. The touted benefits of this device include the elimination of cystourethroscopy for placement of the bulking agent and a reproducible method of bulking agent placement. In the United States, this device currently is under investigation. Yet to be determined is whether injection at the midurethra will be as efficacious as injection at the bladder neck or the equivalent to the varied midurethral slings currently in use.

Key Concept

• Once the mucosa at the 4 o'clock position has expanded to the midline, the technique is repeated again at the 8 o'clock position.
• A 0-, 12-, or 30-degree lens is best for providing a good view of the urethra as well as the injection needle.

Periurethral Injection

Injections also may be performed periurethrally via a needle placed percutaneously lateral to the urethral meatus and parallel to the urethra (see Fig. 12.3). While the needle is placed, the urethra is visualized through a cystourethroscope [17, 18]. Localization of the needle tip may be facilitated by preinjecting the urethra with methylene blue during the periurethral approach [19]. With the periurethral approach, there often is less bleeding, which can improve visualization. There also is less extrusion of the material injected, although this depends on the type of material injected as well. The desired amount of coaptation is the same as when performed via a transurethral technique. After the periurethral block, a 20-gauge spinal needle is placed at the 4 o'clock position into the periurethral tissue within the lamina propria. Urethroscopy is then performed as the needle is further inserted with minimal resistance up to the level of the bladder neck. The needle is then rocked in a horizontal plane to assess the location of the needle tip, ensuring placement at the proper depth. The material is then injected slowly while observing for coaptation similar to the transurethral technique, and the process is repeated at the 8 o'clock position. If material is noted in the lumen of the urethra, the needle is removed and relocated

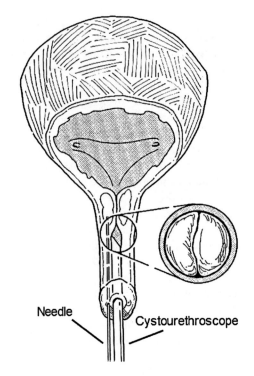

FIG. 12.3. Technique of periurethral approach

to a more anterior position where the injection is repeated again. Once sufficient coaptation is noted, the procedure is ended. A needle with a "bent tip" has been manufactured (Boston Scientific Inc, Natick, MA) to facilitate placement into the proper plane. With advancement of the needle, the tip is brought more medially. These needles were designed to ease the injection of Durasphere™, since a larger bore size (18-gauge) also aids in the passage of the particles.

The differences between the transurethral and periurethral techniques were reviewed by Faerber et al. In their study, they found similar outcomes with no significant differences in adverse events using collagen. Of significance, the amount of material injected was less using a transurethral approach [20]. A prospective, randomized comparison was later performed in women again with no noted differences in efficacy, but a higher rate of urinary retention and also an increased volume of injected material was seen in the periurethral group [21]. It appears that a periurethral approach tends to use larger volumes of material and has been noted to have a longer learning curve than the transurethral approach.

Ultrasound Guidance

Although transurethral and periurethral injections are the most commonly performed, injections also may be performed in females with use of an ultrasound probe [22]. Theoretically, this technique circumvents the passage of instruments through the urethra, which may alter the placement of the bulking agent affecting coaptation. First, a transrectal ultrasound probe with a biopsy port is placed into the vagina. Once the bladder neck has been identified, a needle of the same type for transurethral injection is placed through the port. Longitudinal views by ultrasound are used to determine coaptation of the bladder neck. Studies have demonstrated that three-dimensional ultrasound views may predict long-term outcomes and may provide an objective measure for amount of material to be placed [23]. In later studies with three-dimensional ultrasound, collagen injections were shown to maintain their volume and ultrasound appearance with an associated improved continence and quality of life. It also was found that the most desirable appearance on ultrasound was either a circumferential or horseshoe configuration [24]. Regardless of the technique, coaptation of the urethra is the goal.

Postoperative Care

Immediate postoperative complications are rare. After completion of the procedure, the patient should demonstrate the ability to void. If the patient is in acute urinary retention, most often they will be able to urinate shortly after the periurethral block loses effect. Meanwhile, the patient is usually catheterized with a small 10- to 14-French catheter to relieve the patient's full bladder after cystourethroscopy. An indwelling foley catheter should be avoided since there is a theoretical risk of the bulking agent molding around the catheter and losing its effect, although there is no evidence to support that short-term catheterization decreases the efficacy of intraurethral bulking. If long-term catheterization is necessary, a suprapubic catheter until return of voiding would be best to avoid disrupting the placement of the bulking agent. After injection, treatment with antibiotics is recommended for 2–3 days to avoid urinary tract infections. Many patients will require more than one session to achieve maximal continence.

Different waiting periods are required for each individual bulking agent. Bulking agents such as collagen can be repeated after 1 week (in the original multicenter study a 4-week waiting period was used). Ethylene vinyl alcohol copolymer requires a 3-month wait, allowing for ingrowth of the spongiform material. With polytetrafluoroethylene, a 4-month wait is required, since improved coaptation occurs with time. On repeat injection if erosion is noted, injection into that side should be avoided until re-epithelialization occurs.

Irritative voiding symptoms also may develop after placement of bulking agents. Surprisingly, in a study by Steele et al., 50% of patients were reported to have developed de novo detrusor overactivity [13]. In a study by Cross et al., 28% of patients were found to have de novo urge incontinence without ISD when undergoing urodynamics for posttreatment incontinence [25]. Stothers et al. reported a 12.6% rate of de novo urgency with urge incontinence in 337 women enrolled in a prospective of which 21% failed anticholinergic treatment [26]. Commonly, minor urethral bleeding may occur. If the urethral mucosa becomes disrupted, perforation and extravasation of the bulking agent may occur. An advantage of the periurethral approach involves placement of the bulking agent without disruption of the mucosa.

Key Concept

- If the patient is in acute urinary retention a catheterize with a small 10- to 14-French catheter to relieve the patient's full bladder.

Injectable Agents

Other methods of treatment for SUI include urethropexies, slings, and artificial urinary sphincters. Often bulking agents are compared to these other methods of treatment. What has been demonstrated in some studies is that midurethral slings and Burch urethropexies tend to have higher failure rates in patients with a "fixed urethra" [27, 28]. These patients are better off treated with intraurethral bulking agents, bladder neck slings, or artificial urinary sphincters. Compared to injectable agents, the artificial urinary sphincter and bladder neck slings both involve undergoing a surgical procedure that involves surgical risk as well as the risk of anesthesia, whereas the intraurethral bulking agent involves only local anesthesia and minimal complications.

Comparing the different injectable agents is a difficult task. There are few controlled, long-term studies involving commonly used bulking agents. Even within those rare studies, there are many variables that make it difficult to compare one to another. This is due to the different patients with different severities and etiologies of stress incontinence. Not all studies differentiate the results in patients with and without urethral hypermobility and/or ISD. The procedures themselves have also varied due to different technical factors such as injection technique and instrumentation. Additionally, reported results have been largely subjective rather than objective measures, creating a difficult situation in which to compare data. Variability also exists within the reported outcomes as different criteria have been used to define "cured" or "improved."

Auotologous Materials

Autologous Blood

Autologous blood is readily available and accessible. In a study of 14 women, 30 ml of blood was obtained in a heparinized syringe from the antecubital vein. Continence was achieved after two treatments. Unfortunately, all patients became incontinent again after 10–17 days [18].

Autologous Fat

Autologous fat is another readily available biomaterial. Although not as accessible as blood, it can be obtained easily through liposuction. In 1989, this technique was reported in ten women [29]. In a different study with 1-year follow-up, 0 of 5 men and 5 of 15 women reported improvement [30]. In a study by Santarosa and Blaivas, 83% of 12 women with ISD were subjectively improved, although, at 1 year the results were much lower [31]. Looking at women with urethral hypermobility, Blaivas et al. reported poor results [32]. Even more discouraging in a randomized, double-blind, controlled trial, fat was found to be as effective as the saline control group at 6 months [33].

These poor results are thought to be secondary to fat degradation. After injection, neovascularization never becomes adequate at the fat graft's center leaving only a miniscule amount of viable fat, which may hinder its bulking effect. After 3 weeks, 60% of the fat injected is degraded [34]. Once the fat is reabsorbed, inflammation occurs with resulting fibrosis, which leads to the bulking effect [31]. Although this material is accessible and complications are rare, it has been reported to be associated with systemic embolization and death [33, 35]. Therefore, use of autologous fat as a bulking agent is discouraged.

Biomaterials

Glutaraldehyde Cross-Linked Bovine Collagen (GAX-Collagen)

Of all the injectables, glutaraldehyde cross-linked bovine collagen (GAX-collagen) is probably the most used with the most publications describing its safety and efficacy. Before its use as a bulking agent, bovine dermal collagen was primarily used to make absorbable sutures and hemostatic agents. When used as a bulking agent, bovine collagen is cross-linked with glutaraldehyde to create a stabilized, fibrillar collagen that confers resistance to denaturation by collagenases. It consists of 35% purified bovine collagen in a phosphate buffer. The collagen itself is composed of 95% type I collagen, which is the type found predominately in ligaments and confers structural strength; however, between 1 and 5% is composed of type III collagen, which is the type abundant in vaginal tissue, giving added flexibility [36]. GAX-collagen is prepared by selective hydrolysis of the collagen molecule at the nonhelicoidal amino-terminal and carboxy-terminal segments, also known as telopeptides. This serves two functions. One is to decrease the antigenicity, and the other is to increase resistance to collagenases to increase the durability of the implant [37, 38].

When injecting this material, the surgeon inserts the exact amount needed to achieve the desired effect, since there is no expansion or shrinking after injection. Acting as a matrix, it promotes ingrowth of new collagen within the implant [39]. Since GAX-collagen is both biocompatible and biodegradable, only minimal inflammatory changes occur [40]. After 12 weeks, the collagen starts to degrade, but persists up until 19 months [41]. Despite the fact that GAX-collagen is degraded, it maintains effectiveness in 80% of those who became continent, which is thought to be secondary to the ingrowth of new collagen [42].

In one series, it was reported that 55% of women could achieve continence after one injection session [43]. In a multicenter clinical study involving 127 women with ISD, 88 patients completed 2-year follow-up. At 2 years, 46% of patients were dry and 34% were significantly improved, requiring only a single pad or tissues. Urodynamic studies also revealed a rise of 40 cm H_2O in abdominal LPP. A mean volume of 18.4 ml of GAX-collagen with a mean of 2.1 ($\pm$1.5) treatment sessions were given to those who achieved continence [44]. Other independent studies have supported these results [9, 45, 46]. These reported rates have compared favorably with other treatment modalities for ISD [47]. As time progresses, a noted decline in efficacy has been witnessed. Forty-five percent of elderly women were improved at 24.4 months in a report by Winters et al. Of note in this group, at an average of 7.9 months, 40% required more injections. After additional material was injected, only 42% became continent again [12]. Forty-two patients with ISD were followed at an average of 46 months by Richardson et al. In their series, they reported a 40% dry rate, 43% improved rate, and a 17% rate of failure [48]. At 50 months, Corcos and Fournier reported a cured rate of 30% and improved rate of 40% in 40 women, although four women in the cured group and five women in the improved group required "maintenance" injections [49]. In a study up to 5 years, Gorton et al. reported that only 26% of 53 women reported continued improvement [50].

Few complications have been found with the use of GAX-collagen. In the US clinical trials, 15% developed transient urinary retention, 5% had a urinary tract infection (UTI), and 1% of patients experienced irritative voiding [51]. Rates of de novo urgency and frequency have been reported to range from 10-as high as 50% [13, 49]. There has been no evidence of foreign body response or migration [39]. This is due partly to the small amount of glutaraldehyde in GAX-collagen, which creates minimal immunoreactivity and cytotoxicity

[52]. GAX-collagen is biocompatible and allows fibroblasts to deposit native collagen as well as neovascularization to occur as the implant is degraded over 12 weeks [53]. After 10–19 months all of the implant has completely degraded [40]. Only a mild inflammatory response has been associated after injection [54]. In a report of two postmortem patients having had laryngeal implants of GAX-collagen, an inflammatory response was nearly absent and the implanted collagen was colonized with host cells and new vessels [41]. However, there have been several case reports of sterile abscesses at the injection sites of which some required drainage [35, 55].

One potential hazard of GAX-collagen involves an allergic reaction to the bovine protein, although reduced by cross-linking and skin testing. Approximately 4% of female patients will have a positive skin test, which precludes them from treatment, although many are unlikely to suffer from an allergic reaction [44]. Despite being extraordinarily rare, delayed hypersensitivity has been reported. These have occurred at the skin test site and sometimes have been associated with arthralgia [56]. Currently, there is no evidence to support that GAX-collagen injections are associated with any medical disorder as disorders have been found to occur in even lower rates in the general population [39, 47]. Overall, due to its complete degradation with minimal inflammatory response and lack of migration, GAX-collagen has been the most popular intraurethral bulking agent used to treat incontinence.

Key Concept

- As time progresses, a noted decline in efficacy has been witnessed.
- Approximately 4% of female patients will have a positive skin test, which precludes them from treatment.

Synthetic Materials

Polytetrafluoroethylene (Polytef™)

In 1973, Berg first reported the use of polytetrafluoroethylene (PFTE) in a glycerol paste used on three women with ISD after surgery. These women were treated successfully; however, two women required repeat injection and one patient experienced asymptomatic bacteriuria [57]. Many authors have been able to demonstrate this material's efficacy as a bulking agent [58–63]. Success rates have ranged from 70 to 90% with PFTE [64]. This material also was studied by the Department of Technology Assessment of the American Medical Association and found to be an easily performed, effective treatment with good short-term results [65]. However, longer follow-up has proven otherwise. In one study, a 38% success rate between 21 and 72 months (mean, 49 months) was noted in women [66].

In addition to the shortcomings in long-term efficacy, rates of urinary retention have ranged from 20 to 25% [67]. Transient irritative voiding symptoms may develop in approximately 20% of patients [62]. Urinary tract infection has been reported to occur at a rate of 2% [61].

Of greater concern, the long-term safety profile of this agent has been brought into question. Foreign body reaction with granuloma formation is a known risk [68]. After injection, histiolytic and giant cells are responsible for this reaction. Particles have been found in blood vessels as well as lymphatics. These particles have been thought to elicit an allergic response in some patients, which is believed to be responsible for culture-negative fevers in 25% of patients. Five percent of patients also complain of transient perineal discomfort with spontaneous resolution, which also is thought to be an immune-related phenomenon [67, 69].

Once inside blood vessels or lymphatics, particles can migrate to distant locations. In animal models, PTFE particles have been found in pelvic lymph nodes, lungs, brain, kidneys, and spleen at 1 year [70, 71]. Particle migration to distant sites has been reported in humans as well. First reported by Mittleman and Marraccini in 1983, a PTFE granuloma was found in the lung of a patient 2 years after injection [72]. Claes et al. reported on a patient who was experiencing fevers with biopsy-proven PTFE granulomas in the lung 3 years after PTFE injection [73]. In another field, PTFE was used to inject the larynx for vocal cord paralysis. Twenty months after injection, a granuloma was found in the anterior lobe of the thyroid [74].

Despite granuloma formation, patients rarely have had any clinical consequences. It is the formation of granulomas and their association with cancer that is of more concern. Sarcomas have been induced in rats and mice with material related to PTFE [75]. Hakky et al. reported a chondrosarcoma of the larynx 6 years after treatment of the vocal cords for paralysis, although PTFE has not been linked to carcinogenesis with 30 years of use as a bulking agent for the urethra and larynx [76]. In fact, there have been only reported cases of cancer near PTFE injections sites, but none have demonstrated PTFE as the precipitating factor [77–79]. This risk was reviewed by Dewan. It was concluded that the available evidence did not support PTFE as a carcinogenic agent, but suggested that if a risk existed, it was low [80]. In 1995, Dewan reviewed the risk of both PTFE and Bioplastique in a rat model. A similar incidence of tumors was found in the PTFE, Bioplastique, and control group [81]. Additional late adverse events include fibrosis of the urethra and granuloma balls in the bladder at a rate of 15% [66]. Currently, the US Food and Drug Administration (FDA) is investigating the product to better clarify its safety and efficacy in the treatment of urinary incontinence with ISD and is not available on the market.

Key Concept

- Particle migration with granuloma formation to distant sites has been reported, although patients rarely have had any clinical consequences.

Silicone Polymers (Macroplastique™, Bioplastique™)

Silicone polymers such as Macroplastique™ and Bioplastique™ are made of polydimethylsiloxane macroparticles suspended in a carrier hydrogel consisting of polyvinylpyrrolidone (povidone). The solid particles make up 33% of the total volume and are greater than 100 μm in size. Silicone polymer was first used in 1992 with encouraging short-term follow-up. In 84 patients cure was attained in 82% [81]. Like other agents as time progressed, the cure rate fell to 70% at 14 months [82]. In other studies with Macroplastique™, 19.6% were considered cured and 41.1% significantly improved at 19 months [83]. In another study using the Stamey grading system, as well as the King health questionnaire at 12 months, 57.1% patients considered themselves cured and 19% improved. From the surgeon's subjective grading 38.1% were cured and 28.6% improved. The authors concluded that Macroplastique™ had acceptable outcomes for the patient and the surgeon [84]. To date there has been one prospective, randomized study comparing Macroplastique™ to GAX-collagen in 62 women. The authors concluded that there was no significant objective difference between the two agents at 12 months. The only difference was that the Macroplastique™ group had less volume injected, although pretreatment pad test loss was significantly less in that group [85].

Complications with use of this material included urinary retention at a rate of 5.9–17.5%, urinary frequency at a rate of 0–72.4%, dysuria from 0 to 100%, and UTI 0–6.25% [86]. A study to determine the migratory properties of this material was performed on dogs. Small particles were found in the lungs, kidney, brain, and lymph nodes within 4 months of injection. In comparison, only one large particle was found in the lung without any associated reaction [87]. In a rat model, four sarcomas with Bioplastique group were associated with silicone particles [80]. Given the recent controversy over silicone used in breast implants as well as the possibility of migration, it is unlikely that silicone will become a popular agent for intraurethral injections.

Carbon-coated Zirconium Beads (Durasphere™ and Durasphere EXP™)

Durasphere™, a new synthetic material, was approved by the FDA in 1999. It is composed of pyrolytic carbon-coated zirconium oxide beads in a 2.8% beta-glucan water-based gel. Bulking effect lasts for at least 2 years as the beads are encapsulated into the periurethral tissue. Compared to collagen, it is an inert and nonimmunogenic material eliminating the need for skin testing. However, Durasphere™ can be more technically difficult to inject given its higher viscosity.

Durasphere™ was compared to GAX-collagen in a multicenter, randomized, controlled, double-blind study with follow-up at 1 year. The Durasphere™ group achieved improvement in one Stamey grade or more in 80% of patients compared to 69% of patients in the GAX-collagen group, although the difference did not reach statistical significance. Pad weights at 12 months were equivalent between the two groups. The Durasphere™ group had a sig-

nificantly smaller volume injected and was more successfully treated with a single injection [88]. Although permanent, questions concerning longevity similar to GAX-collagen were brought forth. Panneck et al. noted a decrease in success from 77% at 6 months to 33% at 12 months in a group of 13 women. In their study, one female patient also was noted to have asymptomatic distant particle migration into the regional and distal lymph nodes [89]. Due to intraneedle resistance secondary to bead size, injection of Durasphere™ can be technically difficult. In response to this issue, Madjar et al. used a periurethral approach at a single injection site. With 92% of 46 patients achieving excellent or good coaptation, 65% considered themselves cured or improved at a mean of 9.4 months. Additionally, 50% of 36 patients had 24-h pad test with 8 gm or less of urine [90]. Long-term data have been reported in a multicenter, comparative trial of Durasphere™ and GAX-collagen. Durasphere™ remained effective in 33% of patients at 24 months and 21% at 36 months. Those who received GAX-collagen reported effectiveness in 19% of patients at 24 months and 9% at 36 months. However, when controlled for differences in follow-up time, the time to failure between the two groups did not reach statistical significance. Interestingly, one third of each group felt that treatment was successful [91].

In the trials for FDA approval, the most common adverse events were acute retention (≤7 days) at 13%, dysuria at 12%, UTI at 9%, and hematuria at 6%, and retention >7 days at 6%. Other adverse events occurred at ≤4% [92]. There also have been case reports of sterile abscess formation. In one series, two of four abscesses required incision and drainage [93].

Durasphere's™ beads are much larger than either PFTE or silicone polymers. In spite of their size, there have been reports of migration despite lacking clear evidence [89, 94]. As determined by studies involving polytetrafluorethylene, macrophages are able to phagocytize particles smaller than 80 μm. Once phagocytized, the particles then can be carried to different parts of the body. Since Durasphere ranges from 212 to 500 μm, phagocytosis and therefore migration should not occur. Case reports involving beads found in lymphatics and so forth are likely due to a high-pressure embolization effect, which may displace beads into vascular or lymphatic spaces. Delivery with large particles under low pressure should elimi- nate the risk of embolization. Durasphere-EXP™ is a modification of the original Durasphere™ that should allow lower pressure injection due the smaller bead size (95–550 μm, yet above 80 μm to avoid migration).

Key Concept

- Durasphere™ achieved improvement in one Stamey grade or more in 80% of patients com- pared to 69% of patients in the GAX-collagen group, although the difference did not reach sta- tistical significance.

Ethylene Vinyl Alcohol Copolymer (Tegress™, Uryx™)

Approved by the FDA in 2004, Tegress™ is com- posed of 8% ethylene vinyl alcohol (EVOH) copol- ymer dissolved in dimethyl sulfoxide (DMSO), which is a permanent, hypoallergenic, nonimmu- nogenic implant. It comes prepared in 3 ml glass vials with a 3 ml DMSO-compatible syringe. The material is injected via a 25-gauge needle. Once Tegress™ is exposed to fluid within the tissue, the DMSO diffuses out, causing the precipitation of EVOH into a soft, spongy, hydrophilic material. The time required for the chemical reaction to occur is within 60 s. Care must be taken to avoid contami- nation of this agent with fluid prior to injection. At 1 month, an acute inflammatory response has been noted to be at its greatest. This effect lasts until 3 months when the reaction has become more mild and localized with some resultant mineralization. There has been no evidence of EVOH affecting tissue at remote sites from the injection site. There also has been no evidence of migration.

When EVOH is used as a bulking agent, a dif- ferent technique must be applied. If an excessive amount of material is injected, erosion through the urethral mucosa is likely to occur. In order to decrease the risk of erosion, the manufacturer suggests injecting at a more distal location in the urethra approximately 1.5 cm distal to the bladder neck. Each injection is to take place over 1 min with an additional minute waited to allow the chemical reaction to occur before removing the needle [95]. When the needle is removed, a twist- ing motion often helps to separate the precipitated material off the needle tip and minimize the length

of tail left at the injection site. Injections should not be performed until coaptation is noted, which is dissimilar to many of the other bulking agents. Urethral coaptation may suggest that too much material may have been injected [96].

Currently for EVOH, the only large study is from the trial for FDA approval. A multicenter, prospec- tive, randomized trial was conducted with 177 of 253 women completing follow-up at 12 months compar- ing EVOH to GAX-collagen. The first 16 patients were excluded from the data, since they were the first patients undergoing a new technique. At 12 months, efficacy was assessed by Stamey grade, pad weight, and quality of life questionnaire: 18.4% of patients were dry by Stamey grade of those who received EVOH compared to 16.5% of those who received collagen. The difference between the two groups who had improvement by at least one Stamey grade did not reach clinical significance. In respect to pad weights, 37.8% were dry in the EVOH group com- pared to 32.1% undergoing collagen injection. This study resulted in FDA approval of EVOH [95, 97].

In the trials for FDA approval, EVOH has been shown to have similar rates and severity of adverse events when compared to collagen. The one excep- tion is the rate of material exposure of 16%. During this study, it was noted that the exposure rate was higher with periurethral injection, and therefore is not recommended. Exposed material did not result in any adverse consequences and usually resolved. However, in the authors' experi- ence erosion rates of 37% in women and 41% in men necessitated multiple office visits for several patients with severe dysuria [98, 99]. Other com- mon adverse events included UTI (29%), delayed voiding (18%), dysuria (18%), urinary urgency (14%), and frequency (13%). Interestingly, 9% of patients developed urge incontinence and 8% had worsening of incontinence [95].

Key Concepts

- With EVOH, injections should not be performed until coaptation is noted, which is dissimilar to many of the other bulking agents.

Calcium Hydroxyapatite (Coaptite®)

Approved in December 2005, calcium hydroxya- patite is a synthetic agent that consists of car- boxymethylcellulose in the form of an aquaeous gel. It is the same material found in bone and teeth and has been used in dental work as well as bone healing. Calcium hydroxyapatite is biocompatible, does not encapsulate, and facilitates ingrowth of native tissues. This material also can be identified on radiographic studies as well as ultrasound. Another advantage includes ease of injection of material.

In a study with 1-year follow-up, seven of ten women reported substantial improvement in continence, a 90% decrease in mean pad weight, and increase in mean Valsalva leak point pressure from 39 to 46 cm H_2O [100]. In the data for FDA approval, 158 patients received Coaptite® with a mean follow-up of 11.2 months. No statistical difference was found in change in Stamey grade, pad weight, or quality of life when compared to GAX-collagen as the control [101].

Common adverse events from the FDA data included urinary retention (41%), hematuria (19.6%), dysuria (15.2%), and UTI (8.3%). Changes in voiding occurred with urinary urgency at 7.6%, frequency at 7.0%, and urge incontinence at 5.7%. Two serious adverse events occurred, with one erosion through the vaginal wall that required surgery and dissection into the bladder and another causing tissue bridging of which no surgical correction was needed. Overall, the erosion rate was 1.3% [101].

Key Concept

• No statistical difference was found in change in Stamey grade, pad weight, or quality of life when compared to GAX-collagen as the control.

Future Agents

In patients with minimal urethral–vesical junction mobility, ISD, and a stable bladder with an adequate capacity, intraurethral injections can offer treatment responses similar to those of surgical correction with minimal complications. However, most of these data are short-term with a scarcity of data over 5 years, and the majority of studies followed at much less time. For GAX-collagen, reinjection rates can be as high as 22% at 32 months after having achieved continence [102]. The other injectable agents on the market have much fewer data, and they lack long-term follow-up. For patients who are younger, the cost of reinjection can become significant.

Although numerous injectable agents have entered the market over the last several years, the search for the ideal bulking agents continues. Listed below are some of the current agents undergoing investigation.

Hyaluronic Acid

Made of a water-insoluble complex glycosaminoglycan, which itself is composed of disaccharide units, hyaluronic acid has completed a stage I study [103]. This type of hyaluronic acid is cross-linked, highly biocompatible, as well a nonimmunogenic, making it well tolerated with some longevity before undergoing absorption. The molecules weigh between 8 and 23 million molecular weight. This agent comes dissolved in normal saline to allow ease of injection. Currently, the FDA has given approval to start a stage II multicenter study to compare hyaluronic acid to GAX-collagen.

Hyaluronic Acid and Dextranomer Microspheres

Hyaluronic acid and dextranomer microspheres are complex sugar polymers which are glycosaminoglycan and cross-linked dextran, respectively. Each polymer has its own function. Hyaluronic acid serves as a carrier and is degraded and reabsorbed within 2 weeks, while the dextranomer microspheres function as the bulking agent. The dextranomer microspheres may last up to 4 years due to slow degradation [104]. Similar to collagen with ease of injection, it provides a foundation for fibroblasts to deposit new collagen. Currently, clinical trials in the United States are underway. This agent already is approved in Europe. In the United States, it is only approved for the treatment of vesicoureteral reflux in children in which it has been used extensively. In a study by Stenberg et al., only 3 of 20 patients (15%) failed this treatment and in those who responded, 57% had a sustained response [105]. A new device known as the "implacer" has been studied with this agent as well. This device allows the placement of four syringes of material to be placed via a transurethral technique without cystourethroscopy. Van Kerrebroeck et al. reported a significant decrease in incontinent episodes, with 69% of patients improving on the 6-point perception scale in a study of 42 patients over 1 year [106].

Bioglass

Bioglass is an inert compound derived from calcium oxide, calcium silicone, and sodium oxide. In animal models, it has been demonstrated to elicit a minimal inflammatory response and no toxicity has been found. Similar to other agents, the compound serves as a framework for fibroblasts to deposit collagen to integrate host tissue with the implant [107]. Currently, no human trials have been performed.

Autologous Tissue

Described by Atala et al., intraurethral bulking with autologous chondrocytes could be performed by harvesting chondrocytes from the patient's auricular surface. Tissue engineering then is required to culture and expand these cells and place them in an alginate polymer for insertion into the urethral submucosa [108]. In one study of 32 patients, 16 were dry and 10 improved at 12 months [109]. This technique is to be assessed in a multicenter trial.

Harvesting myoblasts from the biceps muscle is another tissue-engineering concept being considered [110]. Using autologous tissue alleviates problems with biocompatibility. Since these tissues can continue to grow and thrive in their environment, they should maintain longevity as well. An additional advantage of muscle cells is that they differentiate into smooth or striated muscle, which can actively help to improve the mucosal seal. This agent has much promise in the human model [111, 112].

Disadvantages to tissue engineering include cost as well as safety. Enormous expense can be generated from tissue engineering as well as the possibility of stored cells for potentially further treatment. Safety also is a concern, since there is no way to predict how many cells are required upon implantation as well as the potential of mixing specimens in laboratory facilities prior to injection. Further research is needed to investigate this technique before clinical trials can be considered.

Microballoons

The first microballoons were placed via a periurethral approach and had encouraging results [113]. However, trials in the United States were never conducted due to problems in the way the microballoons were delivered. New balloons have been developed that allow for balloon adjustment. These are placed via a periurethral approach as before and currently are being investigated worldwide. The new devices are placed at the level of the bladder neck and are outside the urethra rather than intraurethrally. The balloon then can be filled through a port that is accessible through the labium similar to the pump from an artificial urinary sphincter. In contrast to intraurethral agents, local anesthetic is not sufficient, requiring an operative room with regional or general anesthesia.

Conclusion

Currently, injectable agents are best used for those who are good candidates for successful treatment, those who wish to avoid a surgical procedure, or those who have problematic medical comorbidities that preclude them from undergoing surgical correction. Research continues the search for an effective, inert, nonmigratory, nonimmunogenic material that allows incorporation into native tissue, maintains its shape, and injects with ease. Currently, intraurethral bulking remains an art, as there is no exact measurement or amount of material used for each patient to achieve continence.

References

1. Murless BC. The injection treatment of stress incontinence. J Obstet Gynecol Br Emp 1938; 45:521–524.
2. Quackels R. Deux incontinence apr; ages adenonectomie: Queries par injection de paraffine dans la perin; aaee. Acta Urol Belg 1955; 23:259–262.
3. Sachse H. Treatment of urinary incontinence with sclerosing solutions: Indications, results, complications. Urol Int 1963; 15:225–244.
4. Dmochowski RR, Appell RA. Injectable agents in the treatment of stress urinary incontinence in women: Where are we now? Urology 2000; 56(Suppl 6A):32–40.
5. Crystle CD, Charme LS, Copeland WE. Q-tip test in stress urinary incontinence. Obstet Gynecol 1971; 39:313–315.
6. Appell RA, Ostergard D. Practical urodynamics. Illustr Med Female Urol Ser 1992; 2:4–29.
7. Kreder KJ, Austin JC. Treatment of stress urinary incontinence in women with urethral hypermobility and intrinsic sphincter deficiency. J Urol 1996; 156:1995–198.

8. Smith DN, Appell RA, Winters JC, et al. Collagen injection therapy for female intrinsic sphincter deficiency. J Urol 1997; 152:1275–1278.

9. Herschorn S, Radomski SB, Steele DJ. Early experience with intraurethral collagen injection for urinary incontinence. J Urol 1992; 148:1797–1800.

10. Herschorn S, Radomski SB. Collagen injections for genuine stress urinary incontinence: Patient selection and durability. Int Urogynecol J 1997; 8:18–24.

11. Faerber GJ. Endoscopic collagen injection therapy for elderly women with type I stress urinary incontinence. J Urol 1995; 153:527A.

12. Winters J, Chiverton A, Scarpero H, et al. Collagen injection therapy in elderly women: Long-term results and patient satisfaction. Urology 2000; 55:815–818.

13. Steele AC, Kohli N, Karram MM. Periurethral collagen injection for stress incontinence with and without urethral hypermobility. Obstet Gynecol 2000; 95:322–331.

14. Bent, AE, Foote, J, Siegel S, et al. Collagen implant for treating stress urinary incontinence in women with urethral hypermobility. J Urol 2001; 166(4):1354–1357.

15. Winters JC. Urodynamics in the era of tension-free slings. Curr Urol Rep 2004; 5(5):343–347.

16. O'Connell HE, McGuire EJ. Transurethral collagen therapy in women. J Urol 1995; 154:1463–1465.

17. Appell RA. Injectables for urethral incompetence. World J Urol 1990; 8:208–211.

18. Appell RA. The periurethral injection of autologous blood. Presented at the American Urogynecologic Society annual meeting, Toronto, 1994.

19. Neal ED Jr , Lahaye ME, Lowe DC. Improved needle placement technique in periurethral collagen injection. Urology 1995; 45:865–866.

20. Faerber GJ, Belville WD, Ohl DA, et al. Comparison of transurethral versus periurethral collagen injection in women with intrinsic sphincter deficiency. Tech Urol 1998; 4(3):124–127.

21. Schulz JA, Nager CW, Stanton SL, et al. Bulking agents for stress urinary incontinence: Short-term results and complications in a randomized comparison of periurethral and transurethral injection. Int Urogynecol J Pelvic Floor Dysfunct 2004; 15:261–265.

22. Appell RA. Collagen injections. In: Raz S, ed. Female urology. 2nd ed. Philadelphia: WB Saunders, 1996: 399–405.

23. Defreitas GA, Wilson TS, Zimmern PE, et al. Three-dimensional ultrasonography: An objective outcome to assess collagen distribution in women with stress urinary incontinence. Urology 2003; 62:232–236.

24. Poon CI, Zimmern PE, Defreitas GA, et al. Three-dimensional ultrasonography to assess long-term durability of periurethral collagen in women with stress urinary incontinence due to intrinsic sphincteric deficiency. Urology 2005; 65:60–64.

25. Cross CA, English SF, Cespedes RD, et al. A follow-up on transurethral collagen injection therapy for urinary incontinence. J Urol 1998; 159:106–108.

26. Stothers L, Goldenberg SL, Leone EF. Complications of periurethral collagen injection for stress urinary incontinence. J Urol 1998; 159(3):806–807.

27. Bergman A, Koonings PP, Ballard CA. Negative Q-tip test as a risk factor for failed incontinence surgery in women. J Reprod Med 1990; 34(3):193–197.

28. Segal JL, Vasallo BJ, Kleeman SD, et al. The efficacy of tension-free vaginal tape in the treatment of five subtypes of stress urinary incontinence. Int J Pelvic Floor Dysfunct 2006; 17(2):120–124.

29. Gonzalez de Garibay AS, Castro-Morrondo JM, Castro-Jimeno JM. Endoscopic injection of autologous adipose tissue in the treatment of female incontinence. Arch Esp Urol 1989; 42:143–146.

30. Gonzalez de Garibay AS, Castillo-Jimeno JM, Villanueva-Perez PI. Treatment of urinary stress incontinence using paraurethral injection of autologous fat. Arch Esp Urol 1991; 44:595–600.

31. Santarosa RP, Blaivas JG. Periurethral injection of autologous fat for the treatment of sphincteric incontinence. J Urol 1994; 151:607–611.

32. Blaivas JG, Herwitz D, Santarosa RP, et al. Periurethral fat injection for sphincteric incontinence in women. J Urol 1994; 151:419A.

33. Lee PE, Kung RC, Drutz HP. Periurethral autologous fat injection as treatment for female stress urinary incontinence: A randomized double-blind controlled trial. J Urol 2000; 165: 153–158.

34. Bartynski J, Marion MS, Wang TD. Histopathologic evaluation of adipose autografts in a rabbit ear model. Otolaryngology 1990; 102:314.

35. Sweat SD, Lightner DJ. Complications of sterile abscess formation and pulmonary embolism following periurethral bulking agents. J Urol 1999; 161:93–96.

36. Moalli PA, Shand SH, Zyczynski HM, et al. Remodeling of vaginal connective tissue in patients with pelvic organ prolapse. Obstet Gynecol 2005; 106(5 Pt 1):953–963.

37. DeLustro F, Dasch J, Keefe J, et al. Immune response to allogeneic and xenogeneic implants of collagen and collagen derivatives. Clin Orthop 1990; 260:263–279.

38. McPherson JM, Sawamura S, Armstrong R. An examination of the biologic response to injectable glutaraldehyde cross-linked collagen implants. J Biomed Matter Res 1986; 20:93–97.

39. DeLustro F, Keefe J, Fong AT, et al. The biochemistry, biology, and immunology of injectable collagens: Contigen Bard collagen implant in treatment of urinary incontinence. Pediatr Surg Int 1991; 6:245–251.

40. Canning DA, Peters CA, Gearhart JR, et al. Local tissue reaction to glutaraldehyde cross-linked bovine collagen in the rabbit bladder. J Urol 1988; 139:258–259.

41. Remacle M, Marbaix E. Collagen implants in the human larynx. Arch Otorhinolaryngol 1988; 245:203–209.

42. Appell RA. Collagen injection therapy for urinary incontinence. Urol Clin North Am 1994; 21:177–182.

43. Appell RA. New developments: Injectables for urethral incompetence in women. Int Urogynecol J 1990; 1:117–119.

44. Appell RA, McGuire EJ, DeRidder PA, et-al. Summary of effectiveness and safety in the prospective, open, multicenter investigation of Contigen implant for incontinence due to intrinsic sphincteric deficiency in females. J Urol 1994; 151:418A.

45. Striker P, Haylen B. Injectable collagen for type 3 female stress incontinence: The first 50 Australian patients. Med J Aust 1993; 158:89–91.

46. Swami SK, Eckford SD, Abrams P. Collagen injections for female stress incontinence: Conclusions of a multistage analysis and results. J Urol 1994; 151:479A.

47. Appell RA. Use of collagen injections for treatment of incontinence and reflux. Adv Urol 1992; 5:145–165.

48. Richardson TD, Kennelly MJ, Faerber GJ. Endoscopic injection of glutaraldehyde cross-linked collagen for the treatment of intrinsic sphincteric deficiency in women. Urology 1995; 46:378–381.

49. Corcos J, Fournier C. Periurethral collagen injection for the treatment of female stress urinary incontinence: 4-year follow-up results. Urology 1999; 54:815–818.

50. Gorton E, Stanton S, Monga A, et al. Periurethral collagen injection: A long-term follow-up study. BJU Int 1999; 84:966–971.

51. Bard CR, Inc. PMAA submission to United States Food and Drug Administration for IDE G850010, 1990.

52. Ford CN, Martin CW, Warren TF. Injectable collagen in laryngeal rehabilitation. Laryngoscope 1984; 95:513–518.

53. Stegman S, Chu S, Bensch K, et al. A light and electron microscopic evaluation of Zyderm and Zyplast implants in aging human facial skin: A pilot study. Arch Dermatol 1987; 123:1644–1649.

54. DeLustro F, Condell RA, Nguyen MA, et al. A comparative study of the biologic and immunologic response to medical devices derived from dermal collagen. J Biomed Mater Res 1986; 20:109–120.

55. McLennan MT, Bent AE. Suburethral abscess: A complication of periurethral collagen injection therapy. Obstet Gynecol 1998; 92:650–652.

56. Stothers L, Goldenberg SL. Delayed hypersensitivity and systemic arthralgia following transurethral collagen injection for stress urinary incontinence. J Urol 1998; 159:1507–1509.

57. Berg S. Polytef augmentation urethroplasty: Correction of surgically incurable urinary incontinence by injection technique. Arch Surg 1973; 107:379–381.

58. Politano VA, Small MP, Harper JM, et al. Periurethral Teflon injection for urinary incontinence. J Urol 1974; 111:180–183.

59. Heer H. Die Behandlung der Harnin-kontinenz mit der Teflon-paste. Urol Int 1977; 32:295–302.

60. Lampante L, Kaesler FP, Sparwasser H. Endourethrale submukose Tefloninjektion zur Erzielung von Harninkontinenz. Akt Urol 1979; 10:265–272.

61. Lim KB, Ball AJ, Feneley RCL. Periurethral Teflon injection: A simple treatment for urinary incontinence. Br J Urol 1983; 55:208–210.

62. Schulman CC, Simon J, Wespes E, et al. Endoscopic injection of Teflon for female urinary incontinence. Eur Urol 1983; 9:246–247.

63. Deane AM, English P, Hehir M, et al. Teflon injection in stress incontinence. Br J Urol 1985; 57:78–80.

64. Appell RA. Commentary: Periurethral polytetrafluoroethylene (Polytef) injection. In: Whitehead ED, ed. Current operative urology. Philadelphia: JB Lippincott, 1990:63–66.

65. Cole HM. Diagnostic and therapeutic technology assessment (DATTA). JAMA 1993; 269:2975–2980.

66. Buckley JF, Lingham K, Meddings RN, et al. Injectable Teflon paste for female stress incontinence: Long-term follow-up and results. J Urol 1993; 149:418A.

67. Politano VA. Periurethral polytetrafluoroethylene injection for urinary incontinence. J Urol 1982; 127:439–442.

68. Stone JW, Arnold GE. Human larynx injected with Teflon paste: Histologic study of innervation and tissue reaction. Arch Otolaryngol 1967; 86:550–562.

69. Politano VA. Periurethral Teflon injection for urinary incontinence. Urol Clin North Am 1978; 5:415–422.

70. Malizia AA Jr, Reiman JM, Myers RP, et al. Migration and granulomatous reaction after periurethral injection of Polytef (Teflon). JAMA 1984; 251:3277–3281.

71. Vandenbossche M, Delhobe O, Dumortier P, et al. Endoscopic treatment of reflux: Experimental study

and review of Teflon and collagen. Eur Urol 1994; 23:386.

72. Mittleman RE, Marraccini JV. Pulmonary Teflon granulomas following periurethral Teflon injection for urinary incontinence. Arch Pathol Lab Med 1983; 107:611–612.

73. Claes H, Stroobants D, van Meerbeek J, et al. Pulmonary migration following periurethral polytetrafluoroethylene injection for urinary incontinence. J Urol 1989; 142:821–822.

74. Sanfilippo F, Shelburne J, Ingram P. Analysis of a Polytef granuloma mimicking a cold thyroid nodule 17 months after laryngeal injection. Ultrastruct Pathol 1980; 1:471–475.

75. Oppenheimer BS, Oppenheimer ET, Stout AP, et al. The latent period in carcinogenesis by plastics in rats and its relation to the presarcomatous stage. Cancer 1958; 11:204–213.

76. Hakky M, Kolbusz R, Reyes CV. Chondrosarcoma of the larynx. Ear Nose Throat J 1989; 68:60–62.

77. Lewy RB. Experience with vocal cord injection. Ann Otol Rhinol Laryngol 1976; 85:440–450.

78. Montgomery WW. Laryngeal paralysis – Teflon injection. Ann Otol 1979; 88:647–657.

79. Dewan PA. Is injected polytetrafluoroethylene (Polytef) carcinogenic? Br J Urol 1992; 69:29–33.

80. Dewan PA, Owen AJ, Byard RW. Long-term histological response to subcutaneously injected Polytef and Bioplastique in a rat model. Br J Urol 1995; 76(2):161–164.

81. Buckley JF, Scott R, Meddings, et al. Injectable silicone microparticles: A new treatment for female stress incontinence. J Urol 1992; 147:280A.

82. Buckley JF, Lingham K, Lloyd SN, et al. Injectable silicone macroparticles for female urinary incontinence. J Urol 1993; 149:402A.

83. Radley SC, Chapple CR, MItsogiannis IC, et al. Transurethral implantation of Macroplastique for the treatment of female stress urinary incontinence secondary to intrinsic sphincteric deficiency. Eur Urol 2001; 39:383–389.

84. Tamanini JT, D'Ancona CA, Tadini V, et al. Macroplastique implantation system for female stress urinary incontinence. J Urol 2003; 169:2229–2233.

85. Anders K, Khullar V, Cardozo L, et al. Gax-collagen or Macroplastique. Does it make a difference? Neururol Urodyn 1999; 18:297–298.

86. Ter Meulen PH, Berghmans LC, van Kerrebroeck PE. Systematic review: Efficacy of silicone microimplants (Macroplastique) therapy for stress urinary incontinence in adult women. Eur Urol 2003; 44:573–582.

87. Henly DR, Barrett DM, Weiland TL, et al. Particulate silicone for use in periurethral injections: Local tissue effects and search for migration. J Urol 1995; 153:2039–2043.

88. Lightner D, Calvosa C, Andersen R, et al. A new injectable bulking agent for treatment of stress urinary incontinence: Results of a multicenter, randomized, controlled, double-blind study of Durasphere. Urology 2001; 58:12–15.

89. Pannek J, Brands FH, Senge T. Particle migration after transurethral injection of carbon coated beads for stress urinary incontinence. J Urol 2001; 166:1350–1353.

90. Madjar S, Covington-Nichols C, Secrest CL. New periurethral bulking agent for stress urinary incontinence: Modified technique and early results. J Urol 2003; 170:2327–2329.

91. Chrouser KL, Fick F, Goel A, et al. Carbon coated zirconium beads in beta-glucan gel and bovine glutaraldehyde cross-linked collagen injections for intrinsic sphincteric deficiency: Continence and satisfaction after extended follow-up. J Urol 2004; 171:1152–1155.

92. United States Food and Drug Administration: Durasphere™ Injectable Bulking Agent. Summary of Safety and Effectiveness Data, 1999. www.fda.gov/cdrh/pdf/p980053.html.

93. Madjar S, Sharma AK, Waltzer WC, et al. Periurethral mass formations following bulking agent injection for the treatment of urinary incontinence. J Urol 2006; 175:1408–1410.

94. Ritts RE. Particle migration after transurethral injection of carbon coated beads. J Urol 2002; 167:1804–1805.

95. United States Food and Drug Administration. URYX® Urethral bulking agent – P030030 Part II: Summary of safety and effectiveness data, 2004. http://www.fda.gov/cdrh/PDF3/p030030b.

96. Dmochowski RR, Appell RA. Advancements in minimally invasive treatments for female stress urinary incontinence: Radiofrequency and bulking agents. Curr Urol Rep 2003; 4:350–355.

97. Dmochowski RR. Tegress™ Urethral implant phase III clinical experience and product uniqueness. Rev Urol, 2005; 7(Suppl 1):S22–26.

98. Hurtado EA, McCrery RJ, Appell RA. The safety and efficacy of ethylene vinyl alcohol copolymer as an intra-urethral bulking agent in women with intrinsic urethral deficiency. Int Urogynecol J 2007; 18:869–873.

99. Hurtado EA, McCrery RJ, Appell RA. Complications of ethylene vinyl alcohol copolymer as an intra-urethral bulking agent in men with stress urinary incontinence. Urology 2008; 71:662–65.

100. Mayer R, Lightfoot M, Jung I. Preliminary evaluation of calcium hydroxylapatite as a transurethral bulking agent for stress urinary incontinence. Urology 2001; 57:434–438.

101. United States Food and Drug Administration. Coaptite® implanted device. www.fda.gov/cdrh/mda/docs/p040047.html, 2005.

102. Winters JC, Appell RA. Periurethral injection of collagen in the treatment of intrinsic sphincteric deficiency in the female patient. Urol Clin North Am 1995; 22:673–678.

103. Biomatrix Corporation. Formal report of feasibility study of Hylagel Uro. Corporate white paper. Ridgefield, NJ, June 2000.

104. Stenberg A, Larsson G, Johnson P, et al. DiHA Dextran copolymer, a new biocompatible material for endoscopic treatment of stress incontinent women. Acta Obstet Gynecol Scand 1999; 78:436–442.

105. Stenberg A, Larsson G, Johnson P. Urethral injection for stress urinary incontinence: Long-term results with dextranomer/hyaluronic acid copolymer. Int Urogynecol J Pelvic Dysfunct 2003; 14:335–338.

106. Van Kerrebroeck P, ter Meulen F, Larsson G, et al. Efficacy and safety of a novel system (NASHA/Dx copolymer using the Implacer device) for treatment of stress urinary incontinence. Urology 2004; 64:276–281.

107. Walker RS, Wilson K, Clark AE. Injectable bioglass as a potential substitute for injectable polytetrafluorethylene. J Urol 1992; 148:645–647.

108. Atala A, Cima LG, Kim W, et al. Injectable alginate seeded with chondrocytes as a potential treatment for vesicoureteral reflux. J Urol 1993; 150:745–747.

109. Bent AE, Tutrone RT, McLennan, et al. Treatment of intrinsic sphincter deficiency using autologous ear chondrocytes as a bulking agent. Neurourol Urodyn 2001; 20:157–165.

110. Yokoyama T, Chancellor MB, Watanabe T, et al. Primary myoblast injection into urethra and bladder as a potential treatment of stress urinary incontinence and impaired detrusor contractility: Long-term survival without significant cytotoxicity. J Urol 2000; 161:307.

111. Cannon TW, Lee JY, Somogyi G, et al. Improved sphincter contractility after allogenic muscle-derived progenitor cell injection into the denervated rat urethra. Urology 2003; 62:958–963.

112. Peyromaure M, Sebe P, Praud C, et al. Fate of implanted syngeneic muscle precursor cells in striated urethral sphincter of female rats: Perspectives for the treatment of urinary incontinence. Urology 2004; 64:1037–1041.

113. Pycha A, Klinger CH, Haitel A, et al. 3 years experience with implantable microballoons for the treatment of intrinsic sphincter deficiency. J Urol 2000; 161:307.

Chapter 13
Surgery for Stress Urinary Incontinence: Midurethral Slings

Demetri C. Panayi and Vik Khullar

Introduction

There is a spectrum of urodynamic stress incontinence ranging from women with pure intrinsic sphincter deficiency to women with only hypermobility to women with a mixture of both. Bladder neck slings previously were used in those women where an obstructive procedure was required. However, the introduction of midurethral slings and the concept of "tension-free" placement of these tapes changed this idea significantly. This type of tape appears to be useful in treating women with both intrinsic sphincter deficiency and bladder neck hypermobility.

Various etiologic factors contribute to reducing the ability of the submucosal and muscular layers of the urethra to compress the lumen and therefore function as a sphincter. These factors include trauma, denervation, or devascularization phenomena such as neurological compromise (caused by certain conditions such as sacral agenesis, spinal cord injury, or myelodysplasia), childbirth injury, connective tissue disorders, menopause, or exposure to radiation.

The other management options when considering treating women with this condition include retropubic surgery, bulking agents and artificial urinary sphincters. Slings have better long-term success rates compared to bulking agents [1] and less morbidity when compared to artificial sphincters, which can suffer malfunction or lead to infection and erosion [2]. It also is considered the best procedure in women with coexisting medical problems such as obesity, which increases the risk of operative complications and failure [3].

Pubovaginal slings have been described as a treatment for stress incontinence since the beginning of the twentieth century. The technique of their application and the materials used has varied.

The first descriptions of the suburethral sling procedure occurred in the early 1900s and involved the use of pyramidalis or gracilis muscles or rectus sheath as a suburethral sling with or without plication of the bladder neck. The use of rectus sheath fascia was first described in 1942 by Aldridge, and this was further modified in 1968, when Chasse Moir introduced the gauze hammock procedure.

Until recently slings were considered a second- or third-line procedure in the treatment of stress incontinence; however, since the 1990s it now is considered that a sling procedure is indicated if there is intrinsic sphincter deficiency with or without hypermobility, irrespective of whether the woman has undergone previous incontinence surgery.

Sling materials broadly include *autologous materials,* which include rectus fascia, dermis, and tendons; *allografts* from human cadavers including rectus fascia, dermis, and dura mater; *xenografts* such as porcine or bovine dermis, bovine pericardium, dura, or intestinal submucosa; and *synthetic* materials such as Mersilene and Prolene. The length of the sling can vary from "full length" (>20 cm) to "patch slings" (3–5 cm).

Aldridge originally described the procedure as an active mechanism in that the sling moves with the abdominal wall (to which it is attached via the abdominal aponeurosis) during episodes of increased intra-abdominal pressure; during coughing and sneezing, the sling is drawn anteriorly, therefore increasing intraurethral closure pressure [4]. In this way the sling procedure aims to restore sufficient outlet resistance to the urethra during stress events to prevent leakage without producing obstruction during voiding while also providing some bladder neck support.

Zacharin [5] suggested that the endopelvic fascia and pubourethral ligaments allow effective transmission of increases in intra-abdominal pressure by providing support to the urethra. The sling therefore may be providing support and passive resistance to the urethra in the same manner rather than causing elevation and compression.

In summary, traditional pubovaginal slings attempt to correct hypermobility of the bladder neck and enhance transmission of intra-abdominal pressure provoked by straining.

Slings that are inserted at the midurethral point mainly use synthetic materials. Introduced in 1994, these have grown in acceptance and the tension-free vaginal tape (TVT) is now the most common procedure carried out for incontinence in the world. Originally, Mersilene, a multifilament mesh, and other low-porosity mesh materials were employed until being replaced with polypropylene monofilament mesh tapes because of concerns regarding a high erosion rate with multifilaments [6]. Polypropylene monofilament mesh currently is considered the material of choice (Fig. 13.1).

The principle behind the midurethral approach is that incontinence results from weakening of the existing support structures of the urethra, anterior vaginal wall to the midurethra, and the vagina is connected to the arcus tendinus fasciae pelvis providing support to the midurethra [7].

The midurethral approach is favored because it involves minimal vaginal dissection or alteration of vaginal architecture, and therefore minimal effect on the mobility of the proximal urethra. Many authors believe the proximal urethra to be an important determinant of normal voiding, which can be affected as a complication of continence surgery. Tape insertion is also a relatively easy procedure to technically master and is not associated with the operative morbidity of the Burch colposuspension, nor does it necessitate an abdominal incision as pubovaginal slings do.

The mainstay of midurethral surgery is the TVT, which employs the technique of transvaginal introduction of the synthetic tape that passes retropubically and is exposed through the anterior abdominal wall [8] (Fig. 13.2). However, a transobturator approach recently has been introduced and despite the lack of long-term data has reported similar cure and complication rates with a reduced risk of bladder trauma [9–12]

Mastery of any sling procedure requires intimate understanding of the local anatomy to minimize intraoperative complications and maximize surgical effect.

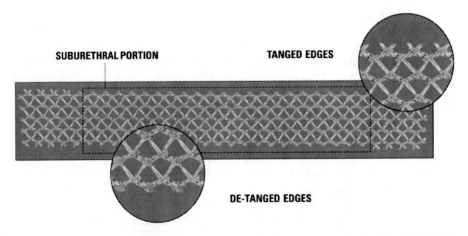

SUBURETHRAL PORTION   TANGED EDGES

DE-TANGED EDGES

FIG. 13.1. The polypropylene mesh used in the Boston Scientific ObTryx System (reproduced with kind permission of Boston Scientific Corporation)

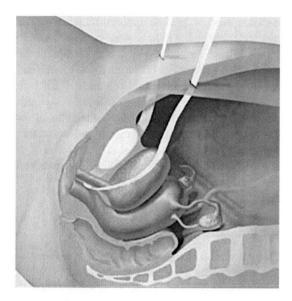

FIG. 13.2. The correct position of the tension-free vaginal tape (reproduced with kind permission of Gynecare/Ethicon)

Patient Selection and Assessment

As with any surgery, prior to a sling procedure, women need a thorough assessment including details of genital and urinary symptoms including incontinence type and severity and symptoms of vaginal prolapse, full obstetric history, any neurological conditions, and previous surgical procedures or exposure to radiation. Examination should involve pelvic floor compartment examination for demonstration of incontinence and assessment of any other pelvic pathology. Investigations should include urinalysis, uroflowmetry, and postvoid residual because all procedures for treatment of incontinence can be complicated by voiding difficulties especially those with preexistent high postvoid residuals or those with prolonged intermittent uroflow patterns. In the cases of these patients, appropriate counseling of this risk and training in intermittent self-catheterization preoperatively is essential.

Further investigations prior to the sling procedure also should include assessment of urethral mobility (video)urodynamics, imaging of the bladder neck, and assessment of urethral resistance via maximal urethral closure pressure or leak point pressure. Leak point pressures of below 60 cm H_2O or maximal urethral closure pressures of below 20 cm H_2O are diagnostic of intrinsic sphincter deficiency. The other benefit of urodynamics is the assessment of detrusor muscle activity, voiding function, and bladder compliance. Patients with history and urodynamic evidence of mixed incontinence present a clinical challenge and use of anticholinergics prior to embarking on midurethral tape procedure may be appropriate.

Patients who have had previous continence surgery or have operative bladder symptoms also should have urodynamic studies and may need cystoscopic assessment of the lower urinary tract prior to insertion of the midurethral tape.

The Tension-Free Vaginal Tape

The Gynecare TVT (Fig. 13.3) system employs a polypropylene mesh tape with a pore size of 75–150 mm. The large pores encourage incorporation into the patient's own tissues; the mesh itself is elastic, and hence moves with the patient's own movements and yet forms a backstop to actions such as coughing, laughing, and sneezing. The knitted monofilament provides resistance to infection. In keeping with the principles of midurethral systems, the TVT attempts to reinforce dysfunctional pubourethral ligaments, enhance connective tissue in the paraurethral area, and create a solid floor beneath the urethra.

This procedure was described by Ulmsten in 1995 [8] as an alternative to the more time-consuming and technically difficult Burch colposuspension. It has shown comparable cure rates as well as shorter operating time and reduced morbidity associated with it [13–17]. The procedure also can be performed under sedation with local anesthesia or spinal anesthesia, thereby reducing the anesthetic risks to the patient.

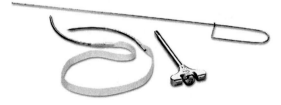

FIG. 13.3. The Gynecare TVT system comprising TVT needles with removable handle, polypropylene tape, and guide (reproduced with kind permission of Gynecare/Ethicon)

Procedure

The TVT was developed as a standardized technique to allow a safe method with the best clinical outcome. The technique described below is prone to variation between individual operators. However, the principles underpinning safe insertion and minimal exposure to complications remain the same.

The procedure is performed with the patient in lithotomy position with no more than 70° of hip flexion. Vaginal examination is performed and via abdominal palpation, the anticipated pathway of the tape is demonstrated. A solution of 100 ml normal saline mixed with 20 ml of 0.25% bupivicaine is used to infiltrate retropubically, with 40 ml of solution infiltrated suprapubically behind the pubic bone 3 cm from the midline. Then 20 ml of the solution is introduced vaginally paraurethrally under the pubic bone on each side. The aim is for the infiltrate to follow the retropubic course of the tape on either side of the midline. The landmarks are the posterior surface of the pubic bone down to the urogenital diaphragm. Further 5 ml of 0.5% xylocaine anesthetic with 1 in 50,000 of adrenaline is introduced into the vaginal mucosa at the midurethral point and paraurethrally up to the urogenital diaphragm. A 2-cm vaginal incision is made beneath the urethra. Through this incision, paraurethral dissection is undertaken bilaterally to the level of the urogenital diaphragm. The TVT needle then is introduced with slow, controlled pressure aimed at the inferior tip of the ipsilateral scapula following the pathway previously hydrodissected with local anesthetic. A wire guide inserted into the urethral foley catheter is used to deviate the bladder to the contralateral side of needle insertion to prevent injury. It is important to remain close to the pubic bone before angling upward and emerging through the skin incision in the abdomen. These are made 2–3 cm either side of the midline. Once the needle emerges through the skin of the anterior abdominal wall, a cystoscopy is performed to identify any bladder trauma. This needle has a removable handle and so it can be used to repeat the procedure on the other side. Some operators perform a cough test, which involves filling the bladder and instructing the patient to cough vigorously so that the tape can be adjusted accordingly. If the patient is under general anesthesia, this is not possible so the tape is adjusted by tightening against an instrument placed between the tape and the midurethral portion. The tape is contained within a plastic sheath, which serves to ease the passage of the tape through the tissues and prevent its contamination. Once final tensioning adjustments have been made, the sheath is removed and the tape is cut flush to the abdominal skin, which is lifted under tension to allow the tape to lie free of the incision and no further tightening occurs. The vaginal skin is closed with absorbable suture and the abdominal incisions can be closed with suture or with glue.

Complications

The advantage of the TVT is that it is minimally invasive, can be carried out under local or spinal anesthesia, and in some units is carried out as a day case procedure. As a result it has a relatively low complication rate when compared to Burch colposuspension, the gold standard treatment for stress incontinence [14, 17].

However, some of the risks associated with continence procedures do apply to TVT. The more common complications include voiding difficulties (7–20%), urgency (1–20%), urinary tract infection, (4–15%), bladder injury (2–5%), hematoma (1–3%), wound infection (1%), bleeding (1–3%), and vaginal (0.7%)/urethral (2.7%) erosion.

Outlet obstruction also can manifest as urinary retention, high postoperative residuals, urgency or worsening of previous urgency. Difficulty in voiding may be associated with increased tension in the tape itself. It is important to remember that the tape is intended to be placed "tension-free" and overzealous tightening of the vaginal tape can lead to voiding difficulties or retention. Obstructive symptoms usually resolve with time. Uncommonly, patients need a repeat procedure to transect, loosen, or remove the tape, or require clean intermittent catheterization. Long-term retention is a rare complication of TVT (0.6–3.8%).

As insertion of the needles into the vagina and through the anterior abdominal wall is performed blindly, one might perceive that there is considerable risk of breaching the abdominal cavity and/or causing serious vascular damage. However, these occurrences are rare, with bowel perforation reported at a very low rate (0.03–0.05%), as is severe vascular injury (0.04–0.08%).

Evidence-Based Clinical Outcome

The majority of recent studies reflect a favorable cure rate compared with Burch colposuspension and other continence procedures [1, 11, 14–21]. Ward et al. [17], in a cohort of 344 patients with 175 undergoing TVT and 169 undergoing Burch, found a cure/improvement rate of 66% in the TVT group after 6-month follow-up compared with 57% in the Burch group. The cure criteria were negative cystometry and negative pad test. At 2 years the same group demonstrated 63% cure rate versus 51% for the Burch group.

Paraiso et al. [16] compared TVT to laparoscopic Burch colposuspension in 72 patients, with cure criteria of urodynamic studies at 1 year and no symptomatic leakage. Thirty-six underwent TVT and 36 underwent laparoscopic Burch colposuspension. They found a cure rate of 97% in the TVT group compared to 81% in patients who underwent the laparascopic Burch.

Rechberger et al. [21] studied 100 patients, 50 of whom underwent TVT and 50 had multifilament intravaginal slingplasty, a modification of TVT. The cure rates at 4–18 months were defined as being free of symptoms of stress incontinence and having negative supine and standing cough stress test. They also defined improvement as having symptomatic stress incontinence but improved from the preoperative state. They found an 88 and 80% cure rate in the TVT and intravaginal slingplasty groups, respectively.

Dietz et al. [19] looked at 106 patients, 69 of whom underwent TVT, while 37 had suprapubic pubic arch sling procedure (SPARC), another modification of TVT. The cure rate at 6 weeks to 18 months was defined as a negative cough stress test and subjective cure of symptoms reported by the patient. There was a 94% cure rate associated with TVT, with a 74% cure rate with patients who had SPARC.

Other authors report similar rates of success: Wang et al. (2003) with an objective cure rate of 82%; Ustun et al. (2003) and Liang et al. (2002) determined an 83% cure rate. There also is considerable long-term evidence to support the use of TVT [18, 22–25].

Transobturator Approach

The theory of the transobturator route is an extension of the principles of the mechanism of action of the TVT. The transobturator approach involves placement of midurethral tape through the obturator membrane (Fig. 13.4). Although there is a lack of long-term data regarding this approach, the current data suggest a comparable continence and complication rate with TVT, with some studies suggesting a reduction in incidence of bladder trauma compared to TVT or colposuspension [9–12, 26].

Procedure

The technique for introduction of the tape is divided into two categories. The "outside-to-in" or "inside-to-out" methods. The description "inside to out" refers to the introduction of the tape from the vaginal incision, with it emerging "outward" or lateral to the thigh folds. The "outside-to-in" method involves the tape entering through an incision lateral to the labia majora and emerging in the vaginal incision.

The inside-to-out tape is the tension-free vaginal tape-obturator (TVT-O) manufactured by Gynecare. The first difference between this tape and the TVT procedure is the positioning of the patient. For all transobturator methods the patient is in lithotomy with 120° hyperflexion. The first step is to mark the exit points of the tape in the lateral thigh folds. Using a marker pen, the exit points of the tape are designated. These are 2 cm lateral to where a line parallel and 2 cm superior to a horizontal line intersects the thigh folds.

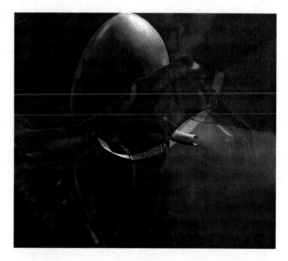

Fig. 13.4. Schematic showing the transobturator route (reproduced with kind permission of Boston Scientific Corporation)

The TVT-O equipment itself consists of the polypropylene mesh with large open-knit pores, which is blue for easy identification, a winged guide along which the helical passers are introduced, and tip tubing that is held allowing the helical passers to be withdrawn.

Once the exit points have been marked and the equipment is assembled and checked, local anesthetic is infiltrated into the vagina and a vaginal incision is made in a similar fashion to the TVT. The dissection, however, is laterally and toward the ischiopubic ramus. A "give" will be felt as the obturator membrane is breached. The metal winged guide then is inserted following the pathway of dissection and passes through the obturator membrane. The helical passers then are introduced along the gutter of the metal guide. Once through the obturator membrane the helical passers are rotated under controlled pressure and turned so their tips emerge at the designated exit points marked at the start of the procedure. The plastic tip tubings are externalized through the skin and then grasped with clamps, allowing the helical passer to be withdrawn by performing the introduction maneuver in reverse. The procedure is repeated on the contralateral side of the patient. The plastic sheath around the tape is removed simultaneously, allowing the tape to be centered correctly and the tension of the tape is adjusted as for a TVT. The vagina then is closed with absorbable suture and the skin over the tape can be glued or sutured.

The "outside-to-in method" is performed with the patient in the same position as inside to out. There are many more systems available for this method, including Monarc (American Medical Systems), Eris (Mentor), and Obtryx™ Transobturator Mid-Urethral Sling System (Boston Scientific) (Fig 13.5). This employs the Advantage™ Mesh, a polypropylene mesh with a detangled suburethral segment with a large pore size >100 mm.

For this method the incision is made on the lateral aspect of the labia majora at the level of the clitoris, posterior to the insertion of the adductor longus muscle tendon and 1–2 cm lateral to the ischopubic ramus. The vaginal incision then is made after infiltration with local anesthetic. The helical introducer then is introduced through the skin directed in a perpendicular fashion to the skin. Once the distinct sensation of breaching the obturator membrane is felt, the helical introducer is rotated medially to

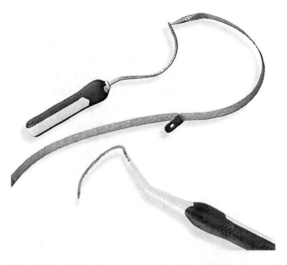

FIG. 13.5. Helical passers and polypropylene tape of the Obtryx transobturator system (reproduced with kind permission of Boston Scientific Corporation)

emerge in the vagina onto the tip of the index finger of the operator, which serves to protect the urethra and allow controlled passage of the helical introducer. Once the tip of the introducer has emerged in the vaginal incision, the operator should verify that a vaginal mucosal "button-hole" has not been created and check the urethra for any trauma. Once this has been confirmed, the tape is attached onto the tip of the introducer using various methods. Once the tape is secured, the helical introducers are rotated back in a reverse fashion and out through the original skin incision. This procedure then is repeated on the contralateral side. The tension of the tape is adjusted using a pair of scissors or clamp between it and the urethra. Because of the much-reduced incidence of bladder injury associated with the obturator approach, cytoscopy is not universally practiced; however, it is good practice to perform cytoscopy following the insertion of the tape. The vagina and skin incisions are closed in a similar fashion to the inside-to-out technique.

Complications

There are similar risks associated with the transobturator approach as there are with the TVT. The risk of bladder injury is reported to be lower than in the retropubic approach, with inside-to-out method using the TVT-O associated with the lowest incidence.

Vaginal tape erosion or exposure in the vagina or bladder remain risks with all synthetic slings. There are two separate processes occurring, although the mechanism is not entirely clear. First is a failure of primary vaginal healing resulting in the tape becoming exposed in the vagina often as a result of infection. Second, there is tape migration, which may be associated with mechanical friction or failure of integration of the tape into the host's tissues. It has been suggested that tapes with larger pore sizes integrate more effectively, and hence are associated with reduced incidence of erosion. Should tape erosion occur, then it may be necessary to remove the tape, especially if a multifilament tape such as ObTape or IVS tape was used.

There appears to be a lower incidence of postoperative voiding dysfunction associated with the transobturator tapes compared to the retropubic tapes. The risk of de novo urgency is reported between 2 and 7%; however, De Tayrac et al. (2004) and Mansoor et al. (2003) found no difference in voiding difficulties or retention between TVT and transobturator tapes with between 1 and 15% rate of voiding obstruction has been reported in the literature.

Other complications associated specifically with transobturator tapes include hematoma or neuropathic trauma leading to postoperative leg or groin pain, which has been observed in 2–15% of cases depending on the study quoted. In all cases, the pain was temporary and usually responded to standard oral analgesia.

91% cure rate after 17 months follow-up. Costa et al. [28] stated an outcome of 80.5% cure rate, with a mean of 7 months follow-up with a cough stress test and questionnaire-based assessment. More recently, a meta-analysis considering studies comparing TVT to the transobturator approach using the "inside-to-out" and "outside-to-in" methods [9] showed that the transobturator approach was associated with similar cure rates and reduced rates of bladder injury and voiding difficulties; however, mesh erosion, vaginal injuries, and leg or groin pain were more common with TVT-O. Mean follow-up in these studies, however, was 7 months and this remains the weakness in the evidence for using the transobturator approach. One recent study by Giberti and co-authors [29] studied 108 women with a mean follow-up of 2 years and reported subjective cure rates and objective of 92 and 80%, respectively.

The potential advantages of the obturator approach make it appear to be an attractive alternative to the TVT. The procedure is shorter and an easier technique to master and it does not involve proximity to the pelvic vasculature or intra-abdominal organs, and therefore does not encumber the risk of their injury. The risks of lower urinary tract injury appear to be less than TVT, and thus do not necessitate cystoscopy, although it remains good practice to perform this procedure after insertion of any tape.

Despite these points for optimism, there needs to be a larger body of evidence to support its clinical effectiveness with long-term follow-up.

Evidence-Based Clinical Outcome

More research is required into the clinical effectiveness of the transobturator tape. The body of evidence is inferior to that which supports the case for the TVT, particularly in terms of long-term data. However, results are encouraging, with clinical effectiveness in the limited numbers of studies comparable to the TVT procedure.

De Tayrac et al. [2004] looked at 61 patients: 31 had TVT and 30 had transobturator suburethral tape (TOT). The definition of cure was negative stress test and symptomatic dryness. The cure rates were 84% for TVT and 90% for TOT after 1-year follow-up. Similarly, Delorme et al. [27] found a

Suprapubic Pubic Arch Sling (SPARC) Procedure

This system is a similarly minimally invasive sling procedure using a loosely knitted self-fixating 4–0 propylene mesh, which is positioned at the midurethra via passing suspension needles "from above" through incisions on the anterior abdominal skin and emerging in the vaginal incision. This is effectively the TVT method using the "outside-to-in" principle. Its mechanism of action mirrors the principles behind all midurethral tapes: forming an anatomical hammock and following the role of the pubourethral ligament and paravaginal structure in supporting the urethra.

As well as the mesh itself, the SPARC equipment (American Medical Systems) is composed of disposable suspension needles, dilator-connectors to which the tape is attached that permit untwisting of the mesh after attachment, a plastic sheath surrounding the mesh, and an absorbable colored tensioning suture knotted at intervals within the mesh sling preventing pretensioning of the mesh when the sheath is withdrawn as well as allowing intra- and postoperative sling adjustment.

Procedure

The SPARC procedure can be performed under general, regional, or local anesthesia. The patient is in the lithotomy position and with the bladder emptied.

The entry points for the suspension needles are located 1.5 cm either side of the midline over the symphysis pubis and it is here that stab incisions are made. A 2–3-cm vaginal incision is made over the area of the midurethra, which can be preceded by infiltration to aid dissection of the plane between the vaginal epithelium and the periurethral fascia. Using scissors this plane is developed to the border of the pubic ramus at the level of the midurethra, creating adequate room for the surgeon's finger to be inserted, thereby allowing controlled passage of the suspension needles through the periurethral fascia and into the vaginal incision.

The suspension needle is passed through the abdominal incisions and downward onto the symphysis pubis before being passed along the superior surface of the bone and downward through the rectus fascia and muscle. It then is rotated along the posterior surface of the bone through the space of Retzius before being guided inferiorly until reaching the endopelvic fascia. Staying in close proximity to the pubic bone minimizes the risk of bowel, blood vessel, bladder, or urethral injury. The finger in the vaginal incision then palpates the needle tip and directs it to the point of perforation of the endopelvic fascia, which is as lateral as possible against the inferior border of the pubic ramus. Once the endopelvic fascia has been breached, the suspension needle tip can be controlled along the dissected plane with the vaginal finger checking that no "button-holing" has occurred. The procedure is repeated on the contralateral side followed by cystoscopy with a filled bladder including careful

inspection of the urethra. The sling is attached to the needle tips with its markings positioned centrally. With this system the connectors snap and click into place before the needles are directed backward into the retropubic space by the surgeon and then upward to be withdrawn through the abdominal skin incisions. The tape can be adjusted in a similar fashion to other slings by inserting a pair of scissors, clamp, or dilator between it and the midurethra and applying traction to its ends. Once satisfactory tension is achieved, the plastic sheaths can be withdrawn and the mesh is cut flush to the skin before the skin is lifted to cover the mesh ends. Closure of the abdominal skin incisions as with the TVT can be with absorbable suture, glue, or steri-strips, and the vagina is closed with absorbable sutures.

Complications

Postoperative de novo urgency and voiding difficulties including urinary retention remain a complication with this system as with all continence procedures. As with other sling procedures, care must be taken to avoid excessive tension applied to the sling intraoperatively; also this system contains a tensioning suture that provides a restraint to sling stretching which may occur during loosening of the sling during the procedure.

Bladder and urethral injury are a recognized complication of this procedure but with an incidence no greater than with TVT. Good technique and cytoscopy during the procedure if injury is suspected are essential. The incidence of bowel or blood vessel injury remains relatively rare.

Tape exposure in the vagina may result from failure of primary wound healing especially as a result of infection, a recognized risk of synthetic sling materials. Tape erosion into the bladder or urethra usually occurs as a result of perforation during the procedure.

Evidence-Based Clinical Outcome

Dietz and co-authors [19] compared SPARC to TVT in 106 women: 69 underwent the TVT procedure and 37 underwent the SPARC procedure. The follow-up of these patients ranged from 6 weeks to 18 months, with cure being defined as negative cough stress test. A cure rate of 94% was reported with TVT and 78% with SPARC.

Primus [30] with a group of 103 women followed up after 1 year reported a cure rate of 84%, where cure was defined as a negative cough stress test and a pad weight test less than 1 g.

Lord et al. [31] had a cohort of 290 women: 147 underwent TVT and 154 had SPARC. He reported similar objective cure rates of stress incontinence symptoms at 6-week follow-up with 97.4% in the TVT group and 97.4% in the SPARC group, but a statistically significantly higher subjective cure rate in the TVT group (87.1% vs. 76.5% for SPARC). He also reported no statistically significant difference between the rates of bladder perforation, hemorrhage, or de novo urgency, although a higher incidence of acute retention was noted with the SPARC system, requiring statistically significantly more adjustments of the tape in theatre.

Gandhi and coauthors [32] in 2006 also reported higher subjective and objective cure rates in TVT compared to SPARC in 122 women in a retrospective study. However, Tseng and co-authors [33], in a randomized study in 2005, reported no statistically significant difference in cure rates, although more bladder injuries occurred with SPARC, which was not statistically significant. They concluded that both procedures were equally effective.

As with the transobturator systems, SPARC's effectiveness, particularly in the long term, does not yet have the evidence base to support it and further study is needed.

Tension-Free Vaginal Tape-Secur (Tvt-S)

This is a smaller device produced by Gynecare (see Fig. 13.6). Its purported advantages over the current sling procedures is that it has all the benefits of a minimally invasive procedure but avoids the nerve structures that may result in postoperative pain, as well as avoiding the discomfort associated with the sites where the tape exits in the abdominal or thigh skin. It also is inserted via a simpler method and can employ the retropubic or transobturator pathways.

In the retropubic pathway due to its size it avoids proximity to the bowel or major vessels by not reaching the region close to the peritoneal cavity. It requires a small skin incision of only 1 cm and minimal paraurethral dissection (Fig. 13.7).

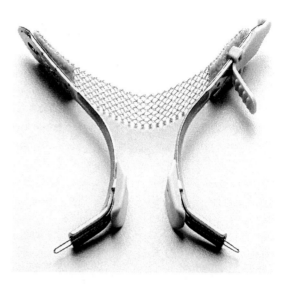

FIG. 13.6. The TVT-Secur system (reproduced with kind permission of Gynecare/Ethicon)

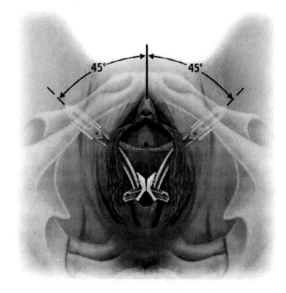

FIG. 13.7. The position of the TVT-Secur system when adopting the retropubic route (reproduced with kind permission of Gynecare/Ethicon)

Following the transobturator route this sling reaches but does not penetrate and emerge from the obturator membrane, and thus it is proposed that the postoperative leg or groin pain associated with TVT-O will be eliminated (Fig. 13.8).

At this stage there is little in the way of evidence to support the effectiveness of this device, and hence its application can only remain in the field of research.

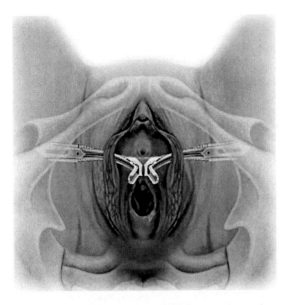

FIG. 13.8. The position of the TVT-Secur system when adopting the transobturator route without passing through the obturator membrane (reproduced with kind permission of Gynecare/Ethicon)

Summary

All midurethral slings apply the same basic mechanism of action by providing suburethral support, and thereby mimicking the function of the pubourethral ligaments and paravaginal tissues. Their mechanism of action stems from the importance of midurethral stabilization, which prevents the separation of the posterior urethral wall from the anterior urethral wall during rotational motion around the inferior portion of the pubic ramus, which appears to be integral to continence. Elevation of the bladder neck, which is the role of pubourethral slings and retropubic urethropexies, may no longer be necessary to achieve continence.

Currently, the TVT is the most common continence procedure carried out worldwide. Of all the synthetic sling procedures it has the largest body of randomized controlled studies supporting its use. It has similar success rates when compared with the gold standard procedure—the Burch colposuspension—with lower operative morbidity associated with it.

The transobturator method is supported by production of many systems of which the majority employ the outside-to-in method. Only the Gynecare TVT-O system uses the inside-to-out approach. The tran-

sobturator method is considered to have a reduced incidence of bladder or urethral injury, particularly the inside-to-out method, with comparable success rates to TVT in the small amount of evidence available regarding its effectiveness. There is limited information regarding the long-term outcome of this method and further study is required.

The SPARC system was proposed to have a reduced incidence of visceral injury, although this has yet to be supported by the literature. What little evidence is available regarding this method reports comparable success rates to TVT; however, data regarding long-term follow-up are awaited.

Female incontinence remains a hotbed for the development of new devices that reduce complication rates and are technically easier to perform with comparable results to traditional procedures. The TVT-Secur is another system involving a considerably small mesh that can be employed via the transobturator pathway where the obturator membrane is not penetrated, or via the retropubic route where its size prevents it from risking bowel or blood vessel injury. Its application remains in the sphere of clinical research until further evidence is gathered to support more widespread use.

References

1. Cody J, Wyness L, Wallace S, et al. Systematic review of the clinical effectiveness and cost-effectiveness of tension-free vaginal tape for treatment of urinary stress incontinence. Health Technol Assess 2003; 7(21):iii1–iii189.
2. Diokno AC. Erosions of the artificial urinary sphincter: Risk factors, outcomes and management. Nat Clin Pract Urol 2006;3(11):580–581.
3. Mukherjee K, Constantine G. Urinary stress incontinence in obese women: Tension-free vaginal tape is the answer. BJU Int 2001; 88(9):881–883.
4. Hilton P. A clinical and urodynamic study comparing the Stamey bladder neck suspension and suburethral sling procedures in the treatment of genuine stress incontinence. Br J Obstet Gynaecol 1989; 96(2):213–220.
5. Zacharin RF. The suspensory mechanism of the female urethra. J Anat 1963; 97:423–427.
6. Andonian S, St-Denis B, Lemieux MC, Corcos J. Prospective clinical trial comparing Obtape(R) and DUPS to TVT: One-year safety and efficacy results. Eur Urol 2007.
7. DeLancey JO. Structural aspects of the extrinsic continence mechanism. Obstet Gynecol 1988; 72 (3 Pt 1):296–301.

8. Ulmsten U, Petros P. Intravaginal slingplasty (IVS): An ambulatory surgical procedure for treatment of female urinary incontinence. Scand J Urol Nephrol 1995; 29(1):75–82.

9. Latthe PM, Foon R, Toozs-Hobson P. Transobturator and retropubic tape procedures in stress urinary incontinence: A systematic review and meta-analysis of effectiveness and complications. BJOG 2007; 114(5):522–531.

10. Liapis A, Bakas P, Giner M, Creatsas G. Tension-free vaginal tape versus tension-free vaginal tape obturator in women with stress urinary incontinence. Gynecol Obstet Invest 2006; 62(3):160–164.

11. Neuman M. TVT and TVT-Obturator: Comparison of two operative procedures. Eur J Obstet Gynecol Reprod Biol 2007; 131(1):89–92.

12. Zullo MA, Plotti F, Calcagno M, et al. One-year follow-up of tension-free vaginal tape (TVT) and transobturator suburethral tape from inside to outside (TVT-O) for surgical treatment of female stress urinary incontinence: A prospective randomised trial. Eur Urol 2007; 51(5):1376–1384.

13. Dean N, Herbison P, Ellis G, Wilson D. Laparoscopic colposuspension and tension-free vaginal tape: a systematic review. BJOG 2006; 113(12):1345–1353.

14. El-Barky E, El-Shazly A, El-Wahab OA, Kehinde EO, Al-Hunayan A, Al-Awadi KA. Tension-free vaginal tape versus Burch colposuspension for treatment of female stress urinary incontinence. Int Urol Nephrol 2005; 37(2):277–281.

15. Kuuva N, Nilsson CG. Tension-free vaginal tape procedure: An effective minimally invasive operation for the treatment of recurrent stress urinary incontinence? Gynecol Obstet Invest 2003; 56(2):93–98.

16. Paraiso MF, Walters MD, Karram MM, Barber MD. Laparoscopic Burch colposuspension versus tension-free vaginal tape: A randomized trial. Obstet Gynecol 2004; 104(6):1249–1258.

17. Ward KL, Hilton P. A prospective multicenter randomized trial of tension-free vaginal tape and colposuspension for primary urodynamic stress incontinence: Two-year follow-up. Am J Obstet Gynecol 2004; 190(2):324–331.

18. Chene G, Amblard J, Tardieu AS, et al. Long-term results of tension-free vaginal tape (TVT) for the treatment of female urinary stress incontinence. Eur J Obstet Gynecol Reprod Biol 2006.

19. Dietz HP, Foote AJ, Mak HL, Wilson PD. TVT and SPARC suburethral slings: A case-control series. Int Urogynecol J Pelvic Floor Dysfunct 2004; 15(2):129–131.

20. Meschia M, Bertozzi R, Pifarotti P, et al. Perioperative morbidity and early results of a randomised trial comparing TVT and TVT-O. Int Urogynecol J Pelvic Floor Dysfunct 2007.

21. Rechberger T, Rzezniczuk K, Skorupski P, et al. A randomized comparison between monofilament and multifilament tapes for stress incontinence surgery. Int Urogynecol J Pelvic Floor Dysfunct 2003; 14(6):432–436.

22. Holmgren C, Nilsson S, Lanner L, Hellberg D. Long-term results with tension-free vaginal tape on mixed and stress urinary incontinence. Obstet Gynecol 2005; 106(1):38–43.

23. Hualde AA, Jimenez CJ, Sarmiento GC et al. [TVT: Our experience five years and six months later]. Actas Urol Esp 2006; 30(2):181–185.

24. Nilsson CG, Kuuva N, Falconer C, Rezapour M, Ulmsten U. Long-term results of the tension-free vaginal tape (TVT) procedure for surgical treatment of female stress urinary incontinence. Int Urogynecol J Pelvic Floor Dysfunct 2001; 12 Suppl 2:S5–S8.

25. Nilsson CG, Falconer C, Rezapour M. Seven-year follow-up of the tension-free vaginal tape procedure for treatment of urinary incontinence. Obstet Gynecol 2004; 104(6):1259–1262.

26. Botros SM, Miller JJ, Goldberg RP, et al. Detrusor overactivity and urge urinary incontinence following trans obturator versus midurethral slings. Neurourol Urodyn 2007; 26(1):42–45.

27. Delorme E, Droupy S, de TR, Delmas V. [Transobturator tape (Uratape). A new minimally invasive method in the treatment of urinary incontinence in women]. Prog Urol 2003; 13(4):656–659.

28. Costa P, Grise P, Droupy S, et al. Surgical treatment of female stress urinary incontinence with a trans-obturator-tape (T.O.T.) Uratape: Short term results of a prospective multicentric study. Eur Urol 2004; 46(1):102–106.

29. Giberti C, Gallo F, Cortese P, Schenone M. Transobturator tape for treatment of female stress urinary incontinence: Objective and subjective results after a mean follow-up of two years. Urology 2007; 69(4):703–707.

30. Primus G. One year follow-up on the SPARC sling system for the treatment of female urodynamic stress incontinence. Int J Urol 2006; 13(11):1410–1414.

31. Lord HE, Taylor JD, Finn JC, et al. A randomized controlled equivalence trial of short-term complications and efficacy of tension-free vaginal tape and suprapubic urethral support sling for treating stress incontinence. BJU Int 2006; 98(2):367–376.

32. Gandhi S, Abramov Y, Kwon C, et al. TVT versus SPARC: Comparison of outcomes for two midurethral tape procedures. Int Urogynecol J Pelvic Floor Dysfunct 2006; 17(2):125–130.

33. Tseng LH, Wang AC, Lin YH, Li SJ, Ko YJ. Randomized comparison of the suprapubic arc sling procedure vs. tension-free vaginal taping for stress incontinent women. Int Urogynecol J Pelvic Floor Dysfunct 2005; 16(3):230–235.

Part IV
Management of Urge Incontinence

Chapter 14
Behavioral Treatments for Urge Incontinence

Howard B. Goldstein and Kristene E. Whitmore

Introduction

Urge urinary incontinence is defined as the involuntary loss of urine accompanied by or preceeded by an urge to urinate [1]. In the normal continent patient, as the bladder fills with urine it will distend, sending afferent signals to the bladder neck and urethra via the sympathetic outflow tracts, leading to contraction of the urethral sphincter and inhibition of the detrusor muscle. Urge incontinence can develop if this delicate neurophysiological pathway is disrupted, leading to uncontrolled detrusor contractions [2]. Treatments for this condition consist of behavioral therapies, medical therapies, and surgical interventions. Over many years behavioral therapies have developed from simple practices such as fluid management and voiding diaries to sophisticated biofeedback techniques with electrical stimulation. Many practitioners consider behavioral therapy as a first-line treatment option for urge incontinence. The Agency for Health Care Policy and Research in 1996 published guidelines for the treatment of urinary incontinence and cited behavioral therapy as a first-line treatment option [3]. Behavioral therapies consist of dietary modification, bladder training, pelvic floor muscle exercises (PFME), biofeedback, functional electrical stimulation (FES), and functional magnetic stimulation (FMS).

Dietary Modification

Anecdotal evidence suggests that reducing bladder irritants such as acidic foods, artificial sweeteners, caffeine, alcohol, or certain fruits may improve urinary incontinence [4]. Research, however, has not demonstrated clear evidence that this is true. Studies examining the role of alcohol with lower urinary tract dysfunction show both no effect and a protective effect [5]. A cross-sectional study of 4,000 men examining the role of food and alcohol in the development of overactive bladder syndrome (OAB) found that alcohol consumption was protective in developing overactive bladder syndrome and that only potatoes appeared to have an association with worsening symptoms [6]. A different cross-sectional study of 6,424 women with stress and urge incontinence/OAB found that there was no association between alcohol consumption and the presence of OAB/urge incontinence [7]. This same study, however, found that smoking, obesity, and consumption of carbonated beverages was associated with OAB/urge incontinence [7].

Caffeine is a xanthine derivative found naturally in coffee beans, tea leaves, and cocoa beans. It is thought to have an excitatory effect on the detrusor muscle and has been shown to cause detrusor contractions on urodynamic testing [8]. Two small studies utilizing psychiatric patients demonstrated that withdrawal of caffeine was associated with a decrease in frequency of incontinent episodes [9, 10]. A study of 41 women with urinary incontinence (stress, urge, and mixed) showed no statistical association between caffeine intake and incontinence [11]. It is difficult to draw any definitive conclusions from the research regarding caffeine intake and its possible association with urge incontinence. Good evidence to suggest that it is associated with urge incontinence and that eliminating it from the diet will improve or cure the condition does not currently exist.

Most patients with urinary incontinence believe that by restricting their fluid intake, they can reduce their incontinence episodes. This often leads to other medical conditions such as dehydration and/or constipation. In a retrospective study of 126 women, Wyman et al. found that there was a weak association between fluid consumption and degree of urinary incontinence [12]. In another study of 128 patients with urinary incontinence (stress, urge, and mixed), Griffiths et al. found that fluid intake was strongly associated with the amount of fluid voided per void and only slightly associated with number of incontinence episodes. They also found that among patients with urge incontinence there was a small association between reducing the amount of evening fluid intake and reducing number of nocturnal enuresis episodes [13]. The evidence does not suggest that reducing fluid intake during the day will improve urge urinary incontinence. There may be a slight improvement in nocturia and nocturnal enuresis in reducing evening fluid intake.

Bladder Training

In a case report in 1966, Jeffcoate et al. first described bladder training as a treatment for urinary incontinence [14]. This therapy relies on the theory that urinary urgency develops first in a patient and this leads to urinary frequency. As this cycle progresses, the patient develops a decreased bladder capacity, which then will lead to detrusor overactivity. The detrusor overactivity then will progress to urge incontinence [15]. If one can break the urinary frequency, then the urgency might stop, which will lead to improvement of the detrusor overactivity and urge incontinence. To accomplish this goal the brain must be trained to ignore the signals from the

detrusor muscle. In our practice we first start with a 3-day voiding diary. The voiding diary will help determine the voiding interval. At the beginning, the patient should be told to void at an interval shorter than their actual interval determined by the voiding diary. If, for example, a patient has a voiding interval of 1 h, then the patient should be instructed to void every 45 min for 1 week and then increase the interval by 15 min each week. At the time that the voiding diary is examined any patterns of incontinent episodes associated with fluid intake or medication times should be examined. If, for example, the patient is ingesting large quantities of fluid before bedtime and then finds that she wakes five to seven times at night to void with some incontinent episodes, then she should be instructed to reduce the fluid intake at night to reduce the nocturia and nocturnal enuresis. The voiding interval should be increased weekly until a normal interval is accomplished. If during the interval the patient has the urge to void, then she should be taught strategies to help ignore the sensation. At this point the patient can use other behavioral therapies to help suppress the desire. Such therapies as deep breathing, quick pelvic floor muscle contractions in succession (quick flicks), meditation, and distraction techniques such as balancing one's checkbook can help suppress the urge (Fig. 14.1). In a study of 123 women with either intrinsic sphincter deficiency ($n = 88$) or urge incontinence ($n = 35$) who received bladder training, there was a 57% reduction in incontinence episodes. In this study the patients underwent urodynamic testing both pre- and posttreatment. Interestingly, after the bladder training therapy the urodynamic testing results remained the same and the bladder capacity on voiding diary did not change after successful bladder training therapy [16]. These findings make one wonder what exactly changes after successful bladder training. Does successful bladder training only affect the brain and its response to detrusor signaling or is there something happening at the level of the detrusor muscle to cause this change? In a study utilizing biofeedback-assisted PFME and urge strategies such as deep breathing for urge incontinence, patients underwent pre- and posttreatment urodynamic testing to assess the treatment's effect on bladder sensation and capacity. Patients reported an 80% reduction in incontinence

STEP	ACTIVITY	COMMENT
1	3 Day Voiding Diary	Obtain number of voids along with volume of fluid intake and medications.
2	Review voiding diary and calculate average voiding interval.	Educate patient on fluid intake and appropriate times to take medications.
3	Set voiding interval 15 minutes less than average voiding interval.	Encourage patient using positive reinforcement. Teach other behavioral techniques such as pelvic floor muscle exercises, deep breathing, etc to overcome urgency between voiding interval.
4	Return to office in 1-2 weeks, review progress, and increase voiding interval by 15 minutes.	Each week increase voiding interval by 15 minutes until a normal interval in achieved.

FIG. 14.1. Pelvic and sexual health institute bladder training program

episodes, yet there were no significant changes in bladder capacity [17].

Cure rates with bladder training have varied from 26 to 90% [18, 19] (Table 14.1). A Cochrane Database meta-). A Cochrane Database meta-analysis conducted in 2003 of all trials evaluating bladder training found that bladder training may be helpful for the treatment of urinary incontinence [20]. There are no standardized bladder-training programs so it is problematic to compare one trial to another. In each study authors often used different programs and added other modalities such as biofeedback or PFME.

Bladder training is a valuable tool for the treatment of urge urinary incontinence. We suggest that it should be used in a multimodal program with other behavioral treatments in order to achieve the greatest success.

Pelvic Floor Muscle Exercises

PFME were first described by Arnold Kegel, an obstetrician and gynecologist, in 1948. He noticed that through exercise he could improve the strength of the pelvic floor muscles, which leads to improved postpartum urinary incontinence. Since his published paper, PFME have become synonymous with Kegel exercises. Kegel applied basic muscle physiology and rehabilitation to the pelvic floor. He noted that inactive, injured muscle will lose approximately 80% of its weight, while active, injured muscle will only lose approximately 20% of its weight [25]. In the postpartum period, by exercising the injured pelvic floor muscles, the degree of muscle wasting could be reduced.

In Kegel's original paper he described the method for identifying the correct muscles for

TABLE 14.1. Randomized control trials for bladder training for urge incontinence.

Author	Study	n	Outcome	P value
Wiseman et al. [21]	BT vs. BT with terodiline	34	56% subjective improvement vs. 44% subjective improvement	NSa
Szonyi et al. [22]	BT vs. BT with oxybutynin	47	44% reduction in leaks per week vs. 82% reduction in leaks per week	NSa
Burgio et al. [23]	BT vs. oxybutynin vs. placebo	169	81% reduction in incontinent episodes vs. 69% reduction in incontinent episodes vs. 39% reduction in incontinent episodes	<0.001
Jarvis et al. [24]	BT vs. imipramine	50	84% subjective improvement vs. 56% subjective improvement	<0.05

aNS Not statistically significant

rehabilitation by placing a finger 1 cm from the introitus immediately inside the pubic rami along the lateral side wall. He described having the patient contract that muscle while simultaneously palpating the abdominal wall to ensure she did not contract the rectus abdominis muscles. He emphasized that the purpose is for the patient to contract the pubococcygeus muscle only [25].

The pubococcygeus muscle is composed of both type 1 (slow twitch) and type II (fast twitch) muscle fibers [26]. Type I fibers are fatigue resistant and depend on oxidative respiration. These fibers can produce muscle contractions over long periods of time, yet they are not extremely forceful. Type II fibers are resistance prone and can function under anaerobic respiration. These fibers can produce forceful contractions but only for short periods of time. In order to reach maximum benefit from PFME, one must exercise and develop both types of muscle fibers. To train the slow twitch fibers, one must have the muscle sustain a contraction with a small force over a long period of time. To train the fast twitch fibers one must contract the muscle with a large force many times, holding for very short periods of time [27]. PFME programs use this knowledge to develop both types of fibers of the levator ani muscles.

Originally it was thought that PFME therapy would benefit only patients with stress incontinence. At the moment the intra-abdominal pressure increases as with a cough or sneeze, the patient can quickly and forcibly contract the levator ani

muscles which will push the urethra against the pubic symphysis, and thus occlude the urethra and prevent any leakage. This type of PFME has been named the "knack" or "stress strategy." The mechanism of action with urge incontinence suggests that when a detrusor contraction occurs the individual contracts her pelvic floor muscles, which leads the central nervous system to send a signal to the pontine micturition center causing inhibition of the detrusor muscle and relaxation of the bladder [28, 29].

The majority of research trials evaluating the efficacy of PFME focus on patients with stress incontinence. The largest well-designed randomized trial of PFME therapy for urge incontinence was conducted by Burgio et al. [22]. In this trial she sampled 197 nondemented patients with urge incontinence who were randomized to PFME with biofeedback, medical therapy (oxybutynin chloride), or placebo. After 8 weeks of therapy the patients were offered combination therapy for another 8 weeks. Combination therapy consisted of medical therapy with PFME and biofeedback. Burgio found an 80.7% reduction in incontinent episodes in the PFME group, a 68.5% reduction of incontinent episodes in the medical therapy group, and a 39.4% reduction in incontinent episodes in the placebo group (all statistically significant) [22]. In a subsequent publication from the original trial focusing on combination therapy, eight patients (12.7%) in the PFME group decided to cross over and continue with combination therapy. These eight patients had a 57.5% reduction of incontinent episodes utilizing PFME therapy. When they crossed over their reduction rate improved to 88.5%, which was statistically significant. Of the patients in the medical therapy arm, 27 (41.5%) decided to cross over and continue with combination therapy. These 27 patients had a 72.7% reduction of incontinence episodes with medical therapy and when combined with PFME it increased to 84.3%, which was statistically significant. This paper demonstrates the effectiveness of PFME for the treatment of urge incontinence and when combined with medical therapy, the reduction in incontinence episodes improves even more [30]. A criticism of this study is that over half of the sample had mixed incontinence. The medical therapy arm was biased for failure as the medication would only address the urge component of the mixed incontinence, whereas the PFME/biofeedback therapy arm was biased for success as this therapy could address both components of the mixed incontinence [31].

In three other randomized controlled trial trials utilizing PFME with mixed incontinence, success rates were reported to range from 54 to 74%. In these studies patients were randomized to PFME or PFME with bladder training, with a control group consisting of no treatment [32–34]. The problem with trials that evaluate the efficacy of PFME is that there are no standardized programs that all authors follow. Each trial has a program unique to that institution and author. Comparing one trial to another is difficult. The authors of the Cochrane Meta-analysis on pelvic floor muscle training describe the problem with research into this modality. They conclude that PFME is a viable first-line therapy for urinary incontinence [35]. The proper number of PFME in a program has not been well established. Various programs range from 45 to 200 exercises. In our practice we have found that prescribing our patients three sets of 15 exercises three times a week has been successful. In a set of 15 contractions we have the patient perform five quick flick contractions (held for 1–2 s) and ten long contractions (held for 6–10 s). This enables us to work both the fast and slow twitch fibers. We have the patient relax the pelvic floor muscles after each contraction for as long as the contraction was held. We instruct our patients that maximum benefit may not be seen until 4–6 months of therapy.

Biofeedback Therapy

In Kegel's original study he found that 30% of women evaluated could not correctly contract her pelvic floor muscles. For these women he used perineometry, utilizing inflatable vaginal probes that could detect the pressure in the vagina, to teach the patient how to correctly contract the pelvic floor muscles [36]. Cardozo et al. described the use of biofeedback for the treatment of detrusor instability. She measured detrusor pressures and recorded them on a chart which then could be converted to an auditory signal the patient could hear. The auditory signal would increase as the pressure rose and decrease as the pressure dropped. The patient also could see the detrusor pressure on the screen and see the rise and fall of pressure. Using this method the patient could both see and hear signals as the detrusor pressure changed. She studied 30 women with this technique and after an average of five 1 h sessions the patients reported a subjective improvement or cure rate of 87% and objective improvement or cure rate of 60% [37].

Biofeedback is an adjunct method used along with PFME to ensure that the patient is contracting the proper muscles. It is based on operant conditioning and is not a treatment in itself. It can take the form of simple verbal feedback during a pelvic exam, vaginal or anal electromyography studies (EMG), or vaginal or anal manometry of the pelvic floor muscles during a pelvic floor muscle contraction (Fig. 14.2). Using visual, tactile, or auditory signals, biofeedback allows the patient to become aware of an unconscious function. Often this information is recorded on a polygraph such that the information can be tracked and observed. Biofeedback therapy has been used in many different specialties such as psychiatry, cardiology, and neurology.

It is estimated that 50% of patients cannot correctly contract their pelvic floor muscles with simple instruction and approximately 25% of those may be worsening their incontinence with the improper pelvic floor muscle contraction or paradoxical contraction of the rectus abdominis muscle [3]. A study of women evaluating the EMG activity of the pelvic floor muscles while also monitoring the EMG activity of the abdominal muscles found concomitant contraction of the pelvic floor muscles and abdominal muscles. This increased intra-abdominal pressure would worsen incontinence in

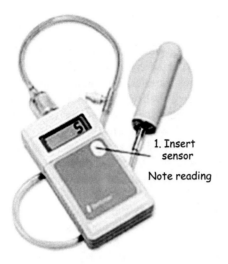

1. Insert sensor

Note reading

Fig. 14.2. Peritron vaginal perineomotry (courtesy of Cardio Design LTD)

the setting of stress or urge incontinence. When the women were told to relax their abdominal muscles while contracting their pelvic floor muscles, the EMG activity showed that their pelvic floor muscles would only produce 25% of its maximum contraction force [38].

In a single-blind, randomized, controlled trial evaluating PFME, PFME with biofeedback and functional electrical stimulation (FES) for patients with overactive bladder and/or urge incontinence, Wang et al. found that there was no difference in subjective improvement and cure rates among the three arms. He also found that the arm receiving PFME with biofeedback had a statistically significant improvement of quality of life, based on scores of the King's Health Questionnaire compared to PFME alone. This study also evaluated pelvic floor muscle strength both before and after treatment. Using this parameter,

the PFME with biofeedback group had the greatest improvement in muscle strength among the three groups (statistically significant) [39].

In a study evaluating which form of biofeedback was superior; Burgio et al. randomized 222 women to anal manometry biofeedback, verbal biofeedback, and a control group consisting of a self-help booklet. All patients had either urge or mixed incontinence. The authors found that there was a 63.1% reduction of incontinence in the anal manometry group, 69.4% reduction in the verbal feedback, and 58.6% reduction in the control group. No statistical significance was found among the three groups [40]. One of the issues this study brings to light is that biofeedback may not be necessary for everyone. Only an estimated 50% of patients will need biofeedback to correctly contract their pelvic floor muscles [3]. Biofeedback should be reserved for patients who fail a traditional PFME program.

The majority of literature on biofeedback relates to patients with stress incontinence. In a review of randomized clinical trials evaluating biofeedback and PFME for the treatment of urge incontinence, Berghman et al. found too few studies to make a conclusion about its efficacy [41] (Table 14.2).

Functional Electrical Stimulation

All of the above therapies require the active participation of the patient. FES is a behavioral therapy that does not require active participation. By using electrical impulses directed to the pelvic nerves, the pelvic floor muscles will contract and potentially lead to their rehabilitation. If setting the FES to a frequency at or below 12 Hz, the pudendal and pelvic nerve stimulation cause an inhibitory effect on the detrusor muscle [42]. FES can be applied

Table 14.2. Randomized control trials of biofeedback therapy for the treatment of urge incontinence.

Author	Study	n	Outcome	P value
Burgio et al. [22]	BF (anal manometry) vs. oxybutynin vs. placebo	190	81% reduction in incontinent episodes vs. 69% reduction in incontinent episodes vs. 39% reduction in incontinent episodes	<0.001
Burgio et al. [40]	BF (anal manometry) vs. PFME coached vs. PFME uncoached (given written instructions)	195	63% reduction in incontinent episodes vs. 69% reduction in incontinent episodes vs. 59% reduction in incontinent episodes	NS[a]

[a]NS Not statistically significant

Table 14.3. Randomized control trials of FES for the treatment of urge incontinence.

Author	Study	n	Outcome	P value
Smith et al. [46]	FES vs. propantheline	38	72% marked improvement vs. 50% marked improvement	NS[a]
Yamanishi et al. [47]	FES vs. sham	60	22% increase in MCC[b] vs. −9% increase in MCC[b]	0.02
Wang et al. [39]	FES vs. BF vs. PFME	103	51% vs. 50% vs. 38% (at least 50% reduction in incontinent episodes)	NS[a]

[a]*NS* Not statistically significant
[b]*MCC* Maximum cystometric capacity

to the pelvic floor via an anal probe, intravaginal probe, or needle electrodes. This therapy can be preformed either in the office or at home. Daily use of FES will make an office-only program impractical. The most common approach to this therapy is an initial office visit to establish correct use of the therapy followed by home use that can be monitored with frequent office visits. This therapy can be used either to allow the patient to identify the pelvic floor muscles and then progress to a PFME program or can be the sole therapy for the patient.

In order for FES to work the proper nerves must be stimulated. As the electrical impulse travels from the device to the target its current will diminish as an inverse square of the distance from the electrical source to the target nerve. Therefore, in an obese patient the distance from the vaginal or anal canal to the nerves may require much higher currents, which can lead to heating of the tissues and pain at the probe site compared to functional magnetic stimulation (FMS) [43].

Many trials have evaluated FES for the treatment of urinary incontinence. It is difficult to compare one trial to another as there are no standardized settings. In each study the current, pulse duration, frequency, and cycle ratio can be different, which may affect the outcome of the therapy. In a randomized, double-blind, placebo-controlled trial of 32 patients with urge incontinence being treated with FES, Yamanishi et al. found that the FES group had a greater cure and improvement rate, increased cystometric capacity, and increased capacity at first desire to void compared to the sham group [44].

In Wang et al., 103 women with overactive bladder and or urge incontinence were randomized to either PFME, biofeedback assisted PFME, or FES. He found that after 12 weeks of therapy 51% of women receiving FES, 50% of women receiving biofeedback-assisted PFME, and 38% of women receiving PFME alone improved or were cured by their treatments. This was not statistically significant [39].

In Brubaker et al., a total of 121 women with either incontinence from detrusor overactivity, stress incontinence, or mixed incontinence were randomized to either FES or sham therapy. In this study, 49.5% of patients were diagnosed with stress incontinence, 23.2% diagnosed with urge incontinence, and 27.3% diagnosed with mixed incontinence. After 8 weeks of therapy the authors found a statistically significant difference between the pre- and posttreatment cures of detrusor overactivity in the FES group and not the sham group. She found a cure rate of 49% in patients with detrusor overactivity [45].

In the proper setting, FES is an effective tool for urge incontinence. If a patient is not able to contract the pelvic floor muscles properly and has failed biofeedback therapy, then it is warranted to introduce FES. In our practice we use it in this setting and then progress to a biofeedback-associated PFME program once the patient can accurately perform pelvic floor muscle contractions. (Table 14.3)

Functional Magnetic Stimulation

Magnetic therapy was first used in the eighteenth century by an Italian physician named Galvani. He used a battery to contract a frog's leg. Since that time magnetic fields have been shown to cause an alignment of electrons that can stimulate an electrical impulse. One of the differences between the generation of magnetic fields and electrical fields is that magnetic fields do not degrade when traveling through tissues. Electrical fields will degrade as they travel through clothing, skin, fat, and bone. Magnetic fields will not. The current required to stimulate the pudendal nerves in an obese patient compared to a very thin patient in magnetic therapy is the same. In FES, the current required to stimulate an obese patient is much greater than a thin patient, thus increasing the likelihood of an adverse reaction to the high current. Functional magnetic stimulation (FMS) often is provided through a coil implanted in a chair that the patient sits on. This therapy can be applied while the patient remains clothed, without the use of any probes or electrode needles. One of the obstacles to providing this therapy is that it cannot be applied in the home. The magnetic chairs currently available are not for home use so the patient must come to the office approximately two times a week for 6 weeks of treatment [43] (Fig. 14.3). Functional magnetic therapy works similarly to FES. At a low current it will cause the stimulation of the pelvic and pudendal nerves, which will lead to a relaxation of the detrusor muscle [48].

In a trial comparing the efficacy of functional magnetic therapy with FES, 32 patients with urge incontinence were randomized to the two therapies. The authors found that although both therapies were efficacious, the functional magnetic therapy sample had an increased cystometric capacity of 106% from baseline compared to an increase of 16% from baseline in the FES group (statistically significant) [47].

In a trial of 24 patients with urge or mixed incontinence who underwent twice weekly treatments for 8 weeks of FMS found that 58% had an objective improvement and 71% had a subjective improvement. Although these findings were significantly different from pretreatment values, the authors did not compare this therapy to any other treatment or placebo so it is difficult to interpret the results [43].

Conclusion

Behavioral treatment for urge incontinence is a viable option. Using the above therapies in a systematic manner can lead to a successful outcome. In our practice we first start with a voiding diary and bladder training (Fig. 14.4). We then

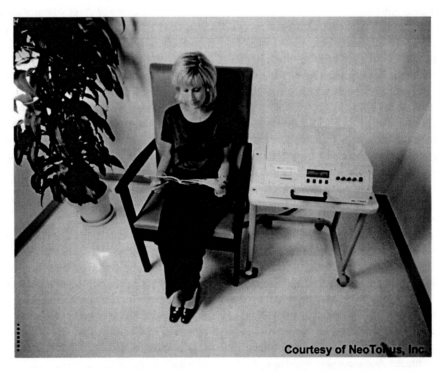

Fig. 14.3. Neocontrol functional magnetic stimulation (courtesy of Neotonus Company)

FIG. 14.4. The Pelvic and sexual health institute behavioral treatment algorithm

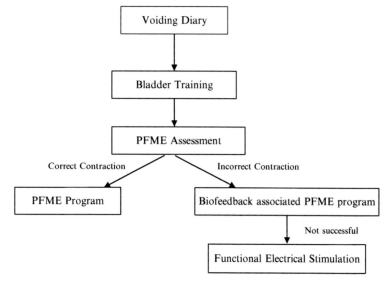

have the patient evaluated by our physical therapist for PFME. If the patient cannot correctly contract and relax the proper muscles, then the patient will undergo biofeedback-assisted PFME. If the patient still cannot properly perform PFME, then we implement FES. We do not use FMS since it cannot be performed in the home and the goal of our programs is for the patients to undergo a home regimen with periodic office visits to monitor success. After 2–3 weeks of FES we then revert back to biofeedback-assisted PFME. We also teach the patient behavioral strategies to resist the urgency such as deep breathing techniques, not running to the bathroom, doing 5–10 quick flick PFME, and sitting when the urgency occurs. We have found that our algorithm has been successful for the treatment of urge incontinence.

References

1. Abrams P, Cardoza L, Fall M, et al. The standardization of terminology of lower urinary tract dysfunction: Report from the standardization sub-committee of the international continence society. Neurourol Urodynman 2002; 21: 167–178.

2. De Groat WC. A neurologic basis for the overactive bladder. Urology 1997; 50(Sup 6A): 36–52.

3. Fantyl JA, Newman DK, Colling J, et al. Urinary incontinence in adults: Acute and chronic management. Clinical practice guideline no 2, 1996 update. Rockville (MD): US Department of Health and Human Services, Public Health Services, Agency for Health Care Policy and Research; March 1996.

4. Wyman J. Management of urinary incontinence in adult ambulatory care population. Annu Rev Nurs Res 2000; 18: 171–194.

5. Roe B, Doll H. Lifestyle factors and continence status: Comparison of self-report data from a postal survey in England. J Wound Ostomy Continence Nurs 1999; 26(6): 312–313.

6. Dallosso H, Matthews R, McGrother C, et al. The association of diet and lifestyle factors with the onset of overactive bladder: A longitudinal study in men. Public Health Nutr 2004; 7(7): 885–891.

7. Dallosso HM, McGrother CW, Matthews RJ, et al. The association of diet and other lifestyle factors with overactive bladder and stress incontinence: A longitudinal study in women. BJU Int 2003; 92: 69–77.

8. Creighton SM, Stanton SL. Caffeine: Does it affect your bladder? Br J Urol 1990; 66: 613–614.

9. James JE, Sawczuk D, Merrett S. The effect of chronic caffeine consumption on urinary incontinence in psychogeriatric inpatients. Psychol Health 1989; 3: 297–305.

10. Edelstein BA, Keaton-Brasted C, Burg MM. Effects of caffeine withdrawal on nocturnal enuresis, insomnia, and behavior restraints. J Consult Clin Psychol 1984; 52: 857–862.

11. Tomlison BU, Dougherty MC, Pendergast JF, et al. Dietary caffeine, fluid intake, and urinary incontinence in older rural women. Int Urogynecol J 1999; 10: 22–28.

12. Wyman JF, Elswick RK, Wilson MS, et al. Relationship of fluid intake to voluntary micturitions and urinary

incontinence in women. Neurourol Urodyn 1991; 10: 463–473.

13. Griffiths DJ, McCracken PN, Harrison GM, et al. Relationship of fluid intake to voluntary micturition and urinary incontinence in geriatric patients. Neurourol Urodyn 1993; 12: 1–7.

14. Jeffcoate T, Francis W. Urinary incontinence in the female. Am J Obstet Gynecol 1966; 94: 604–618.

15. Burgio KL. Current perspectives on management of urgency using bladder and behavioral training. J Am Acad Nurse Pract 2004; 16(10): 4–7.

16. Fantl JA, Wyman JF, McClish DK, et al. Efficacy of bladder training in older women with urinary incontinence. JAMA 1991; 265(5): 609–613.

17. Goode PS, Burgio KL, Locher JL, et al. Urodynamic changes associated with behavioral and drug treatment of urge incontinence in older women. J Am Geriatr Soc 2002; 50:808–16.

18. Hu TW, Igou JF, Kaltreider DL, et al. A clinical trial of a behavioral therapy to reduce urinary incontinence in nursing homes. JAMA 1989; 261: 2656–2662.

19. Jarvis GJ, Millar DR. Controlled trial of bladder drill for detrusor instability. BMJ 1980; 281: 1322–1323.

20. Wallace SA, Roe B, Williams K, et al. Bladder training for urinary incontinence in adults (Cochrane Review). In: the Cochrane Library. Aberdeen, UK: John Wiley and Sons, Ltd; 2004;2.

21. Wiseman PA, Malone-Lee J, Rai GS. Terodiline with bladder retraining for treating detrusor instability in elderly people. BMJ 1991; 302: 994–996.

22. Szonyi G, Collas DM, Ding YY, et al. Oxybutynin with bladder retraining for detrusor instability in elderly people: A randomized controlled trial. Age Ageing 1995; 24: 287–291.

23. Burgio KL, Locher JL, Goode PS, et al. Behavioral vs. drug treatment for urge urinary incontinence in older women: A randomized controlled trial. JAMA 1998; 280(23): 1995–2000.

24. Jarvis GJ. A controlled trial of bladder drill and drug therapy in the management of detrusor instability. Br J Urol 1981; 53: 565–566.

25. Kegel, AH. Progressive resistance exercises in the functional restoration of the perineal muscles. Am J Obstet Gynecol 1948; 56:238–248.

26. Gosling JA, Dixon JS, Critchley HOD, et al. A comparative study of the human external sphincter and the periurethral levator ani muscles. Br J Urol 1981; 53: 35–41.

27. American College of Sport's Medicine. Guidelines for exercise testing and prescription, 2nd ed. Philadelphia: Lea and Febiger, 1993.

28. Messelink EJ. The overactive bladder and the role of the pelvic floor muscles. Br J Urol 1999; 83(S2): 31–35.

29. Shafik A, Shafik IA. Overactive bladder inhibition in response to pelvic floor muscle exercises. World J Urol 2003; 20(6): 374–377.

30. Burgio KL, Locher JL, Goode PS. Combined behavioral and drug therapy for urge incontinence in older women. J Am Geriatr Soc 2000; 48(4): 370–374.

31. Bo K, Berghmans LCM. Nonpharmacologic treatments for overactive bladder-pelvic floor exercises. Urology 2000; 55(Suppl 5A): 7–11.

32. Burns P, Pranikoff K, Nochajski M, et al. Treatment of stress incontinence with pelvic floor exercises and biofeedback. J Am Geriatr Soc 1990; 38: 341–344.

33. Obrien J, Austin M, Sethi P, et al. Urinary incontinence: Prevalence, need for treatment, and effectiveness of intervention by nurse. BMJ 1991; 303: 1308–1312.

34. Lagro-Janssen ALM, Debruyne FMJ, Smits AJA, et al. The effects of treatment of urinary incontinence in general practice. Fam Pract 1992; 9: 284–289.

35. Hay-Smith EJC, Dumoulin C. Pelvic floor muscle training versus no treatment, or inactive control treatments, for urinary incontinence in women. Cochrane Database Syst Rev 2006; 1: CD005654.

36. Kegel AH. Stress incontinence of urine in women: Physiological treatment. J Int Col Surg 1956; 25: 487–499.

37. Cardozo LD, Abrams PD, Stanton SL, et al. Idiopathic bladder treated by biofeedback. BJU 1978; 50(7): 521–523.

38. Neumann P, Gill V. Pelvic floor and abdominal muscle interaction: EMG activity and intra-abdominal pressure. Int Urogynecol J 2002; 13: 125–132.

39. Wang AC, Wang Y, Chen M. Single-blind, randomized trial of pelvic floor muscle training, biofeedback-assisted pelvic floor muscle training, and electrical stimulation in the management of overactive bladder. Urology 2004; 63: 61–66.

40. Burgio KL, Goode PS, Locher JL, et al. Behavioral training with and without biofeedback in the treatment of urge incontinence in older women. JAMA 2002; 288(18): 2293–2299.

41. Berghmans LC, Hendricks HJ, de Bie RA, et al. Conservative treatment of urge urinary incontinence: A systematic review of randomized clinical trials. BJU Int 2000; 85: 254–263.

42. Amaro JL, Gameiro MO, Padovani CR. Effect of intravaginal electrical stimulation on pelvic floor muscle strength. Int Urogynecol J 2005; 16: 355–358.

43. Chandi DD, Groenendijk PM, Venema PL. Functional extracorporeal magnetic stimulation as a treatment for female urinary incontinence: "The chair." BJU Int 2004; 93: 539–542.

44. Yamanishi T, Yasuda K, Sakakibara R, et al. Randomized, double-blind study of electrical stimulation for urinary incontinence due to detrusor overactivity. Urology 2000; 55: 353–357.
45. Brubaker L, Benson J, Bent A, et al. Transvaginal electrical stimulation for female urinary incontinence. Am J Obstet Gynecol 1997; 173(3): 536–540.
46. Smith JJ. Intravaginal stimulation randomized trial. J Urol 1996; 155: 127–130.
47. Yamanishi T, Sakakibara R, Uchiyama T, et al. Comparative study of the effects of magnetic versus electrical stimulation on inhibition of detrusor overactivity. Urology 2000; 56: 777–781.
48. Goldberg RP, Sand PK. Electromagnetic pelvic floor stimulation for urinary incontinence and bladder disease. Int Urogynecol J 2001; 12: 401–404.

Chapter 15
Pharmacotherapy of Urgency Incontinence

Martin C. Michel

Introduction

Urgency urinary incontinence (UUI) occurs in about one third of patients with overactive bladder (OAB), and hence is present in about 5% of the general adult population [1, 2]. As discussed elsewhere in this book, its prevalence increases with age [1, 2]. The prevalence of OAB is above average among patients seeing a physician for any reason, ie, irrespective of their urinary symptoms [3], or in residents of nursing homes. Pharmacotherapy is the mainstay of management of UUI patients. While the following focuses on patients with incontinence, it should be noted that continent OAB patients may have quantitatively similar symptoms and distress [4]. While the effects of medical treatment have been poorly explored in continent compared to incontinent OAB patients, limited data suggest that most of the following also is applicable to the continent OAB population [4, 5].

Underlying Concepts

Medical treatment of UUI in principle could work on various levels involved in the control of bladder function including the sensory mechanisms, the smooth muscle cell, and the central nervous system. Several recent reviews have discussed potential sites of action and the involved mechanisms in great detail [6–10]. Currently used approaches are limited largely to the use of muscarinic acetylcholine receptor antagonists. Their use is based on the idea that muscarinic receptors are the physiologically most

relevant receptors in mediating bladder contraction. Although the bladder of humans and various animal species expresses much more M_2 than M_3 muscarinic receptors, bladder contraction occurs largely if not exclusively via the M_3 subtype [11], an observation that is supported by studies with M_3 receptor knockout mice [12]. Nevertheless, M_2 receptors also can contribute to bladder contraction, and their role may increase under some pathological conditions [7]. While original concepts have focused largely on muscarinic receptors on the bladder smooth muscle cells, it now is apparent that the urothelium not only expresses such receptors [13] but also may be a mediator of the therapeutic effects of muscarinic antagonists [14]. The relative roles of urothelium versus smooth muscle in the effects of muscarinic antagonists currently are under investigation. Moreover, an additional site of action in the central nervous system has been proposed [15].

Available Drugs and Their Properties

Many muscarinic receptor antagonists are now available for clinical use, some of them in multiple pharmaceutical formulations. These include immediate-release (IR), extended-release (XL), and transdermal (TD) formulations of oxybutynin [16–19] and IR and XL formulations of tolterodine [19, 20]. Other drugs have been in clinical use in selected countries such as propiverine [21]. More recently additional drugs were introduced, after having been available in few countries for a long time, and/or have been made available on a wider scale. These include darifenacin [22, 23], solifenacin [23, 24], and trospium [23, 25]. Moreover, additional muscarinic receptor antagonists such as fesoterodine, which is metabolized to the same active compound as tolterodine, are currently in late stages of clinical development [26].

The various muscarinic receptor antagonists differ in their affinity profile for subtypes of muscarinic receptors (Table 15.1). In this regard propiverine, tolterodine, and trospium have very similar affinity for all subtypes of muscarinic receptors; oxybutynin and solifenacin are moderately selective for M_3 relative to M_2 receptors; and darifenacin is selective for M_3 relative to M_2 and, to a lesser extent, to M_1 receptors. All these drugs

have been shown to inhibit the contraction of isolated bladder strips elicited by muscarinic receptor antagonist in vitro and also to inhibit nonvoiding contractions of the urinary bladder in animal models of OAB. While some drugs have been better documented in this regard than others, there is little reason to believe that any of them should behave qualitatively differently in the bladder compared to the others.

The pharmacokinetic properties of the various muscarinic antagonists vary considerably and have been reviewed comprehensively for most agents [28]. A summary including the corresponding information for the newer agents is presented in Table 15.2. Based on their affinity for the target receptors and their pharmacokinetic properties, the various drugs also differ in their recommended therapeutic

TABLE 15.1. Muscarinic receptor subtype affinity of clinically used antagonists[a].

	M_1	M_2	M_3	M_4	M_5
Darifenacin	7.3	46	0.79	46	9.6
Oxybutynin	1.0	6.7	0.67	2.0	11.0
Propiverine	230	347	175	154	364
Solifenacin	25	125	10	?[b]	?
Tolterodine	3.0	3.8	3.4	5.0	3.4
Trospium	0.75	0.65	0.50	1.0	2.3

[a]Drug affinities are given in nmole/liter, with a smaller value representing a higher affinity, and are based on [7, 27]. Note that some drugs (eg, oxybutynin, tolterodine) form active metabolites in vivo, but their affinities are similar to those of the respective parent compound
[b]?, affinity not reported

TABLE 15.2. Key pharmacokinetic properties and standard doses of clinically used muscarinic receptor antagonists[a].

	t_{max} (h)b	$t_{1/2}$ (h)	Oral bioavailability (%)	Elimination route	Dosage
Darifenacin	7	3	15–19	Hepatic, CYP 2D6 and 3A4	1×7.5–15 mg
Oxybutynin IR	0.5–1	2–4	2–11	Hepatic, CYP 3A4	3–4×2.5–5 mg
Oxybutynin XL	5	16	–[c]		2–3×5 mg
Propiverine	2	15	40	Hepatic, CYP 3A4	3–4×5–10 mg
Solifenacin	4–6	45–55	88	Hepatic, CYP 3A4	1×5–10 mg
Tolterodine IR	1–2	3	–[d]	Hepatic, CYP 2C9,	2×2 mg
Tolterodine XL	4	6–8		2D6 and 3A4	1×4 mg
Trospium	5–6	20	10	Renal, >50% in active form	2×20 mg

[a]For details see [17–22, 24, 25, 28, 29]
[b]t_{max}, time to reach maximal plasma concentration after oral administration; $t_{1/2}$: elimination half-life
[c]The oral bioavailability of the XL formulation is increased by about 50% for the parent compound, whereas that of the active metabolite is decreased by about 30%
[d]Absolute bioavailability dependent on genotype for CYP 2D6 ranging from 26% in extensive metabolizers to 91% in poor metabolizers. Note that t_{max} and $t_{1/2}$ are not applicable to the TD formulation of oxybutynin, which has the same elimination route; the standard dosing is one patch (delivering 3.9 mg/day) every 3–4 days [16]

doses (Table 15.2). In this context it also should be considered that some muscarinic antagonists undergo extensive metabolism and that in some cases such metabolites may contribute to the observed clinical effects of said drugs in a relevant manner [30, 31].

Considerations for the Interpretation of Clinical Data

The interpretation of the available data on the clinical effects of muscarinic antagonists in OAB is complicated by a number of factors that differ markedly among reported studies. One set of important variables relates to the characteristics of the patient population being investigated. For example, patients previously being treated for this condition may respond differently from those who are treatment-naïve. This is exemplified by studies with oxybutynin TD where, starting from similar baseline values of about 30 incontinence episodes per week, two studies in unselected patients reported median reductions by 18 episodes [32], whereas one in known oxybutynin responders found median reductions by 25 episodes [33]. Another patient-related difference among studies is the question of continent versus incontinent patients. As the development programs for most drugs have used the number of incontinence episodes as the primary endpoint, their pivotal studies were based solely on incontinent patients. In contrast, the development program for solifenacin has used the number of micturitions as the primary endpoint, and accordingly has included both continent and incontinent patients. However, recent studies indicate that muscarinc receptor antagonists also are effective relative to placebo in continent patients [5] and that continent and incontinent patients will respond similarly to a muscarinic antagonist if their baseline symptoms are similar [4]. Other patient-related variables possibly differing among studies are patient gender and age (see below) and the recruitment via specialists (urologists, urogynecologists) versus general practitioners, but little information is available with regard to the latter.

Reported treatment efficacies, and particularly differences between active treatment and placebo, also in part will depend on how they have been assessed. For example, the inclusion criteria of most randomized controlled trials (RCT) specify certain minimum values for the parameter, which also is used as the primary or secondary endpoint. This introduces a single-sided regression-to-the-mean phenomenon, which can contribute to the apparently large "placebo responses" typically seen in OAB studies. Moreover, both shorter (eg, 3 days) and longer (eg, 7 days) versions of micturition diaries are used to assess episode frequencies of OAB symptoms. Although values from both types of diaries are reasonably correlated, the use of 3-day diaries for measuring inclusion criteria as well as outcome parameters aggravates the single-sided regression-to-the-mean phenomenon. Thus, studies using 3-day diaries generally have reported large responses to both placebo and active treatments than those using 7-day diaries [34]. Thus, the symptom improvement in response to placebo only partly represents a "true" placebo effect under such conditions. While the relative magnitude of the placebo in the total treatment response to incontinence medications already appears large [35], it may even be underestimated. Thus, the "baseline" response symptoms reported in OAB studies typically are measured after a single-blind placebo run-in periods. While few data have been published on OAB, experience from studies in male patients with lower urinary tract symptoms suggestive of benign prostatic hyperplasia suggests that considerable symptom improvement may occur already during such run-in periods [36]. Hence, the reported effects of active treatment in such studies may actually overestimate the component attributable to the active ingredient.

As baseline symptoms can vary considerably among patients, it is necessary to consider the impact of analyzing absolute versus percent changes and of changes of means versus those of medians. The practical implications of absolute versus percent changes is easily seen when it is considered that a reduction of incontinence episodes by five per week means a lot for a patient with a baseline value of five (this patient becomes dry) but probably only a little for someone with 26 episodes per week (this patients continues to wet herself three times a day). Accordingly, it was found that calculations of percent changes yield more consistent measures of treatment effects [37]. Since baseline episode frequencies of OAB symptoms in the population do not exhibit a Gaussian distribution, the calculation of mean values, which assumes such distribution, is not sound on a theoretical basis and median values may be more robust. This has practical implications as, eg, studies reported consistently greater reductions of urgency episodes with placebo or solifenacin treatment if the data were analyzed based on medians rather than means [23]. Accordingly, the FDA now routinely requests that submissions for approval are based on an analysis of medians rather than means.

Another issue related to the proper statistical analysis of clinical OAB studies concerns secondary subgroup analyses. For various reasons, trial costs being an important one, the number of patients in a controlled study typically is predefined to yield sufficient statistical power to answer the primary question, ie, whether the study drug is better than placebo or a comparator drug. If secondary analyses are performed, eg, comparing old and young, male and female, or more and less severely afflicted patients, group sizes become smaller, and hence the statistical power decreases. If such secondary analyses fail to find significant differences among subgroups, there always is the possibility that this may reflect a false-negative result due to insufficient statistical power. Similarly, studies are mostly powered to detect differences in efficacy, ie, something that can be measured in each patient. This means that they often are underpowered to detect differences in tolerability, particularly if the focus is on specific side effects that occur only in a minority of patients. Unfortunately, the vast majority of studies on OAB treatment fail to state for which type of difference they have been powered.

Another biometrical issue is the analysis of OAB-related symptom scales. For example, the validated "Urgency Perception Scale" gives the three options "usually able to finish what I'm doing before going to toilet," "usually able to hold until I reach toilet," and "usually not able to hold urine" [38, 39]. Frequently these are scored as 1, 2, and 3, respectively, and then group means before and after treatment are calculated. However, such averaging implies that two patients going from the most severe to the medium score are statistically the same as two going from the medium to the least severe group or as one going from most to least severe and one not changing. Obviously, this does not fit clinical reality, and distribution histograms of patients in the various subgroups before and after treatment are a more appropriate representation of such data [4]. Similar considerations obviously apply to other OAB rating scales.

Another consideration is that both the desired and the adverse effects of muscarinic receptor antagonists are dose-dependent. Hence, a drug with an improved efficacy/tolerability ratio may appear to have fewer side effects for a given level of efficacy or to be more efficacious for a given level of side effects. This relationship is highlighted by a recent study comparing the solifenacin with tolterodine XL [40]. In this study solifenacin appeared to have greater efficacy than tolterodine XL, but a closer inspection of the data showed that this occurred at the expense of more adverse events. In other words, apparently the dose of solifenacin in this study relative to its half-maximally effective dose was higher than that of tolterodine XL. In this vein it appears conceivable that medications allowing the use of multiple doses allow greater flexibility in identifying the optimal dose for a given patient.

A final general consideration relates to the comparison of RCT with real-life practice (RLP) studies. Contrary to common belief it cannot be said that one type of study is scientifically superior to the other. Rather, each study type has distinct advantages and disadvantages, which need to be kept in mind in the interpretation of the respective data. Particularly in a condition that is characterized by considerable treatment responses to placebo, only RCT involving a placebo arm can prove whether a given active treatment indeed is superior to placebo. However, in the field of muscarinic receptor antagonists the power of placebo-controlled studies should not be overestimated, as recent research shows that a considerable fraction of patients in such studies can guess correctly whether they are on active treatment or placebo [41], which effectively may unintentionally at least partly unblind such studies. On the other hand, RCT also have several disadvantages. As explained above their reports frequently ignore symptom improvements during the placebo run-in period, and the use of the same parameter as inclusion and efficacy criterion introduces a single-sided regression-to-the-mean phenomenon. Moreover, such studies typically have stringent inclusion and exclusion criteria that question the applicability of the results to the general patient population presenting to a physician. On the other hand, RLP studies do not allow statements on the efficacy of a drug specifically attributable to its active ingredient. However, they avoid biases due to inclusion and exclusion criteria, placebo run-in phases, and artificial cutoffs for being eligible for treatment. This also may explain why treatment efficacies reported from RLP studies often exceed those from RCT (Fig. 15.1). Moreover, RLP studies frequently are performed on much larger groups of patients than RCT, and hence are statistically better powered to allow for subgroup comparisons. In other words, RCT have high internal validity but limited external validity, whereas RLP studies have lower internal but possibly higher external validity. Thus, RLP studies reflect what physician and patient realistically can expect from a drug in daily practice, whereas RCT establish how much of this response is indeed due to the active ingredient of such medication.

Clinical Experience with Muscarinic Receptor Antagonists

Numerous placebo-controlled, double-blind randomized clinical trials (RCT) have shown that muscarinic receptor antagonists relieve symptoms of OAB [34, 35, 44]. Comprehensive reviews have been published previously that summarize the clinical data with darifenacin [22], oxybutynin IR [45], oxybutynin XL [17], oxybutynin TD [16], propiverine [21], solifenacin [24], tolterodine IR [20], tolterodine XL [19], and trospium [25]. Readers are referred to these publications for more details on individual drugs.

Based on requirements of the regulatory authorities, such studies primarily have looked at the frequency of incontinence episodes or, more recently, of micturitions. In this regard a focus on incontinence episodes neglects the fact that two thirds of all OAB patients are continent [1, 2] and that continent OAB can impair the quality of life (QoL) of the afflicted patients to a similar degree as incontinent OAB [4]. Interestingly, measurements of treatment efficacy based on urgency or nocturia only have emerged in recent years [23]. Moreover, there is an ongoing debate whether the impact of urgency for the patient is best assessed by counting episode numbers or by one of several OAB rating scales [38, 39, 46, 47] or concepts such as "warning

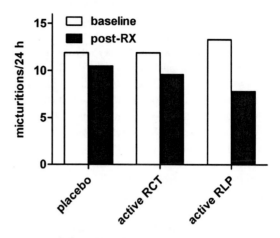

solifenacin frequency

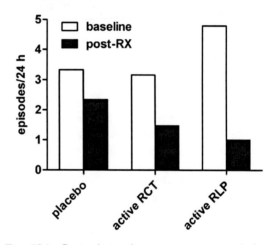

tolterodine XL incontinence

FIG. 15.1. Comparison of treatment responses during randomized controlled trials (RCT) and real-life practice (RLP) studies. Data are shown at baseline and after treatment (post-RX) and are based on data from the pivotal registration RCT [34, 42] and RLP performed in Germany [4, 43]. For each drug the response parameter defined as the primary endpoint in the pivotal RCT was used

time" [48] or "urgency-free interval" [49]. Recent data based on factor-analysis demonstrate that both related rating scales explain a considerably greater fraction of data variance than episodes of classic OAB symptoms [50]. Urodynamic measurements such as volume-to-first-contraction also have been used to measure the efficacy of muscarinic receptor antagonists [35], but have not been the primary endpoint of registration studies.

In 2003, a meta-analysis of the efficacy and tolerability of muscarinic receptor antagonists in the treatment of OAB was published by the Cochrane collaboration, which largely was based on studies with the IR formulations of oxybutynin, propiverine, tolterodine, and trospium [35]. This meta-analysis reported only moderate efficacy compared to placebo, eg, an improvement of leakage episodes by 0.56 per day and of micturitions by 0.59 per day. Newer studies using XL formulations of oxybutynin or tolterodine as well as newer agents tend to report a somewhat greater but still only moderate advantage over placebo [34, 44]. This apparently moderate efficacy of muscarinic receptor antagonists relative to placebo has sparked a debate about the usefulness. However, even if a major part of the effects of such medications occurs independently of their active ingredients, the overall effect in daily clinical practice is considerable (Fig. 15.1).

In general, muscarinic receptor antagonists can be considered to be a safe class of drugs. Side effects are dominated by those to be expected based on their mechanism of action and relate to the blockade of muscarinic receptors in the salivary glands (dry mouth), the gastrointestinal tract (constipation), and the eye (blurred vision, accommodation disorders). Although most muscarinic receptor antagonists used in the treatment of OAB also will block M_2 receptors, a subtype relevant for the control of heart rate [51], clinically relevant heart rate elevations surprisingly have not been a prominent feature of such drugs [52, 43]. Similarly, it is interesting to note that muscarinic antagonists in the treatment of OAB apparently do not promote urinary retention [35]. However, drugs blocking M_1 receptors in the central nervous system may have adverse effects on cognitive function [53]. While central nervous system effects, particularly cognitive side effects, have not been reported often in the treatment of OAB, this may represent an underreporting, since physicians treating OAB may not always carefully test cognitive function.

As outlined above, there is considerable heterogeneity among patient populations under investigation and methods of data analysis and presentation among studies. This makes it very difficult to perform meaningful indirect comparison among the various muscarinic receptor antagonists. On the other hand, numerous studies have reported on randomized, double-blind studies directly comparing

muscarinic receptor antagonists. In the interpretation of such studies it should be considered that the minimum difference in incontinence episodes noticeable by a patient in a QoL assessment tool is three episodes per week [54]. Most direct comparative studies have profiled agents against oxybutynin IR. Such studies were performed for oxybutynin XL [55, 56], oxybutynin TD [33], darifenacin [52], propiverine [57], tolterodine IR [58, 59], tolterodine XL [60], and trospium [61, 62]. Across the board these studies show that oxybutynin IR has a worse efficacy/tolerability ratio than any other approach including XL and TD formulation of oxybutynin. Such findings have been substantiated by smaller clinical pharmacological studies on salivation [63], central nervous effects [64], sleep [65, 66], and ocular effects [67], confirming that oxybutynin IR despite its wide use probably is the least suitable treatment option for OAB patients.

For clinical comparisons among the muscarinic receptor antagonists with better efficacy/tolerability ratios, most studies have profiled drugs against either of the two tolterodine formulations, most likely because tolterodine is the international market leader. In comparison with tolterodine, IR studies were presented for darifenacin [68], oxybutynin XL [69–71], oxybutynin TD [32], propiverine [72], and solifenacin [73, 74]. More recently, data also have been presented for comparisons with tolterodine XL for oxybutynin XL [75] or solifenacin [40]. Although many of these studies have reported minor differences in efficacy and/or tolerability among drugs (not surprisingly always in favor of the company sponsoring the study), the overall evidence does not suggest that any of these drugs is superior to the others for general use by a clinically relevant margin.

Treatment Strategy

A rational basis for a differential use of the various agents mainly is based on factors of convenience, eg, the need for a single pill per day and, more importantly, aspects related to safety and tolerability. For example, trospium is the only drug that is largely excreted by the kidneys in its active form (Table 15.2); this may be beneficial in patients with impaired liver function but disadvantageous in those with impaired renal function. In patients where even minor adverse effects on cognitive function would be disadvantageous, a drug with a well-documented lack of effect on cognitive function such as darifenacin may deserve preferential attention [76]. Tolterodine and trospium also appear to lack major adverse effects on cognitive function [64–66].

Moreover, potential differences in the efficacy and tolerability among patient groups have to be considered. In this regard, experimental and clinical evidence indicate that men and women respond similarly to the treatment with muscarinic antagonists [77]. Nevertheless, the vast majority of all current prescriptions of muscarinic antagonists are for women. This may at least partly reflect concerns regarding the use of such drugs in men with enlarged prostate glands, although the validity of such concerns has been questioned recently [78]. Another factor to be considered is patient age. Despite a reduced muscarinic receptor expression in the aged bladder [79], treatment responses to muscarinic receptor agonists remain largely unchanged in the elderly [77, 80]. However, it may be necessary to adapt the dose of some drugs in the elderly in order to accommodate age-related alterations of pharmacokinetics, eg, with trospium.

A major fraction of patients with OAB/UUI concomitantly have stress urinary incontinence, ie, mixed incontinence. Duloxetine is the only proven medication to treat stress urinary incontinence [81]. Both muscarinic receptor antagonists [46, 82] and duloxetine [83] have shown efficacy in women with mixed incontinence. However, at present little information is available about how these two approaches behave in direct comparison and/or what the role of a possible combination treatment might be. In the absence of such data, it appears prudent to base the initial treatment decision in mixed incontinence patients on the predominant character of the symptoms.

Finally, after the best possible treatment has been chosen and administered, the question arises about how long a given drug needs to be administered. While there is no evidence to suggest that the OAB syndrome will "heal" spontaneously on drug treatment, the clinical experience suggests that not all patients have a degree of symptoms requiring long-term treatment. This was exemplified by a study in which patients, who had successfully responded to a 3-month treatment with a mus-

carinic antagonist, were systematically withdrawn; within a 1-month observation thereafter, only 35% of patients requested to be put back on treatment [84]. While more data is clearly required in this regard, it appears that not all OAB patients will require continuous treatment.

Conclusions and Future Directions

Muscarinic receptor antagonists have proven useful in the treatment of OAB, but there clearly is room for improved treatment modalities with regard to efficacy and/or tolerability, particularly in patients refractory to muscarinic antagonists [85]. Therefore, a variety of options currently are under investigation to expand our therapeutic approaches. Among these the use of botulinum toxin, which prevents acetylcholine release in the bladder probably has advanced most [86, 87]. While the promising reports and the availability of this drug make it tempting to use it, the published evidence is not yet sufficient to support its routine clinical use. Moreover, botulinum toxin has not been registered as a medication to treat OAB in any major country, and hence can be considered only as an off-label use. Other approaches in various stages of investigation include β_3-adrenoceptor agonists [88], agonists of VR1 vanilloid receptors such as resineferatoxin [89], potassium channel openers [90], and neurokinin receptor antagonists [91]. However, clinical data, particularly studies comparing their efficacy and safety to those of muscarinic receptor antagonists, remain to be reported before any of these can be considered a viable alternative for clinical use.

References

1. Milsom I, Abrams P, Cardozo L, et al. How widespread are the symptoms of an overactive bladder and how are they managed? A population-based prevalence study. BJU Int 2001; 87(9):760–766.
2. Stewart WF, van Rooyen JB, Cundiff GW, et al. Prevalence and burden of overactive bladder in the United States. World J Urol 2003; 20:327–336.
3. Goepel M, Hoffmann J, Piro M, et al. Prevalence and physician awareness of symptoms of urinary bladder dysfunction. Eur Urol 2002; 41(3):234–239.
4. Michel MC, de la Rosette JJMCH, Piro M, Schneider T. Comparison of symptom severity and treatment

response in patients with incontinent and continent overactive bladder. Eur Urol 2005; 48(1):110–115.

5. Abrams P, Swift S. Solifenacin is effective for the treatment of OAB dry patients: A pooled analysis. Eur Urol 2005; 48:483–487.

6. Abrams P, Andersson K-E, Buccafusco JJ, et al. Muscarinic receptors: Their distribution and function in body systems, and the implications for treating overactive bladder. Br J Pharmacol 2006; 148:565–578.

7. Hegde SS. Muscarinic receptors in the bladder: From basic research to therapeutics. Br J Pharmacol 2006; 147(Suppl. 2):S80–S87.

8. Peters SLM, Schmidt M, Michel MC. Rho kinase: A target for treating urinary bladder dysfunction? Trends Pharmacol Sci 2006; 27(9):492–497.

9. Andersson K-E, Arner A. Urinary bladder contraction and relaxation: Physiology and pathophysiology. Physiol Rev 2004; 84:935–986.

10. Andersson K-E, Wein AJ. Pharmacology of the lower urinary tract: Basis for current and future treatments of urinary incontinence. Pharmacol Rev 2004; 56(4):581–631.

11. Schneider T, Fetscher C, Krege S, Michel MC. Signal transduction underlying carbachol-induced contraction of human urinary bladder. J Pharmacol Exp Ther 2004; 309(3):1148–1153.

12. Matsui M, Motomura D, Karasawa H, et al. Multiple functional defects in peripheral autonomic organs in mice lacking muscarinic acetylcholine receptor gene for the M3 subtype. Proc Natl Acad Sci USA 2000; 97(17):9579–9584.

13. Wuest M, Kaden S, Hakenberg OW, et al. Effect of rilmakalim on detrusor contraction in the presence and absence of urothelium. Naunyn-Schmiedeberg's Arch Pharmacol 2005; 372(3):203–212.

14. Chess-Williams R. Muscarinic receptors of the urinary bladder: Detrusor, urothelial and prejunctional. Auton Autacoid Pharmacol 2002; 22:133–145.

15. Kono M, Nakamura Y, Ishiura Y, et al. Central muscarinic receptor subtypes regulating voiding in rats. J Urol 2006; 175(1):353–357.

16. Davila GW. Transdermal oxybutynin: A new treatment for overactive bladder. Expert Opin Pharmacother 2003; 4(12):2315–2324.

17. Michel MC. A benefit-risk assessment of extended-release oxybutynin. Drug Saf 2002; 25(12):867–876.

18. Andersson K-E, Chapple CR. Oxybutynin and the overactive bladder. World J Urol 2001; 19(5):319–323.

19. Rovner ES, Wein AJ. Once-daily, extended-release formulations of antimuscarinic agents in the treatment of overactive bladder: A review. Eur Urol 2002; 41(1):6–14.

20. Clemett D, Jarvis B. Tolterodine. A review of its use in the treatment of overactive bladder. Drugs Aging 2001; 18(4):277–304.

21. Madersbacher H, Mürtz G. Efficacy, tolerability and safety profile of propiverine in the treatment of the overactive bladder (non-neurogenic and neurogenic). World J Urol 2001; 19:324–335.

22. Haab F. Darifenacin for the treatment of overactive bladder. Women's Health 2005; 1(3):331–343.

23. Michel MC, de la Rosette JJMCH. Role of muscarinic receptor antagonists in urgency and nocturia. BJU Int 2005; 96(Suppl. 1):37–42.

24. Payne CK. Solifenacin in overactive bladder syndrome. Drugs 2006; 66(2):175–190.

25. Rovner ES. Trospium chloride in the management of overactive bladder. Drugs 2004; 64(21):2433–2446.

26. Cole P. Fesoterodine, an advanced antimuscarinic for the treatment of overactive bladder: A safety update. Drugs Future 2004; 29(7):715–720.

27. Guay DRP. Clinical pharmacokinetics of drugs used to treat urge incontinence. Clin Pharmacokin 2003; 42(14):1243–1285.

28. Wuest M, Weiss A, Waelbrock M, et al. Propiverine and metabolites: Differences in binding to muscarinic receptors and in functional models of detrusor contraction. Naunyn-Schmiedeberg's Arch Pharmacol 2006; 374(2):87–97.

29. Michel MC, Hegde SS. Treatment of the overactive bladder syndrome with muscarinic receptor antagonists – A matter of metabolites? Naunyn-Schmiedeberg's Arch Pharmacol 2006; 374(2):79–85.

30. Dmochowski RR, Nitti V, Staskin D, et al. Transdermal oxybutynin in the treatment of adults with overactive bladder: Combined results of two randomized clinical trials. World J Urol 2005; 23:263–270.

31. Davila GW, Daugherty CA, Sanders SW. A short-term, multicenter, randomized double-blind dose titration study of the efficacy and anticholingeric side effects of transdermal compared to immediate release oral oxybutynin treatment of patients with urge urinary incontinence. J Urol 2001; 166(1):140–145.

32. Michel MC, Oelke M, Zinner N. Novel muscarinic antagonists to treat incontinence and/or overactive bladder. Drug Discov Today Ther Strateg 2005; 2(1):1–6.

33. Herbison P, Hay-Smith J, Ellis G, Moore K. Effectiveness of anticholinergic drugs compared with placebo in the treatment of overactive bladder: Systematic review. Br Med J 2003; 326(7394):841–844.

34. Chapple CR, Wyndaele JJ, Nordling J, et al. Tamsulosin, the first prostate-selective α_{1A}-adrenoceptor antagonist. A meta-analysis of two randomized, placebo-controlled multicentre studies in

patients with benign prostatic obstruction (symptomatic BPH). Eur Urol 1996; 29:155–167.

35. Landis JR, Kaplan S, Swift S, Versi E. Efficacy of antimuscarinic therapy for overactive bladder with varying degrees of incontinence severity. J Urol 2004; 171(2):752–756.

36. Freeman R, Hill S, Millard R, et al. Reduced perception of urgency in treatment of overactive bladder with extended-release tolterodine. Obstet Gynecol 2003; 102(3):605–611.

37. Cardozo L, Coyne KS, Versi E. Validation of the urgency perception scale. BJU Int 2005; 95:591–596.

38. Chapple CR, Martinez-Garcia R, Selvaggi L, et al. A comparison of the efficacy and tolerability of solifenacin succinate and extended release tolterodine at treating overactive bladder syndrome: results of the STAR trial. Eur Urol 2005; 48:464–470.

39. DuBeau CE, Khullar V, Versi E. "Unblinding" in randomized controlled drug trials for urinary incontinence: Implications for assessing outcomes when adverse effects are evident. Neurourol Urodyn 2005; 24(1):13–20.

40. Chapple C, Khullar V, Gabriel Z, Dooley JA. The effects of antimuscarinic treatments in overactive bladder: A systematic review and meta-analysis. Eur Urol 2005; 48(1):5–26.

41. Yarker YE, Goa KL, Fitton A. Oxybutynin. A review of its pharmacodynamic and pharmacokinetic properties, and its therapeutic use in detrusor instability. Drugs Aging 1995; 6(3):243–262.

42. Khullar V, Hill S, Laval K-U, et al. Treatment of urge-predominant mixed urinary incontinence with tolterodine extended release: A randomized, placebo-controlled trial. Urology 2004; 64(2):269–275.

43. Zinner N, Harnett M, Sabounjian L, et al. The overactive bladder-symptom composite score: A composite symptom score of toilet voids, urgency severity and urge urinary incontinence in patients with overactive bladder. J Urol 2005; 173(5):1639–1643.

44. Cardozo L, Dixon A. Increased warning time with darifenacin: A new concept in the management of urinary urgency. J Urol 2005; 173(4):1214–1218.

45. Khullar V, Hill S, Solanki J, Barr A. Tolterodine increases the urgency-free time interval: A sensory or motor effect? http://www.continet.org/publications/2004/PDF/0172.PDF. 2004. 23–11–2005.

46. Michel MC, Oelke M, Goepel M, et al. Relationships among symptoms, bother, and treatment satisfaction in overactive bladder patients.Neurourol Urodyn 2007;26:190–195.

47. Dhein S, van Koppen CJ, Brodde O-E. Muscarinic receptors in the mammalian heart. Pharmacol Res 2001; 44(3):161–182.

48. Chapple CR, Abrams P. Comparison of darifenacin and oxybutynin in patients with overactive bladder: Assessment of ambulatory urodynamics and impact on salivary flow. Eur Urol 2005; 48(1):102–109.

49. Michel MC, Wetterauer U, Vogel M, de la Rosette JJMCH. Cardiovascular safety of solifenacin in routine clinical use. Urology 2006; 68:71–72.

50. Ancelin ML, Artero S, Portet F, et al. Non-degenerative mild cognitive impairment in elderly people and use of anticholinergic drugs: Longitudinal cohort study. Br Med J 2006; 332:455–458.

51. Homma Y, Koyama N. Minimally clinically important change in urinary incontinence detected by a quality of life assessment tool in overactive bladder syndrome with urge incontinence. Neurourol Urodyn 2006; 25(3):228–235.

52. Anderson RU, Mobley D, Blank B, et al. Once daily controlled versus immediate release oxybutynin chloride for urge urinary incontinence. J Urol 1999; 161(6):1809–1812.

53. Versi E, Appell R, Mobley D, et al. Dry mouth with conventional and controlled-release oxybutynin in urinary incontinence. Obstet Gynecol 2000; 95(5):718–721.

54. Madersbacher H, Halaska M, Voigt R, et al. A placebo-controlled, multicentre study comparing the tolerability and efficacy of propiverine and oxybutynin in patients with urgency and urge incontinence. BJU Int 1999; 84(6):646–651.

55. Abrams P, Freeman R, Anderström C, Mattiasson A. Tolterodine, a new antimuscarinic agent: As effective but better tolerated than oxybutynin in patients with overactive bladder. Br J Urol 1998; 81:801–810.

56. Malone-Lee J, Shaffu B, Anand C, Powell C. Tolterodine: Superior tolerability than and comparable efficacy to oxybutynin in individuals 50 years old or older with overactive bladder: A randomized controlled trial. J Urol 2001; 165(5):1452–1456.

57. Homma Y, Paick JS, Lee JG, Kawabe K. Clinical efficacy and tolerability of extended-release tolterodine and immediate-release oxybutynin in Japanese and Korean subjects with an overactive bladder: A randomized, placebo-controlled trial. BJU Int 2003; 92:741–747.

58. Madersbacher H, Stöhrer M, Richter R, et al. Trospium chloride versus oxybutynin: A randomized, double-blind, multicentre trial in the treatment of detrusor hyperreflexia. Br J Urol 1995; 75:452–456.

59. Halaska M, Ralph G, Wiedemann A, et al. Controlled, double-blind, multicentre clinical trial to investigate long-term tolerability and efficacy of trospium chloride in patients with detrusor instability. World J Urol 2003; 20:392–399.

60. Chancellor MB, Appell RA, Sathyan G, Gupta SK. A comparison of the effects on saliva output of oxybutynin chloride and tolterodine tartrate. Clin Ther 2001; 23(5):753–760.

61. Todorova A, Vonderheid-Guth B, Dimpfel W. Effects of tolterodine, trospium chloride, and oxybutynin on the central nervous system. J Clin Pharmacol 2001; 41:636–644.

62. Diefenbach K, Donath F, Maurer A, et al. Randomised, double-blind study of the effects of oxybutynin, tolterodine, trospium chloride and placebo on sleep in healthy young volunteers. Clin Drug Invest 2003; 23(6):395–404.

63. Diefenbach K, Arold G, Wollny A, et al. Effects on sleep of anticholinergics used for overactive bladder treatment in healthy volunteers aged >50 years. BJU Int 2005; 95:346–349.

64. Altan-Yaycioglu R, Yaycioglu O, Akova YA, et al. Ocular side-effects of tolterodine and oxybutynin, a single-blind prospective randomized trial. Br J Clin Pharmacol 2005; 59(5):588–592.

65. Romanzi L, DelConte A, Kralidis G. Impact of darifenacin versus tolterodine on incontinence episodes in patients with overactive bladder. Obstet Gynecol 2005; 105:88S.

66. Sussman D, Garely A. Treatment of overactive bladder with once-daily extended-release tolterodine or oxybutynin: The antimuscarinic clinical effectiveness trial (ACET). Curr Med Res Opin 2002; 18(4):177–184.

67. Diokno AC, Appell RA, Sand PK, et al. Prospective, randomized, double-blind study of the efficacy and tolerability of the extended-release formulations of oxybutynin and tolterodine for overactive bladder: Results of the OPERA trial. Mayo Clin Proc 2003; 78:687–695.

68. Sand PK, Miklos J, Ritter H, Appell R. A comparison of extended-release oxybutynin and tolterodine for treatment of overactive bladder in women. Int Urogynecol J 2004; 15:243–248.

69. Jünemann K-P, Halaska M, Rittstein T, et al. Propiverine versus tolterodine: Efficacy and tolerability in patients with overactive bladder. Eur Urol 2005; 48:478–482.

70. Chapple CR, Arano P, Bosch JLHR, et al. Solifenacin appears effective and well tolerated in patients with symptomatic idiopathic detrusor overactivity in a placebo- and tolterodine-controlled phase 2 dose-finding study. BJU Int 2004; 93(1):71–77.

71. Chapple CR, Rechberger T, Al-Shukri S, et al. Randomized, double-blind placebo- and tolterodine-controlled trial of the once-daily antimuscarinic agent solifenacin in patients with symptomatic overactive bladder. BJU Int 2004; 93(3):303–310.

72. Appell RA, Sand P, Dmochowski R, et al. Prospective randomized controlled trial of extended-release oxybutynin chloride and tolterodine tartrate in the treatment of overactive bladder: Results of the OBJECT Study. Mayo Clin Proc 2001; 76: 358–363.

73. Kay G, Crook T, Rekeda L, et al. Differential effects of the antimuscarinic agents darifenacin and oxybutynin ER on memory in older subjects. Eur Urol 2006; 50:317–326.

74. Michel MC, Schneider T, Krege S, Goepel M. Do gender or age affect the efficacy and safety of tolterodine? J Urol 2002; 168(3):1027–1031.

75. Chapple CR, Roehrborn CG. A shifted paradigm for the further understanding, evaluation, and treatment of lower urinary tract symptoms in men: Focus on the bladder. Eur Urol 2006; 49(4):651–659.

76. Schneider T, Hein P, Michel-Reher M, Michel MC. Effects of ageing on muscarinic receptor subtypes and function in rat urinary bladder. Naunyn Schmiedebergs Arch Pharmacol 2005; 372(1):71–78.

77. Zinner NR, Mattiasson A, Stanton SL. Efficacy, safety, and tolerability of extended-release once-daily tolterodine treatment for overactive bladder in older versus younger patients. J Am Geriatr Soc 2002; 50:799–807.

78. Michel MC, Oelke M. Duloxetine in the treatment of stress urinary incontinence. Womens Health 2005; 1(3):345–358.

79. Michel MC, de la Rosette JJMCH, Piro M, Goepel M. Does concomitant stress incontinence alter the efficacy of tolterodine in patients with overactive bladder? J Urol 2004; 172(2):601–604.

80. Bump RC, Norton PA, Zinner NR, Yalcin I. Mixed urinary incontinence symptoms: Urodynamic findings, incontinence severity, and treatment response. Obstet Gynecol 2003; 102(1):76–83.

81. Choo M-S, Song C, Kim JH, et al. Changes in overactive bladder symptoms after discontinuation of successful 3-month treatment with an antimuscarinic agent: A prospective trial. J Urol 2005; 174(1):201–204.

82. Sahai A, Khan MS, Arya M, et al. The overactive bladder: Review of current pharmacotherapy in adults. Part 2: Treatment options in cases refractory to anticholinergics. Exp Opin Pharmacother 2006; 7(5):529–538.

83. Sahai A, Khan M, Fowler CJ, Dasgupta P. Botulinum toxin for the treatment of lower urinary tract symptoms: A review. Neurourol Urodyn 2005; 24(1):2–12.

84. Schurch B. Botulinum toxin for the management of bladder dysfunction. Drugs 2006; 66(10):1301–1318.

85. Michel MC, Vrydag W. α1-, α2-, and β-Adrenoceptors in the urinary bladder, urethra and prostate. Br J Pharmacol 2006; 147(Suppl. 2):S88–S119.

86. Avelino A, Cruz F. TRPV1 (vanilloid receptor) in the urinary tract: Expression, function and clinical applications. Naunyn Schmiedebergs Arch Pharmacol 2006; 373:287–299.

87. Chapple CR, Patroneva A, Raines SR. Effect of an ATP-sensitive potassium channel opener in subjects with overactive bladder: A randomized, double-blind, placebo-controlled study (ZD0947IL/0004). Eur Urol 2006; 49:879–886.

88. Sellers DJ, Chapple CR, Hay DPW, Chess-Williams R. Depressed contractile responses to neurokinin A in idiopathic but not neurogenic overactive human detrusor muscle. Eur Urol 2006; 49(3):510–518.

89. Maruyama S, Oki T, Otsuka A, et al. Human muscarinic receptor binding characteristics of antimuscarinic agents to treat overactive bladder. J Urol 2006; 175(1):365–369.

90. Croom KF, Keating GM. Darifenacin in the treatment of overactive bladder. Drugs Aging 2004; 21(13):885–892.

91. van Kerrebroeck P, Kreder K, Jonas U, et al. Tolterodine once-daily: Superior efficacy and tolerability in the treatment of overactive bladder. Urology 2001; 57(3):414–421.

Chapter 16
Alternative Therapies for Urinary Urgency Incontinence: Acupuncture and Herbology

Sarit O. Aschkenazi and Peter K. Sand

Background

Urinary urgency is defined by the International Continence Society as a sudden and compelling desire to pass urine that is difficult to defer [1]. In both sexes the symptoms tend to increase as one ages, but in women they are more often associated with urge urinary incontinence (UUI). The overactive bladder syndrome (OAB) is defined as urgency usually accompanied by urinary frequency and nocturia, with or without UUI, and is widely prevalent among women, affecting nearly 17% of the overall female population [2]. Symptoms and signs of urgency and UUI become more evident after menopause, increasing with advancing age [3]. It is estimated that the number of American women aged 65 years and older will double in the next 25 years to more than 40 million women by 2030 [4], which will further increase the already high cost of OAB to society and impairment of quality of life for the individual [5]. Up to 39% of new admissions to long-term care facilities report having urinary incontinence, of which nearly two thirds had objectively documented involuntary bladder contractions [6].

Effective first-line treatments for the OAB syndrome are nonsurgical, such as pharmacotherapy, behavioral therapy, and pelvic floor electrical stimulation. Behavior modification includes fluid and dietary changes, bladder drill entailing scheduled voiding to restore normal cortical control over micturition, and exercises to strengthen the pelvic floor muscles for patients with mixed incontinence. The combination of these behavioral treatment modalities may improve symptoms by 75–80% [7].

Antimuscarinic pharmacotherapy has become the mainstay for persistent OAB symptoms [5]. Goode et al. [8] found that objective bladder capacity improved significantly with antimuscarinic therapy compared to a group receiving behavioral therapy [8], but nocturia was better treated by combined behavioral therapy and pharmacological treatment [9]. There is evidence that the placebo effect plays a major role in the treatment of UUI [10]. Overall reduction in UUI with placebo alone is believed to reach about 40% [11]. As effective as antimuscarinic drugs may be, they fail to adequately resolve symptoms in a substantial number of cases, and their use is frequently limited by side effects. The elderly are especially susceptible to serious anticholinergic CNS side effects such as significant memory impairment and hallucinations [12]. Although significant CNS reactions are not common, it generally is encouraged to avoid prescription of antimuscarinic medications that cross the blood–brain barrier in the elderly whenever possible [13].

For nonresponders to these interventions, and as first-line therapy for selected cases, a variety of nonpharmacological alternatives with documented efficacy have been developed. The potential benefits of complementary therapies are that they have few, if any, adverse effects compared with antimuscarinic pharmacotherapy [14]. Acupuncture generally is well tolerated and is an increasingly popular complement to standard therapy for a variety of medical ailments and as primary therapy for select cases.

Other modalities include pelvic floor electrical stimulation (PFES) using vaginal or rectal probes and neuromodulation. This involves either the implantation of a sacral quadripolar electrode and neurostimulator or transcutaneous posterior tibial nerve stimulation in the office, which have been offered for recalcitrant OAB symptoms. Medicare reimbursement is available in the United States for PFES and neuromodulation, which make them affordable treatment options for women with OAB symptoms [5] not responding to behavioral and antimuscarinic pharmacotherapy. The mechanism of action for PFES, for example, is suggested to be stimulation of skeletal muscle contractions of the levator ani and urethral and anal sphincters with reflexive relaxation of the detrusor [5]. PFES is reported to completely resolve UUI in 20% of women and improve symptoms in 37% [15].

Mechanisms of Action for Acupuncture

The mechanisms of action for acupuncture have been studied extensively to explain the its pain-relieving effects. Controlled clinical trials demonstrate that acupuncture has a clinically relevant pain-relieving effect on certain forms of chronic nociceptive pain [16]. One human study indicated that acupuncture activates CNS endorphin systems, decreasing pain sensation. Further support comes from experimental studies in animals indicating that acupuncture partially works through the endorphinergic system [17]. Urodynamic studies show that opiate antagonists may increase intravesical pressure, decrease bladder capacity, and lower urethral closure pressure [18]. Central b-endorphins are increased by acupuncture, potentially exerting an inhibitory effect on the pontine micturition center, leading to increased bladder storage. It has been shown that there may be similarities between the physiology of muscle training and acupuncture, suggesting that acupuncture can simulate pelvic floor muscle training [16].

Peripheral circulation is increased with both acupuncture and transcutaneous electrical nerve stimulation in humans and animal models. Various studies have demonstrated this effect in ischemic skin flaps [19], the parotid gland [20] in patients with Raynaud's syndrome [21] and in the uterine artery in infertile women [22]. Elevated blood pressure can be treated with electroacupuncture through central sympathetic inhibition and evidence of increased levels of b-endorphin in the cerebrospinal fluid [16]. One study showed significant improvement in menopausal hot flashes after a series of electroacupuncture treatments and suggested that acupuncture is a viable alternative treatment of vasomotor symptoms in postmenopausal women [23]. Acupuncture stimulation has been known to cause periurethral EMG excitation [24]. Somatovisceral reflexes have been studied and reviewed by Sato [25]. He demonstrated that in anesthetized animals stimulation of the perineal area induced bladder function changes and sphincter activity that could be both excitatory and inhibitory. The responses were segmentally organized. The authors concluded that stimulation of the skin, muscle, and/or joints that are innervated by afferent nerve fibers entering the sacral spinal cord segments could modulate bladder and sphincter muscle reflex responses.

Reviewing the Evidence

Several studies have investigated the efficacy of acupuncture in the treatment of lower urinary tract complaints and chronic pelvic pain [26]. Stimulation of the posterior tibial nerve has been shown to activate the third sacral nerve roots that innervate the pelvic floor. Chang was the first to report a prospective sham-controlled study of posterior tibial acupuncture (SP-6) for the treatment of OAB symptoms [27] in 52 women. Bladder capacity in the treated subjects increased in 88.5% compared to 23.1% of control subjects. In women with initial detrusor overactivity, 65% experienced complete resolution of their symptoms compared to 23% of controls. In the long-term follow-up of these subjects [28], which averaged 66.2 months, women needed a mean of 4.8 repeat treatments to treat recurrent symptoms. The authors' conclusion was that posterior tibial nerve acupuncture at SP-6 was beneficial, but required repeated treatment sessions for long-term symptom relief.

Recently, a well-planned, randomized, sham-controlled trial was published on acupuncture treatment for OAB with UUI [29]. Eighty-seven percent of the 85 women enrolled completed all aspects of the study. Subjects were assigned randomly to either receive acupuncture at SP-6 or a sham acupuncture treatment designed to promote relaxation. The primary endpoint was the number of incontinence episodes on a 3-day diary after 4 weeks of acupuncture treatment. Secondary endpoints were urinary frequency, urgency, maximum cystometric capacity, voided volumes, and quality of life metrics. Subjects were evaluated before and after treatment by urodynamic testing, a 3-day voiding diary, a urogenital distress inventory and incontinence impact questionnaire, and validated quality-of-life inventories. In both the sham and treatment groups there were significant decreases in incontinence episodes (40% in the sham group and 59% in the active treatment group). In the treatment group there was a significant reduction in urinary frequency (14%) and urgency (30%) and a 13% increase in both maximum voided volume and cystometric capacity ($P = 0.01$). Both groups showed improved urinary distress inventory and incontinence impact questionnaire scores, with a 54% decrease in the treatment group and a 34% decrease in the sham group that was better in the active treatment group ($P < 0.001$). The authors concluded that in women with OAB symptoms, 4 weekly bladder-specific acupuncture treatments at SP-6 caused significant symptom improvement compared with sham acupuncture needle placement.

Philp et al. [30] performed a small, uncontrolled study and found that lower extremity acupuncture produced significant improvement in 77% of 20 women with idiopathic detrusor overactivity. Acupuncture was used to treat 20 children with nocturnal enuresis and detrusor overactivity [31]. Nocturnal enuresis completely resolved in 11 (55%) subjects and improved in 7 (35%).

Yuksek et al. [32] aimed to assess the efficacy of acupressure for treating nocturnal enuresis compared with oxybutynin. Acupressure was administered to 12 children by their parents, who had been taught the technique. Pressure was applied at 16 acupuncture points including SP-6. Twelve control children received 0.4 mg/kg oxybutynin. Parents were asked to record incidences of bed-wetting and subjects and/or their parents completed a questionnaire 15 days and 1, 3, and 6 months after the start of treatment. Complete and partial responses after 6 months of treatment were seen in 83.3 and 16.7%, respectively, of subjects treated with acupressure and in 58.3 and 33.3%, respectively, of children who received oxybutynin. They concluded that nocturnal enuresis could be partially treated by oxybutynin, but acupressure could be an alternative nondrug therapy. Acupressure has the advantages of being noninvasive, painless, and cost-effective.

Following the success of peripheral acupuncture near the posterior tibial nerve, a commercially available device for treatment of the OAB became available.

The Stoller afferent nerve stimulator (SANS) conveys a fine electrical current through a needle electrode inserted adjacent to the nerve. The largest observational study of this device [33] was performed on only 15 patients with OAB. Complete resolution of symptoms was noted in 46.7%, significant improvement was noted in 20.0%, and a third did not have any improvement. Urodynamic testing showed posttreatment resolution of bladder instability in 76.9%. The maximum cystometric capacity and bladder volume at normal desire to void increased from 197 to 252 ml ($P = 0.008$) and from 133 to 188 ml ($P = 0.002$), respectively. Subjects who responded had mean total daily urinary frequency and nocturia decrease from 16.1 to 4.4 ($P = 0.002$) and 8.3 to 1.4 ($P = 0.002$), respectively. There were no adverse effects or complications attributed to the electroacupuncture treatment.

Conclusion

It is important to be acquainted with acupuncture as a complementary treatment modality for UUI and OAB symptoms that are inadequately treated with conventional pharmacotherapy and behavior modification. After reviewing the literature available on this treatment modality, it seems that there are preliminary data to indicate that acupuncture may be regarded as a potential treatment option with a safe treatment profile. The preliminary accumulated data indicate that acupuncture may provide short term but significantly effective symptom relief. Additional research in larger study cohorts should be performed to further investigate what appears to be a safe treatment modality. It may prove especially useful for women who do not tolerate the side effects elicited by antimuscarinic pharmacotherapy.

Herbology

Background

Many women turn to natural medicines for the treatment of lower urinary tract symptoms when conventional therapies fail to achieve sufficient relief. There is some limited literature about herbal medications that may ameliorate irritable bladder symptoms. Most of the data are anecdotal and do not rely on blinded, randomized controlled trials but rather on descriptive case reports, case controlled studies, and uncontrolled observational studies. The paucity of data makes it impossible to provide information that reliably indicates the degree of efficacy and safety of herbal remedies; the mechanism of action and active ingredients in these herbal remedies also are poorly understood.

In this chapter we describe just a few of the myriad of herbal products that are being used for the treatment of lower urinary tract symptoms as well as many unrelated ailments and symptoms. We will review what is known about popular, folklore herbal therapies that are purchased by patients "over-the-counter." The herbal treatments described here were chosen because some evidence exists to suggest that they may provide some treatment benefit. It should be emphasized, however, that insufficient scientific data are available to recommend these herbal treatments as effective therapies.

Finally, a mention will be made of an FDA approved treatment for lower urinary tract symptoms that consists of bladder installations with dimethylsulfoxide (DMSO). This chemical, when used intravesically, has been tested in well-constructed research studies and is approved by the FDA for the treatment of urinary urgency, frequency, and nocturia associated with interstitial cystitis. None of the treatments discussed should be used during pregnancy and lactation.

Bladderwort

Bladderwort, or *Utricularia vulgaris*, is a plant belonging to the Lentibulariaceae plant family [34–36] (Fig. 16.1).Species belonging to the bladderwort plant family are carnivorous. The plant grows in ponds and marshes. The stems spread out widely and have threadlike leaves up

to 3 in long. The bladderwort does not root to the ground: It is free-floating, with most of the plant hanging in the water near the bottom. It floats to the top when it is ready to flower. The flower and the stalk can stretch up to 2feet above the water. Attached to the leaves are tiny bladders, or pouches, about 1/8 in. wide. The bladders have an opening surrounded by tiny hairs. They release slimy mucus, which smells sweet and lures small insects such as mosquito larvae and water fleas. When the insect gets close enough to touch the hairs, the bladder sucks it inside. Once the insect is trapped inside the bladder, the plant secretes chemicals that break its prey, allowing nutrients to be absorbed into the plant. Greater bladderwort may have over 500 bladders on it and can eat thousands of prey every day.

No data or references from clinical studies were found to support the usage of bladderwort in the treatment of lower urinary tract symptoms. However, anecdotally, bladderwort has been described to have diuretic, antispasmodic, and anti-inflammatory effects and has been used to treat disorders of the lower urinary tract, especially conditions involving complaints of urgency and UUI. It also is used for kidney stones and urinary tract

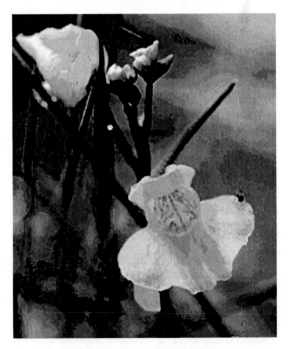

Fig. 16.1. Bladderwort, *Utricularia vulgaris*

infections. It had been used to promote weight loss and to stimulate gall-bladder secretions. Topically, bladderwort is used for burns and skin and mucous membrane inflammation. It is prepared as a tea for treatment of urinary symptoms.

There are insufficient data about the safety and effectiveness of bladderwort. It should not be recommended for usage during pregnancy and lactation. Insufficient reliable information is available about the possible mechanism of action and active ingredients.

For its diuretic effects, bladderwort is administered as a tea. There are no data on efficacy, and therefore it is impossible to make a recommendation regarding the most suitable dose. The tea is prepared by steeping 2 g of dried bladderwort leaf in 100 ml of boiling water for 10–15 min and then straining [35]. As a tea it also can be used as a mouthwash. As a topical agent, it is recommended for its anti-inflammatory effects, as well as application in cleansers, cosmetic, and medical packs.

Pumpkin Seed Oil

Pumpkin seed oil also is known by its scientific names, *Cucumis pepo* and *Cucurbita galeottii*; *Cucurbita mammeata* is a plant belonging to the Cucurbitaceae plant family [35, 36]. Seeds of autumn squash (*Cucurbita maxima*) and Canadian pumpkin (crooked neck squash, *Cucurbita moschata*) have properties similar to *Cucurbita pepo* seed [37]. It has been used for dysuria secondary to bladder irritation and for the treatment of pyelonephritis. Pumpkin seed oil has been described as exhibiting a diuretic effect. Animal research also suggests that it might improve bladder and urethral function [38] and bladder irritability. Another constituent, cucurbitin, has antihelminthic effects and has been used for treating intestinal worms. The concentration of cucurbitin varies significantly among *Cucurbita* species [36]. In men, it has been described for the treatment of benign prostatic hyperplasia.

There is insufficient reliable information available about the safety and effectiveness of pumpkin seed oil. It should not be recommended for usage during pregnancy and lactation. There are insufficient data about its interaction with other herbs and or medications.

TABLE 16.1. Nutritional content of raw pumpkin seeds.

Pumpkin seeds, raw 0.25 cup 186.65 calories

Nutrient	Amount	Nutrient density
Manganese	1.04 mg	5.0
Magnesium	184.58 mg	4.5
Phosphorus	405.03 mg	3.9
Tryptophan	0.11 g	3.3
Iron	5.16 mg	2.8
Copper	0.48 mg	2.3
Vitamin K	17.73 µg	2.1
Zinc	2.57 mg	1.7
Protein	8.47 g	1.6

The roasted pumpkins seeds are considered to be a delicious snack food, but it is recommended that one not consume greater amounts than that found in food or supplements. The therapeutic part of the pumpkin is the seed. Pumpkin seeds contain fatty oil, protein, and carbohydrates (Table 16.1) [39]. Pumpkin seeds also are rich in carotenoids, including lutein, carotene, and beta-carotene [36]. The seed oil is rich in unsaturated fatty acids, including 47% linoleic acid, 29% oleic acid, 14% palmitic acid, and 8% stearic acid. The oil also is rich in vitamin E, including both gamma-tocopherol and alpha-tocopherol (3 mg/100 g) [38]. The enzyme acyl-coenzyme A oxidase (ACOX) is present in the pumpkin seed. This enzyme catalyzes fatty acid oxidation, specifically the oxidation of fatty acid CoA esters with 4–10 carbon atoms [40].

Bladderwrack

Bladderwrack, is known also by its scientific names, *Fucus vesiculosus* and *Ascophyllum nodosum* [33, 34]. Another *Fucus* species is black tang, also know as bladder *Fucus*, blasentang, cutweed *Fucus*, kelp, kelp-ware, knotted wrack, marine oak, meereiche, quercus marina, rockweed, rockwrack, schweintang, seawrack, tang, and varech. These belong to the plant Fucaceae family(Fig. 16.2).

Bladderwrack is used orally for genitourinary disorders. It is described as being used for thyroid disorders, iodine deficiency, lymphadenoid goiter, myxedema, obesity, arthritis, rheumatism, arteriosclerosis, digestive disorders, heartburn, constipation, bronchitis, emphysema, anxiety, and decreased immunity and to increase energy. Topically, bladderwrack

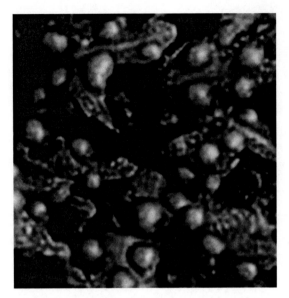

Fig. 16.2. Bladderwrack or *Fucus vesiculosus*. It is a brown seaweed that grows along the northern coasts of the Atlantic and Pacific oceans and Baltic sea

is used for skin diseases, burns, aging skin, and insect bites. When used orally, bladderwrack can contain high concentrations of iodine and heavy metals [41]. Ingesting more than 150 mg of iodine per day can cause hyperthyroidism or exacerbate existing hyperthyroidism. Heavy metal poisoning also has been reported [42].

Bladderwrack is likely unsafe during pregnancy and lactation when used orally and should be avoided [43]. There is insufficient information available about the effectiveness of bladderwrack for any of its described uses.

Bladderwrack is a brown seaweed. It may be confused with bladderwort. The plant contains high concentrations of iodine, which is present in varying amounts. It also can contain heavy metals such as arsenic and cadmium. Bladderwrack also is a source of fiber, vitamin B12, and minerals such as iron [43]. Preliminary clinical research suggests bladderwrack might extend the menstrual cycle and have antiestrogenic effects in premenopausal women. It also may increase progesterone levels [44]. Research suggests that extracts of bladderwrack also might have antibacterial, anti-HIV, and antioxidant activity [45, 46].

Fucoidan, a sulfated polysaccharide derivative of bladderwrack, seems to be active against a variety of viruses including the herpes virus, HIV, and cytomegalovirus [47]. Other research suggests that fucoidan might decrease fertility by preventing the binding of sperm to ova [48] and should be avoided in women trying to conceive. In premenopausal women, bladderwrack seems to lower 17-beta-estradiol levels and to increase progesterone levels in a dose-dependent manner [49].

Fucoidan also seems to stimulate the activity of transforming growth actor (TGF)-beta to increase fibroblast proliferation, which suggests it might be useful for wound healing [50]. Available data suggest that fucoidan also has anticoagulant, fibrinolytic, and antiplatelet adhesion effects [51]. Other studies suggest that it might have antiangiogenic and antineoplastic activity [52]. Topical administration of bladderwrack extract might reduce skin thickness and other signs of aging [52].

Theoretically, concomitant use of bladderwrack with herbs that affect platelet aggregation might increase the risk of bleeding [52]. These herbs include angelica, clove, danshen, fenugreek, feverfew, garlic, ginger, ginkgo, *Panax* ginseng, poplar, red clover, turmeric, and others. Bladderwrack seems to have anticoagulant effects. It can increase activated prothrombin time (aPTT) test results due to the heparinlike activity of one of its constituents (12,797) [52]. Theoretically, taking bladderwrack with antiplatelet or anticoagulant drugs might increase the risk of bruising and bleeding. These drugs include aspirin; clopidogrel; nonsteroidal anti-inflammatory drugs, such as diclofenac, ibuprofen, naproxen, warfarin, and heparin; and low-molecular-weight heparins such as dalteparin and enoxaparin.

Bladderwrack contains significant amounts of iodine, which might exacerbate hyper- or hypothyroidism [53] with prolonged use. Bladderwrack might increase serum TSH levels and might interfere with the results of thyroid function tests using radioactive iodine uptake [43]. Some medications can result in additive hypothyroid activity when used concomitantly with bladderwrack and may cause hypothyroidism [43]. These medications, which include methenamine mandelate, methimazole, potassium iodide, and others, should not be used concomitantly with bladderwrack. Bladderwrack should be avoided in people sensitive to iodine [43].

There is no recommended typical dosage. In a case report, heavy metal poisoning was described, where arsenic poisoning occurred with ingestion of a contaminated kelp product [54]. Another case of arsenic-related poisoning occurred with bladder-wrack ingestion of 400 mg tid for 3 months which resulted in renal tubular necrosis and interstitial fibrosis [55].

In another report, a 39-year-old obese woman developed palpitations and syncope after taking a weight loss supplement containing a combination of bladderwrack, dandelion, and boldo for 3 weeks. The patient was found to have a prolonged QT-interval on ECG and frequent episodes of sustained polymorphic ventricular tachycardia [56]. It is not clear whether bladderwrack, another ingredient, or the combination of ingredients was responsible for this adverse effect.

Teas

Teas have a long history of use, dating back to China approximately 5,000 years ago. The tea plant is native to Southeast Asia, with India and Sri Lanka being the major producers of black and green tea. Turkish traders reportedly introduced tea to Western cultures in the sixth century. By the eighteenth century, tea was commonly consumed in England, where it became customary to drink tea at 5 p.m. Black tea reached the Americas with the first European settlers in 1492.

Tea varieties reflect the growing region, district, form, and the processing method of the leaves resulting in black, green, or oolong tea. Drying the leaves of *Camellia sinensis* produces the black tea [33, 34]. Teas long have been used to treat a myriad of ailments. Teas have been used to prevent kidney stones, to induce smooth muscle relaxation, and as diuretics. Green, black, and oolong tea are all derived from the same plant, *Camellia sinensis*, which is a perennial evergreen shrub. All teas are a source of caffeine, a methylxanthine that relaxes smooth muscle, promotes diuresis in the kidney, stimulates the central nervous system, and increases heart rate. One cup of tea contains approximately 50 mg of caffeine, compared to coffee, which contains up to 175 mg of caffeine per cup. Tea also contains polyphenols (catechins, anthocyanins, phenolic acids), tannin, trace elements, and vitamins (Fig. 16.3).

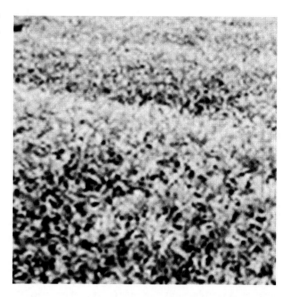

FIG. 16.3. Tea shrub, *Camellia sinensis*. Tea is made from the dried leaves of *Camellia sinensis*, an evergreen shrub. Green tea, black tea, and oolong tea are all made from the same plant

Chamomile

Chamomile is a common tea that has an applelike smell and taste [33, 34]. The name "chamomile" is derived from the Greek kamai melon, which means ground apple. It has become a popular home remedy for many conditions. Chamomile most often is used for bladder irritation, vaginitis, the common cold, diarrhea, ulcers, and in extreme cases oral mucositis. It exerts an effect as a smooth muscle relaxant and provides relief for skin and stomach discomfort.

However, there is not enough scientific evidence to recommend chamomile for any health problems. Although many uses for this tea have been tested in humans and other animals, safety and efficacy have not always been proven. It is crucial to emphasize that some of the conditions for which it is used can lead to significant morbidity if not effectively treated and patients should be evaluated by a qualified health care provider.

It is recommended not to consume chamomile tea for 2 weeks before surgery, dental, or diagnostic procedures that entail a bleeding risk. It also is advised to use chamomile sparingly if driving or operating machinery. It should be avoided during pregnancy and lactation because of the paucity of information regarding its effect on the fetus and neonate.

There is a cross-sensitivity with related plants such as aster, chrysanthemum, mugwort, ragweed, or ragwort, and people allergic to these plants should avoid chamomile. Possible adverse effects of this tea include allergic conjunctivitis, skin rash, vomiting when consumed in large quantities, breathing difficulties, blood pressure changes, easy bruising, confusion, drowsiness, and pruritis. Adverse reactions have been described with concomitant use of alcohol, barbiturates, benzodiazepines, anticoagulants, raloxifene, tamoxifen, sedatives, narcotics, and herbs or supplements with similar effects.

Chamomile dosing and route of administration have been extremely varied. For adults (18 years and older) use has been through consuming tea, infusions, liquid extracts, tinctures, capsules, tablets, pastes, plasters, ointments, douches, mouth rinses, and alcoholic extracts. There are not enough scientific data available to recommend the usage for children and adolescents younger than 18.

Sweet Sumach

Sweet sumach also is known as aromatic sumac, fragrant sumac, polecatbush, skunkbrush and squawbush. Its scientific name is *Rhus aromatica*, belonging to the family of Anacardiaceae. Sweet sumach belongs to the same family as poison ivy and can cause similar dermal reactions [57]. This plant has been used orally for urinary urgency, frequency, urinary incontinence, and nocturnal enuresis. The applicable part of sweet sumach is the root bark. This species of sumach, usually growing about 4 ft high, was introduced into England as an ornamental shrub in 1759. The bark is used in tanning. The wood exudes a peculiar odor and is used by the Native-Americans in Arizona, California, and New Mexico for making baskets (Fig. 16.4).

There is very little scientific information about this product and insufficient reliable information available about the safety and effectiveness of sweet sumach. It should be avoided during pregnancy and lactation.

Not enough reliable information is available regarding the possible mechanism of action and active ingredients. Adverse reaction to topical application of sweet sumach can cause contact allergic dermatitis in susceptible individuals [1].

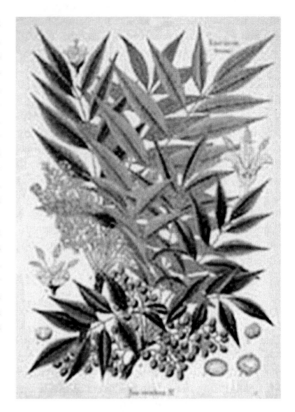

FIG. 16.4. Sweet sumach also known as *Rhus aromatica*

Goldenrod

Goldenrod also is known as Aaron's rod, Canadian goldenrod, early goldenrod, european goldenrod and woundwort. Its scientific names are *Solidago virgaurea* (European goldenrod), *Solidago canadensis* (Canadian goldenrod), and *Solidago gigantea* (early goldenrod). The goldenrods belong to the family of Asteraceae/Compositae. The pharmaceutically active part of goldenrod is the above-ground part of the plant. Goldenrods are very common wildflowers throughout Europe and North America. Over 50 species of goldenrod are known and most of them are very similar and difficult to tell apart. All goldenrods are late bloomers, flowering in late summer into the fall. Most species have spectacular displays of bright yellow flowers, which are clustered on long stalks. Most goldenrods have long, narrow leaves. Some species' leaves have smooth edges and some are toothed. Goldenrods vary in height, with 6 feet being the tallest (*Solidago gigantean*). Some, such as *Solidago Canadensis*, have pleasant odors. Goldenrods are extremely important to other wildlife, especially insects (Fig. 16.5)..

Goldenrod is classified as a diuretic but without increased electrolyte excretion [58]. The anti-inflammatory and aquaretic effects of goldenrod may be due to their saponin and flavonoid constituents. Goldenrod also might have bacteriostatic activity. This plant is used orally as a diuretic. It is thought to have anti-inflammatory and antispasmodic effects. It also is used orally to alleviate symptoms of gout, arthritis, eczema, and other skin conditions. Goldenrod also is used for acute exacerbations of pulmonary tuberculosis, diabetes mellitus, hepatomegaly, hemorrhoids, internal bleeding, allergic rhinitis, asthma, and prostatic hypertrophy. It is recommended that it be taken with copious amounts of fluids to increase urine flow in order to treat and prevent lower urinary tract disorders, such as urinary tract infections (UTIs) [59], urinary calculi, and urolithiasis. Topically, goldenrod is used as a mouth rinse for gingival inflammation and pharyngitis and to improve wound healing. There is insufficient reliable information available about the safety and effectiveness of goldenrod, and it should be avoided in pregnancy and lactation.

Orally, goldenrod may cause an allergic reaction in individuals sensitive to the Asteraceae/Compositae family. Some members of this family include ragweed, chrysanthemums, marigolds, and daisies.

Its use is contraindicated with concomitant congestive heart failure or renal impairment because of the considerable fluid shifts that it may cause. Theoretically, goldenrod might increase sodium retention and worsen hypertension [59].

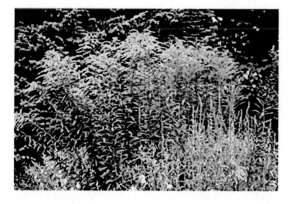

FIG. 16.5. Goldenrod

There is not enough evidence to recommend dosages and how much should be administered. Attention should be given to avoid confusion with mullein (*Verbascum densiflorum*; also referred to as goldenrod). Early goldenrod, European goldenrod, and Canadian goldenrod are used interchangeably.

Dimethylsulfoxide

Dimethylsulfoxide is an industrial solvent, which also is known as dimethyl sulfoxide, dimethyl sulphoxide, dimethylis sulfoxidum, methyl sulphoxide, NSC-763, SQ-9453, and sulphinybismethane. It is FDA approved for intravesical instillation to treat urinary frequency, urgency, and nocturia in interstitial cystitis patients.

Orally, DMSO has been used for the management of amyloidosis and related symptoms. Topically, DMSO has been used to decrease pain and speed the healing of wounds and burns. It has been reported to treat acute musculoskeletal injuries, headache, inflammation, arthritis, tic douloureux, cataracts, glaucoma, retinal degeneration, bunions, calluses, fungus toenails, asthma, and cancer, and to flatten raised keloid scars.. It also used topically to prevent tissue necrosis after extravasation with antineoplastic agents, to treat osteoarthritis, rheumatoid arthritis, scleroderma, and amyloidosis.

Topically it also has been used for reducing skin flap ischemia following surgery, for complex regional pain syndromes, as a vehicle in combination with idoxuridine to decrease the development of inflammatory reactions and lesions associated with herpes zoster infection, and to decrease the pain associated with postherpetic neuralgia. Intravenously, DMSO also has been used to manage symptoms associated with secondary amyloidosis and to lower intracranial hypertension.

An aqueous 50% solution of DMSO is FDA approved for intravesical use in the treatment of interstitial cystitis [58], and it also seems to decrease symptoms associated with chronic inflammatory bladder disease [60].

DMSO may be unsafe when used topically, especially when industrial-grade DMSO is used for self-treatment. This is not of the same quality of that used for medical purposes, since it may contain impurities. DMSO readily penetrates the skin and enhances the absorption of impurities and other substances, which may be hazardous to health [61]. DMSO also is reported to decrease the pain associated with postherpetic neuralgia [62]. Trigeminal herpes zoster has been noted to be most responsive [63]. There is insufficient reliable information available about the DMSO's effectiveness for its other suggested applications. Due to the paucity of reliable information available, it is recommended to avoid using DMSO in pregnancy and lactation.

The mechanism of action of DMSO is partially understood. DMSO is a highly polar solvent, which penetrates the skin easily when concentrated (80–100%) and has a large volume of distribution after administration [64]. It metabolizes to dimethyl sulfone and dimethyl sulfide, the latter causing a strong odor. DMSO's analgesic effect is attributed to slowing the conduction of capsaicin-sensitive nerve fibers [65]. During bladder instillations, it might cause the release of nitrogen oxide from afferent neurons [66], which acts as a peripheral neurotransmitter in the function of the lower urinary tract. DMSO also is associated with mast cell degranulation, accounting for the occurrence of eosinophilia and hypersensitivity reactions with its use.

DMSO may selectively dissolve collagen fibers, sparing to a large extent the elastic fibers [67]. It is thought to stabilize lysosomal membranes and cause vasodilatation. Its anti-inflammatory, cryopreservative, cryoprotective, anti-ischemic, and possible radioprotective activity [68] are attributed to the presence of a free hydroxyl radical with scavenging properties

DMSO exerts antimicrobial activity [68] by altering RNA structures essential for bacterial protein synthesis. It inhibits acetyl-cholinesterase activity, causing lowered cardiovascular vagal effects and increased response to nerve and muscle stimulation of skeletal, smooth, and cardiac muscle [68]. In vitro, DMSO increases levels of prostaglandin-E1 (PGE1) and cyclic-AMP, which reduce platelet aggregation, and decrease fibrinogen and thromboxane A2 secretion, all of which protect against ischemic injury [69].

Intravesical instillation of DMSO may cause adverse reactions such as hematuria due to a chemical cystitis, bladder discomfort, or detrusor overactivity [70]. A garliclike odor may emanate orally and transdermally with all routes of administration, which can be very bothersome and lead to discontinuation of treatment. Rare hypersensitivity reactions leading to anaphylaxis can happen with all application modes. Due to the high absorption of DMSO, an extensive list of systemic adverse effects has been described with topical use, including sedation, headache, dizziness, drowsiness, nausea, vomiting, diarrhea, constipation, anorexia, erythema, pruritus, burning, blistering, drying and scaling skin, dry or sore throat, cough, dry nasal passages, dyspnea, worsening of bronchial asthma, and an influenzalike syndrome [71–75].

In addition to the adverse effects listed above, intravenous administration has the potential of causing fluid overload, electrolyte disturbances, especially hypernatremia, increased serum osmolality and creatinine, and a diuresis. Hematologic changes include hemolysis with hematuria and eosinophilia. Reported, but rare, central nervous system side effects include confusion, lethargy, disorientation, agitation, dysarthria, hypoactive reflexes, decreased consciousness, and encephalopathy. Cardiovascular symptoms include vasodilation, hypotension, chest pain, sinus tachycardia, and weakness [76, 77], DMSO may potentiate the action of numerous medications in animals [67]. Topical DMSO can increase insulin effect and should be used with extreme caution in patients with diabetes mellitus [65]. Elevated serum osmolality can occur in patients with increased intracranial pressure. Due to reported hepatotoxicity with DMSO intravenous administration, it is recommended to check liver and renal function tests every 6 months [70].

References

1. Abrams P,Cardozo L,Fall M et al.The standardization of terminology in lower urinary tract function: Report from the Standardization Sub-committee of the International Continence Society. Neurouol Urodyn 2002;21:167–178.
2. Stewart W, Herzog R, Wein A, et al. The prevalence and impact of overactive bladder in the US: Results from the NOBLE program. Neurourol Urodyn 2001;20:406–408.
3. Stewart WF, Van Rooyen JB, Cundiff GW, et al. Prevalence and burden of overactive bladder in the United States. World J Urol 2003;20:327–336.
4. US Census Bureau. US interim projections by age, sex, race, and Hispanic origin. Available at: http://

www.census.gov/ipc/www/usinterimproj,November 2006–12–05.

5. Fantl JA,NewmanDK,CollingJ, et al. Urinary incontinence in adults: Acute and chronic management 1996. Rockville, MD: US Department of Health and Human Services.

6. Ouslander J, Leach G, Abelson S, et al. Simple versus multichannel cystometry in the evaluation of bladder function in an incontinent geriatric population. J Urol 1988;140:1482–1486.

7. Burgio KL, Locher JL, Goodle PS, et al. Behavioral vs. drug treatment for urge urinary incontinence in older women: A randomized controlled trial. J Am Geriatr Soc 2000;48:370–374.

8. Goode PS, Burgio KL, Locher JL, et al. Urodynamic changes associated with behavioral and frug treatment of urge incontinence in olderwomen. J Am Geriatr Soc 2002;50:808–816.

9. Martin C. Michel, Jean J.M.C.H. de la Rosette. Role of muscarinic receptor antagonists in urgency and nocturia. BJU Int 2005;96(Suppl. 1):37–42.

10. Khullar V, Hill S, Laval KU, et al. Treatment of urge-predominant mixed urinary incontinence with tolterodine extended release: A randomized placebo-controlled trial. Urology, 2004;64:269–274.

11. Teunissen TA, de Jonge A, van Weel C, et al. Treating urinary incontinence in the elderly—Conservative therapies that work: A systematic review. J Fam Pract 2004;53:25–30.

12. Tsao J. Transient memory impairment and hallucinations associated with tolterodine use. N Eng J Med 2003;349:2274–2275.

13. Beers M. Explicit criteria for determining potentially inappropriate medication use by the elderly: An update. Arch Intern Med 1997;157:1531–1536.

14. Flaherty JH, Takahashi R. The use of complementary and alternative medical therapies among older persons around the world. Clin Geriatr Med 2004;20:179–200.

15. Appell RA. Electrical stimulation for the treatment of urinary incontinence. Urology 1998;51:S24–S26.

16. Bergström K, Christer P, Carlsson O, et al. Improvement of urge- and mixed-type incontinence after acupuncture treatment among elderly women – A pilot study. J Auton Nerv Syst 2000;79(2–3):173–180.

17. Andersson S, Lundeberg T. Acupuncture—From empiricism to science: Functional background to acupuncture effects in pain and disease. Med Hypotheses 1995;45(3):271–281.

18. Chai TC, Steers WD. Neurophysiology of micturition and continence in women. Int Urogynecol J Pelvic Floor Dysfunct 1997;8(2):85–97.

19. Jansen G, Lundeberg T, Kjartansson J, et al. Acupuncture and sensory neuropeptides increase cutaneous blood flow in rats. Neurosci Lett 1989;97(3):305–309.

20. Blom M, Lundeberg T, Dawidson I, et al. Effects on local blood flux of acupuncture stimulation used to treat xerostomia in patients suffering from Sjogren's syndrome. J Oral Rehabil 1993;20(5):541–548.

21. Appiah R, Hiller S, Caspary L, et al. Treatment of primary Raynaud's syndrome with traditional Chinese acupuncture. J Intern Med 1997;241(2):119–124.

22. Stener-Victorin E, Waldenstrom U, Andersson SA, et al. Reduction of blood flow impedance in the uterine arteries of infertile women with electroacupuncture. Hum Reprod 1996;11(6):1314–1317.

23. Wyon Y, Wijma K, Nedstrand E, et al. A comparison of acupuncture and oral estradiol treatment of vasomotor symptoms in postmenopausal women. Climacteric 2004;7(2):153–164.

24. Morrison JF, Sato A, Sato Y, et al. Long-lasting facilitation and depression of periurethral skeletal muscle following acupuncture-like stimulation in anesthetized rats. Neurosci Res 1995;23(2):159–169.

25. Sato A. Somatovisceral reflexes. J Manipulative Physiol Ther 1995;18(9):597–602.

26. Dale R. The origins and future of acupuncture. Am J Acupunct 1982; 10:101–120.

27. Chang PL. Urodynamic studies in acupuncture for women with frequency, urgency and dysuria. J Urol 1988;140:563–566.

28. Chang PL, Wu CJ, Huang MH. Long-term outcome of acupuncture in women with frequency, urgency and dysuria. Am J Chin Med 1993;21(3–4):231–236.

29. Emmons SL, Otto L. Acupuncture for overactive bladder: A randomized controlled trial. Obstet Gynecol 2005;1066(1):138–143.

30. Philp T, Shah PJR, Worth PHL. Acupuncture in the treatment of bladder instability. Br J Urol 1988;61:490–493.

31. Minni B, Capozza N, Creti G, et al. Bladder instability and enuresis treated by acupuncture and electro-therapeutics: Early urodynamic observations. Acupunct Electrother Res 1990;15(1):19–25.

32. Yuksek. MS. Erdem. AF. Atalay C, et al. Acupressure versus oxybutynin in the treatment of enuresis. J Int Med Res 2003;31(6):552–556.

33. Klingler HC, Pycha A, Schmidbauer J, et al. Use of peripheral neuromodulation of the S3 region for treatment of detrusor overactivity: A urodynamic-based study. Urology 2000;56(5):766–771.

34. http://www.naturaldatabase.com.

35. http://www.naturalstandard.com.

36. Gruenwald J, Brendler T, Jaenicke C. PDR for herbal medicines, 1st ed. Montvale, NJ: Medical Economics Company, 1998.

37. Foster S, Tyler VE, Tyler's honest herbal, 4th ed. Binghamton, NY: Haworth Herbal Press, 1999.

38. Zhang X, Ouyang JZ, Zhang YS, et al. Effect of the extracts of pumpkin seeds on the urodynamics of rabbits: An experimental study. J Tongji Med Univ 1994;14:235–238.

39. Younis YM, Ghirmay S, al-Shihry SS. African *Cucurbita pepo* L.: Properties of seed and variability in fatty acid composition of seed oil. Phytochemistry 2000;54:71–75.

40. De Bellis L, Gonzali S, Alpi A, et al. Purification and characterization of a novel pumpkin short-chain acyl-coenzyme A oxidase with structural similarity to acyl-coenzyme A dehydrogenases. Plant Physiol 2000;123:327–334.

41. Baker DH. Iodine toxicity and its amelioration. Exp Biol Med (Maywood) 2004;229:473–478.

42. Pye KG, Kelsey SM, House IM, et al. Severe dyserythropoeisis and autoimmune thrombocytopenia associated with ingestion of kelp supplement. Lancet 1992;339:1540.

43. Phaneuf D, Cote I, DumasP, et al. Evaluation of the contamination of marine algae (seaweed) from the St. Lawrence River and likely to be consumed by humans. Environ Res 1999;80:S175–S182.

44. Skibola CF. The effect of *Fucus vesiculosus*, an edible brown seaweed, upon menstrual cycle length and hormonal status in three pre-menopausal women: A case report. BMC Complement Altern Med 2004;4:10.

45. Ruperez P, Ahrazem O, Leal JA. Potential antioxidant capacity of sulfated polysaccharides from the edible marine brown seaweed *Fucus vesiculosus*. J Agric Food Chem 2002;50:840–845.

46. Beress A, Wassermann O, Tahhan S, et al. A new procedure for the isolation of anti-HIV compounds (polysaccharides and polyphenols) from the marine alga *Fucus vesiculosus*. J Nat Prod 1993;56:478–488.

47. Baba M, Snoeck R, Pauwels R, et al. Sulfated polysaccharides are potent and selective inhibitors of various enveloped viruses, including herpes simplex virus, cytomegalovirus, vesicular stomatitis virus, and human immunodeficiency virus. Antimicrob Agents Chemother 1988;32:1742–1745.

48. Patankar MS, Oehninger S, Barnett T, et al. A revised structure for fucoidan may explain some of its biological activities. J Biol Chem 1993;268:21770–21776.

49. Skibola CF. The effect of *Fucus vesiculosus*, an edible brown seaweed, upon menstrual cycle length and hormonal status in three pre-menopausal women: A case report. BMC Complement Altern Med 2004;4:10.

50. O'Leary R, Rerek M, Wood EJ. Fucoidan modulates the effect of transforming growth factor (TGF)-beta1 on fibroblast proliferation and wound repopulation in in vitro models of dermal wound repair. Biol Pharm Bull 2004;27:266–270.

51. Durig J, Bruhn T, Zurborn KH, et al. Anticoagulant fucoidan fractions from *Fucus vesiculosus* induce platelet activation in vitro. Thromb Res 1997;85:479–491.

52. Koyanagi S, Tanigawa N, Nakagawa H, et al. Oversulfation of fucoidan enhances its anti-angiogenic and antitumor activities. Biochem Pharmacol 2003;65:173–179.

53. Food and Nutrition Board, Institute of Medicine. Dietary reference intakes for vitamin A, vitamin K, arsenic, boron, chromium, copper, iodine, iron, manganese, molybdenum, nickel, silicon, vanadium, and zinc. Washington, DC: National Academy Press, 2002. Available at: http://www.nap.edu/books/0309072794/html/.

54. Pye KG, Kelsey SM, House IM, et al. Severe dyserythropoeisis and autoimmune thrombocytopenia associated with ingestion of kelp supplement. Lancet 1992;339:1540.

55. Conz PA, La Greca G, Benedetti P, et al. *Fucus vesiculosus*: A nephrotoxic alga? Nephrol Dial Transplant 1998;13:526–527.

56. Agarwal SC, Crook JR, Pepper CB. Herbal remedies – How safe are they? A case report of polymorphic ventricular tachycardia/ventricular fibrillation induced by herbal medication used for obesity. Int J Cardiol 2006;106:260–261.

57. Foster S, Duke JA. The Peterson field guide to medicinal plants: Eastern and Central North America. Boston, MA: Houghton Miffin, 1990.

58. Robbers JE, Tyler VE. Tyler's herbs of choice: The therapeutic use of phytomedicinals. New York, NY: The Haworth Herbal Press, 1999.

59. Wichtl MW. Herbal drugs and phytopharmaceuticals. Bisset NM,ed. Stuttgart: Medpharm GmbH Scientific Publishers, 1994.

60. Barker SB, Matthews PN, Philip PF, et al. Prospective study of intravesical dimethyl sulphoxide in the treatment of chronic inflammatory bladder disease. Br J Urol 1987;59(2):142–144.

61. Prior D, Mitchell A, Nebauer M, et al. Oncology nurses' experience of dimethyl sulfoxide odor. Cancer Nurs 2000;23:134–140.

62. MacCallum FO, Juel-Jensen BE. Herpes simplex virus skin infection in man treated with idoxuridine in dimethyl sulphoxide. Results of double-blind controlled trial. Br Med J 1966;2:805–807.

63. Wildenhoff KE, Esmann V, Ipsen J, et al. Treatment of trigeminal and thoracic zoster with idoxuridine. Scand J Infect Dis 1981;13:257–262.

64. Brayton CF. Dimethyl sulfoxide (DMSO): A review. Cornell Vet 1986;76:61–90.

65. Evans MS, Reid KH, Sharp JB. Jr. Dimethylsuloxide (DMSO) blocks conduction in peripheral nerve C fibers: a possible mechanism of analgesia. Neurosci Lett 1993;150(2):145–148.

66. Birder LA, Kanai AJ, de Groat WC. DMSO: Effect on bladder afferent neurons and nitric oxide release. J Urol 1997;158:1989–1995.

67. Jacob SW, Herschler R. Pharmacology of DMSO. Cryobiology 1986;23:14–27.

68. Brayton CF. Dimethyl sulfoxide (DMSO): A review. Cornell Vet 1986;76:61–90.

69. de la Torre JC. Role of dimethyl sulfoxide in prostaglandin-thromboxane and platelet systems after cerebral ischemia. Ann N Y Acad Sci 1983;411:293–308.

70. Martindale W. Martindale the extra pharmacopoeia. London: Pharmaceutical Press, 1999.

71. Rosenstein ED. Topical agents in the treatment of rheumatic disorders. Rheum Dis Clin North Am 1999;25:899–918.

72. Merlini G. Treatment of primary amyloidosis. Semin Hematol 1995;32:60–79

73. Trice JM, Pinals RS. Dimethyl sulfoxide: A review of its use in the rheumatic disorders. Semin Arthritis Rheum 1985;15:45–60.

74. Juel Jensen BE,MacCallum FO,Mackenzie AM, et al. Treatment of zoster with idoxuridine in dimethyl sulphoxide. Results of two double-blind controlled trials. Br Med J 1970;4:776–780.

75. Williams HJ, Furst DE, Dahl SL, et al. Double-blind, multicenter controlled trial comparing topical dimethyl sulfoxide and normal saline for treatment of hand ulcers in patients with systemic sclerosis. Arthritis Rheum 1985;28:308–314.

76. Marshall LF, Camp PE, Bowers SA. Dimethyl sulfoxide for the treatment of intracranial hypertension: A preliminary trial. Neurosurg 1984;14(6):659–663.

77. Wolf P, Simon M. Dimethyl sulphoxide (DMSO) induced serum hyperosmolality. Clin Biochem 1983;16(4):261–262.

Chapter 17
Sacral Nerve Stimulation for Neuromodulation of the Lower Urinary Tract

Dennis J.A.J. Oerlemans and Philip E.V. Van Kerrebroeck

Introduction

Chronic types of lower urinary tract dysfunction, including urgency incontinence (UI) and urgency–frequency (UF) and nonobstructive urinary retention (UR), still present a therapeutic challenge. Most patients initially are treated with conservative therapies including bladder retraining, pelvic floor exercises, and biofeedback. In the majority of patients this standard regimen is supported with pharmacological therapy (anticholinergics). However, approximately 40% either do not achieve an acceptable level of therapeutic benefit or remain completely refractory to treatment. Alternative surgical procedures such as bladder transsection, transvesical phenol injection of the pelvic plexus, augmentation cystoplasty, and even urinary diversion have been advocated for these chronic conditions. However, these procedures have variable efficacy and have been associated with significant morbidity and risk. Therefore, research into the use of electrical current for the treatment of lower urinary tract dysfunction has been initiated.In 1878, Saxtorph reported intravesical electrostimulation in patients with an acontractile bladder and complete urinary retention [50]. He inserted a special catheter with a metal electrode transurethrally. Years later, Ascoli and Katona applied electrostimulation in patients with chronic neurogenic retention and neurogenic overactivity [1, 39]. In the field of urology electric currents were and are used particularly in the bladder, the pelvic floor muscles, and the sacral roots [6, 7, 20]. Stimulation of the sacral nerves was developed to electrically empty the bladder and later poststimulus voiding was developed [10, 22, 36, 37]. Brindley developed an electrode for long-term stimulation of the spinal roots and it was implanted in the first patient in 1972 [9]. Electrodes were implanted in the first paraplegic patients since 1978, using direct stimulation [11]. A study by Nashold et al. in 1971 reported on a successful implantation of a neural prosthesis in the sacral segment of the spinal cord [47]. The implant was used to activate voiding in a patient with spinal cord injury. Jonas and Tanagho tried to improve this prosthesis, since this type of stimulation resulted not only in bladder contractions but in urinary sphincter contractions as well [36, 37]. Later, Tanagho and Schmidt demonstrated that the stimulation of sacral root S3 generally modulates detrusor and sphincter action and could be used in clinical practice [53, 62–64]. After two decades of experimentation with sacral root stimulation, finally in October 1997, sacral neuromodulation for treatment of refractory UI was approved by the Food and Drug Administration in the United States. More then 25,000 patients have undergone sacral nerve stimulation (SNS) since then.

The stimulation of afferent nerve fibers by electrical current modulates reflex pathways involved in the filling and evacuation phase of the micturition cycle through spinal circuits mediating somatovisceral interactions within the sacral spinal cord. SNS is proposed to activate or "reset" the somatic afferent inputs that play a pivotal role in the modulation of sensory processing and micturition reflexpathways in the spinal cord [25, 43].

Because beneficial effects can be demonstrated at intensities of stimulation that do not activate movements of striated muscle, the afferent system is the most likely to be affected [65]. Fowler et al. demonstrated that the anal sphincter reaction seen by acute testing is the result of an afferent-mediated response [26].

UR and dysfunctional voiding can be resolved by inhibition of the guarding reflexes. Detrusor overactivity can be suppressed by one or more pathways, ie, direct inhibition of bladder preganglionic neurons, as well as inhibition of interneuronal transmission in the afferent limb of the micturition reflex [43].

Recent research with PET studies indicates that at the level of the brain, the activity of centers in the paraventricular gray involved in activation or inhibition of the micturition reflex can be enhanced or reduced by SNS. This results in up- or down-grading of lower urinary tract activity [2, 4, 19]. Blok et al. reported on the acute and chronic effects of SNS on the brain in patients with UI. They registered differences between newly and chronically implanted patients in brain areas involved in sensory and motor learning. No differences were seen in regional cerebral blood flow (rCBF) in areas that are part of the micturition reflex. Changes in rCBF were seen in specific areas: areas known to be involved in micturition and areas involved in awareness and awakeness. Acute SNS modulates sensorimotor learning areas and these become less active during chronic SNS [4].

Selecting Patients for SNS

All patients who have symptoms of voiding dysfunction and who cannot be helped by other measures should be considered for SNS. Patient selection begins with a careful history, physical examination, routine urine tests, and, very importantly, the voiding diaries. Voiding diaries are a valuable instrument during the selection of patients and must be filled out carefully. Urodynamics are used to identify the patients with detrusor overactivity with or without urinary leakage or UR. Koldewijn et al. studied predictors of success in 100 test stimulation patients and did not find any [42]. Scheepens et al. studied the data from 211 patients who underwent a test stimulation [percutaneous nerve evaluation (PNE)] to determine the clinical parameters that

can enhance the prediction of PNE success. They found that intervertebral disk prolapse (IPD) surgery, duration of complaints, neurogenic bladder dysfunction, and UI were found to be significant predictive factors. IPD surgery can compromise the sacral root function and therefore can cause UI and UR [48, 70]. In this study patients who underwent IPD surgery had a 3.7 times higher chance on a positive test. Patients with UI responded 2.51 times better to the PNE test. Both found duration of complaints for more then 7 months and neurogenic bladder dysfunction were to be negative predictors of success. However, a PNE remains necessary to evaluate a patient's chance of permanent implant success objectively [52].

Cohen et al. recently published a study on motor versus sensory response. They concluded that a good motor response during implantation was a predictive factor (in 95% of successfully treated patients) for success, while a sensory response was not. Electrodes were implanted in all of these patients under local anesthesia but with intravenous sedation, and therefore the sensory perception of these patients may be unreliable [14].

Although not clearly reported before, it is known that a substantial number of the patients selected for SNS therapy have a history of psychological dysfunction and/or sexual abuse in the past. Weil et al. reported that special attention is needed for this group of patients [68]. They noted that patients with a history of psychological disorders, who had a good response during temporary test stimulation, had a far greater chance of lack of maintaining effect after permanent implantation. Of these patients, 82% showed a poor result after definitive implantation compared to 28% of the patients without a history of psychological disorders. Besides this lack of effect, 25% of the reoperations were done in this group, most of them with no effect. Psychological testing or psychiatric evaluation in case of doubt was advised before implantation of a permanent system.

A study by Everaert et al. showed similar findings [24]. In this study the two-stage procedure was compared with the single-stage procedure. In the two-stage implant group there were no failures during the first stage while in the single-stage procedure three patients had an immediate failure. They suggested that these results might be strongly influenced by psychological factors. Mental disorders were not related to objective or subjective success, but these cofactors surely interfere with symptomatology and therewith coinfluencing the results of therapy.

Technique of Sacral Neuromodulation

SNS incorporates a temporary test stimulation procedure that allows patients and physicians to assess SNS over a trial period [54]. This test stimulation, also known as a PNE test, is conducted as an outpatient procedure. Preferably it is performed under local anesthetic and comprises two steps: acute testing and the home evaluation phase. The original technique was described by Schmidt [54]. A test needle is inserted into the third sacral foramen to stimulate the sacral root (Fig. 17.1). Lead migration is a known complication of this test; other complications are technical failures or pain [57].

Some patients who fail a PNE test are still good candidates for SNS therapy. For these reasons a two-stage implant technique was developed [34]. With this technique a permanent electrode is implanted and connected to an external stimulator (Fig. 17.2). Less lead migration and a longer test period made it possible to separate nonresponders from technical failures. Using this two-stage implant technique eight of ten patients who failed a PNE test had a good result with SNS therapy and were implanted with a permanent system. A less invasive technique in com-

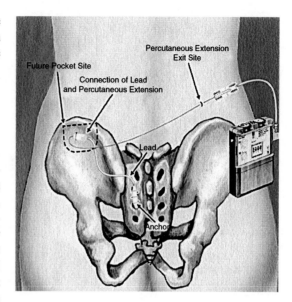

FIG. 17.2. Permanent electrode connected to an external stimulator

bination with a new designed self-anchoring lead made it possible to test patients with this two-stage technique [59, 60]. This "tined lead" has four sets of self-anchoring tines and made a minimally invasive percutaneous placement possible. The procedure can be performed under local anesthesia, requiring no additional incision and no additional anchoring. Besides these advantages this way of implantation made it possible to test the sensitive responses during implantation and it resulted in a reduction of operating time. The tined lead-staged implant technique is used widely in Europe and the United States [61].

The acute phase, whether a PNE or tined lead procedure is performed, is used to test the neural integrity, and therefore sensory and motor responses should be obtained during this test. The motor responses are important to identify the right sacral root. Typical S3 stimulation results in bellows movement of the pelvic floor, plantar flexion of the great toe, and paresthesia in the rectum, perineum, scrotum, or vagina. Stimulation of the other sacral roots results in different motor responses: S2 gives clamp movement or twisting and pinching of the anal sphincter and plantar flexion, with lateral rotation of the entire foot; S4 stimulation results in bellows motion of the pelvic floor, no lower extremity activity, and a sensation of pulling in the rectum [16].

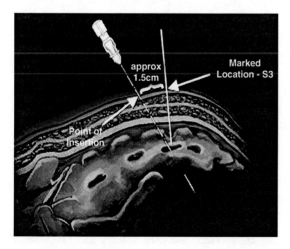

FIG. 17.1. Test needle inserted in the third sacral foramen

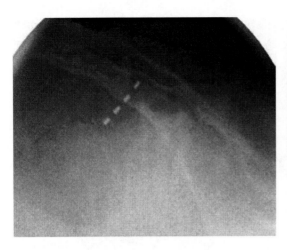

Fig. 17.3. Lateral X-ray of a permanent lead passing through the sacral foramen

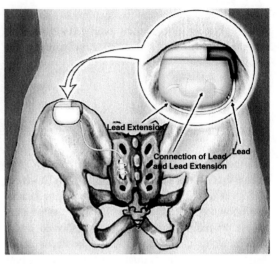

Fig. 17.4. Permanent pulse generator connected to the electrode

It can be difficult to palpate the bony landmarks, necessary to identify the right puncture place, in obese patients. Fluoroscopy then can be used for S3 localization. More importantly, the use of lateral imaging helps to determine the depth required for implanting the S3 lead (Fig. 17.3). The use of fluoroscopic localization of S3 allowed the introduction of tined S3 lead and transformed the placement of a lead from an open procedure to a completely percutaneous one [59, 60]. The widely adopted percutaneous use of a tined lead approach abandoned the need for fixation of the lead by methods such as bone anchors.

If the patient's symptoms improve at least more than 50%, then the patient is a candidate to undergo the stage II or permanent step in which the permanent implantable pulse generator (IPG) is implanted in the soft tissue of the buttock of the patient (Fig. 17.4).

Relatively low amplitudes (0–3.0 V) are sufficient for stimulation of the somatic nerve fibers and to minimize the potential for nerve damage due to overstimulation. Within the recommended stimulation parameters (210 μs, 10–16 Hz) continuous stimulation is possible without pain sensation.

Unilateral or Bilateral Stimulation

Although temporary and chronic SNS can result in significant permanent clinical improvement, some patients improve only partially or temporarily

[5, 69]. For these patients several methods have been developed to improve the results [59–61]. The most widely accepted method to test a patient for SNS therapy is unilateral stimulation. In some clinics bilateral stimulation has been suggested as a method to obtain better results [8, 32]. The bilateral innervation of the bladder is the basis for this type of intervention [21, 33]. Animal studies were performed to find a scientific basis for the application of bilateral stimulation. Schultz-Lampel et al. suggest that bilateral SNS can be a more effective technique for voiding dysfunction [56]. They conclude that bilateral stimulation may be more effective at lower stimulation intensities with positive side effects such as longer stimulator battery life and less potential nerve damage.

The only prospective randomized crossover trial to compare unilateral approach with bilateral sacral nerve stimulation was performed by Scheepens et al. [51]. In this study, 33 patients with chronic voiding dysfunction underwent unilateral as well as bilateral test stimulation to assess the possible advantages of bilateral stimulation. All patients were stimulated during at least 72 h in a unilateral and a bilateral setting with a washout period of at least 48 h between these two test periods. Standardized voiding records were used and urine was measured using standard measuring cups. They analyzed results for 12 patients with UI and for 13 patients with nonobstructive UR.

They did not find any significant differences comparing the results for unilateral with bilateral stimulation. Although two patients of the retention group started voiding during bilateral stimulation, while during unilateral stimulation they were still in complete retention. The reason for this result could be that with bilateral stimulation sufficient sacral nerve afferents are stimulated to achieve a marked effect at the central level.

In conclusion unilateral stimulation should be performed before bilateral sacral stimulation is considered. However, a bilateral test stimulation could be indicated when a unilateral test fails [40, 51]. Further research with clinical follow-up could identify suitable patients for bilateral sacral nerve stimulation.

Clinical Results

In 1999, a prospective randomized study was published in which the results of SNS therapy for UI were evaluated [55]. In total, 76 patients were treated in a multicenter trial: 34 patients received the implant and received chronic stimulation for 6 months, after which they completed a therapy evaluation test (on vs. off); 42 patients in a delay group were treated with standard medical therapy for 6 months and were offered implantation after this period. After 6 months the number of daily incontinence episodes, the number of daily replaced diapers, and the severity of incontinence were significantly reduced in the stimulation group. In the stimulation group, 16 patients (47%) were completely dry and 10 patients (29%) showed a greater than 50% reduction in incontinence episodes. In the delay group (controls) the average incontinence episodes increased during 6 months of conservative therapy from 2.63.5 heavy episodes at baseline to 3.9±3.8 heavy episodes a day at 6 months. After 18 months the efficacy appeared to be sustained. During the therapy evaluation at 6 months the stimulation group returned to baseline symptoms when stimulation was stopped.

Hassouna et al. reported in 2000 on the treatment of UF symptoms with SNS therapy [29]. In total, 51 patients—a stimulation group of 25 patients and a control group of 26 patients—enrolled in this multicenter trial. All the patients had been tested with a PNE test and showed satisfactory responses. The stimulation group received implant directly after this test and the control group received implant after a 6-months delay period. Statistically significant improvements were seen in the stimulation group for diary parameters as: number of voids daily (16.9±9.7 to 9.3±5.1), volume per void (118±74 to 226±124 ml), and degree of urgency (rank 2.2±0.6 to 1.6±0.9). In the control group no significant changes were seen. After 6 months the stimulation group had an evaluation test and urinary symptoms returned to baseline when stimulation was turned off. After reactivation of the stimulation sustained efficacy was seen at 12 and 24 months.

A report of use of SNS in UR was published in 2001 by Jonas et al. A total of 177 patients with UR refractory to conservative therapy were enrolled in this multicenter trial between 1993 and 1998 [38]. Thirty-seven patients were assigned to treatment and 31 to the control group. At 6 months the stimulation group showed 69% elimination of catheterization and an additional 14% with greater than 50% reduction in catheter volume per catheterization. Temporary inactivation (3 days) of SNS therapy resulted in significant increase in residual volume. The effectiveness of SNS therapy was sustained for 18 months after implantation.

The first medium-term follow-up results of the above mentioned patient series were published in 2000 [57]. Results were reported for 1.5 to 3 years of follow-up. Of 41 UI patients, 59% showed a greater than 50% reduction in leaking episodes, with 46% of the patients being completely dry after 3 years. After 2 years of follow-up, 56% of the UF patients showed a greater than 50% reduction in voids per day. In the retention group, 70% of 42 patients showed a greater than 50% reduction in catheter volume per catheterization.

During the MDT-103 trial in 89 patients, depression and health-related quality of life (HRQOL) were assessed [17]. Patients were divided into a direct implant group and a delayed implant group. At baseline they noted detectable levels of depression in 73% of all patients. After 3 months patients in the implanted group had a significant improvement in depression scores. The improved scores remained at the 6- and 12-month visits. The scores on the SF-36 questionnaire, a questionnaire to investigate pain, vitality, physical functioning, social functioning, and mental health, increased in the implant group for role-physical, pain, and social functioning. This study demonstrated the serious impact that unresolved voiding dysfunction has on quality of life. SNS was associated with significant improvement in depression and HRQOL.

Recently, the 5-year follow-up results of patients included in the trial in order to obtain FDA approval were analyzed. Of 163 patients enrolled, 152 have received implants. Of the 163 patients, 103 (64%) had UI, 28 (17%) UF, and 31 (19%) UR. Voiding diaries were collected annually over 5 years. For UI patients, the mean number of leaking episodes per day declined from 9.6 ± 6.0 to 3.9 ± 4.0. For UF patients, mean voids per day decreased from 19.3 ± 7.0 to 14.8 ± 7.6. Mean volume voided per void increased from 92.3 ± 52.8 to 165.2 ± 147.7 ml. In the UR group the average number of catheterizations per day decreased from 5.3±2.8 at baseline to 1.9±2.8 at 5 years postimplant. No life-threatening or irreversible adverse events occurred. Of 152 patients, 102 experienced 31 device-related and 240 therapy-related adverse events. Among these therapy-related events, the most frequently reported event was new pain or undesirable change in stimulation (60 times in 41 patients). Pain at the implant site or related to the implanted pulse generator (IPG) was the second-most reported event (40 times in 30 patients). However, an important finding in this study is the high correlation between the 1- and 5-year success rates. Of the implanted patients, 84% with UI, 71% with UF, and 78% with UR continued to have a successful outcome at 5-year follow-up if they were successful at 1 year [41].

Different groups have published their long-term results in recent years [18, 23, 67]. They all conclude that SNS therapy is safe and effective.

Complications

Most studies mentioned in the clinical results section reported on complications during SNS. Siegel et al. summarized the complications in patients who were included in the original trials of SNS [57]. The complications were divided into PNE-related complications and implant-related problems. Of the 914 test stimulation procedures done on the 581 patients, 181 adverse events occurred in 166 of these procedures (18.2% of the 914 procedures). The vast majority of complications were related to lead migration (108 events, 11.8% of procedures).

Technical problems and pain represented 2.6 and 2.1% of the adverse events, respectively. For the 219 patient who underwent implantation of the permanent system, the following adverse events were seen during follow-up: pain at neurostimulator site (15.3%), new pain (9%), suspected lead migration (8.4%), transient electric shock (5.5%), pain at lead site (5.4%), adverse change in bowel function (3.0%), and some less frequent events such as technical problems, device problems, change in menstrual cycle, and others. Surgical revisions of the implanted neurostimulator or lead system were performed in 33.3% of cases (73 of 219 patients) to resolve an adverse event. Mostly this was done to relocate the stimulator because of pain or because of suspected lead migration. No serious adverse events, side effects, or permanent injury were reported.

Recently our long-term follow-up results with complication rates were published [67]. Of 149 patients analyzed, 107 had overactive bladder symptoms and 42 had urinary retention. Mean follow-up was 64.2 (SD = 38.5) months. In the whole group 194 adverse events occurred. Six patients had infection in their implanted system; one was explanted for infection. Most events could be solved by giving advice or by reprogramming the stimulator. In all, 129 reoperations have been performed and 21 patients had their system explanted. The most frequent surgical procedures performed were repositioning of the IPG, revision of the electrode because of suspected lead migration, and reoperation for parameter change in patients implanted with the Itrell-I IPG (the first model used for SNS). Analysis of the data shows a striking difference in the incidence of reoperations, but small differences in subjective results in the groups of patients implanted before or after 1996, suggesting that a proactive approach toward adverse events is worthwhile. In our experience with the tined lead implantation we see a clear decrease in reoperation rate [66]. Of 39 patients implanted with the tined lead, van Voskuilen et al. described seven severe adverse events on medium term, three of whom needed a reoperation. Three patients could be treated with one or two reprogramming sessions. Three patients had a reoperation to reposition the IPG after complaints of pain. These three patients had good results afterward. One patient with an incomplete spinal cord lesion had no benefit of the implanted system.

Of 161 patients implanted with the tined lead between July 2002 and September 2004, Hijaz et al. described the complications seen in their institute [31]. They had three categories for complications: infections, mechanical problems, and response-related dysfunction. In total they reported 17 explantations (10.5%). Eight explantations were done due to infection and seven due to loss of effect. In 26 (16.1%) patients they performed a revision after these patients presented with a decrease in clinical response. The reasons for revision were mechanical (lead) problems, IPG site discomfort, lead migration, and infectious causes. The complication rates show a decrease over the years mainly due to technical and procedural improvements.

Gaynor-Krupnick et al. as well as Hijaz and Vasavada presented an algorithm for evaluation and managing of a malfunctioning neuromodulation system [27, 30].

Expanding Indications

With the widespread use, incidental improvements were published for other pathological conditions. Use of SNS for other off-label applications have been reported for treatment of interstitial cystitis, chronic pelvic pain, pediatric voiding dysfunction, and neurogenic lower urinary dysfunction seen in multiple sclerosis.

Long-term results for the use of SNS in neurogenic UI patients were presented by Chartier-Kastler [13]. The results for nine patients were shown with a mean follow-up of 43.6 months. All patients had significant clinical improvement and five (56%) patients were completely dry. The number of leakages per day went from an initial 7.3 to 0.3 (at last follow-up). Frequency improved after implantation from 16.1 to 8 voids per day and the mean volume per void increased from 115 to 249 ml.

In 2000, the first papers were published with positive results with the use of SNS in interstitial cystitis [12, 71]. Comiter evaluated the effect of SNS therapy for interstitial cystitis in a prospective study in 2003 [15]. Seventeen of 25 patients were implanted with a permanent system. After a mean follow-up of 14 months there were significant improvements in daytime frequency and nocturia, which improved from 17.1 to 8.7 and 4.5 to 1.1, respectively ($P < 0.01$). Mean voided volume increased from 111 to

264 ml ($P < 0.01$). Average pain score decreased from 5.8 to 1.6 points on a scale of 0 to 10 ($P < 0.01$). Interstitial Cystitis Symptom and Problem Index scores decreased from 16.5 to 6.8 and 14.5 to 5.4, respectively ($P < 0.01$).

In 2001 Siegel et al. implanted ten patients with chronic pelvic pain [58]. These patients all had a history of at least 6 months of pelvic pain refractory to conventional treatment without a primary complaint of voiding dysfunction. After 9 months of follow-up nine of ten patients had a decrease in most severe pain scores; after a median follow-up of 19 months six of ten patients reported significant improvement in pain symptomatology.

After the clinical implication of SNS therapy for voiding dysfunction, Matzel, together with Schmidt and Tanagho, started to investigate SNS therapy in bowel dysfunction [44, 45]. In a prospective, nonrandomized, multicenter study 37 patients underwent a test stimulation with SNS therapy for fecal incontinence [46]. Thirty-four patients were implanted with a permanent system. The effect on incontinence was assessed by daily bowel habit diaries and a disease-specific quality of life questionnaire. The frequency of incontinent episodes per week decreased from 16.4 to 3.1 at 12 months and to 2.0 at 24 months for both urge and passive incontinence. The mean number of incontinence episodes per week, staining, and pad use declined significantly, too. Quality of life improved significantly in ASCRS scales,;in the SF-36 scales only social functioning improved significantly.

Jarrett et al. did a systematic review of SNS for fecal incontinence and constipation [35]. They reported total continence in 41–75% of the patients and 75–100% experienced improvement in the incontinence symptoms. The results for patients treated with SNS for constipation discussed in this review seem promising, but limited data are available at this time.

The results of SNS therapy in children with neurogenic bladder dysfunction are described by Guys et al. [28]. Forty-two children with neurogenic bladder dysfunction, mainly due to spina bifida, were enrolled in this prospective, randomized controlled trial. Twenty-one patients were treated conservatively while the other 21 patients were treated with SNS therapy. After 12 months no significant better results were seen in the group treated with SNS. The authors stated that probably the intervention group was too small or the bladder dysfunction in these patients too severe.

During routine follow-up patients may report improved sexual functioning after implant. Pauls et al. recently reported a pilot study to determine whether sacral neuromodulation has an effect on the patient's subsequent sexual function [49]. Eleven patients with a permanent system implanted were questioned about their sexual function before and after implantation. With SNS therapy sexual frequency and Female Sexual Function Index (FSFI) increased significantly. No correlation was found between improvement in urinary symptoms and FSFI scores.

Conclusions

After years of experimental therapy, initiated by Tanagho and Schmidt, SNS now is a widely used therapy. Although the mechanisms of action are still not fully understood, the therapy has been proven effective in the long term. Due to the less invasive technique and other technical improvements, it is expected that complication rates will further decrease within the coming years. The expanding use of SNS therapy in fields other than urology probably will result in FDA approval for gastrointestinal indications.Further research, possibly with the help of animal models, has to be performed to understand in a more precise way the mechanism of SNS therapy. Other goals in research could be patient selection (finding ways to identify the best candidates), the effect of SNS in combined (urological/gynecological/gastroenterological) pathology, and the effect of bilateral versus unilateral stimulation.

References

1. Ascoli R. 1965. [Treatment of neurogenic bladder]. Acta Urol Belg 33:76–83.
2. Blok BF. 2002. Central pathways controlling micturition and urinary continence. Urology 59(5 Suppl 1):13–17.
3. Blok BF, Groen J, Veltman D, Bosch R. 2003. Brain plasticity and urge incontinence: PET studies during the first hours of sacral neuromodulation. Neurourol Urodyn 22:490–491.
4. Blok BF, Groen J, Bosch JL, et al. 2007. Different brain effects during chronic and acute sacral neuromodulation in urge incontinent patients with implanted neurostimulators. BJU Int 99:700–700.
5. Bosch JL, Groen J. 2000. Sacral nerve neuromodulation in the treatment of patients with refractory motor urge incontinence: Long-term results of a prospective longitudinal study. J Urol 163(4):1219–1222.
6. Boyce WH, Lathem E, Hunt LD. 1963. Research related to the development of an artificial electrical stimulator for the paralyzed human bladder: A review. Trans Am Assoc Genitourin Surg 55:81–91.
7. Boyce WH, Lathem JE, Hunt LD. 1964. Research related to the development of an artificial electrical stimulator for the paralyzed human bladder: A review. J Urol 91:41–51.
8. Braun P, Seif C, Scheepe J, et al. 2002. [Chronic sacral bilateral neuromodulation. Using a minimal invasive implantation technique in patients with disorders of bladder function]. Urologe A 41(1):44–47.
9. Brindley GS. 1972. Experiments directed towards a prosthesis which controls the bladder and the external sphincter from a single site of stimulation. Proc Biol Eng Soc 46th Meeting, Liverpool.
10. Brindley GS. 1977. An implant to empty the bladder or close the urethra. J Neurol Neurosurg Psychiatry 40(4):358–369.
11. Brindley GS. 1993. History of the sacral anterior root stimulator, 1969–1982. Neurourol Urodyn 12(5):481–483.
12. Chai TC, Zhang C, Warren JW, Keay S. 2000. Percutaneous sacral third nerve root neurostimulation improves symptoms and normalizes urinary HB-EGF levels and antiproliferative activity in patients with interstitial cystitis. Urology 55(5):643–646.
13. Chartier-Kastler EJ, Ruud Bosch JL, Perrigot M, et al. 2000. Long-term results of sacral nerve stimulation (S3) for the treatment of neurogenic refractory urge incontinence related to detrusor hyperreflexia. J Urol 164(5):1476–1480.
14. Cohen BL, Tunuguntla HS, Gousse A. 2006. Predictors of success for first stage neuromodulation: Motor versus sensory response. J Urol 175(6):2178–2180; discussion 2180–2171.
15. Comiter CV. 2003. Sacral neuromodulation for the symptomatic treatment of refractory interstitial cystitis: A prospective study. J Urol 169(4):1369–1373.
16. Daneshgari F. 2006. Applications of neuromodulation of the lower urinary tract in female urology. Int Braz J Urol 32(3):262–272.
17. Das AK, Carlson AM, Hull M. 2004. Improvement in depression and health-related quality of life after

sacral nerve stimulation therapy for treatment of voiding dysfunction. Urology 64(1):62–68.

18. Dasgupta R, Wiseman OJ, Kitchen N, Fowler CJ. 2004. Long-term results of sacral neuromodulation for women with urinary retention. BJU Int 94(3):335–337.

19. Dasgupta R, Critchley HD, Dolan RJ, Fowler CJ. 2005. Changes in brain activity following sacral neuromodulation for urinary retention. J Urol 174(6):2268–2272.

20. Dees JE. 1965. Contraction of the urinary bladder produced by electric stimulation. Preliminary report. Invest Urol 15:539–547.

21. Diokno AC, Davis R, Lapides J. 1973. The effect of pelvic nerve stimulation on detrusor contraction. Invest Urol 11(3):178–181.

22. Eidelberg E, Bors E, Woodbury CM, Brigham A. 1974. Effect of electrical stimulation of dorsal and ventral spinal cord roots on the cat's urinary bladder. Urol Int 29(5):375–381.

23. Elhilali MM, Khaled SM, Kashiwabara T, et al. 2005. Sacral neuromodulation: Long-term experience of one center. Urology 65(6):1114–1117.

24. Everaert K, Kerckhaert W, Caluwaerts H, et al. 2004. A prospective randomized trial comparing the 1-stage with the 2-stage implantation of a pulse generator in patients with pelvic floor dysfunction selected for sacral nerve stimulation. Eur Urol 45(5):649–654.

25. Fall M, Lindstrom S. 1991. Electrical stimulation. A physiologic approach to the treatment of urinary incontinence. Urol Clin North Am 18(2):393–407.

26. Fowler CJ, Swinn MJ, Goodwin RJ, et al. 2000. Studies of the latency of pelvic floor contraction during peripheral nerve evaluation show that the muscle response is reflexly mediated. J Urol 163(3):881–883.

27. Gaynor-Krupnick DM, Dwyer NT, Rittenmeyer H, Kreder KJ. 2006. Evaluation and management of malfunctioning sacral neuromodulator. Urology 67(2):246–249.

28. Guys JM, Haddad M, Planche D, et al. 2004. Sacral neuromodulation for neurogenic bladder dysfunction in children. J Urol 172(4 Pt 2):1673–1676.

29. Hassouna MM, Siegel SW, Nyeholt AA, et al. 2000. Sacral neuromodulation in the treatment of urgency-frequency symptoms: A multicenter study on efficacy and safety. J Urol 163(6):1849–1854.

30. Hijaz A, Vasavada S. 2005. Complications and troubleshooting of sacral neuromodulation therapy. Urol Clin North Am 32(1):65–69.

31. Hijaz A, Vasavada SP, Daneshgari F, et al. 2006. Complications and troubleshooting of two-stage sacral neuromodulation therapy: A single-institution experience. Urology 68(3):533–537.

32. Hohenfellner M, Schultz-Lampel D, Dahms S, et al. 1998. Bilateral chronic sacral neuromodulation for treatment of lower urinary tract dysfunction. J Urol 160(3 Pt 1):821–824.

33. Ingersoll EH, Jones LL, Hegre ES. 1957. Effect on urinary bladder of unilateral stimulation of pelvic nerves in the dog. Am J Physiol 189(1):167–172.

34. Janknegt RA, Weil EH, Eerdmans PH. 1997. Improving neuromodulation technique for refractory voiding dysfunctions: Two-stage implant. Urology 49(3):358–362.

35. Jarrett ME, Mowatt G, Glazener CM, et al. 2004. Systematic review of sacral nerve stimulation for faecal incontinence and constipation. Br J Surg 91(12):1559–1569.

36. Jonas U, Tanagho EA. 1975. Studies on the feasibility of urinary bladder evacuation by direct spinal cord stimulation. II. Poststimulus voiding: A way to overcome outflow resistance. Invest Urol 13(2):151–153.

37. Jonas U, Heine JP, Tanagho EA. 1975. Studies on the feasibility of urinary bladder evacuation by direct spinal cord stimulation. I. Parameters of most effective stimulation. Invest Urol 13(2):142–150.

38. Jonas U, Fowler CJ, Chancellor MB, et al. 2001. Efficacy of sacral nerve stimulation for urinary retention: Results 18 months after implantation. J Urol 165(1):15–19.

39. Katona F. 1975. Stages of vegetative afferentation in reorganization of bladder control during intravesical electrotherapy. Urol Int 30(3):192–203.

40. Kerrebroeck van PE, Scheepens W, de Bie R, Weil E. 2005. European experience with bilateral sacral neuromodulation in patients with chronic lower urinary tract dysfunction. Urol Clin North Am 32(1):51–57.

41. Kerrebroeck van PE, Voskuilen van AC, Heesakkers JPFA, et al. 2007. Five-year results of sacral neuromodulation therapy for urinary voiding dysfunction: Outcomes of prospective, worldwide clinical study. J Urol 178:2029–2034.

42. Koldewijn EL, Rosier PF, Meuleman EJ, et al. 1994. Predictors of success with neuromodulation in lower urinary tract dysfunction: Results of trial stimulation in 100 patients. J Urol 152(6 Pt 1):2071–2075.

43. Leng WW, Chancellor MB. 2005. How sacral nerve stimulation neuromodulation works. Urol Clin North Am 32(1):11–18.

44. Matzel KE, Schmidt RA, Tanagho EA. 1990. Neuroanatomy of the striated muscular anal continence mechanism. Implications for the use of neurostimulation. Dis Colon Rectum 33(8):666–673.

45. Matzel KE, Stadelmaier U, Hohenfellner M, Gall FP. 1995. Electrical stimulation of sacral spinal nerves for treatment of faecal incontinence. Lancet 346(8983):1124–1127.

46. Matzel KE, Kamm MA, Stosser M, et al. 2004. Sacral spinal nerve stimulation for faecal incontinence: Multicentre study. Lancet 363(9417):1270–1276.

47. Nashold BS Jr , Friedman H, Boyarsky S. 1971. Electrical activation of micturition by spinal cord stimulation. J Surg Res 11(3):144–147.

48. O'Flynn KJ, Murphy R, Thomas DG. 1992. Neurogenic bladder dysfunction in lumbar intervertebral disc prolapse. Br J Urol 69(1):38–40.

49. Pauls RN, Marinkovic SP, Silva WA, et al. 2006. Effects of sacral neuromodulation on female sexual function. Int Urogynecol J Pelvic Floor Dysfunct 17(1):27–29.

50. Saxtorph M. 1878. Stricture urethrae – Fistula perinee – Retentio urinae. Clinsk Chirurgi, Gyldendalske Fortag Copenhagen: 265–280.

51. Scheepens WA, de Bie RA, Weil EH, van Kerrebroeck PE. 2002a. Unilateral versus bilateral sacral neuromodulation in patients with chronic voiding dysfunction. J Urol 168(5):2046–2050.

52. Scheepens WA, Jongen MM, Nieman FH, et al. 2002b. Predictive factors for sacral neuromodulation in chronic lower urinary tract dysfunction. Urology 60(4):598–602.

53. Schmidt RA, Bruschini H, Tanagho EA. 1979. Sacral root stimulation in controlled micturition. Peripheral somatic neurotomy and stimulated voiding. Invest Urol 17(2):130–134.

54. Schmidt RA, Senn E, Tanagho EA. 1990. Functional evaluation of sacral nerve root integrity. Report of a technique. Urology 35(5):388–392.

55. Schmidt RA, Jonas U, Oleson KA, et al. 1999. Sacral nerve stimulation for treatment of refractory urinary urge incontinence. Sacral Nerve Stimulation Study Group. J Urol 162(2):352–357.

56. Schultz-Lampel D, Jiang C, Lindstrom S, et al. 1998. Neurophysiologische Effekte unilateraler und bilateraler sakraler Neuromodulation. Aktuel Urol 29:354–360.

57. Siegel SW, Catanzaro F, Dijkema HE, et al. 2000. Long-term results of a multicenter study on sacral nerve stimulation for treatment of urinary urge incontinence, urgency-frequency, and retention. Urology 56(6 Suppl 1):87–91.

58. Siegel S, Paszkiewicz E, Kirkpatrick C, et al. 2001. Sacral nerve stimulation in patients with chronic intractable pelvic pain. J Urol 166(5):1742–1745.

59. Spinelli M, Giardiello G, Arduini A, van den Hombergh U. 2003a. New percutaneous technique of sacral nerve stimulation has high initial success rate: preliminary results. Eur Urol 43(1):70–74.

60. Spinelli M, Giardiello G, Gerber M, Arduini A, van den Hombergh U, Malaguti S. 2003b. New sacral neuromodulation lead for percutaneous implantation using local anesthesia: Description and first experience. J Urol 170(5):1905–1907.

61. Spinelli M, Weil E, Ostardo E, et al. 2005. New tined lead electrode in sacral neuromodulation: Experience from a multicentre European study. World J Urol 23(3):225–229.

62. Tanagho EA, Schmidt RA. 1982. Bladder pacemaker: Scientific basis and clinical future. Urology 20(6):614–619.

63. Tanagho EA, Schmidt RA. 1988. Electrical stimulation in the clinical management of the neurogenic bladder. J Urol 140(6):1331–1339.

64. Tanagho EA, Schmidt RA, Orvis BR. 1989. Neural stimulation for control of voiding dysfunction: A preliminary report in 22 patients with serious neuropathic voiding disorders. J Urol 142(2 Pt 1):340–345.

65. Vodusek DB, Light JK, Libby JM. 1986. Detrusor inhibition induced by stimulation of pudendal nerve afferents. Neurourol Urodyn 5(4):381–389.

66. Voskuilen van AC, Oerlemans DJ, Weil EH, et al. 2006a. Medium-term experience of sacral neuromodulation by tined lead implantation. BJU Int 99:107–110.

67. Voskuilen van AC, Oerlemans DJ, Weil EH, et al. 2006b. Long term results of neuromodulation by sacral nerve stimulation for lower urinary tract symptoms: A retrospective single center study. Eur Urol 49(2):366–372.

68. Weil EH, Ruiz-Cerda JL, Eerdmans PH, et al. 1998. Clinical results of sacral neuromodulation for chronic voiding dysfunction using unilateral sacral foramen electrodes. World J Urol 16(5):313–321.

69. Weil EH, Ruiz-Cerda JL, Eerdmans PH, et al. 2000. Sacral root neuromodulation in the treatment of refractory urinary urge incontinence: A prospective randomized clinical trial. Eur Urol 37(2):161–171.

70. Yamanishi T, Yasuda K, Sakakibara R, et al. 1998. Detrusor overactivity and penile erection in patients with lower lumbar spine lesions. Eur Urol 34(4):360–364.

71. Zermann DH, Weirich T, Wunderlich H, et al. 2000. Sacral nerve stimulation for pain relief in interstitial cystitis. Urol Int 65(2):120–121.

Chapter 18
Peripheral Neuromodulation for the Treatment of Overactive Bladder

Anurag K. Das

Overactive bladder (OAB) is a common syndrome defined by the International Continence Society [1] as "urgency with or without urge incontinence, usually with frequency and nocturia, in the absence of other pathologic or metabolic conditions to explain these symptoms." Most cases of OAB are idiopathic and many respond to behavioral modification or antimuscarinic medications. However, it is not uncommon for patients to not respond to these interventions and to be classified as having refractory OAB symptoms. One such refractory case is illustrated below.

Case 1. A 46-year-old white female presents with complaints of urinary urge incontinence. She leaks in moderate amounts generally on her way to the bathroom, but also with changes in position such as getting out of a chair or bed. She has been tried on various combinations of anticholinergic and tricyclic medications with mild improvement, but the medications further worsened her constipation, which already is a significant problem for her. She has been taught guarding maneuvers, behavioral modification, and pelvic floor rehabilitation without satisfactory improvement in her symptoms. Past medical history is otherwise unremarkable and past surgical history is remarkable for appendectomy and hysterectomy (for large fibroids). There is no history of back problems or neurological disease. Physical examination is unremarkable and urogenital examination reveals a normal meatus, minimal cystourethrocele, and normal neurological examination including normal perianal sensation and rectal sphincter tone.

Voiding diary reveals a functional bladder capacity of 300 ml, average voided volume of ~160 ml, and two to three moderate volume leakage episodes daily. Urodynamic studies in the standing position at a fill rate of 60 ml/min with room temperature sterile contrast material reveal phasic detrusor overactivity starting at volumes of 160–180 ml with moderate volume leakage. Bladder is normally oriented and the patient is able to void to completion with low voiding pressures.

Although this patient responded to some degree to anticholinergic therapy, she could not tolerate it due to side effects especially constipation. Although frequency–urgency syndromes and urge incontinence are quite common and many patients can be adequately managed with combinations of behavioral therapy, pelvic floor rehabilitation, and pharmaceutical therapy, a significant minority of patients do not respond adequately to these measures or cannot tolerate the side effects and desire further treatment. Options generally are limited and require major surgical procedures such as augmentation cystoplasty, which often can result in incomplete emptying and need for intermittent catheterization, an alternative not acceptable for many such patients. While sacral neuromodulation (SNS) has been used in the treatment of refractory OAB with reasonable success rates in appropriately selected patients and is addressed in detail elsewhere, for many patients it represents a more invasive treatment option than they would like. Prior to considering sacral neuromodulation, which is more invasive and significantly more expensive, patients can consider tibial nerve stimulation, a relatively inexpensive minimally invasive procedure working in a retrograde manner to effect sacral nerve root function. In this chapter, I will review the history, indications, and mechanism of action, techniques, and outcomes of tibial nerve stimulation as a model for peripheral neuromodulation.

History

The use of electrical stimulation for treatment of various disorders has a long and colorful history. Electrical stimulation was used for such disease processes as excess libido and, of course, depression. Caldwell [2] used electrical stimulation of the pelvic floor using implanted electrodes in an attempt to treat stress urinary incontinence and also attempted to treat neurogenic incontinence with an implantable stimulator. With advances in cardiac pacing and the improved understanding and miniaturization of electronic instruments, interest in neuromodulation of bladder function was revived in the 1970s and 1980s. The Department of Urology at the University of California, San Francisco, led by Drs. Richard Schmidt and Emil Tanagho, was instrumental in performing some of the early work and laying the foundation for the use of sacral neuromodulation for the treatment of refractory voiding dysfunction. Dr. Edward McGuire [3], in the early 1980s, first reported using tibial stimulation with a patch electrode, while Dr. Marshall Stoller, in the late 1980s, pioneered the use of tibial nerve stimulation with the percutaneous Stoller afferent neurostimulation (SANS) method.

Mechanism of Action

The mechanism of action of peripheral nerve stimulation (PNS) is not completely understood. It is probable that stimulation of the tibial nerve causes retrograde modification of S3 nerve root function. This may be similar to sacral neuromodulation, and as Chancellor and DeGroat [4, 5] have suggested may improve somatic afferent inhibition of sensory processing in the spinal cord. Since the S2–4 nerve roots provide the primary autonomic (parasympathetic through the pelvic nerve) and somatic (pudendal nerve) innervation to the blad-

der, urethra, and pelvic floor, this processing somehow helps in the treatment of OAB by "inhibiting" these nerve roots. Further data to support the view that afferent pathways play a role in SNS-related symptom improvement come from Fowler [6, 7], who suggests neuromodulation affects afferent pathways probably through mediating changes in spinobulbospinal pathways to the pontine micturition center. Because visceral afferents require higher stimulation amplitudes, it is more likely that somatic afferents play a more important role in the mechanism involved, and thus the term "somatic afferent inhibition."

Indications

Peripheral neuromodulation has been used for the treatment of refractory urge incontinence, refractory urinary frequency–urgency syndromes, or refractory OAB syndrome, depending on one's preference, in controlled trials. Generally, patients who have failed or could not tolerate more conservative therapies, such as behavioral modification, pelvic floor rehabilitation (including pelvic floor biofeedback/muscular vaginal electrical stimulation), and anticholinergic/antimuscarinic medications, are given a trial of percutaneous peripheral neuromodulation. It is important to remember that patients with neurological disease have been excluded from most of the trials, and thus there are few data that patients with neurological diseases may respond well to this modality. All patients being considered for PNS should have a complete history and physical examination including a genital, rectal, and neurological examination. These patients should perform accurate voiding diaries and undergo urodynamic studies to confirm the diagnosis and ascertain they are suitable candidates. These patients should have failed or could not tolerate more conservative therapies such as behavioral modification and/or appropriate medications.

PNS Procedure

The procedure is fairly straightforward. It is performed with the patient sitting in a frog-legged position with the soles of the feet touching. The medial aspect of the malleolus is palpated and a sensitive pressure point is identified approximately three finger breadths cephalad. This point is about a fingerbreadth posterior to the edge of the tibia. A 34-gauge, solid stainless steel needle is advanced through the skin with the aid of an overlying plastic cylinder that is about 3 mm shorter than the needle. Once the skin is pierced the cylinder is removed, and the needle is advanced approximately 3–4 cm. The needle trajectory is 60° from a perpendicular line along the length of the tibia, advanced toward the patient's head (Fig. 18.1). Needles may be placed bilaterally in a similar fashion.

A grounding pad is placed over the medial aspect of the calcaneus. A stimulator is then connected to the needle and the ipsilateral ground pad (Fig. 18.2). Stimulation is titrated from 0 to 10 mA with a pulse width of 200 ms at a frequency of 20 Hz. Proper needle placement is confirmed with great toe flexion and/or fanning of ipsilateral digits two through five. The therapeutic session is 30 min long and sessions may be carried out weekly.

Results

The results of a large multicenter study on patients with urge incontinence and frequency–urgency were reported by Govier et al. [8]. Fifty-three patients who met study entry criteria were treated for a total of 12 weeks; 47 patients

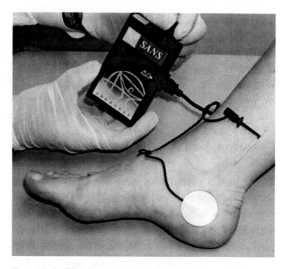

FIG. 18.2. Tibial neurostimulation (picture courtesy of Drs. P. Rosenblatt and N. Kohli)

finished the trial and were evaluable. Overall, the patients achieved a 35% reduction in daytime and nighttime urge incontinence or leak episodes during the 12-week treatment period ($P < 0.05$). Of the patients completing the trial, 71% were classified by the investigators as having achieved treatment success after 12 weeks. Success was defined as at least a 25% reduction in daytime and/or nighttime frequency. No serious or unanticipated adverse events were reported, and no adverse events resulted in patient discontinuation from the study. There were three events that met the definition of a primary safety endpoint adverse event, including moderate throbbing pain at the needle site, moderate right foot pain, and stomach discomfort. All events resolved spontaneously and did not preclude further treatment. Although the defined criteria for a successful outcome in this trial can be debated, there certainly appeared to be some defined improvement in patient symptoms and in quality of life indicators with minimal patient risk.

Another study reported by Amarenco [8] utilized acute posterior tibial nerve stimulation with surface electrodes to study changes in urodynamic parameters in patients with detrusor overactivity including neurogenic detrusor overactivity. Mean first involuntary detrusor contraction volume increased from 163±96 ml to 232±115 ml during posterior tibial nerve stimulation, while

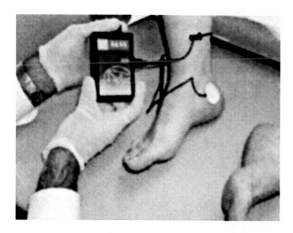

FIG. 18.1. Needle placement for tibial nerve stimulation (SNS) (picture courtesy of Drs. P. Rosenblatt and N. Kohli)

maximum cystometric capacity increased from 221±130 to 277±118 ml. Both results were statistically significant at <0.0001. Other more limited studies by Pannek [10] and Karademir [11] show similar results.

Conclusions

Tibial nerve stimulation may be considered an alternative for patients with urinary frequency–urgency or urge incontinence who have not responded to behavioral modification, biofeedback, and pelvic floor rehabilitation. Some may argue that this modality may be worth trying in patients with OAB even prior to considering anticholinergic medication, but larger-scale, longer-term trials are needed prior to making such a determination. However, it is clear that a significant number of patients with OAB symptoms either do not respond to or cannot tolerate the side effects of current anticholinergics, and it is not unreasonable to try these patients on peripheral neuromodulation such as tibial nerve stimulation. Unfortunately, there also are many limitations to such peripheral neuromodulation, including insurance coverage issues in the United States, and the requirement for the patient to make periodic visits for needle placement and stimulation as an implantable neuroprosthesis is not currently available. If such an implantable neurostimulator system becomes available and further long-term data can show lasting improvement in patient symptoms and quality of life indicators, peripheral neuromodulation may develop a much larger following as this approach offers patients and physicians alike a less invasive and less expensive treatment option compared to sacral neuromodulation.

References

1. Abrams P, Cardozo L, Fall M, et al. The standardisation of terminology of lower urinary tract function: report from the Standardisation Sub-committee of the International Continence Society. Neurourol Urodyn 2002;21:167–178.
2. Caldwell KP. The electrical control of sphincter incompetence. Lancet 1963;2:174–175.
3. McGuire EJ, Zhang SC, Horwinski ER, Lytton B. Treatment of motor and sensory detrusor instability by electrical stimulation. J Urol 1983;129(1):78–79.
4. Leng WW, Chancellor MB. How sacral nerve stimulation neuromodulation works. Urol Clin North Am 2005;32(1):11–18.
5. Yoshimura N, Seki S, Chancellor MB, et al. Targeting afferent hyperexcitability for therapy of the painful bladder syndrome. Urology 2002;59(5 Suppl 1):61–67.
6. Fowler CJ. The perspective of a neurologist on treatment-related research in fecal and urinary incontinence. Gastroenterology 2004;126(1 Suppl 1): S172–S174.
7. Fowler CJ, Swinn MJ, Goodwin RJ, et al. Studies of the latency of pelvic floor contraction during peripheral nerve evaluation show that the muscle response is reflexly mediated. J Urol 2000;163(3):881–883.
8. Govier FE, Litwiller S, Nitti V, et al. Percutaneous afferent neuromodulation for the refractory overactive bladder: Results of a multicenter study. J Urol 2001;165(4):1193–1198.
9. Amarenco G, Ismael SS, Even-Schneider A, et al. Urodynamic effect of acute transcutaneous posterior tibial nerve stimulation in overactive bladder. J Urol 2003;169(6):2210–2215.
10. Pannek J, Nehiba M. [Initial results of Stoller peripheral neuromodulation in disorders of bladder function]. Urologe A 2003;42(11):1470–1476.
11. Karademir K, Baykal K, Sen B, et al. A peripheric neuromodulation technique for curing detrusor overactivity: Stoller afferent neurostimulation. Scand J Urol Nephrol 2005;39(3):230–233.

Chapter 19
Surgery for Urge Urinary Incontinence: Cystoplasty, Diversion

Petros Sountoulides and M. Pilar Laguna

Introduction and Indications for the Surgical Treatment of Urge Incontinence

Detrusor Overactivity

Detrusor overactivity (DO) is characterized by involuntary detrusor contractions during the filling phase and is associated with urgency or urge incontinence. Urge urinary incontinence (UUI) is the complaint of involuntary leakage accompanied by or immediately preceded by urgency [1]. Patients with severe DO are distressed by urinary incontinence and often are desperate for treatment. The vast majority of patients suffering from overactive bladder and UUI can be treated successfully using a combination of pharmacological therapy, behavioral management, and lifestyle adjustments. During the last decades the evolution in understanding the pathophysiology of the irritative-storage symptoms, along with the widespread adoption of urodynamics, have centered treatment on drugs that modulate the cholinergic control of detrusor contractions during the storage phase. This has resulted in competitive nonselective muscarinic antagonists having dominated the field of overactive bladder (OAB) treatment during the last few years.

Bladder training, pharmacotherapy, transcutaneous electrical nerve stimulation, or S3-neuromodulation and lately botulinum toxin type-A injections are considered to be the major contemporary treatment alternatives for OAB-related incontinence. Consequently, the treatment of the OAB-related urge incontinence has to follow a stepwise fashion, starting with the minimal invasive and least harmful therapy and escalating to major surgery.

Surgical treatment for intractable nonneuropathic OAB incontinence therefore is reserved for those who have failed an adequate trial of these measures. However, resolution to surgery which may involve transposition of intestinal segments into the urinary tract (eg, augmentation enterocystoplasty) should be the outcome of adequate counseling and complete and thorough urological–urodynamic evaluation, given the associated risks and complications of these largely invasive surgical procedures.

Neurogenic Bladder Dysfunction

Neurogenic bladder dysfuntion (NBD) usually is the result of congenital or acquired disorders including myelodysplasia, multiple sclerosis, detrusor hyperreflexia, spinal cord injury, sacral agenesis, cerebral palsy, and previous pelvic operations such as hysterectomy. In the context of NBD the clinical picture is complicated further by additional problems related to bladder overactivity, including detrusor contraction and varying degrees of bladder outflow obstruction [2].

NBD can present clinically in a number of ways including frequency, urgency, urinary incontinence, intermittency, urinary retention, or urinary tract infections. Before the era of clean intermittent self-catheterization (CISC) [3], many patients with NBD had their urine diverted by means of an ileal conduit when conservative measures failed.

Now, NBD is a major indication for augmentation cystoplasty or urinary diversion in women [4, 5]. The main indications for such surgery in this group of patients include intractable incontinence, deteriorating renal function, and high-pressure bladders [6].

Surgical Techniques for the Management of Urge Incontinence

In recent years the mainstay of contemporary therapy for urge incontinence has been augmentation cystoplasty, most usually using the "clam" technique [2]. Surgical options that have been added to the options for the management of urge incontinence in recent years include bladder auto-augmentation, sacral neuromodulation, and lately bladder augmentation using tissue engineering.

It is the purpose of this chapter to focus mainly on the role of augmentation cystoplasty, autoaugmentation, and urinary diversion for the contemporary management of urge incontinence associated with DO and NBD. However, the current position of open or transurethral bladder denervation techniques also will be briefly discussed (Table 19.1).

Denervation Techniques

Escalating from the least invasive techniques to major procedures for the treatment of urge incontinence one has to comment on the various denervation techniques that have been described. The aim of denervation is to interrupt the micturition reflex and therefore reduce involuntary detrusor contractions.

Both open and endoscopic denervation techniques have been used for the treatment of OAB and neurogenic detrusor overactivity over the years. Transvaginal or transurethral ablation of the afferent postganglionic nerve fibers by the use of injectable phenol or ethanol were plagued, however, by serious complications, such as vesicovaginal fistulas and detrusor acontractility [7, 8].

Subtrigonal injection of a neurolytic chemical agent, phenol, in an aqueous solution of 5–6%, has been described for denervation. Initial short-term results were encouraging, reporting response rates between 58 and 83% [9, 10], but were not reproduced by subsequent studies with longer follow-up. In fact, the procedure led to disappointing results with sustained benefit in the long-term, progressively declining from 16% (at 6 months) to 0% (after 4 years) [11–13].

The technique has significant complications, including bladder ulcers, abscesses, fistula formation, urinary retention, and significant hematuria. The routine use of transvesical phenol injection no longer can be supported because of its high complication rate together with the fact that it produces unreliable and short-lived results.

Ingelman–Sundberg Bladder Denervation Procedure

The Ingelman–Sundberg procedure for the treatment of urge incontinence associated with detrusor overactivity originally was introduced by the surgeon with the same name in 1959 [14]. It is an open denervation procedure, which aims at disrupting the innervation from the inferior hypogastric plexus to the bladder. This is accomplished by extensive dissection near the cervix via a transvaginal

TABLE 19.1. Results of the most frequent surgical techniques for management of urge incontinence.

Technique	Results	Remarks
Ingelman-Sundberg denervation	54–64% cure urge incontinence 14% partial response	Follow-up 1 year to mean of 44 months
Clam enterocystoplasty	Continence in NBD 72–90% Continence in DO 70–90%	Results are less satisfactory in women
Bladder autoaugmentation	80% Continence improvement in children	No/or up to 40% increase in bladder capacity
	63% Continence improvement in adults	23–45% of children require enterocystoplasty Few studies in adults

approach and division of the preganglionic pelvic nerves in this region.

Patient Selection and Evaluation

Female patients with urge incontinence who had failed conservative therapy were candidates for the Ingelman–Sundberg procedure and initially were subjected to subtrigonal infiltration with a local anesthetic in order to predict the outcome of the open denervation procedure.

The anesthetic block was given with the patient on a cystoscopy table, and 10 ml of 0.25% bupivacaine were injected using a 22-gauge spinal needle in different areas of the region of the trigone via a transvaginal approach. Then the patient's response during the action of bupivacaine (6–24 h) was evaluated. Patients who reported significant benefit from the injection of the local anesthetic, interpreted as marked decrease or complete resolution of urge incontinence episodes, were offered a transvaginal open bladder denervation [15].

Technique and Complications

An inverted-U vaginal incision is made in the anterior vaginal wall over the bladder trigone, while the patient is in the dorsal lithotomy position under regional or general anesthesia. A foley catheter of 14–16 Ch can be placed in order to facilitate identification of the trigone and retraction of the bladder. The vaginal epithelium and perivesical fascia are dissected off the trigone, while the plane of dissection is kept within the serosal layer of the bladder. Sharp and blunt dissection are limited to the lateral and posterior borders of the bladder in order to obtain access to the terminal branches of the pelvic nerve and divide them. After the pelvic nerve plexuses have been dissected, the vaginal mucosa is reapproximated with a running 2–0 chromic and a povidone iodine-soaked vaginal pack is placed.

The entire procedure does not take more than 15 min and blood loss is minimal. The urethral catheter and vaginal pack are removed the next morning and the patient is discharged after confirming that she is voiding freely. Complications include transient retention or voiding dysfunction, while theoretically there is a risk of inadvertent injury to the bladder or ureter in case the dissection extends beyond the serosal layer of the bladder. However, in experienced hands there were no complications whatsoever related to this procedure [15].

Results

Initial results from case series were encouraging, with the majority of patients with detrusor overactivity incontinence either cured or improved [16]. A modification of this technique with limited vaginal dissection yielded a 64% cure rate of urge incontinence at a mean follow-up of more than 1 year and reduced morbidity [17](level 4 evidence).

Longer-term results (mean 44 months) of the modified Ingelman–Sundberg technique in a series of 28 patients revealed a 54% success rate with cessation of all urge incontinence episodes, while another 14% showed partial response, demonstrating at least 50% decrease in urgency and urge incontinence episodes [18]. However, the lack of randomized controlled trials or even comparative studies regarding the efficacy and durability of the original or modified Ingelman–Sundberg procedures limits the ability to draw more substantiated conclusions.

Enlargement (Augmentation) Cystoplasty

Augmentation cystoplasty is a procedure during which the bladder is enlarged (augmented) by incorporating a selected gastrointestinal segment as a patch into the native bladder. Augmentation cystoplasty in the canine model was first described in 1888 [19]. Enterocystoplasty was first performed in humans by von Mikulicz in 1899 [20], and later popularized by Couvelaire [21] for the treatment of the small contracted tuberculous bladder. Bladder-augmenting, pressure-reducing sphincter cystoplasty procedures were introduced later for the treatment of refractory detrusor overactivity-related incontinence [22, 23] as well as for patients with NBD usually caused by spinal cord injury, multiple sclerosis, and myelodysplasia [24, 25].

The therapeutic goal for the patients with urge incontinence is to provide adequate urinary storage by creating a low-pressure reservoir with convenient, voluntary, and complete emptying while preserving renal function and continence [26]. The principle underlying any form of augmentation cystoplasty is that by dividing a functionally overactive bladder and interpositioning an intestinal segment it is possible to create a bladder with an increased functional capacity and a lower end filling pressure.

Among the factors that enhanced the adoption of bladder augmentation techniques for the treatment of urge incontinence, the introduction of clean intermittent catheterization as a safe and effective method of emptying the bladder was marginal [3]. Additionally, the consequent wide adoption of urodynamics proved beyond any doubt that in the patient with NBD, a high-pressure lower urinary tract potentially can cause upper tract dilatation, renal dysfunction, and insufficiency [27].

Surgical Options: Which Bowel Segment to Use?

Theoretically every portion of the gastrointestinal tract, as well as the ureter, has been used for bladder augmentation [28]. The choice of intestinal segment is a matter of preference of the surgeon, as it does not appear to be an important factor for predicting success or complications, with the exception of jejunum, which quickly fell into disrepute because of particular problems with water reabsorption [29]. However, no single segment has been proved ideal for bladder augmentation, as each is associated with unique properties and possible complications [30].

The *cecum* can be used as a detubularized patch in conjunction with the terminal ileum as an ileocecoplasty, and it has advantages in cases where cystoplasty is part of undiversion [31]. However, the use of cecum for augmentation cystoplasty is avoided because of the high incidence of diarrhea and malabsorption associated with resection of the ileocecal valve, and the fact that cecocystoplasties produce 50% more mucus than ileocystoplasties [26, 32].

The *sigmoid* is the usual alternative to ileum for a simple augmentation. The sigmoid has the advantages of a thick muscular wall, large lumen size, and abundant mesentery, ensuring adequate neobladder capacity [33, 34]. Furthermore, sigmoid cystoplasty appears to have significantly less postoperative bowel dysfunction than ileocystoplasty [35]. The disadvantages of sigmoid cystoplasty are the higher risk of UTI (secondary to colonic bacteria) and a theoretically higher long-term risk of malignancy [26]. Therefore and

for these reasons its use is not encouraged and is restricted in cases where the ileum has a very short mesentery or is unavailable. The *stomach* occasionally has been used for bladder augmentation as an alternative to enterocystoplasty in situations where bowel was unavailable or unsuitable. Stomach theoretically could be an ideal material for bladder augmentation because it is easy to mobilize, is well-vascularized, and produces less mucus than bowel. Furthermore, it secretes hydrochloric acid which has a bactericidal action (asymptomatic bacteriuria is seen in only 20–30% of patients) [36, 37]. However, contemporary indications of gastrocystoplasty are limited to the occasional patient who is predisposed to stone formation or has a history of pelvic irradiation. Complications specific to gastrocystoplasty include mainly the "hematuria–dysuria" syndrome due to gastric acid secretions. This syndrome consists of bladder/urethral pain, hematuria in the absence of infection, and skin excoriation, which represents a serious complication seen in up to 36% of patients after gastric augmentation [30]. Other complications include peptic ulceration of the bladder, perforation of the gastric segment due to peptic ulcer, and hypergastrinemia with consequent metabolic alkalosis [38–41].

Complications associated with partial gastrectomy include "dumping" syndrome and exacerbation of pre-existing peptic ulcer disease or gastroesophageal reflux, while there also is the risk of malignancy in the gastric patch. The combination of these problems, but particularly the hematuria–dysuria syndrome, have reduced the use of stomach for augmentation, except as a last resort when no other alternatives are available [26].

Ileum has been used to form a bladder cup [42] or to create a simple form of cystoplasty when used as a detubularized segment [23]. Although bowel contractions cannot be completely abolished, detubularization of the ileum is important to prevent peristaltic waves [43]. Moreover, detubularized ileum is preferable to sigmoid colon because its tissue properties demonstrate better compliance and ensure the creation of a lower pressure reservoir [44].

Patient Selection and Evaluation

A complete evaluation of both upper and lower urinary tracts with detailed estimation of bladder and sphincter function is fundamental to the success of any bladder augmentation procedure. Renal ultrasonography and radionuclide scan together with serum creatinine measurement will suffice for evaluating renal function, while the lower urinary tract is evaluated with filling and voiding videourodynamics and cystourethroscopy. Additional studies such as electromyography may be required for the evaluation of patients with specific neurological lesions.

In urge incontinence associated with NBD, sphincteric function should be assessed in order to exclude the presence of a dyssynergic sphincter, which could be managed by simultaneous sphincterotomy. Patients with an underactive sphincter and a normal urethra may be managed synchronously with augmentation cystoplasty and an artificial urinary sphincter (AUS) or periurethral bulking agent (Teflon, collagen, autologous fat) or colposuspension in females [43]. The AUS can be inserted during the same session with augmentation cystoplasty in neuropathic patients [26] with no increased risk of infection [45, 46], while implantation of just the cuff of the AUS initially may prove adequate in achieving continence [47].

In the few patients who will fail to achieve a critical balance between voiding efficacy and continence, resorting to clean intermittent self-catheterization (CISC) may be necessary. It has been estimated that more than one third of patients with DO urge incontinence will need to perform CISC in the long-term after augmentation cystoplasty [48]. Therefore, the willingness and manual dexterity to perform CISC should be preoperatively assessed in all patients who are candidates for the procedure [15].

In the case of urge incontinence associated with NBD, preoperative evaluation of the upper urinary tracts is necessary in order to exclude the presence of hydronephrosis and the risk of renal insufficiency resulting from the transmission of high back pressures from a reduced compliance bladder toward the upper urinary tract. Therefore, the combination of enterocystoplasty with other reconstructive procedures not only safeguards continence but also can be effective in reducing the risk of reflux, associated infection, and upper tract pressure-related injury.

Contraindications

The presence of impaired renal function is a more controversial relative contraindication. In this case the re-absorption of urea and electrolytes from the bowel segment may lead to decompensation of renal function and renal insufficiency. Although there is evidence that augmentation in the presence of an already impaired creatinine clearance is associated with progressive decline in renal function, correction of the bladder abnormality in patients with even endstage renal failure has provided continence without adding a further negative effect in the rate of decline in renal function [26].

The issue of CISC already has been discussed; unwillingness or inability to perform CISC may render the option of augmentation cystoplasty inappropriate. An alternative option in these cases is the formation of a continent diversion with a catheterizable abdominal stoma using the Mitrofanoff technique or other variations, which could be managed even by patients with poor dexterity due to neurological impairment [48, 49].

Some indications for creating an abdominal stoma include women with spasticity of the lower extremities because of neurological conditions, patients whose native urethra is obstructed or damaged, and those with refractory sphincteric incontinence or fistulas. Although a continent catheterizable stoma may prove to be effective, stomal complications are seen in almost half of the patients [50].

Moreover, continent diversion with the use of a Mitrofanoff stoma is associated with a higher incidence of mucus retention within the bladder, which probably accounts for the higher incidence of stone formation in these patients. This is the reason why some surgeons choose to place the Mitrofanoff stoma as low as possible on the abdominal wall, to aid the siphon effect during bladder catheterization [29].

Another contraindication, although not an absolute one, to bowel substitution cystoplasty is the presence of a severely irradiated bladder with the possibility of compromised sphincter function. The presence of intrinsic bowel disease, eg, Crohn's disease, may affect the choice of the substitution segment, while in cases of short gut syndrome or previous radiotherapy the additional removal of the bowel segment might prove disastrous [26]. Liver function tests and arterial blood gases also should be checked preoperatively to rule out hepatic failure, which could be aggravated by ammonia resorption through the bowel used in cystoplasty [43].

The extremely poor results that have been demonstrated in cases of severely diseased and fibrotic bladders due to interstitial cystitis have led authors to consider interstitial cystitis a contraindication for any form of enterocystoplasty [50].

The "Clam" Ileocystoplasty

Different procedures for ileocystoplasty have been described, including the bladder augmentation technique proposed by Leng et al. [51], where a detubularized U- or S- or W-shaped ileal flap is interpositioned into an anterior wall-based cystotomy. However, the most frequently performed variation of enterocystoplasty is the "clam shell" ileocystoplasty, originally introduced by Bramble in 1982 and later popularized by Mundy and Stephenson [22], will be discussed in more detail in this chapter [23].

The "clam" enterocystoplasty, which is a simple augmentation ileocystoplasty, actually was developed in order to overcome certain problems that were faced with previously used augmentation techniques. Previous experience with simple augmentation cystoplasties without bladder resection, like the Goodwin "cup-patch" procedure [42, 52], had shown that with these procedures the bladder was actually "augmented" into a low-pressure and a high-pressure compartment. This way, unstable detrusor contractions would lead to the evacuation of the high-pressure compartment to the low-pressure (patch) compartment, thus leading to the formation of a bladder diverticululum.

The rationale of the "clam" procedure is that bladder augmentation by ileum interposition is combined with deactivation of the detrusor by extensively "bivalving" it. In this way when the two parts of the reconstructed "clam bladder" contract synchronously, the risk of diverticulating the intervening U-shaped patch of ileum is minimized. Another plausible mechanism for improvement with the "clam" procedure involves mainly the reduction of intravesical pressure rather than the accomplished increase of bladder volume, since the incorporated bowel segment remains relaxed while the bladder contracts.

During clam ileocystoplasty the bladder is divided almost completely by a coronal or sagittal incision, which is carried down to the bladder base within 1.5 cm of the internal urethral meatus, just anterior to the ureteric orifice on each side. This way the bivalved bladder resembles an open scallop or clam, hence the term "clam shell" configuration [53].

Although there functionally is no difference whether the bisecting incision is sagittal or coronal, some authors have found the sagittal incision to be technically simpler [54]. A technical point of vital importance is that both ends of the incision are extended right down to the bladder base to ensure deactivation of the overactive detrusor.

An isolated, about 25-cm-long segment of ileum, located 25–40 cm from the ileocecal valve, is ideal for bladder augmentation as it produces the least metabolic consequences. The ileal segment then is incised along its antimesenteric border, detuburarized, and patched to the open bladder. The ileal patch can be sutured into the bladder defect with a single layer of continuous vicryl [53] or a single interrupted layer of 3–0 PGA suture. An important technical point in this step of the procedure is to take care not to obstruct the ureteric ostium by including it in the anastomotic suturing.

Adequate bladder drainage after augmentation cystoplasty is of utmost importance during the early postoperative phase. For this reason a 19F Jackson-Pratt fenestrated tube [55] or a 22F to 24F catheter must be placed as a suprapubic catheter [15] along with a large-bore urethral catheter to ensure optimum bladder drainage. Furthermore, the use of sling-suture-retained catheters is preferred over balloon-retained urethral catheter by some authors, since inadvertent traction upon a self-retained catheter may result in disastrous disruption of the anastomotic suture line between bowel and bladder.

Intraoperatively the anastomotic suture line can be tested by clamping the foley catheter while infusing saline into the suprapubic catheter. Postoperatively, continuous normal saline irrigation (2 liter/day) can be administered in order to prevent catheter blocking by mucus or blood clots. Continuous irrigation is usually stopped the following day and replaced by catheter flushing twice daily [55]. Patients usually are discharged home a week or more after the operation with both draining catheters in place. The suprapubic catheter usually is removed on the 12th day and the urethral catheter is removed 2 weeks postoperatively (Fig. 19.1).

Modifications of the "clam" ileocystoplasty have been described, like the star incision of the bladder as

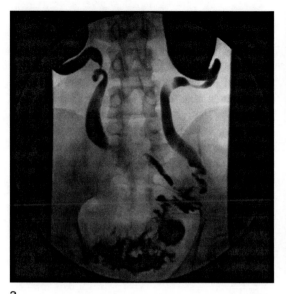
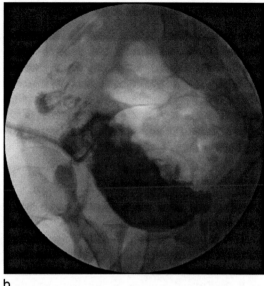

a   b

Fig. 19.1. Pretransplantation clam enterocistoplasty with ileum in a young man with terminal kidney insufficiency because of a NBD (spina bifida), with ureteral obstruction at the bladder level and low-capacity, low-compliance bladder unsuitable for ureter reimplantation. (a) Cystography in the perioperative period. (b) Anterograde study via nephrostomy drains showing the large dilated kidney pelvis, the tortuous and dilated ureter, and the passage of the contrast to the isoperistaltic ileal loop (ileal chimney)

a modification of sagittal cystotomy. This variation has been described in pediatric patients with NBD with small, thick-walled bladders with diminished capacities and poor compliance [56]. However, it never proved to be superior to conventional clam shell cystoplasty in terms of efficacy, and furthermore thoughts were raised that additional cystotomies might compromise blood supply in these patients. Another alternative is the "McGuire" modification of the hemi-Kock procedure of a transverse "smile" incision, which is fashioned 3 cm above the ureteral orifices, creating an anteriorly based detrusor flap [57].

Follow-Up After Augmentation Cystoplasty

Lifelong follow-up of patients after augmentation cystoplasty is crucial in achieving and maintaining satisfactory results, while guarding the patient from the long-term complications associated with these procedures. Adequate bladder emptying is monitored by residual urine measurement and ultrasonography of the upper tracts biannually for the first 2 years and then annually.

Uroflowmetry is not included in the routine follow-up of patients after augmentation cystoplasty. Alternatively, patients may undergo videourodynamics every 6 months after augmentation to document the presence of a good-capacity, low-pressure bladder that empties well with low residual volume. Urodynamic studies have shown that contractility and compliance after augmentation remains unchanged or even deteriorates in about half of patients with neuropathic dysfunction, possibly because intrinsic bowel dysfunction reduces bowel compliance in these patients [58].

Should voiding problems occur, a simple voiding cystourethrogram (VCUG) or even better, an ultrasound VCUG is the investigation of choice for the evaluation of insufficient voiding. This examination can reliably locate the site of a possible outlet obstruction (bladder neck, urethra) and provide information for appropriate management.

While isotope renography is indicated in cases of possible obstruction of the upper tracts, annual isotopic measurement of the GFR is suggested by some authors [26]. Annual flexible cystoscopy is commenced 5–10 years after augmentation.

Complications and Their Management

Early complications include those cardiovascular, thromboembolic, respiratory, and gastrointestinal complications associated with any major abdominal surgery. Augmentation cystoplasty is reported to have 0–2.7% mortality, with higher mortality rates and higher complication rates reported in the earlier series where augmentation was part of urinary undiversion [31, 59] (Table 19.2).

Bowel-Related Complications

Complications after augmentation enterocystoplasty can be significant, mounting up to a rate of 20–22% in some series [57, 60]. Complications associated with bowel are distinguished from those that are inherent to any gastrointestinal surgery and result from the disruption of the gastrointestinal tract and those that arise from the resultant chronic contact of a bowel segment with urine. Early bowel-related complications include small bowel leak, ileus, or bowel–bladder anastomotic leak and fistula formation. Late gastrointestinal complications include adhesion formation, chronic bowel obstruction, or alterations in bowel habits [55].

Any technique of augmentation cystoplasty requires access to the peritoneal cavity, and this carries a considerable risk of postoperative intestinal obstruction from adhesions. Although the exact incidence of this complication is not known, it was estimated to occur in about 10% of pediatric patients undergoing ileocystoplasty [61].

The onset of irregularity in bowel habits, particularly frequency and diarrhea, is one debilitating long-term complication, with significant effect on the patient's quality of life [62]. Up to 25–30% of patients experience long-term problems of increased bowel frequency and troublesome diarrhea, while a quarter of patients with NBD have increased fecal incontinence after enterocystoplasty [35, 63]. The pathogenesis of postaugmentation diarrhea is not clear. A reduction in small bowel absorption may account partly for the increased frequency and diarrhea, although patients with an ileocystoplasty rarely have >30 cm of ileum resected [26]. On the other hand, there is a clear association of detrusor instability with irritable bowel syndrome in up to 30% of patients [64], implying that there might be a common intrinsic disorder of smooth muscle and nerve supply accounting for both the bladder and bowel problems.

Metabolic Disturbance

The incorporation of a bowel segment into the bladder leads to the exposure of the absorptive surface of the small intestine to urine metabolites. This results to a certain degree in reabsorption of water, sodium, hydrogen ions, ammonium, and chloride and increased loss of potassium and bicarbonate into the urine [65, 66].

This chronic effect may lead to the disturbance of the acid–base balance and the development of hyperchloremic metabolic acidosis in ileo- and colocystoplasty. However, this complication is almost always mild or even subclinical and only in rare symptomatic cases requires oral bicarbonate therapy [29, 67]. Chronic metabolic acidosis causes mobilization of calcium carbonate from

TABLE 19.2. Complications of augmentation cystoplasty.

	Early	Late
Bowel related	Intestinal leak	Intestinal adhesions
	Ileus	Intestinal obstruction
	Bowel-bladder leak	Alteration bowel habits
	Fistula	Possible vitamin B12 deficiency
Bowel/urine contact related	–	Hyperchloremic acidosis
		Growth reduction (children)
		Mucus formation
		Malignant transformation
		Bladder perforation
		Bladder stone formation
		Voiding dysfunction
Intrinsic to bladder disorder	UTI	UTI
	Bacteriuria	Bacteriuria

bone and may lead to orthopedic problems or growth reduction in the pediatric population [68]. However, ileum, unlike colon, can reabsorb urinary calcium and may be less prone to this problem.

Vitamin B12 deficiency may occur in case large segments of terminal ileum are used, and long-term follow-up for hematological sequela of this event is mandatory [69].

Mucus Formation

Mucus buildup in the augmented bladder after enterocystoplasty is a problem that also arises from the interposition of small bowel into the bladder and has been reported by as many as 81% of patients [55]. The average daily mucus production from both ileum and colon when used as a cystoplasty segment is 35–40 g, and this amount does not reduce substantially over time, despite a time-related villous atrophy of the intestinal patch mucosa [26].

Mucus has been implicated in stone formation since it binds calcium from the urine and is thought to act as nidus for calculi formation in the augmented bladder [70], although there is little actual evidence of this [71]. On the contrary, mucus may have a protective role to the bowel epithelium, from contact with urinary carcinogens and other substances.

Preventive measures include proper patient instruction to perform weekly or even daily bladder wash out [15, 72]. Oral ranitidine can reduce the amount of mucus produced [73], while instillation of water-soluble N-acetylcysteine into the bladder also has been suggested for dissolving mucus [74].

Urinary Tract Infections

The problem of recurrent urinary tract infections (UTIs) after augmentation cystoplasty has a critical impact on the patient's perceived view of the outcome after the procedure, owing to the added morbidity of recurrent infection and long-term antibiotic treatment. Patients with NBD urge incontinence and high-pressure urine storage or with significant residual urine volumes already have a high incidence of severe symptomatic UTI before surgical treatment with bladder augmentation [75]. In cases of NBD requiring CISC to empty the bladder, nearly half of the patients already suffer from chronic or recurrent UTIs [76], while in most cases the problem does not seem to respond to antibiotic prophylaxis [77].

Although recurrent bacteriuria can be found in more than 75% of patients after augmentation cystoplasty [26], the incidence of symptomatic UTI is lower [62, 78]. Bacteriological data from patients who underwent the clam cystoplasty revealed that 84% of patients on CISC had positive cultures, while bacteriuria was present even in 60% of patients who voided spontaneously [79]. Predisposing factors to the development of UTIs apart from the high bacterial content of bowel include large residual volumes, the presence of mucus, and the need for CISC. In the follow-up of a group of 48 patients (35 with DO) who underwent clam enterocystoplasty, 37% suffered from recurrent UTIs requiring frequent antibiotic treatment more than 1 year after surgery [55].

Therefore, a rigorous strategy of early detection and elimination of infection is of great importance in the follow-up of these patients. However, after enterocystoplasty, despite the continued need for CISC, there are fewer episodes of symptomatic UTI, especially in the patients with NBD, probably owing to the beneficial effect of lowering the intravesical pressure. Therefore, the incidence of significant infective complications after cystoplasty seems to mirror that seen in patients with an ileal conduit or indwelling urinary catheters [29].

Malignant Transformation

The first reports of malignancies occurring in enterocystoplasties came in the early 1970s [80, 81]. Several reports on the occurrence of tumors after bladder augmentation procedures followed [82–85]. Ileocystoplasty carries a low, although significant risk of malignancy [86] while cancers arising within augmented bladders are aggressive and associated with significant mortality [87].In particular, tumors arising after ileocystoplasty usually are located at the enterovesical anastomosis or on the intestinal side of the bladder augmentation [88]. Since the intact ileum rarely undergoes malignant transformation, it was considered possible that urine stasis due to the longer period of urine storage within the augmented bladders together with the large area of juxtaposition between transitional bladder and enteric epithelium may permit formation of carcinogens and malignant transformation of epithelial cells [87].

The etiology of malignant transformation in augmented bladders is probably multifactorial. The fact that most cases occur in adults with other potential risk factors makes it difficult to determine the exact independent risk associated with bladder augmentation.

On the other hand, the most common contemporary indication for augmentation cystoplasty is in children and adolescents with a NBD, the majority of whom have no risk factors for bladder cancer [89]. It seems reasonable to believe therefore that bladder augmentation may be an independent risk factor for the development of malignancy.

The majority of tumors have been adenocarcinoma of the bowel or bladder [87] or squamous cell carcinomas, although cases of transitional cell carcinoma (TCC) also have been reported. Soergel et al. found TCC to develop in 1.2% of cases after bladder augmentation within a mean time of 19 years [89].

One of the etiological factors for malignant transformation was postulated to be the elevated levels of urinary nitrosamines [90]. The basic idea is that nitrates, which are normally excreted in the urine, are degraded to nitrites by colonic bacteria. Nitrites then react with urinary secondary amines to form N-nitrosamines. These compounds have the capability of carcinogenic activity, and therefore may act as tumor initiators [87]. Urinary tract infection and chronic inflammation of the urothelium are known to be associated with an increased risk of bladder tumor formation [82, 87], while the presence of high levels of N-nitrosamines correlates strongly with heavy bacterial growth on urine culture in ileal cystoplasties [91]. On the other hand, inflammatory bladder diseases not associated with bacterial infection such as tuberculosis appeared to be associated with a significant risk of late bladder tumor formation. There were cases of primarily adenocarcinomas that originated near the anastomosis after augmentation enterocystoplasties, most of which were performed on small contracted bladders due to genitourinary tuberculosis [88, 92–95].

The etiology of these augmentation tumors probably is related to chronic inflammation, wound healing, and malignancy. A possible explanation why these tumors usually arise near the anastomotic area is that the products of inflammation and healing may act as tumor promoters [96]. Tumor development can be initiated with the aid of certain growth factors such as the basic fibroblast growth factor, which is thought to originate from the bowel mucosa and has been shown to be elevated in the urine of patients with enterocystoplasty [97]. Although the exact role of elevated levels of urinary basic fibroblast growth factor in the malignant potential of clam enterocystoplasty is still uncertain, there is clear evidence that no relationship exists between bacteriuria and basic fibroblast growth factor levels in these patients [97].

Surveillance and Follow-Up Tactics

There is an issue as to what should be the appropriate surveillance for malignancy formation for patients after bladder augmentation. Also, the time between cystoplasty and the occurrence of tumor is highly variable [98–100]; therefore, lifelong surveillance is mandatory.

Initial recommendations focused on elimination of urinary infection and suggested annual cystoscopic surveillance [53]. However, it seems unlikely that every patient with an enterocystoplasty is at high risk of developing a life-threatening tumor, and malignancy in augmented bladders is still considered to be a rare event [89, 92]. Moreover, as the clam tumors described in the literature have presented within a latency period of 5–29 years (mean 18 years) [87], some authors suggest that lifelong cystoscopic follow-up should start no earlier than 3 years [48] or even 10 years after initial surgery [26, 89]. However, the fact that the most of these tumors present incidentally and only a few are detected by screening emphasizes the need to develop methods of early identification of the patients at risk of tumor formation [101].

In this direction, the presence of genetic instability at the enterovesical anastomosis in patients who had undergone a clam ileocystoplasty was tested using fluorescent in situ hybridization (FISH). The results of this study indicated that morphologically normal tissue obtained from the enterovesical anastomosis displays evidence of chromosomal instability that may predispose to tumor formation [101].

However, polysomy, which is known to be an unfavorable prognostic marker and is associated with rapid progression of a cancer [102–104], was not identified in any of the biopsies taken from the enterovesical anastomosis. Further studies are required to establish the clinical significance of the FISH test in predicting the occurrence of tumor after enterocystoplasty [101]. Although there are suggestions that urine cytology should be routinely assessed in the follow-up of patients [43], the presence of chronic bacterial infection and the resultant infective changes in the bladder mucosa render urine cytology unreliable for the diagnosis of malignancy in augmented bladders [95].

Perforation

Spontaneous perforation of the augmented bladder may occur in 5–10% of patients [105], and is associated with significant (>25%) mortality [106, 107]. Perforation is more common in patients with NBD [48, 108], in patients with recurrent UTI or AUS implantation, and in those using CISC due to infrequent or traumatizing bladder catheterization [14, 105, 107–112]. The perforation site is thought to be located at the anastomotic suture line between the bowel and the native bladder [26]; however, this is not always the case [107, 110, 111, 113].

Bladder overdistension due to clot retention or obstruction from mucus and the resultant high intravesical pressures can cause transient localized microvascular occlusion and local ischemia [111, 112, 114]. This may lead to the creation of an ischemic scar tissue, which can easily rupture after an abrupt increase in pressure [115].

However, other experimental studies support that it is the increased capacity of the enterocystoplasty bladder and increased wall tension, which diminish wall thickness, that lead to perforation [116]. Another possible reason is that repeated bladder infections may lead to chronic inflammatory changes, weakening of the bladder walls, and perforation [108].

Bladder perforation is a feared complication because in cases of delayed diagnosis peritonitis may result in severe shock, rapid deterioration, and death [105]. Abdominal pain is usually the first symptom and is accompanied by fever. However, the presentation is variable with shoulder pain due irritation of the diaphragm from intraperitoneal urine being the presenting symptom [106]. Diagnostic delay is more of a problem in neurologically impaired patients, who due to altered sensation may develop peritonitis and intra-abdominal abscesses without the signs and symptoms of acute abdomen [108,

117].In cases of intra-abdominal perforation of an augmented bladder, signs and symptoms of acute abdomen prevail, necessitating abdominal exploration, regardless of the results of imaging studies [113]. Ultrasound and CT usually reveal urinary extravasation either into the local pelvic tissues or the peritoneal cavity [118]. Routine cystography may give false-negative results in cases of suspected augmented bladder perforation and should not be relied on for the establishment of diagnosis of perforation [112], although others think that a careful cystogram under fluoroscopic control and multiple films of the filled and drained bladder may prove helpful [119].Once major extravasation has not been detected on cystography or ultrasound and there is no evidence of acute abdomen, conservative management with catheter drainage and antibiotics can lead to successful resolution in more than half the cases [29, 115]. Although in patients on CISC whose urine are a priori infected, conservative management may prove inadequate [26].

Stone Formation

Lower urinary tract stones are common after augmentation cystoplasty and seem to occur with increasing frequency as the follow-up lengthens. The incidence of stones forming in enterocystoplasties is reported to range from 13 to 30% in contemporary series [26, 71, 78, 120].

Stones can cause bladder irritation and patients may present with incontinence, hematuria, or urinary tract infection, although they are usually found on routine follow-up ultrasound of patients who have had an augmentation cystoplasty [29]. It already has been noted that patients with an augmented bladder that is emptied through the urethra by "natural" voiding seldom (~2%) form a stone [26]. On the contrary, stones occur five times more often in patients with augmented bladders who were on CISC via the urethra and ten times as common in patients with Mitrofanoff abdominal stomas, implicating stasis to be an important factor in stone formation [121].

Risk factors for stone formation include urine stasis, immobilization, the presence of intravesical foreign bodies such as staples or mesh, or the choice of the intestinal segment used for reconstruction. It is known that gastrocystoplasties are rarely complicated by stones [122].

The proposed enhancing role of mucus in stone formation in reconstructed bladders [120] is not actually evidence-based. Although washouts of mucus are widely recommended for the prevention of stones, it may be that the only advantage is to clear fragments of "sand" before a stone can be formed [71].

In patients with an enterocystoplasty the risk of forming stones, especially triple phosphate stones, is mainly attributed to the high incidence of recurrent urinary tract infections usually from urea-splitting bacteria [120]. Moreover, metabolic changes induced may accentuate the risk of forming oxalic or phosphate calcium stones. These include moderate to severe hypocitraturia [123], hypercalciuria and mild hyperoxaluria, hyperuricosuria, and a low urinary magnesium excretion [71].

Regarding treatment, some form of endoscopic or open surgical procedure is necessary since stones in intestinal reservoirs are not amenable to medical treatment, may act as a nidus for infection, and have a tendency to enlarge if left in situ. Any intervention contemplated must be tailored to the size of the stone and the type of bladder augmentation performed; however, patients with large or multiple stones and those with no urethral access require open surgery for removal [121].

Voiding Dysfunction

One of the major problems of patients undergoing enterocystoplasty is the high incidence of postoperative voiding dysfunction. A priori clam cystoplasty in particular, by dissecting the detrusor causes some degree of outflow obstruction. In the majority of cases, however, the urethra sphincter mechanism fails to adjust to the creation of a low-pressure bowel substitution cystoplasty, and patients are unable to void sufficiently. As a result most patients have to strain to empty their bladder, while succeeding in effectively voiding by abdominal straining make take up to 2–3 months for some patients [53].

In a cohort of patients it was estimated that in around 20% [53] voiding will be sufficient only after a rebalancing procedure is undertaken in order to reduce the urethra closure pressure while taking care not to create urethral incompetence. Rebalancing is usually accomplished by either a bladder neck incision for male patients, or an Ottis

sphincterotomy or a combination of the two. Some authors used to perform a bladder neck incision routinely in all patients who had bladder augmentation [22], sparing only young men who wish to preserve ejaculation.

In cases where these rebalancing procedures are not undertaken in due time or in case these procedures fail to achieve effective voiding, then the patients will have to resort to self-catheterization. CISC may be required for as short as a few weeks after the operation during the "balancing" stage. However, in general, insufficient voiding and the need for CISC increase with time [58, 124].

Several other factors may contribute to insufficient voiding and the need for CISC after a bladder augmentation procedure, including previous operations or the presence of underactive detrusor in spinal cord injury patients [25]. Moreover, the significant decrease in voiding pressures recorded in urodynamic evaluations of patients after enterocystoplasty, together with an increase in total bladder capacity, are factors further contributing to the establishment of voiding dysfunction and obviating the need for CISC [55, 124, 125].

It is only logical that patients with NBD have a higher chance of requiring CISC after bladder augmentation, most probably because the underlying neurogenic pathology generally interferes with adequate sphincter and pelvic floor muscle relaxation. In studies of long-term outcome results after enterocystoplasty for urge incontinence, routine CISC was necessary for 60–75% of neuropathic patients [26, 55].

The need for CISC after augmentation for DO-related urge incontinence is variable, depending to some degree on the patient's tolerance of residual urine. In arecent series, CISC was postoperatively necessary for 6–39% of patients [26, 124].

Technically, a bladder augmentation procedure that requires CISC is considered a simple urethra-cystoplasty and not a sphincter-cystoplasty and some patients may actually be quite pleased with the result [53].

Results of Enterocystoplasty

The majority of publications regarding the results of enterocystoplasty for the treatment of adults with nonneurogenic urge incontinence are either small case series or observational studies with short- or longer-term follow-up (level 4 evidence). There is a lack of randomized controlled trials comparing either clam cystoplasty or other bladder augmentation procedure for the treatment of nonneurogenic DO. Furthermore, it is difficult to draw general conclusions concerning the clinical outcome in patients withDO, mainly due to the heterogeneity of the populations treated with most series including varying numbers of NBD patients.

NBD Patients

Results for neuropathic bladder patients were promising, with patient's satisfaction and continence rates escalating from 72 [55, 126] to over 90% in recent series [26, 127]. Medium- to long-term follow-up showed a sustained improvement in continence exceeding 90% in neuropathic patients [55, 79].

DO Patients

In general, the outcome in patients with DO-related urge incontinence is highly unpredictable. Most series show a sustained improvement in continence exceeding 70 or even 90% in recent series [26, 54, 124, 128].

On the other hand, there had been results on female patients undergoing augmentation cystoplasty for nonneurogenic urge incontinence that were far from optimal. Merely half the patients (53%) were completely continent, while 39% were not pleased and another 18% were still suffering from incontinence postoperatively. An important reason for these results may be the fact that more than half of the patients suffered from associated interstitial cystitis [129].

However, detrusor instability after augmentation cystoplasty for urge incontinence seems to persist in 30% of cases postoperatively [54, 55, 125, 128]. The long-term efficacy of the operation in maintaining continence in patients with intractable DO was evaluated in studies with 38 months to 8 years follow-up (level 4), with results varying from moderate to satisfactory [55, 79, 130].

Results of Augmentation Cystoplasty in Women

There are a few studies evaluating the results of augmentation cystoplasty solely on female patient groups, which include patients who also have undergone some form of bladder neck procedure [129, 131]. In one study on women with NBD-related incontinence, a modified rectus fascial sling procedure was combined with augmentation ileocystoplasty, achieving a 95.2% success rate (patients dry under CIC) [131]. However, others have challenged the hypothesis that augmentation of the bladder alone is inadequate for achieving continence in women with NBD [132]. Ileocystoplasties were performed on 16 patients with myelodysplasia without any additional bladder neck procedures, with continence achieved in all but one [132].

In a study on women with nonneurogenic urge incontinence, augmentation ileocystoplasty was combined with a modified Burch urethrovesical suspension and yielded a 53% success rate (defined as complete continence) and a 25% rate of occasional leaks. However, 39% of patients required regular CIC postoperatively [129]. In conclusion, only one of two women undergoing augmentation enterocystoplasty seems to be satisfied with the procedure in the long-term.

Future Options

Nonpharmacological options for the future management of OAB include tissue engineering, which is seen as an emerging therapy. This is best illustrated by growing bladder tissue on scaffolds for use in augmentation cystoplasty. This greatly simplifies the procedure by eliminating the need for a bowel anastomosis [133].

Tissue engineering currently is being explored in order to provide an alternative to enterocystoplasty to avoid the use of bowel segments. These techniques have been using cultured native urothelial tissues [134], fetal tissues, as well as collagen matrices overgrown with transplanted cells. Early results in animals using the bladder acellular matrix graft with and without urothelial and smooth muscle cell seeding were promising [135, 136]. Recent results from patients who underwent autologous bladder transplantation with tissue engineering were successful in terms of bladder compliance, while none of the usual complications associated with enterocystoplasty were encountered [137]. Other alternatives being developed are small intestinal submucosa as a scaffold for normal urothelial and detrusor ingrowth and progressive percutaneous dilatation for bladder tissue expansion [138]; again, promising early results were reported in animal studies.

Laparoscopic augmentation cystoplasty recently has emerged as a possible alternative to its open counterpart. The first bladder augmentation accomplished entirely by laparoscopy was a gastrocystoplasty performed in a 17-year-old girl with a poorly compliant bladder [139] and a small series of laparoscopically assisted enterocystoplasties with exteriorization of the bowel to facilitate bowel-to-bowel reanastomosis and ileal patch construction followed [140, 141]. The first case of ileal cystoplasty performed completely by laparoscopy was described in a 31-year-old woman with NBD due to spinal cord injury [142]. Longer-term results on larger series are needed in order to evaluate the pros and cons of laparoscopy in bladder augmentation procedures.

Conclusions on Augmentation Cystoplasty

In patients with intractable urge incontinence with a severe negative impact on quality of life or in high-pressure neurogenic bladders with a high risk of damage to the upper urinary tract, augmentation cystoplasty offers a considerable chance of cure. However, it is a major abdominal intervention with significant and potentially severe complications and by no means is a "fit and forget" procedure. Rather, it requires lifetime commitment, careful patient selection, and even more careful selection of the appropriate procedure for the individual patient.

Despite the problems encountered with certain procedures of augmentation cystoplasty, on balance it has been a much better form of management of urge incontinence in patients with bladder neuropathy or high-pressure detrusor contractions than the alternative options of rectal diversion, indwelling catheter, or external urinary diversion [29]. Enterocystoplasty has successfully stood the test of time in restoring storage function by achieving a low-pressure bladder reservoir, despite the significant incidence of complications and reinterventions.

Although there is no single type of bladder augmentation appropriate for all cases, in carefully selected, adequately counseled, and highly motivated patients, the "clam" ileocystoplasty has been proved a valuable and effective treatment option for severe intractable urge incontinence associated with DO and NBD.

Bladder Autoaugmentation

The theoretically appealing idea of augmenting the bladder without the interpositioning of bowel segments has been attempted in a number of ways. Materials that have been used as grafts patched onto the bladder include both synthetic (Teflon, silicone) and natural tissues (omentum, peritoneum, dura) [143–146]. However, results from the use of these materials were disappointing due to the high incidence of adverse effects and complications encountered.

Detrusor Myectomy–Myotomy

The urothelium-lined augmentation of the bladder (autoaugmentation) by excision of the detrusor was described initially in experimental studies in dogs [147]. Its clinical application initially was introduced by Cartwright and Snow as an alternative to enterocystoplasty in seven children with poorly compliant bladders, four of whom were neurologically impaired [148].

The surgical goal can be accomplished by either incision (detrusor myotomy) or excision (detrusor myectomy) of part of the detrusor muscle over the dome of the bladder, leaving the underlying bladder urothelium intact [147]. No difference was noted between detrusor myectomy versus simple detrusor myotomy on urodynamic, radiological, and pathological analysis in animal models [149] and in a small series of 12 pediatric patients with NBD [150]. In another study of 30 patients with refractory DO, detrusor myectomy was successful in as many as 80% of patients after at least 2 years of follow-up; however, more than half of the patients required CIC [151].

Either way, by excision of the detrusor sparing the mucosa, a large epithelial bladder mucosal "bulge" or "artificial diverticulum" is created. This pseudodiverticulum is composed of bladder urothelium, collagen, and some scarce detrusor muscle bundles. The pseudodiverticulum expands during bladder filling, thereby increasing the storage capacity of the bladder, while decreasing storage pressures [2]. Excision of part of the detrusor potentially decreases the number and magnitude of uninhibited detrusor contractions [15, 30]. On the other hand, the emptying contraction of the remaining detrusor is reduced, rendering CISC inevitable, especially for patients with neuropathic bladder dysfunction.

Therefore, autoaugmentation of the bladder by detrusorectomy in theory resembles the patch graft techniques, with the difference being that instead of suturing on an exogenous graft material to act as a framework for tissue regeneration, an expandable epithelial bulge is created instead [147].

One major advantage that makes autoaugmentation attractive over enterocystoplasty is the avoidance of use of bowel and the concomitant complications arising from the interposition of bowel into the bladder and interruption of the GI tract. In autoaugmentation the patient's own bladder is used, no suture line is created, and no graft harvest is required, while the approach is extraperitoneal and therefore suitable for patients with prior abdominal surgery [48]. Operative and recovery time as well as hospital stay are less with autoaugmentation procedures compared to enterocystoplasty resulting in a lower incidence of morbidity [2, 15, 148].

Autoaugmentation does not preclude augmentation cystoplasty either at the operative setting or in the future should it be necessary [147, 148]. While autoaugmentation presents certain attractive features, there is evidence in support of a decreased efficacy in increasing bladder capacity and reducing detrusor overactivity compared to cystoplasty [2, 152]. Disadvantages of the procedure include the development of fibrous tissue around the pseudodiverticulum and the regrowth of the detrusor muscle, possible reasons for the decreased durability of the results achieved with this technique over time [2, 48, 152].

Fibrous tissue ingrowth also may be a possible cause of the increased incidence of bladder rupture following detrusor myotomy in experimental studies [2, 116]. In addition, a higher incidence for use of CISC following autoaugmentation has been reported compared to augmentation cystoplasty [26].

Autoaugmentation with the Use of Demucosalized Gastrointestinal Segments

In initial series there also was a concern regarding the blood perfusion of the diverticulum and the possibility of ischemic necrosis due to the removal of a large portion of the detrusor with its blood supply [147]. Furthermore, the development of adhesions

and fibrotic tissue between the diverticulum and the surrounding tissues was considered to be a cause for the poor urodynamic long-term results seen in many patients [153–155].

Therefore and despite the fact that the highly vascular lamina propria was considered adequate to provide sufficient blood perfusion [147], attempts were made to improve blood supply and create a biological backing for the diverticulum, resembling the protective effects of the elastic nature and contractile properties of the normal detrusor. In this direction a number of variations of the original technique, some of them incorporating the use of various demucosalized intestinal segments on preserved urothelium, were introduced. Gastrointestinal segments used in human and animal studies in combination with detrusor myectomy included gastric muscle, colon, and peritoneum while technical adaptations using rectus abdominis muscle also have been described [153, 156–162]. This technique has the advantage of preventing contact between urine and bowel segments, while preserving native urothelium [163].

Surgical Technique

The patient is placed in the lithotomy position and a Foley catheter is inserted. A Pfannensteil or lower midline incision is made and the bladder is recovered after retraction of the rectus muscle. The anterior wall of the bladder is identified and the peritoneum swept away or dissected off the bladder dome [148]. The bladder is filled with saline via the foley catheter and intravesical pressure is maintained to 20 cmH$_2$O during the procedure in order to facilitate dissection. A transverse incision is made at the intersection of the anterior wall and dome of the bladder. The incision should gently divide all the layers of the bladder musculature until the gray-blue of the bladder mucosa is visualized [15]. After the detrusor has been divided and the mucosa is exposed, the remaining detrusor fibers overlying the urothelium are gently spread apart using a hemostat or carefully dissected using Church scissors. Dissection between the detrusor and the bladder urothelium continues laterally in each direction up to the level of the vesical pedicles, until the entire bladder dome and nearly half of the detrusor have been stripped away from the urothelium [148]. In case a mucosal tear is inadvertly made during dissection, it can be oversewn using 4–0 or 5–0 absorbable sutures. When the dissection has finished, an omental flap can be drawn out through a small incision in the peritoneum and mobilized to cover the anterior bladder wall [15, 152]. Interpositioning and securing of omentum between the serosal side of the bladder mucosa and the perivesical fat and peritoneum potentially facilitates distention of the created diverticulum while protecting against perivesical fibrosis [152].

The result is the creation of a large 8- to 12-cm diameter disk of bladder mucosa, after the flaps of the detrusor overlying the urothelium are dissected free and excised. This way rehealing of the detrusor with development of scar tissue is prevented. In the original technique described by Cartwright and Snow bilateral psoas hitches were performed; however, in later series this was not deemed necessary [164].

When the procedure is complete, a thin large bladder diverticulum bulging as the bladder is filled is created. The created diverticulum continues to expand postoperatively and bladder enlargement develops relatively slowly over a period of several months, which accounts for the incremental symptomatic and urodynamic improvement noted in many patients.

Routinely drainage is not the rule; however, a small Penrose drain can be left in the perivesical space for safety reasons [148]. Care should be taken to avoid inadvertent creation of a cystostomy during dissection of the muscle from the mucosa. In case this occurs, however, the retropubic space should be drained [15].

Routinely the foley catheter is removed after a follow-up cystogram showing no extravasation is performed on the 5–7th postoperative day [148, 152]. Some authors in more recent series remove the bladder catheter on the first postoperative day in neurologically intact patients, allowing them to void spontaneously. For most patients with spinal cord injury and children with myelodysplasia, initiation of a CISC program is warranted.

In most studies follow-up with urodynamics is scheduled for 3 and 6 months after surgery and yearly thereafter. Results in continence should be obvious shortly after the autoaugmentation procedure. If improvement in symptoms is not significant during the first 4–6 weeks after surgery, repeat urodynamic evaluation is required.

An alternative surgical approach that has been recently explored is laparoscopic bladder autoaugmentation [165–167]; however, comments on this technique cannot be made in the event that data are scarce and come from case reports with inadequate numbers of patients and follow-up. Most recently the first case report of detrusor myotomy using the da Vinci surgical robot in a man with NBD and normal bladder capacity [168] appeared. The excellent results achieved in terms of symptoms provide preliminary evidence of the feasibility and efficacy of robotics for bladder autoaugmentation.

Results of Autoaugmentation

The majority of studies on bladder autoaugmentation concentrate on children with neurological dysfunction. Initial results of autoaugmentation in seven pediatric patients with NBD were promising in terms of continence, with six children remaining continent and three no longer requiring CISC [148]. The same group in a subsequent study with a follow-up of more than 2 years reported that 80% of patients were continent, although a significant increase in bladder capacity was not the rule [169]. Detrusorectomy with the addition of a demucosalized patch of gastric muscle to the created bladder diverticulum showed initially favorable results in another series of four children with neurogenic incontinence [156].

Results from a study on pediatric patients with NBD and low-capacity bladders who underwent vesicomyotomy showed a mean increase in bladder capacity of 40%, with a 33% decrease in mean leak-point pressure [150]. However, long-term results of the procedure in children with poorly compliant bladders secondary to myelomeningocele were not encouraging [154, 155].In the study by Marte et al. during a follow-up of 6.6 years, five of the eleven children had to undergo ileocystoplasty because of recurrent urinary tract infection, high-grade VUR, and incontinence [155]. Similarly, results from MacNeily et al. with a follow-up of 75 months revealed that in 12 patients (71%) autoaugmenation failed due to upper tract deterioration and ongoing incontinence, while four patients (23.5%) required enterocystoplasty [154].

Although there have been encouraging results in terms of improvement in bladder capacity for children with myelomeningocele [170], these have been attributed to somatic bladder growth rather than surgical success [154]. Results of these studies further underline the issue of proper patient selection for this procedure, with patients with poorly compliant bladders and an initial capacity of greater than 75% of that expected for age gaining the most benefit from the operation [170].

Recently Perovic et al. reported improvement in symptoms and bladder capacity [161, 162] in children with small-capacity, low-compliance neurogenic bladders. The authors performed a rectus muscle hitch by dissecting both rectus muscles from the fascial sheath, preserving their blood supply, and suturing them to the edges of the detrusor as backing material for the pseudodiverticulum.

Urothelium-preserving procedures incorporating demucosalized gastric muscle and colon have yielded satisfactory results in terms of bladder capacity and compliance in clinical studies of children with neurogenic bladder [156, 163, 171–173]. On the contrary, results of autoaugmentation covered with a peritoneal flap in animal [174] and human studies [159] were inferior to those of conventional autoaugmentation gastrocystoplasty.

These procedures, apart from being technically demanding, are not suitable for small fibrotic bladders, do not seem to be more efficacious than conventional autoaugmentation, and lack long-term results of significant numbers of patients. On the other hand, they have the advantage of sparing the long-term sequalae of enterocystoplasty.

There is a relative lack of studies regarding autoaugmentation in the adult population with and without neurological impairment. A relatively large case series of 29 adult patients aged 14–64 years, most of whom had NBD-related incontinence, revealed that during a follow-up of 7 years after autoaugmentation, half of the patients managed to void without significant residuals, while the other half required CISC. Bladder compliance and capacity also were improved [164].

As previously stated, there is little evidence of the efficacy of autoaugmentation in adults with DO-related incontinence. In a small series of five patients with urge incontinence, results of autoaugmentation were disappointing. Four patients continued to sustain involuntary detrusor contractions resulting in incontinence at 3-month urodynamic and clinical evaluation [175] (level 4 evidence). In a series with 1-year follow-up, symptomatic and urodynamic improvement was evident in 63% of patients, with better results noted in those with idiopathic detrusor instability (12 of 17 cured or improved) [152].Results from Westney et al. on a heterogeneous group of 30 patients who underwent autoaugmentation and were followed-up for 42 months with urodynamic studies revealed that 63% of the patients faired well in terms of increase in bladder compliance and resolution of DO [15]. The authors' observation that the most favorable and consistent outcomes following autoaugmentation were noted in patients with refractory DO and spinal cord injury were in agreement with results from previous studies [176, 177].

Complications of Autoaugmentation

Autoaugmentation seems to be associated with fewer and less severe complications compared to bladder augmentation techniques incorporating the use of bowel. A study comparing autoaugmentation to enterocystoplasty revealed that 3% of patients undergoing detrusorectomy suffered serious complications compared to 22% in the enterocystoplasty group [177].

Theoretically there is a greater risk of bladder perforation following autoaugmentation, owing to the thinness of the mucosa in the created pseudodiverticulum, as has been shown in experimental studies in rats [116]. In clinical practice, however, even in early series, there were no cases of catheter-induced perforation, despite the fact that all patients were put on CISC immediately after the foley catheter was removed [148].

Early postoperative urine extravasation was another frequent complication in an early series (33% incidence in the initial series by Cartwright and Snow [148]); however, extravasation resolved uneventfully after 2–3 weeks of continuous bladder catheterization. In a recent series, however, of 49 patients who underwent detrusor myectomy there was only one case of extraperitoneal bladder leak [15]. Recurrent UTIs following autoaugmentation were usual in early series and were attributed to the presence of large residuals requiring CISC [148, 152].

Conclusions on Bladder Autoaugmentation

There is evidence suggesting that the symptomatic improvement obtained with autoaugmentation—the increase in bladder capacity and the reduction in voiding pressures—are far less pronounced than those produced by enterocystoplasty [55, 123,

178]. However, although a definite advantage of this technique is the lower incidence of morbidity compared with enterocystoplasty, there is a question as to the limited efficacy of the procedure and the possibility that the results achieved may not be maintained in the longer term. Probably this is one of the reasons why this technique has never gained wide acceptance in practice. At the end of the day, and despite the lack of data and the low level of evidence (level of evidence 4) autoaugmentation can be considered to be a viable treatment option for carefully selected patients with drug-refractory urge incontinence, leaving the alternative of enterocystoplasty for the nonresponders.

Urinary Diversion

Contemporary urinary diversion is a rare treatment option almost exclusively reserved for patients with NBD-related incontinence, for those patients with intractable incontinence or severe pelvic pain who are unsuitable for or have failed other surgical measures [179]. However, under certain circumstances, urinary diversion may prove to be better than enterocystoplasty when intractable DO is associated with severe pelvic pain [180] (Fig. 19.2).

Urinary diversion in patients with NBD can be either continent or conduit (noncontinent) diversion. Continent cutaneous urinary diversion requires the creation of a catheterizable stoma that is implanted either into the native bladder or into an intestinal neobladder (Fig. 19.3). For the majority of patients with neurological lesions, some form of bladder augmentation procedure is undertaken during the same session. The rare patient requiring continent diversion for intractable incontinence usually is unable to self-catheterize through the urethra due to a nonaccessible meatus, severe urethral stricture, or pain. Moreover, most neurologically impaired patients would find it easier to catheterize a continent abdominal stoma instead of their native urethra..

Construction of a continent conduit can be managed by using the ileum or colon as in the Yag–Monti procedure, the appendix as in the Mitrofanoff procedure, or even occasionally the ureter. Techniques that create a relatively small-bore outlet, such as the ones mentioned previously, currently are being used more commonly mainly because of the lower incidence of adverse effects. Despite the fact that continence rates exceeding 80% have been reported with these techniques, these results come with a relatively high incidence of complications.

One major complication, ranging from 12 to 30% of cases, is stomal stenosis, which is more common when an umbilical stoma is created. Results from early series with long-term follow-up of the Mitrofanoff procedure in children revealed the most frequent complications requiring surgical revision to be stomal stenosis and persistent leakage [181].

Incontinent conduit diversion became an even more rare treatment option for patients with NBD and urge incontinence, since the introduction of CISC. However, these procedures still may be viable alternative options for patients with intractable incontinence who are not able to perform CISC, have failed previous surgery, and are not indicated for (short bowel syndrome) or refuse continent diversion or bladder augmentation.

Diversion options considered depend on the individual case and include the classic Bricker ileal conduit urinary diversion or an ileovesicostomy "bladder chimney" procedure [182–184]. In case a conduit diversion is created there is a question as to whether a cystectomy also should be performed. Cystectomy is strongly considered in patients with a history of chronic infections due to the high risk of pyocystis if the bladder is left in situ [48].

In ileovesicostomy a 15- to 20-cm segment of terminal ileum is isolated. The proximal 6–8 cm of this segment is opened on the antimesenteric border. The dome of the bladder is opened widely in a transverse manner and the proximal portion of the bowel is sutured onto the bladder. The distal portion of the ileum remains tubularized and becomes the stoma. Recently laparoscopic ileovesicostomy for NBD has been described as an acceptable alternative to the open procedure [185].

As urinary diversion is a surgical option limited to selected patients with urge incontinence, there is a reasonable lack of evidence relative to its efficacy for DO incontinence (level 4 evidence). Results from series with reasonable follow-up render incontinent cutaneous ileovesicostomy a useful alternative for neurologically impaired adult patients with urge incontinence who are unwilling or unable to perform CISC [182, 183, 186], with urethral continence achieved in over 70% of patients in a recent series [187]. Furthermore, ileovesicostomy

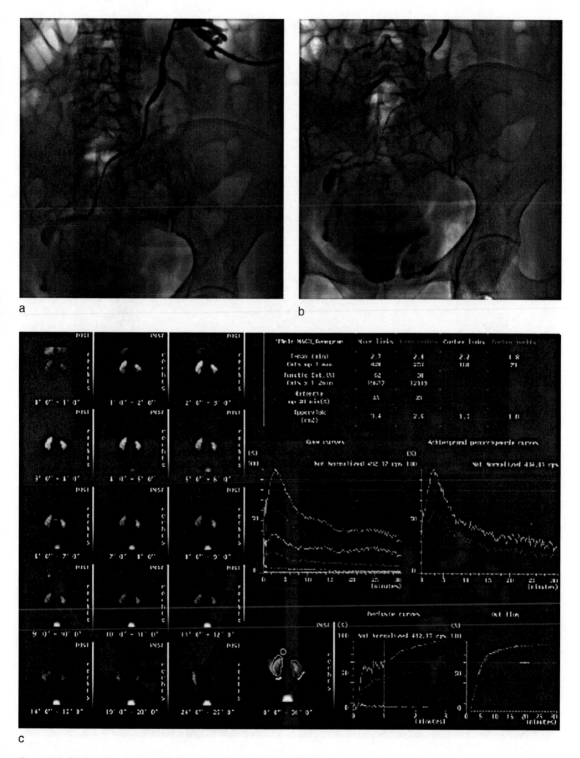

FIG. 19.2. Mainz II pouch, anal diversion. Nephrodrain left because of pyelonephritis. (**a**) After resolution of the infective process, contrast flows down to the rectal pouch. (**b**) Filling of the Mainz II pouch. (**c**) Nuclear scan showing good efflux of both kidneys after resolution of the pyelonephritis

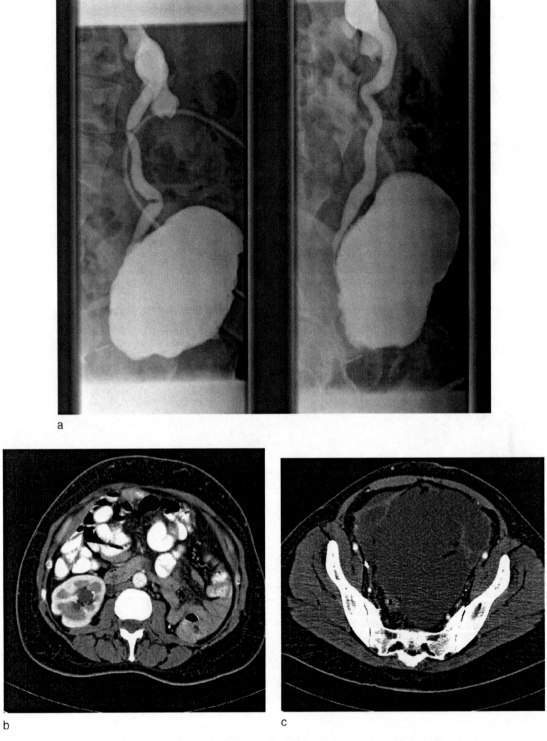

Fig. 19.3. Kock continent cutaneous derivation because of urge incontinence and nephrectomy, left. (a) After stricture of the Mitrofanoff (umbilical stoma), right, reflux developed. (b) CT scan in the same patient showing slight dilatation of the right kidney. (c) CT scan showing the enormous capacity pouch occupying the small pelvis

can provide a safe and effective alternative for urinary drainage while preserving the upper urinary tracts in patients with detrusor hyperreflexia [188]. Complications of incontinent conduit diversions include upper urinary tract infections, stone formation, gastrointestinal sequlae (ileus, fistula), stomal stenosis, and anastomotic ureteroileal stricture [184, 188–191]. However, there is no doubt that any form of urinary tract reconstruction is preferable over indwelling catheter placement in terms of complications [182], quality of life, and sexual function especially for women with NBD-related incontinence [192].

References

1. Abrams P, Cardozo L, Fall M, et al. The standardisation of terminology of lower urinary tract function: Report from the Standardisation Sub-committee of the International Continence Society. Neurourol Urodyn 2002; 21:167–178.
2. Chapple CR, Bryan NP. Surgery for detrusor overactivity. World J Urol 1998; 16:268–273.
3. Lapides J, Diokno AC, Silber SJ, Lowe BS. Clean intermittent self-catheterisation in the treatment of urinary tract disease. J Urol 1972; 107:458461.
4. Fontaine E, Bendaya S, Desert JF, et al. Combined modified rectus fascial sling and augmentation ileocystoplasty for neurogenic incontinence in women. J Urol 1997; 157:109112.
5. Linder A, Leach G, Raz S. Augmentation cystoplasty in the treatment of neurogenic bladder dysfunction. J Urol 1983; 129:491493.
6. Nabi G, Cody J, Dublin N, et al. Urinary diversion and bladder reconstruction/replacement using intestinal segments for intractable incontinence or following cystectomy. Cochrane Database Syst Rev 2003, Issue 1. Art. No.: CD003306. doi:10.1002/14651858. CD003306.
7. Harris RG, Constantinou CE, Stamey TA. Extravesical subtrigonal injection of 50 percent ethanol for detrusor instability. J Urol 1988; 140:111116.
8. McInerney PD, Vanner TF, Matenhelia S, Stephenson TP. Assessment of the long term results of subtrigonal phenolisation. Br J Urol 1991; 67:586587.
9. Blackford HN, Murray K, Stephenson TP, Mundy AR. Results of transvesical infiltration of the pelvic plexuses with phenol in 116 patients. Br J Urol 1984; 56(6):647649.
10. Cameron-Strange A, Millard RJ. Management of refractory detrusor instability by transvesical phenol injection. Br J Urol 1988; 62(4):323325.
11. Chapple CR, Hampson SJ, Turner-Warwick RT, Worth PH. Subtrigonal phenol injection. How safe and effective is it? Br J Urol 1991; 68(5):483486.
12. Rosenbaum TP, Shaw PJ, Worth PH. Trans-trigonal phenol failed the test of time. Br J Urol 1990; 66(2):164169.
13. Wall LL, Stanton SL. Transvesical phenol injection of pelvic nerve plexuses in females with refractory urge incontinence. Br J Urol 1989; 63(5):465468.
14. Ingelman-Sundberg A. Partial denervation of the bladder: A new operation for the treatment of urge incontinence and similar conditions in women. Acta Obstet Gynecol Scand 1959; 38:487502.
15. Westney OL, McGuire EJ. Surgical procedures for the treatment of urge incontinence. Techniq Urol 2001; 7(2):126132.
16. Hodgkinson CP, Drukker BH. Infravesical nerve resection for detrusor dyssynergia. The Ingelman-Sundberg operation. Acta Obstet Gynecol Scand 1977; 56(4):401408.
17. Cespedes RD, Cross CA, McGuire EJ. Modified Ingelman-Sundberg bladder denervation procedure for refractory urge incontinence. J Urol 1996; 156(5):17441477.
18. Westney OL, Lee JT, McGuire EJ, et al. Long-term results of Ingelman-Sundberg denervation procedure for urge incontinence refractory to medical therapy. J Urol 2002; 168(3):10441047.
19. Tizzoni G, Foggi A. Die wiederhestellung der harnblase. Centralbl F Chir 1888; 15:921923.
20. von Mikulicz J. Zur Operation der angeborenen Blasenpalte. Zentralb Chir 1899; 26:641–648.
21. Couvelaire R. La petite vessie des tuberculeux genitourinaires: Essai de classification, places et variantes des cysto-intestinoplasties. J Urol (Paris) 1950; 56:381434.
22. Mundy AR, Stephenson TP. "Clam" ileocystoplasty for the treatment of refractory urge incontinence. Br J Urol 1985; 57(6):641646.
23. Bramble FJ. The treatment of adult enuresis and urge incontinence by enterocystoplasty. Br J Urol 1982; 54:693696.
24. Lockhart JL, Bejany D, Politano VA. Augmentation cystoplasty in the management of neurogenic bladder disease and urinary incontinence. J Urol 1986; 135:969971.
25. Sidi AA, Becher EF, Reddy PK, et al. Augmentation enterocystoplasty for the management of voiding dysfunction in spinal cord injury patients. J Urol 1990; 143:8385.
26. Greenwell TJ, Venn SN, Mundy AR. Augmentation cystoplasty. BJU Int 2001; 88:511525.
27. McGuire EJ, McGuire R, Woodside JR, Borden TA. Upper tract deterioration in patients with myelodysplasia

and detrusor hypertonia: A follow up study. J Urol 1983; 129:823826.

28. Hendren WH. Historical perspective in the use of bowel in urology. Urol Clin N Am 1997; 24:703–713.

29. Gough JW. Enterocystoplasty. BJU Int 2001; 88:739743.

30. Duel BP, Gonzalez R, Barthold JS. Alternative techniques for augmentation cystoplasty. J Urol 1998; 159:9981005.

31. Whitmore WF, Gittes RF. Reconstruction of the urinary tract by cecal and ileocecal cystoplasty: Review of a 15-year experience. J Urol 1983; 129:494498.

32. Murray K, Nurse DE, Mundy AR. Secreto-motor function of intestinal segments used in lower urinary tract reconstruction. Br J Urol 1987; 60:532535.

33. Hendren WH, Hendren RB. Bladder augmentation: Experience with 129 children and young adults. J Urol 1990; 144:445453.

34. Mitchell ME, Piser JA. Intestinocystoplasty and total bladder replacement in children and young adults. J Urol 1987; 138:579.

35. N'Dow J, Leung HY, Marshall C, et al. Bowel dysfunction after bladder reconstruction. J Urol 1998; 159:14701475.

36. Ngan JH, Lau JL, Lim ST, et al. Long-term results of antral gastrocystoplasty. J Urol 1993; 149:731734.

37. Adams MC, Mitchell ME, Rink RC. Gastrocystoplasty: An alternative solution to the problem of urological reconstruction in the severely compromised patient. J Urol 1988; 140:11521156.

38. Plawker MW, Rabinowitz SS, Etwark DJ, et al. Hypergastrinaemia, dysuria-hematuria and metabolic alkalosis: complications associated with gastrocystoplasty. J Urol 1995; 154:546549.

39. Reinberg Y, Manivel JC, Froemming C, et al. Perforation of the gastric segment of an augmented bladder secondary to peptic ulcer disease. J Urol 1992; 148:369371.

40. Tiffany P, Vaughan ED Jr, Manon D, et al. Hypergastrinaemia following antral gastrocystoplasty. J Urol 1986; 136:692695.

41. Bogaert GA, Mevorach RA, Kim J, Kogan BA. The physiology of gastrocystoplasty: Once a stomach, always a stomach. J Urol 1995; 154:546–549.

42. Goodwin WE, Winter CC, Baker WF. 'Cup patch' technique of ileocystoplasty for bladder enlargement or partial substitution. Surg Gynecol Obstet 1959; 108:240244.

43. Cranidis A, Nestoridis G. Bladder augmentation. Int Urogynecol J 2000; 11:33–40.

44. Radomski SB, Herschorn S, Stone AR. Urodynamic comparison of ileum vs. sigmoid in augmentation cystoplasty for neurogenic bladder dysfunction. Neurourol Urodyn 1995; 14:231237.

45. Theodorou C, Plastiras D, Moutzouris G, et al. Combined reconstructive and prosthetic surgery in complicated lower urinary tract dysfunction. J Urol 1997; 157:472474.

46. Gonzalez R, Nguyen DH, Koleilat N, et al. Compatibility of enterocystoplasty and the artificial urinary sphincter. J Urol 1989; 142:502504.

47. Catto JW, Natarajan V, Tophill PR. Simultaneous augmentation cystoplasty is associated with earlier rather than increased artificial urinary sphincter function. J Urol 2005; 173:12371241.

48. Wagg A, Majumdar A, Toozs-Hobson P, et al. Current and future trends in the management of overactive bladder. Int Urogynecol J 2007; 18:81–94.

49. Woodhause CRD, Macneily AE. The Mitrofanoff principle: Expanding upon a versatile technique. Br J Urol 1994; 74:447–453.

50. Blaivas JG, Weiss JP, Desai P, et al. Long-term follow-up of augmentation enterocystoplasty and continent diversion in patients with benign disease. J Urol 2005; 173:1631–1634.

51. Leng WW, McGuire EJ. Reconstructive surgery for urinary incontinence. Urol Clin North Am 1999; 26(1):6180.

52. Goodwin WE, Turner CC. Results of ileocystoplasty. J Urol 1958; 80:461466.

53. Bramble FJ. The clam cystoplasty. Br J Urol 1990; 66:337341.

54. Kockelbergh RC, Tan JB, Bates CP, et al. Clam enterocystoplasty in general urological practice. Br J Urol 1991; 68(1):3841.

55. Hasan ST, Marshall C, Robson WA, Neal DE. Clinical outcome and quality of life following enterocystoplasty for idiopathic detrusor instability and neurogenic bladder dysfunction. Br J Urol 1995; 76:551557.

56. Keating MA, Ludlow JK, Rich MA. Enterocystoplasty: The star modification. J Urol 1996; 155:17231725.

57. Flood HD, Malhotra SJ, O'Connell HE, et al. Long-term results and complications using augmentation cystoplasty in reconstructive urology. Neurourol Urodyn 1995; 14(4):297309.

58. McInerney PD, DeSousa N, Thomas PJ, et al. The role of urodynamic studies in the evaluation of patients with augmentation cystoplasties. Br J Urol 1995; 76:475478.

59. Gonzales R, Sidi AA, Zhang G. Urinary undiversion: Indications, technique and results in 50 cases. J Urol 1986; 136:1316.

60. Mast P, Hoebeke P, Wyndaele JJ, et al. Experience with augmentation cystoplasty: A review. Paraplegia 1995; 33(10):560564.

61. Krishna A, Gough DCS, Fishwick J, Bruce J. Ileocystoplasty in children. Assessing safety and success. Eur Urol 1995; 31:6267.

62. Khoury JM, Timmons SL, Corbel L, Webster GD. Complications of enterocystoplasty. Urology 1992; 40:914.

63. Singh G, Thomas DG. Bowel problems after enterocystoplasty. Br J Urol 1997; 79:328332.

64. Whorwell PJ, Lupton EW, Endura D, et al. Bladder smooth muscle dysfunction in patients with irritable bowel syndrome. Gut 1986; 27:10141017.

65. Nurse DE, Mundy AR. Metabolic complications after cystoplasty. Br J Urol 1985; 63:165170.

66. McDougal WS. Metabolic complications of urinary intestinal diversion. J Urol 1992; 147:11991208.

67. Brkovic D, Linke J, Jakse G, Bauss F. Changes in bone structure after augmentation cystoplasty in chronic uraemic rats. BJU Int 2005; 95:10661070.

68. Mundy AR, Nurse DE. Calcium balance, growth and skeletal mineralisation in patients with cystoplasties. Br J Urol 1988; 140:853855.

69. Steiner MS, Morton RA, Marshall FF. Vitamin B12 deficiency in patients with ileocolic neobladders. J Urol 1993; 149:255257.

70. Khoury A, Salomon M, Doche R et al. Stone formation following augmentation cystoplasty: The role of intestinal mucous. J Urol 1997; 58:40.

71. Woodhouse CRJ, Robertson WG. Urolithiasis in enterocystoplasties. World J Urol 2004; 22:215–221.

72. Clayman RV. Preventing reservoir calculi after augmentation cystoplasty and continent urinary diversion: The influence of an irrigation protocol. J Urol 2005; 173:866867.

73. George VK, Gee JM, Wortley MI, et al. The effect of ranitidine on urine mucus concentration in patients with enterocystoplasty. Br J Urol 1992; 70:3032.

74. Gillon G, Mundy AR. The dissolution of urinary mucus after cystoplasty. Br J Urol 1989; 63:372374.

75. Krishna A, Gough DCS. Evaluation of augmentation cystoplasty in childhood with reference to vesico-ureteric reflux and urinary infection. Br J Urol 1994; 74:465468.

76. Wyndaele JJ, Maes D. Clean intermittent self-catheterisation: A 12 year follow-up. J Urol 1990; 143:906908.

77. Maynard F, Diokno A. Urinary infection and complications during clean intermittent catheterisation following spinal cord injury. J Urol 1984; 132:943946.

78. Kreder KJ, Webster GD. Management of the bladder outlet in patients requiring enterocystoplasty. J Urol 1992; 147(1):3841.

79. Fenn N, Conn IG, German KA, Stephenson TP. Complications of clam enterocystoplasty with particular reference to urinary tract infection. Br J Urol 1992; 69(4):366368.

80. Smith P, Hardy GJ. Carcinoma occurring as a late complication of ileocystoplasty. Br J Urol 1971; 43:576579.

81. Leedham PW, England HR. Adenocarcinoma developing in an ileocystoplasty. Br J Surg 1973; 60:158160.

82. Golomb J, Klutke CG, Lewin KJ, et al. Bladder neoplasms associated with augmentation cystoplasty. Report of 2 cases and literature review. J Urol 1989; 142:377380.

83. Gregoire M, Kantoff P, DeWolf WC. Synchronous adenocarcinoma and transitional cell carcinoma of the bladder associated with augmentation: Case report and review of the literature. J Urol 1993; 149:115–118.

84. Gepi-Attee S, Ganabathi K, Abrams PH, MacIver AG. Villous adenoma in augmentation colocystoplasty: A case report and discussion of the pathogenesis. J Urol 1992; 147:128130.

85. Shokeir AA, Shamaa M, el-Mekresh MM, et al. Late malignancy in bowel segments exposed to urine without fecal stream. Urology 1995; 46:657–661.

86. Ali-El-Dein B, El-Tabey N, Abdel-Latiif M, et al. Late uro-ileal cancer after incorporation of ileum into the urinary tract. J Urol 2002; 167:84–88.

87. Filmer RB, Spencer JR. Malignancies in bladder augmentation and intestinal conduits. J Urol 1990; 143(4):671678.

88. Stone AR, Davis N, Stephenson TP. Cancer associated with augmentation cystoplasty. Br J Urol 1987; 60:236238.

89. Soergel TM, Cain MP, Misseri R, et al. Transitional cell carcinoma of the bladder following augmentation cystoplasty for the neuropathic bladder. J Urol 2004; 172, 1649–1652.

90. Stewart M. Urinary diversion and bowel cancer. Ann R Coll Surg Eng 1986; 68:98102.

91. Nurse DE, Mundy AR. Assessment of the malignant potential of cystoplasty. Br J Urol 1989; 64:489.

92. Barrington JW, Fulford S, Griffiths D, Stephenson TP. Tumors in bladder remnant after augmentation enterocystoplasty. J Urol 1997; 157:482486.

93. Fernandez-Arjona M, Herrero L, Romero J, et al. Synchronous signet ring cell carcinoma and squamous cell carcinoma arising in an augmented ileocystoplasty. Case report and review of the literature. Eur Urol 1996; 29:125128.

94. Gitlin JS, Wu XR, Sun TT, et al. New concepts of histological changes in experimental augmentation cystoplasty: Insights into the development of neoplastic transformation at the enterovesical and gastrovesical anastomosis. J Urol 1999; 162:10961100.

95. Lane T, Shah J. Carcinoma following augmentation ileocystoplasty. Urol Int 2000; 64:3132.

96. Ames BN, Gold LS. Too many rodent carcinogens: Mitogenesis increases mutagenesis. Science 1990; 249:970.

97. Barrington JW, Fraylin L, Fish R, et al. Elevated levels of basic fibroblast growth factor in the urine of clam enterocystoplasty patients. J Urol 1996; 156:468.

98. Carr LK, Herschorn S. Early development of adenocarcinoma in a young woman following augmentation cystoplasty for undiversion. J Urol 1997; 157:22552256.

99. Yoshida T, Kim CJ, Konishi T, et al. Adenocarcinoma of the bladder 19 years after the augmentation ileocystoplasty: Report of a case. Nippon Hinyokika Gakkai Zasshi 1998; 89:54–57.

100. Koizumi S, Johnin K, Kataoka A, et al. Adenocarcinoma occurring 37 years after augmentation ileocystoplasty for tuberculous bladder atrophy: Report of a case. Hinyokika Kiyo 1997; 43: 743–745.

101. Ivil KD, Doak SH, Jenkins SA, et al. Fluorescence in-situ hybridisation on biopsies from clam ileocystoplasties and on a clam cancer. Br J Cancer 2006; 94:891895.

102. Milsom I, Abrams P, Cardozo L, et al. How widespread are the symptoms of an overactive bladder and how are they managed? A population-based prevalence study. BJU Int 2001; 87:760.

103. Krause FS, Feil G, Bichler KH, et al. Clinical aspects for the use of DNA image cytometry in detection of bladder cancer: A valuable tool? DNA Cell Biol 2003; 22:721–725.

104. Deliveliotis C, Georgoulakis J, Skolarikos A, et al. DNA ploidy as a prognostic factor in muscle invasive transitional cell carcinoma of the bladder. Urol Res 2005; 33:3943.

105. De Voogt HD, Rather P, Beyer-Boon ME. Urinary cytology. New York: Springer, 1997:5561.

106. Rushton HG, Woodard JR, Parrot TS, et al. Delayed bladder rupture after augmentation enterocystoplasty. J Urol 1988; 140:344346.

107. Couillard DR, Vapnec JM, Rentzepis MJ, et al. Fatal perforation of an augmentation cystoplasty in an adult. Urology 1993; 42:585588.

108. Elder JS, Snyder HM, Hulbert WC, et al. Perforation of the augmented bladder in patients undergoing clean intermittent catheterization. J Urol 1988; 140:11591162.

109. Anderson PA, Rickwood AM. Detrusor hyperreflexia as a factor in spontaneous perforation of augmentation cystoplasty for neuropathic bladder. Br J Urol 1991; 67:210212.

110. Reisman EM, Preminger GM. Bladder perforation secondary to clean intermittent catheterization. J Urol 1989; 142:1316—1317.

111. Sheiner JR, Kaplan GW. Spontaneous bladder rupture following enterocystoplasty. J Urol 1988; 140(2):1157–1158.

112. Crane JM, Scherz HS, Billman GF, Kaplan GW. Ischemic necrosis: A hypothesis to explain the pathogenesis of spontaneously ruptured enterocystoplasty. J Urol 1991; 146:141144.

113. Bauer SB, Hendren WH, Kozakewich H, et al. Perforation of the augmented bladder. J Urol 1992; 148(2):699703.

114. Rosen MA, Light JK. Spontaneous bladder rupture following augmentation entoerocystoplasty. J Urol 1991; 146:12321234.

115. Essig KA, Sheldon CA, Brandt MT, et al. Elevated intravesical pressure causes hypoperfusion in canine colocystoplasty: A fluorometric assay. J Urol 1991; 146:551553.

116. Slaton JW, Kropp KA. Conservative management of suspected bladder rupture after augmentation enterocystoplasty. J Urol 1994; 152:713715.

117. Rivas DA, Chancellor MB, Huang B, et al. Comparison of bladder rupture pressure intestinal bladder augmentation (ileocystoplasty) and myomyotomy (autoaugmentation) Urology 1996; 48:4046.

118. Rogers CJ, Barber DB, Wade WH. Spontaneous bladder perforation in paraplegia as a late complication of augmentation enterocystoplasty: Case report. Arch Phys Med Rehab 1996; 77: 11981200.

119. Glass RB, Rushton HG. Delayed spontaneous rupture of augmented bladder in children: Diagnosis with sonography and CT. AJR Am J Roentgenol 1992; 158:833–835.

120. Braverman RM, Lebowitz RL. Perforation of the augmented urinary bladder in nine children and adolescents: Importance of cystography. Am J Roentgenol 1991; 157:10591063.

121. Blyth B, Ewalt DH, Duckett JW, Snyder HM. Lithogenic properties of enterocystoplasty. J Urol 1992; 148:575577.

122. Nurse DE, McInerney PD, Thomas PJ, Mundy AR. Stones in enterocystoplasties. Br J Urol 1996; 77:684–687.

123. DeFoor W, Minevich E, Reeves D, et al. Gastrocystoplasty: Long-term follow-up. J Urol 2003; 170:1647–1650.

124. Franco I, Levitt SB. Urolithiasis in the patient with augmentation cystoplasty: Pathogenesis and management. AUA Update 1997;XVII:Lesson 2, 1015.

125. Edlund C, Peeker R, Fall M. Clam ileocystoplasty: Successful treatment of severe bladder overactivity. Scand J Urol Nephrol 2001; 35(3):190–195.

126. Sethia KK, Webb RJ, Neal DE. Urodynamic study of ileocystoplasty in the treatment of idiopathic detrusor instability. Br J Urol 1991; 67(3):286290.

127. McRae P, Murray KH, Nurse DE, et al. Clam enterocystoplasty in the neuropathic bladder. Br J Urol 1987; 60(6):523525.

128. Beier-Holgersen R, Kirkeby LT, Nordling J. Clam ileocystoplasty. Scand J Urol Nephrol 1994; 28:5558.

129. Kayigil O, Atahan O, Metin A. Experiences with clam ileocystoplasty. Int Urol Nephrol 1998; 30(1):4548.

130. Awad SA, Al-Zahrani HM, Gajewski JB, Bourque-Kehoe AA. Long-term results and complications of augmentation ileocystoplasty for idiopathic urge incontinence in women. Br J Urol 1988; 81(4): 569573.

131. Kayigil O, Aytaç B, Çakar KS, Metin A. Clam ileocystoplasty in adult nocturnal enuresis. Int Urol Nephrol 2001; 32:647–649.

132. Fontaine E, Bendaya S, Desert JF, et al. Combined modified rectus fascial sling and augmentation ileocystoplasty for neurogenic incontinence in women. J Urol 1997; 157:109112.

133. Cher ML, Allen TD. Continence in the myelodysplastic patient following enterocystoplasty. J Urol 1993; 149:11031106.

134. Wein AJ. Diagnosis and treatment of the overactive bladder. Urology 2003; 62:2027.

135. Fraser M, Thomas DF, Pitt E, et al. A surgical model of composite cystoplasty with cultured urothelial cells; a controlled study of gross outcome and urothelial phenotype. BJU Int 2004; 93:609616.

136. Yoo JJ, Meng J, Oberpenning F, et al. Bladder augmentation using allogenic bladder submucosa seeded with cells. Urology 1998; 51:221225.

137. Piechota HJ, Gleason CA, Dahms SE, et al. Bladder acellular matrix graft: In vivo functional properties of regenerated rat bladder. Urol Res 1999; 27:206213.

138. Atala A, Bauer SB, Soker S, et al. Tissue engineering autologous bladders for patients needing cystoplasty. Lancet 2006; 376:12411246.

139. Satar N, Yoo JJ, Atala A. Progressive dilation for bladder tissue expansion. J Urol 1999; 162: 829831.

140. Docimo SG, Moore RG, Adams J, et al. Laparoscopic bladder augmentation using stomach. Urology 1995; 46:565–569.

141. Hedican SP, Schulam PG, Docimo SG. Laparoscopic assisted reconstructive surgery. J Urol 1999; 161:267–270.

142. Gill IS, Rackley RR, Meraney AM, et al. Laparoscopic enterocystoplasty. Urology 2000; 55:178181.

143. Meng MV, Anwar HP, Elliott SP, Stoller ML. Pure laparoscopic enterocystoplasty. J Urol 2002; 167:1386.

144. Kelami A, Dustmann HO, Ludtke-Handjery A, et al. Experimental investigations of bladder regeneration using Teflon-felt as a bladder wall substitute. J Urol 1970; 104:693.

145. Goldstein MD, Dearden LC. Histology of omentoplasty of the urinary bladder in the rabbit. Inv Urol 1966; 3:460.

146. Kelami A. Lyophilized human dura as a bladder wall substitute: Experimental and clinical results. J Urol 1971; 105:518.

147. Telly O. Segmental cystectomy with peritoneoplasty. Urol Int 1970; 25:236.

148. Cartwright PC, Snow BW. Bladder autoaugmentation: Partial detrusor excision to augment the bladder without the use of bowel. J Urol 1989; 142:10501053.

149. Cartwright PC, Snow BW. Bladder autoaugmentation: Early clinical experience. J Urol 1989; 142:505508.

150. Johnson HW, Nigro MK, Stothers L, et al. Laboratory variables of bladder autoaugmentation in an animal model. Urology 1994; 44:260.

151. Stothers L, Johnson H, Arnold W, et al. Bladder autoaugmentation by vesicomyotomy in the pediatric neurogenic bladder. Urology 1994; 44:110.

152. Kumar SP, Abrams PH. Detrusor myectomy: Long-term results with a minimum follow-up of 2 years. BJU Int 2005; 96:341.

153. Swami KS, Feneley RC, Hammonds JC, Abrams P. Detrusor myectomy for detrusor overactivity: A minimum 1-year follow-up. Br J Urol 1998; 81:6872.

154. Donald HN, Mitchell ME, Mark H, et al. Demucosalised augmentation gastrocystoplasty with bladder autoaugmentation in pediatric patients. J Urol 1996; 156:206209.

155. MacNeily AE, Afshar K, Coleman GU, Johnson HW. Autoaugmentation by detrusor myotomy: Its lack of effectiveness in the management of congenital neuropathic bladder. J Urol 2003; 170:1643.

156. Marte A, Di Meglio D, Cotrufo AM, et al. A long-term follow-up of autoaugmentation in myelodysplastic children. BJU Int 2002; 89(9):928931.

157. Dewan PA, Stefanek W. Autoaugmentation gastrocystoplasty: Early clinical results Br J Urol 1994; 74(4):460464.

158. Close CE. Autoaugmentation gastrocystoplasty. BJU Int 2001; 88(7):757761.

159. Dewan PA, Lorenz C, Stefanek W, Byard RW. Urothelial lined colocystoplasty in a sheep model. Eur Urol 1994; 26(3):240246.

160. Oge O, Tekgul S, Ergen A, Kendi S. Urothelium-preserving augmentation cystoplasty covered with a peritoneal flap. BJU Int 2000; 85:802805.

161. Close CE, Dewan PA, Ashwood PJ, et al. Autoaugmentation peritoneocystoplasty in a sheep model BJU Int 2001; 88(4):414–417.

162. Perovic SV, Djordjevic ML, Kekic ZK, Vukadinovic VM. Detrusorectomy with rectus muscle hitch and backing. J Pediatr Surg 2003; 38:1637.

163. Perovic SV, Djordjevic ML, Kekic ZK, Vukadinovic VM. Bladder autoaugmentation with rectus muscle backing. J Urol 2002; 168(4 Pt 2):18771880.

164. Dewan PA. Autoaugmentation demucosalized enterocystoplasty. World J Urol 1998; 16:255.

165. Stohrer M et al.: Bladder auto-augmentation— An alternative for enterocystoplasty: Preliminary results. Neurourol Urodyn 1995; 14:1123.

166. Ehrlich RM, Gershman A. Laparoscopic seromyotomy (auto-augmentation) for non-neurogenic neurogenic bladder in a child: Initial case report. Urology 1993; 42:175.

167. Poppas DP, Uzzo RG, Britanisky RG, Mininberg DT. Laparoscopic laser assisted autoaugmentation of the pediatric neurogenic bladder: Early experience with urodynamic follow-up. J Urol 1996; 155:1057.

168. McDougall EM, Clayman RV, Figenshau RS, et al. Laparoscopic retropubic auto-augmentation of the bladder. J Urol 1995; 153:123–126.

169. Mammen T, Balaji KC. Robotic transperitoneal detrusor myotomy: Description of a novel technique. J Endourol 2005; 19(4):476–479.

170. Snow BW, Cartwright PC. Bladder autoaugmentation. Urol Clin North Am 1992; 23:323–331.

171. Skobejko-Wlodarsa L, Strulak K, Nachulewicz P, Szymkiewicz C. Bladder autoaugmentation in myelodysplastic children. Br J Urol 1998; 81:114.

172. Cartwright PC, Snow BW. Autoaugmentation cystoplasty. In: Dewan P, Mitchell M, eds. Bladder augmentation. London: Arnold, 2000:83–91.

173. Nguyen DH, Mitchell ME, Horowitz M, et al. Demucosalized augmentation gastrocystoplasty with bladder autoaugmentation in pediatric patients. J Urol 1996; 156:206–209.

174. Dewan PA, Ehall H. Autoaugmentation gastrocystoplasty: Patient selection, outcome, and ongoing research. Dialogues Pediatr Urol 1999; 22:35.

175. Dewan PA, Close CE, Byard RW, et al. Enteric mucosal regrowth after bladder augmentation using demucosalized gut segments. J Urol 1997; 158:1141.

176. Close CE, Dewan PA, Ashwood PJ, et al. Autoaugmentation peritoneocystoplasty in a sheep model. BJU Int 2001; 88:414.

177. Meulen PH, Heesakkers JP, Janknegt RA. A study on the feasibility of vesicomyotomy in patients with motor urge incontinence. Eur Urol 1997; 32(2):166–169.

178. Stohrer M, Kramer G, Goepel M, et al.: Bladder autoaugmentation in adult patients with neurogenic voiding dysfunction. Spinal Cord 1997; 35:456.

179. Leng WW, Blalock HJ, Fredriksson WH, et al. Enterocystoplasty or detrusor myectomy? Comparison of indications and outcomes for bladder augmentation. J Urol 1999; 161:858.

180. Gurocak S, De Gier RPE, Feitz W. Bladder augmentation without integration of intact bowel segments: Critical review and future perspectives. J Urol 2007; 177:839844.

181. Natarajan V, Singh G. Urinary diversion for incontinence in women. Int Urogynecol J Pelvic Floor Dysfunct 2000; 11:180–187.

182. Appell RA. Surgery for the treatment of overactive bladder. Urology 1998; 51:27–29.

183. Liard A, Séguier-Lipszyc E, Mathiot A, Mitrofanoff P. The Mitrofanoff procedure: 20 years later. J Urol 2001; 165(6 Pt 2):2394–2398.

184. Leng WW, Faerber G, Del Terzo M, McGuire EJ. Long-term outcome of incontinent ileovesicostomy management of severe lower urinary tract dysfunction. J Urol 1999; 161(6):1803–1806.

185. Rivas DA, Karasick S, Chancellor MB. Cutaneous ileocystostomy (a bladder chimney) for the treatment of severe neurogenic vesical dysfunction. Paraplegia 1995; 33(9):530–535.

186. Atan A, Konety BR, Nangia A, Chancellor MB. Advantages and risks of ileovesicostomy for the management of neuropathic bladder. Urology 1999; 54(4):636–640.

187. Hsu TH, Rackley RR, Abdelmalak JB, et al. Laparoscopic ileovesicostomy. J Urol 2002; 168(1):180181.

188. Gudziak MR, Tiguert R, Puri K, et al. Management of neurogenic bladder dysfunction with incontinent ileovesicostomy. Urology 1999; 54(6):1008–1011.

189. Tan HJ, Stoffel J, Daignault S, et al. Ileovesicostomy for adults with neurogenic bladders: Complications and potential risk factors for adverse outcomes. Neurourol Urodyn 2008; 27:238–243.

190. Gauthier AR Jr, Winters JC. Incontinent ileovesicostomy in the management of neurogenic bladder dysfunction Neurourol Urodyn 2003; 22(2):142–146.

191. Hétet JF, Rigaud J, Karam G, et al. Complications of Bricker ileal conduit urinary diversion: Analysis of a series of 246 patients. Prog Urol 2005; 15(1):2329.

192. Watanabe T, Rivas DA, Smith R, et al. The effect of urinary tract reconstruction on neurologically impaired women previously treated with an indwelling urethral catheter J Urol 1996; 156(6):1926–1928.

Chapter 20
Botulinum Toxin: An Effective Treatment for Urge Incontinence

Arun Sahai, Mohammad Shamim Khan, and Prokar Dasgupta

Introduction

Overactive bladder (OAB) is a syndrome characterized by urgency with or without urgency incontinence but usually accompanied by frequency and nocturia. The majority of patients have proven detrusor overactivity (DO), but treatment often is instigated without this knowledge by community practitioners based on symptoms alone. The pathophysiology of DO and the pharmacological options for treating patients with this disorder has been the focus of considerable research in recent years.

Therapeutic options are split into initial treatment and specialized therapy. Initial treatment encompasses lifestyle interventions, "bladder training," and the use of oral anticholinergics. Pharmacotherapy in most individuals is still the first-line treatment. Drugs used in OAB act peripherally, with most currently available drugs (anticholinergics) acting on muscarinic receptors. Unfortunately, anticholinergics are associated with troublesome side effects including dry mouth, constipation, blurred vision, drowsiness, and tachycardia and their use is limited because of this and also because patients become refractory to their beneficial effects. In the past these patients were managed with augmentation cystoplasty or urinary diversion. More recently other options have been developed and include sacral neuromodulation and injections of botulinum toxin (BTX) into the bladder (Fig. 20.1). The use of the latter in the lower urinary tract currently is unlicensed and at present experimental, but it appears to be extremely promising. This will be the focus of this chapter, explaining its possible mechanism of action and clinical aspects of its use in the management of urinary tract disorders.

Botulinum Toxin

BTX is a neurotoxin produced by the gram-positive anaerobic spore-producing organism *Clostridium botulinum* (Fig. 20.2). It is one of the most poisonous naturally occurring toxins known to mankind [2]. Its effects range from food poisoning known as "botulism" to an acute and symmetrical paralysis. The severity of its toxic effects ranges from mild weakness to respiratory failure, coma, and death. Seven distinct botulinum neurotoxins (A–G) have been isolated [3]. Types A and B presently are used in clinical medicine, but several other types are the subject of ongoing research.

Currently two pharmaceutical companies market botulinum toxin-A (BTX-A) in the USA and UK. BTX-A has been marketed as BOTOX® in the USA (Allergan Ltd) and as DYSPORT® in the UK (Ipsen Ltd). Its toxicity is measured in mouse units (mU), which is "the amount fatal to 50% of a batch of Swiss Webster mice" [4]. One unit of BOTOX® (Allergan, Ltd, USA) is considered equivalent to 3–4 units of DYSPORT® (Ipsen, Ltd, UK). This is an important point to keep in mind when analyzing different studies, so as not to inadvertently utilize incorrect doses. Botulinum toxin type B (BTX-B) is commercially available as MYOBLOC® in the US (Elan Pharmaceuticals, Inc) and NEUROBLOC® in Europe (Elan Pharma International Ltd).

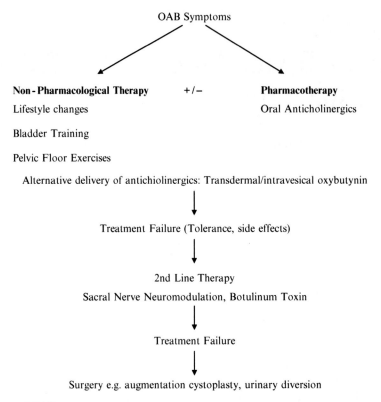

FIG. 20.1. Treatment of OAB

Mechanism of Action and Rationale for Therapeutic Use

The neurotoxin binds to peripheral cholinergic terminals and inhibits acetylcholine release at the neuromuscular junction. Four steps are involved in this process: binding, translocation, cleavage, and inhibition of transmitter release, resulting in blockage of synaptic transmission and flaccid paralysis in the target muscle ensues. Affected nerve terminals do not degenerate and function can be recovered by axonal sprouting and formation of new synaptic contacts [5]. The current view is that the new axons have the ability to form functional sprouts since they contain all the apparatus necessary for exocytosis [6]. However, in a distinct second phase sprouts eventually degenerate and synaptic activity returns in the original nerve terminals [7]. The time required to recover function after BTX paralysis depends on toxin type and type of nerve terminal. The process takes approximately 2–4 months at the mammalian neuromuscular junction and considerably longer in autonomic neurons, in some cases more than a year [8].

BTX is made within the bacterial cytosol and released as a 150-kDa polypeptide chain. Proteolytic cleavage results in a 100-kDa heavy chain and a 50-kDa light chain that remains linked by a noncovalent protein interaction and a disulfide bond essential for neurotoxicity [9, 10]. Once the neurotoxin is released, it diffuses to cholinergic terminals where it binds to as yet unknown receptors on the membrane surface. Once bound, the toxin is internalized inside endocytic vesicles and binds to the lipid bilayer of the vesicle. The heavy chain is thought to play a key role in translocating the light chain into the cytosol, which occurs after the cleavage of the disulfide bond between them. The light chain contains metalloprotease zinc-binding units that have the ability to cleave three soluble N-ethylmaleimide-sensitive factor attachment protein receptors (SNARE) proteins within the nerve terminal [11]. BTXs B, D, F, and G cleave vesicle-associated membrane protein (VAMP)/Synaptobrevin, A and E cleave synaptosomal-associated protein-25 (SNAP-25), and C cleaves both SNAP-25 and syntaxin [12]. As the

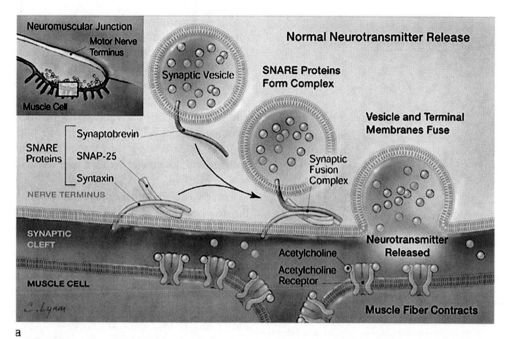

a

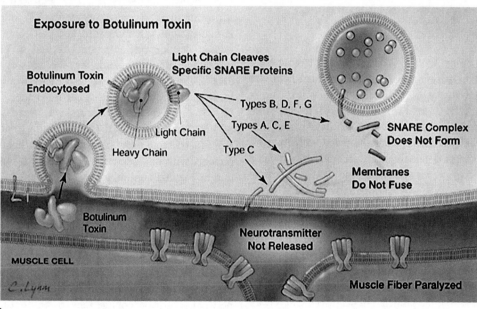

b

FIG. 20.2. Mechanism of action of BTX at the neuromuscular junction. Source [1]

SNARE proteins are essential for normal vesicular transport and fusion, botulinum neurotoxins are able to prevent the release of acetylcholine (ACh) at the presynaptic membrane (Fig. 20.3).

Over 35 years ago, Carpenter reported the effects of acute BTX poisoning in an in vitro rat bladder model [13]. His study showed a marked loss of contraction of the bladder with an associated decrease in ACh release from motor nerve stimulation. Smith reported on the effects of BTX-A on ACh and norepinephrine release from the bladder and urethra of rats, respectively [14]. Rat bladders or urethras were injected with either BTX or sham treatment (normal saline) and the rats were sacrificed

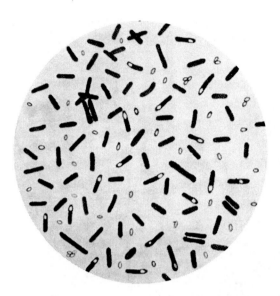

FIG. 20.3. Photomicrograph of *Clostridium botulinum* stained with Gentian violet. Source: http://phil.cdc.gov/phil/details.asp; Centers for disease control and prevention – Public Health Image Library (PHIL)

at either 5 or 30 days. The rat bladder and urethral strips then were isolated and an electrical field was applied to the strips at different frequencies. During 20-Hz electrical field stimulation, ACh release from bladder strips treated with BTX 5 days earlier was significantly reduced when compared with controls. Norepinephrine release from urethral strips treated 30 days prior with BTX during 20-Hz electrical stimulation also was significantly reduced compared with controls. No significant inhibitory effects were found at lower levels of electrical stimulation frequency. ACh release was not affected in 30-day BTX pre-treated rat bladders at 20 Hz nor was norepinephrine release affected by 5 day BTX pretreated rat urethral strips at 20 Hz. From this the authors concluded that the clinical effects of BTX may vary dependent on the anatomical site of injection in the lower urinary tract and the frequency of nerve activity. They postulated that BTX may be more effective at higher stimulation frequencies. This may be of potential clinical significance in cases such as DO and detrusor sphincter dyssynergia where the abnormal nerve hyperactivity affecting the bladder and external sphincter may be inhibited while preserving normal tonic control of bladder and external urethral function, and thus facilitating normal voiding.

Adenosine triphosphate (ATP), a purinergic neurotransmitter, is believed to be coreleased with ACh from parasympathetic cholinergic nerve terminals [15, 16]. It has been postulated that ATP via purinergic mechanisms contributes a significant amount to unstable contractions in IDO [17, 18]. Studies on guinea pig [19, 20] and rat [21, 22] bladder strips have shown that BTX is able to impair both ACh and ATP release, suggesting that its use in treating patients with idiopathic detrusor overactivity (IDO) is well justified.

There has been much excitement recently about the exact mechanism of action of BTX, particularly in the bladder. It is believed to have an effect on the afferent and efferent arms of the micturition reflex and an alternative hypothesis to the long-believed mechanism of action of efferent blockade alone has been proposed [23]. These bladder afferent neurons have several types of receptors, namely vanilloid, purinergic (P2X), neurokinin, and receptors for nerve growth factor (NGF). The neurotransmitters acting at these receptors, namely ATP, substance P, neurokinin A, nitric oxide, and calcitonin gene-related peptide (CGRP), are believed to play an important role in modulating the sensory afferents in the human detrusor, especially in diseased bladder states. The density of substance P and CGRP immunoreactive nerves was increased by 82% in patients with IDO, suggesting that there is an increase in these types of afferent neurons in patients with this condition [24]. In a rat model of chromic spinal cord injury and neurogenic detrusor overactivity (NDO), BTX-A significantly reduced the abnormal distension-evoked urothelial release of ATP [25]. BTX-A also significantly reduced the evoked release of CGRP compared to controls from isolated rat bladders [26]. In a rat bladder pain model, following acetic acid instillation, a significant improvement was demonstrated in the interval between detrusor contractions in those that had received BTX-A with reduced CGRP release from the bladder [27]. The toxin also has been shown to reduce ATP and capsaicin-induced DO in a rat model [28]. Apostolidis et al. have proposed that the primary peripheral effect of BTX-A involves the inhibition of ACh, ATP, and substance P release as well as a downregulation in the expression of capsaicin and purinergic receptors [29]. Studies of bladder biopsies taken at 4 and 16 weeks following intradetrusor BTX-A injections have shown a reduced expression of TRPV1 and P2X$_3$ in the suburothelium of patients with NDO and IDO [30]. Both these sensory receptors are upregulated in IDO and NDO and their levels by 16 weeks normalize to that of controls following administration of 200 and 300 U of BTX-A (BOTOX®, Allergan, Ltd).

Further evidence in support of the afferent mechanism of action comes from a proposed antinociceptive effect separate to its neuromuscular action. Welch et al. has reported that neurotransmitter release from rat dorsal root ganglia was inhibited by various isoforms of BTX [31]. Another group reported on the inhibitory effect of BTX on the release of radioactive-labeled glutamate from rat dorsal root ganglia [32]. In vivo studies have shown that pretreatment with BTX significantly reduced pain in a formalin-induced inflammatory rat model at 5 and 12 days postinjection [33]. This was associated with a reduction in glutamate release from primary afferent terminal and C-fos expression (usually expressed with neuronal stimuli) compared with controls. It was presumed that if a peripheral pain mediator such as glutamate release could be reduced, peripheral sensitization would be blocked, which would indirectly reduce central sensitization [34]. Additional evidence comes from Jankovic and Schwartz in their human study, treating patients with cervical dystonia [35]. They documented that pain improved, soon after injection with BTX, before a reduction in muscle spasm could be detected, implying that a mechanism other than flaccid paralysis of the muscle caused by the toxin may be involved.

As afferent mechanisms may be important in the pathophysiology of DO, the excellent therapeutic efficacy of BTX may be explained in part by this proposed dual mechanism of action. In addition, due to its antinociceptive effect seen in animal models there is a potential for treating conditions such as interstitial cystitis and painful bladder syndrome whether accompanied by DO or not, although this needs further clinical study.

Applications in Medicine and Urinary Tract

The fact that local injection of the toxin into striated muscle can induce paralysis has spurred researchers to investigate its effects in muscle overactivity. Autonomic effects are also observed, as it blocks acetylcholine release in all parasympathetic and at postganglionic sympathetic neurons. There is growing interest in the therapeutic application of BTX to treat overactive smooth muscle conditions and disorders where there is abnormal activity due to excessive postganglionic sympathetic activity such as hyperhidrosis.

BTX currently is licensed for use in cervical dystonia, strabismus, blepharospasm, hemifacial spasm, glabellar wrinkles, focal spasticity including dynamic equines foot deformity due to pediatric cerebral palsy, and severe primary axillary hyperhidrosis not adequately managed with topical agents. It has received a lot of media attention recently for its cosmetic potential in reducing facial wrinkles and rejuvenating facial appearances. Only in recent years has the urology community looked into the potential benefit of this toxin in the urinary tract.

BTX is not currently licensed for use in the urinary tract. Much of the preliminary work carried out to date has focused on intradetrusor injections and treating DO and symptoms of OAB. It has been used, however, with success in treating detrusor sphincter dyssynergia following external sphincter injections and its application has expanded to include prostatitis, chronic prostatic/pelvic pain, benign prostatic hyperplasia, chronic retention, as well as other aspects of voiding dysfunction [36–38]. The rest of this chapter will focus on the use of BTX to treat DO and OAB.

OAB and Detrusor Overactivity

Botulinum Toxin-A

Neurogenic Detrusor Overactivity

The application of BTX-A in DO was pioneered by Brigitte Schurch [39]. Urodynamically proven NDO patients with spinal cord injury who emptied their bladder with clean intermittent self-catheterization (CISC) were recruited into their preliminary study. Patients were injected with either 200 or 300 U of BTX-A (BOTOX®) into the bladder at 30 different sites using a rigid cystoscope. The trigone was spared to avoid the potential complication of vesicoureteric reflux (VUR). At 6-week follow up, 17 of the 19 patients were completely continent based on subjective analysis of their voiding diaries. Two patients who remained incontinent had moderate improvement in symptoms and had received the lower dose of toxin at 200 U. Ten patients managed to reduce the dose, while seven patients discontinued anticholinergic medication all together. Urodynamics confirmed significant increases in mean cystometric capacity (MCC) from a mean value of 296.3–480.5 ml and a decrease in maximum detrusor voiding pressure (MDVP) from 65.6 to 35.0 cm H_2O. At 16 and 36 weeks postinjection 11 patients had been followed up and showed ongoing improvement in bladder function. Seven patients remained continent and in four, mild incontinence was observed which was attributed to bladder infection. No side effects were observed. The effect of injections lasted for at least 9 months, longer than the duration of efficacy reported when the toxin had been injected into the external urethral sphincter. This is attributed to the different mode of action of BTX on different types of muscle in the bladder and external sphincter.

Its efficacy in treating NDO in further small open-labeled studies has been confirmed using 300 or 400 U (BOTOX®) in patients with spinal cord injury [40–42] or multiple sclerosis [43]. Its use in NDO and poorly compliant bladders also had favorable outcome, although an improvement in compliance did not necessarily equate to continence and vice versa [42, 44]. Significant increases in MCC and reflex volume as well as a decrease in MDVP also have been reported in the largest retrospective study consisting of 200 patients with NDO, at 6 and 36 weeks following injection of 300 U (BOTOX®) [45]. Continence was achieved in 132 of 180 patients with 48 reporting some improvement with incontinence. Kuo recently has conducted a comparative study in patients with NDO with either cerebral vascular accident (CVA) or a suprasacral spinal cord lesion. Both groups were injected with 200 U (BOTOX®) [46]. Although reflex volume and MCC increased in those with CVA, large postvoid residuals (PVRs) were noted with little change in incontinence. Overall, however a successful result (either continence or a subjective improvement in incontinence) was noted in 50% in those with CVA compared with 92% in the spinal cord injury group.

More recently several studies have shown that DYSPORT® also has a place in managing NDO [47–49]. Ruffion et al. reported a "good success" defined as no leakage following treatment with either 500 or 1,000 U BTX-A (DYSPORT®) in 76% of patients

[50]. A dose of 1,000 U had a significantly longer median duration of action, but one case of generalized muscle weakness was reported for 1 month. Grosse et al. assessed long-term efficacy with repeat injections of BOTOX® and DYSORT® [51], where the majority of NDO patients assessed had up to four repeat injections without any loss of therapeutic efficacy. There was no statistically significant change in interval between injections (average 9–11 months). The authors concluded that the optimal dose of DYSPORT® for this indication would be 750 U. Finally, Patki et al. in their series of 37 spinal cord injury patients concluded that 1,000 U was effective in treating NDO, with improvements in quality of life (QOL) scores and urodynamic parameters and additionally 50% of patients being able to stop anticholinergic medication [52]. However, two cases of transient muscle weakness were observed with this dose.

Until recently there had been a lack of level I evidence based on randomized, placebo-controlled trials to further validate the use of BTX in this setting. However, in 2005, Schurch reported the first double-blind, randomized placebo-controlled trial involving 59 NDO patients who were randomized to receive in a 1:1:1 ratio, 200 or 300 U BTX-A (BOTOX®) or placebo [50]. Patients were followed up at 2, 6, 12, 18, and 24 weeks. The results are summarized in Table 20.1. The primary endpoint of incontinence episodes decreased significantly at all time points except at 12 and 18 weeks in the 200-U group. Interestingly, when compared with placebo, improvements only reached statistical significance in the 300-U group at 2 and 6 weeks and in the 200-U group at 24 weeks. Patients receiving BTX-A at either dose showed significant improvement in quality of life as assessed by the incontinence quality of life (I-QOL) questionnaire administered at all follow-up timepoints. No severe adverse events were reported. The most common reported adverse event was urinary tract infection in 22% of the patients. They concluded that 200 or 300 U was equally efficacious. Surprisingly, anticholinergic use remained similar in the study and no data were reported on urinary urgency or PVR.

BTX-A versus Resiniferatoxin

Resiniferatoxin (RTX) is extracted from a cactus-like plant called *Euphorbia resinifera* and is an analogue of capsaicin [51]. Both capsaicin and RTX

TABLE 20.1. Summary of results from a double-blind, randomized placebo-controlled trial of BTX-A in patients with NDO.

Variable/time point (weeks)	300 u BTX-A (n = 19)	200 u BTX-A (n = 19)	Placebo (n = 21)
Incontinence episodes			
Baseline	2.8 (1.86)	1.9 (1.78)	3.0 (3.29)
2	−1.3 (1.39)[a]	−1.0 (1.67)[b]	−0.2 (1.02)
6	−1.5 (2.33)[a]	−0.9 (1.84)[b]	−0.2 (1.45)
12	−1.2 (1.66)[b]	−0.9 (2.14)	−0.3 (1.46)
18	−1.2 (1.16)[b]	−0.8 (2.75)	−0.3 (1.59)
24	−0.9 (1.34)[b]	−1.1 (1.92)[a]	−0.1 (1.09)
MCC (mL)			
Baseline	293.6	260.2	254.6
2	479.6 (186.1)[a,b]	482.5 (215.8)[a,b]	282.0 (27.4)
6	462.7 (169.1)[a,b]	448.8 (182.1)[a]	299.6 (45.0)
24	398.2 (92.9)[b]	440.9 (174.2)[a,b]	301.0 (41.6)
RDV (mL)			
Baseline	254.8	169.1	202.4
2	198.1 (8.6)	306.9 (135.3)[b]	206.7 (4.3)
6	268.5 (96.0)[b]	234.2 (47.3)	244.6 (42.6)
24	305.4 (72.4)	327.4 (144.6)[a,b]	226.4 (23.5)
MDP (cm H_2O)			
Baseline	92.6	77.0	79.1
2	41.0 (−66.3)[a,b]	31.6 (−52.9)[a,b]	71.4 (−7.7)
6	45.9 (−62.2)	40.1 (−44.4)[a,b]	69.0 (−10.1)
24	55.2 (−35.5)[a,b]	48.8 (−38.7)[a,b]	80.6 (−1.4)

Source [50]. Mean values (mean change from baseline)
[a]Statistically significant within-group changes from baseline and versus placebo
[b]Statistically significant changes versus placebo

are vanilloids, adopting the vanillyl moiety, and act at the transient receptor potential channel or vanilloid subfamily member-1 (TRPV1) receptor. Vanilloid receptors are predominantly present on C-fiber bladder afferents and upon activation by vanilloids initially excite but subsequently desensitize the C-fibers [52]. This formed the basis of treatment with these compounds as this abnormal spinal micturition reflex can be blocked by their administration, reversibly [53]. Their use at present is experimental. Giannantoni et al. reported on a randomized trial of RTX versus BTX-A in 25 patients with NDO secondary to spinal cord injury [54]. Patients were randomized to receive either O.6 mM RTX in 50 ml of normal saline or 300 U of BTX-A (BOTOX®). Follow-up consisted of voiding diary assessment and urodynamic studies at 6, 12, and 18 months. RTX (n = 13) was found to reduce incontinence episodes and reduce the need for catheterization compared with baseline values at all follow-up timepoints. Continence was achieved in five patients. There was a significant increase in the uninhibited detrusor contraction threshold and in MCC. The average number of RTX instillations per patient was 8.6±1.9 with a mean time between instillations of 51.6±8.2 days. In the BTX arm, the number of incontinence episodes and catheterization frequency was significantly reduced at all follow-up timepoints. At 6 and 12 months, nine patients were dry and this reduced to 6 by 18 months. Urodynamics revealed a significant increase in the uninhibited detrusor contraction threshold and in MCC and a significant decrease in maximum pressure of uninhibited detrusor contractions (MDP) compared to baseline values. Patients required a mean number of 2.1±0.7 treatments, with the mean time between treatments being 6.8±1.5 months. When comparing the two treatments there was a significant decrease in incontinence episodes using BTX compared with RTX at all timepoints. There was a significant increase in the uninhibited detrusor contractions threshold and in MCC with a significant decrease in MDP in the BTX treatment group compared with RTX at 6, 12, and 18 months. Certainly in this subgroup of patients BTX treatment appears to be superior to RTX in terms of clinical and urodynamic benefit.

Idiopathic Detrusor Overactivity

After successful trials of BTX-A in NDO patients, Rapp et al. reported on the use of 300 U (BOTOX®) of BTX-A in patients with OAB who were predominantly nonneurogenic in origin [55]. Thirty-five patients were initially assessed and 21 patients (60%) showed either complete resolution or improvement of their symptoms at 3 weeks. Overall there was a significant improvement in quality of life as assessed by the Urogenital Distress Inventory (UDI-6) and the Incontinence Impact Questionnaire (IIQ-7). Twenty-four patients completed the study at 6 months of which 14 were initial responders at 3 weeks. Of these 14 patients quality of life also was significantly improved at 6 months. Mean daily pad usage significantly reduced in those with urge incontinence from 3.9 to 1.8 per day. Side effects were minimal with mild hematuria, dysuria, and pelvic pain reported in seven patients. A major drawback of this study was the lack of urodynamics performed prior to injections to confirm DO.

Smith et al. have reviewed their experience of using BTX-A in the lower urinary tract over a 6-year period [56]. In their series, 38 patients underwent bladder injections for either NDO or IDO. Between 100 and 300 U of BTX-A (BOTOX®) was injected, although the exact dose given for the various indications was not stated. They employed 30–40 injections in patients with NDO and ten injections for those with IDO. The technique included injecting the trigone. Data presented were pooled for analysis in both NDO and IDO. Improvements were seen at 6 months in MCC, maximal voiding pressure, pad usage, and urinary frequency. There was no significant increase in PVR, a potential concern in patients with OAB and IDO. An excellent response was perceived (on a 3-point scale: excellent, fair response, no improvement) by approximately 50% of the patients with NDO and IDO. Kuo et al. reported on suburothelial injections of 200 U in 20 patients with nonneurogenic detrusor activity (IDO or following transurethral resection of prostate) restoring continence in nine patients, with improvement in eight,

and failure in three at 3 months [57]. Six patients developed transient urinary retention and ten had a PVR of >250 ml at 2 weeks. Overall, 15 (75%) had difficulty voiding and incomplete emptying in the follow-up period; six required clean intermittent self-catheterization (CISC).

Significant reductions in frequency and nocturia and an increase in MCC at 4 and 12 weeks following 100 U BTX-A (BOTOX®) have been reported in females with IDO [58]. PVR was increased at 4 weeks but only two patients required CISC and this was only for 1 week. At 4 weeks 18/26, 12 weeks 16/20, and at 36 weeks 1/5 were continent. Using the King's Health Questionnaire (KHQ) significant subjective improvement in all urge-related parameters was seen at 4 and 12 weeks. Thirty-one percent of women developed urinary tract infections and there were two non-responders.

Symptomatic improvement with BTX-A is a consistent finding from other uncontrolled studies in patients with OAB [59, 60]. Popat and colleagues compared the response to 200 U in IDO with 300 U in NDO and concluded that each provided significant benefit, although the percent reduction in urgency in the NDO group was better compared with the IDO group at 4 and 16 weeks postinjection [61]. The same group when analyzing QOL following BTX-A treatment in NDO and IDO patients found significant benefit when using the UDI-6 and IIQ-7 short forms [62]. On the whole improvement in QOL correlated with improvements in OAB symptoms but not with urodynamic changes.

In order to combat the risk of developing high PVR in patients with IDO a recent study compared bladder injections with bladder and urethral sphincter injections in combination in 44 predominantly female patients [63]. Those with a residual of ³15 ml at baseline were given the sphincteric injection since it was felt they were more prone to developing higher residuals following BTX. Between 200 and 300 U were administered in total with 50–100 U given in the external sphincter. Improvements in frequency, pad usage, and urodynamic parameters were observed and in 86% of cases patients were willing to undergo repeat procedures. Significant reduction in incontinence questionnaires using the short form Urogenital Distress Inventory (UDI-6), Symptom Severity Index, and Symptom Impact Index also were seen for up to 6 months. These positive results were similar for both groups, but a significant PVR at 4 weeks was seen in those with bladder injection alone compared to combination treatment. The development of de novo stress incontinence in those who received sphincteric injections was not proven. Pad usage at 4 weeks was similar in both groups and when assessing the incontinence questionnaires regarding this aspect, although more patients answered in favor of stress symptoms in the combination group, this did not reach statistical significance. No significant side effects were reported.

The largest series to date recruited 100 patients with symptoms of OAB and were treated with 100 U of BTX-A (BOTOX®) [64]. Fifty-four patients had IDO and the remainder sensory urgency (OAB syndrome but without DO on urodynamic studies). Significant improvements in symptomology and urodynamic parameters were seen. Increases in MCC and first desire to void correlated with decreases in daytime frequency and nocturia. Efficacy was quoted as 6±2 months; however, only 20 patients were assessed fully at 9 months. QOL as assessed by the KHQ improved at 4 and 12 weeks in all urge related items. Ninety percent experienced improvement in at least one KHQ domain. Nineteen patients developed voiding

dysfunction following injections (PVR >150 ml) but only four patients required CISC. Eight patients were deemed to have failed treatment (no clinical or urodynamic benefit). All of these had a low detrusor compliance (<10 ml/cm H_2O) and had maximum bladder capacities of <100 ml due to bladder wall fibrosis as assessed by detrusor biopsies. Repeat injections in these cases did not change outcome.

The first randomized placebo-controlled trial in patients with IDO refractory to anticholinergics was recently reported [65] involving the use of 200 U or placebo (normal saline) administered using a flexible cystoscopic technique under local anesthetic. Thirty-four patients were randomized: 16 to BTX-A and 18 to placebo. Baseline characteristics were comparable with an almost equal mix of males and females. The primary endpoint, MCC, increased significantly, and improvement in symptoms, urodynamic, and QOL parameters using the UDI-6 and IIQ-7 was seen in patients in the BTX-A group compared with placebo (see Table 20.2–20.4). Four weeks after treatment, continence was restored in 2 of 16 (12.5%) of those in the placebo group and 8 of 16 (50%) in the BTX-A group who were incontinent at baseline. By 12 weeks, all patients in the placebo group were again incontinent. In the BTX-A group,

TABLE 20.2. Summary of results from a double-blind, randomized placebo-controlled trial of BTX-A in patients with IDO.

Mean value	BTX-A	Placebo	Difference between means (95% Cl)	P
Frequency				
Baseline	15.44	14.33		NS
4 weeks	7.93 (–7.51)	13.30 (–1.03)	–5.37 (–8.82 to –3.78)	<0.0001
12 weeks	9.25 (–6.19)	13.19 (–1.14)	–3.94 (–7.05 to –1.55)	0.0033
Urgency				
Baseline	11.69	7.31		0.0008
4 weeks	2.48 (–9.21)	6.02 (–1.29)	–3.54 (–6.56 to –1.30)	0.0047
12 weeks	3.50 (–8.19)	6.39 (–0.92)	–2.89 (–6.84 to 0.50)	0.0878
Urgency incontinence				
Baseline	4.98	3.91		NS
4 weeks	1.90 (–3.08)	3.17 (–0.74)	–1.27 (–3.79 to –0.23)	0.0284
12 weeks	1.48 (–3.50)	3.20 (–0.71)	–1.72 (–3.78 to –0.63)	0.0076

Frequency – number of micturitions per day; urgency – defined as the sudden desire to pass urine which cannot be deferred; urgency incontinence – defined as urinary leakage associated with urgency. NS = Nonsignificant. Voiding diary data. Source [65] Mean number of daily OAB symptoms following BTX-A treatment (mean change from baseline). Numbers refer to an average of 3 days

TABLE 20.3. Summary of results from a double-blind randomized placebo-controlled trial of BTX-A in patients with IDO.

Mean value	BTX-A	Placebo	Difference between means (95% Cl)	P
MCC (ml)				
Baseline	181.81	198.06		NS
4 weekst	313.25 (+131.44)	168.56 (−29.50)	144.69 (100.95 to 215.75)	<0.0001
12 weeks	263.88 (+82.06)	168.17 (−29.89)	95.71 (47.47 to 172.45)	0.0011
MDP (cm H_2O)				
Baseline	85.06	78.67		NS
4 weeks	34.69 (−50.38)	75.22 (−3.44)	−40.53 (−61.48 to −28.99)	<0.0001
12 weeks	43.81 (−41.25)	78.67 (−0.00)	−34.86 (−55.12 to −24.16)	<0.0001
PVR (cm H_2O)				
Baseline	44.06	22.50		NS
4 weeks	96.13 (+52.06)	31.39 (+8.89)	64.74 (7.30 to 94.18)	0.0235
12 weeks	51.19 (+7.13)	22.50 (−0.00)	28.69 (−24.20 to 58.31)	0.4056
RDV (mL)				
Baseline	124.25	122.53		NS
4 weeks	217.32 (+93.07)	100.89 (−21.64)	116.43 (62.77 to 169.23)	0.0001
12 weeks	147.33 (+23.08)	93.11 (−29.42)	54.22 (7.60 to 99.25)	0.0238

Urodynamic data. Source [65] Urodynamic parameters following BTX-A treatment (mean change from baseline). MCC = Maximum cystometric capacity; MDP = maximum detrusor pressure during filling cystometry; PVR = postvoid residual; RDV = reflex detrusor volume NS = Nonsignificant

TABLE 20.4. Summary of results from a double-blind, randomized placebo-controlled trial of BTX-A in patients with IDO.

Mean value	BTX-A	Placebo	Difference between means (95% Cl)	P
IIQ-7				
Baseline	18.31	14.78		NS
4 weeks	6.00 (−12.31)	10.67 (−4.11)	−4.67 (−10.99 to −0.78)	0.0253
12 weeks	7.94 (−10.38)	15.39 (+0.61)	−7.45 (−13.92 to −2.50)	0.0063
UDI-6				
Baseline	10.75	9.50		NS
4 weeks	5.60 (−5.15)	9.00 (−0.50)	−3.40 (−6.17 to −2.08)	0.0003
12 weeks	5.13 (−5.63)	10.00 (+0.50)	−4.87 (−7.83 to −2.96)	<0.0001

QOL data. Source [65] Quality of life after BTX-A treatment (mean change from baseline). IIQ-7 = Incontinence impact questionnaire short form; UDI-6 = Urogenital Distress Inventory short form; lower scores indicate better QOL. NS = Nonsignificant

50% remained continent at 12 and 24 weeks. Following BTX-A, urinary frequency had normalized in 57, 44, and 36% of patients at 4, 12, and 24 weeks, respectively. In the placebo group, only 11% showed frequency normalization at 4 and 12 weeks. Unblinding took place after 12 weeks and data from the open labeled extension study suggested the beneficial effects of BTX-A lasted at least for 24 weeks. No major complications were noted. Six patients, all in the BTX-A group, had symptomatic >150 ml residual volume at follow-up and were taught CISC.

Pediatric Use

The first published series recruited 17 children (mean age 10.8 years) with myelomeningocoele (MMC) and NDO resistant to anticholinergic medication [66]. BTX-A was injected at 12 U/kg (BOTOX®) to a maximum of 300 U. Significant increases in mean reflex volume (95 vs. 201.45 ml), MCC (137.53 vs. 215.25 ml), and detrusor compliance (20.39 vs. 45.18 ml/cm H_2O) with decreases in MDP (58.94 vs. 39.75 cm H_2O) were observed. No side effects were reported and the beneficial effects lasted up to

6 months. A similar study in 15 patients with MMC and NDO confirmed clinical and urodynamic benefit in patients, with a mean durability of the effect of the toxin for 10.5 months [67]. After repeat injection of the same dose similar beneficial results were reproduced. Twenty patients with MMC or sacral agenesis were injected with 100–300 U of BTX-A at 5 U/kg in another recent study [68]. Sixty-five percent were continent after the first injection and this was associated with significant increases in MCC and a reduction in MDP. Treatment appeared to last for 6–9 months and no adverse effects were reported. Seven patients showed no response and in six despite another injection, no improvement was seen. Recently one study has shown the potential benefits in children (mean age 10.8 years) with IDO refractory to anticholinergics [69]. Assessment was based on 15 patients with at least a 6-month follow-up. After one injection of 100 U (BOTOX®) nine patients had no evidence of urgency or urgency incontinence, three patients a partial response, and no change in three. Eight patients maintained good efficacy even at 12 months follow-up. Four patients were reported to have temporary dysfunctional characteristics on postinjection uroflowometry, of which one girl required temporary CISC. One boy was assumed to have developed VUR since he had loin pain on voiding, although this was never substantiated by micturating cystourethrogram.

It is important to point out that little is known of the long-term effects of repeated injections in children. However, Schulte-Baukloh et al. reported on ten children (all of whom had three injections and four children had five injections) who had repeat injections of BTX-A, following on from their preliminary series [66, 70]. Even after five injections, clear urodynamic benefit was observed with no evidence of drug tolerance. The effect on MDP seemed to be better after the third or fifth injections in contrast to after their first. Of major concern, however, was the observation that baseline detrusor compliance after the treatment effect began wearing off appeared to progressively decrease over time, from 21.7 to 10.3 ml/cm H_2O following the first to after the fifth injection.

Botulinum Toxin-B

BTX-B recently has been used to treat a patient with multiple sclerosis who had NDO resistant to anticholinergics [71]. Before treatment, urody-

namics confirmed severe DO. A dose of 5,000 U (MYOBLOC®) was given initially in ten different sites into the bladder. Symptoms began improving within 24 h and urodynamics 2 months later showed no evidence of DO. The effect of injection lasted approximately 4 months. Following from this case 15 female patients with IDO were recruited to a dose escalation study to determine the efficacy of BTX-B (MYOBLOC®) [72]. The duration of response was dose-related, with maximal benefit lasting approximately 3 months in patients receiving 10,000 or 15,000 U. All but one patient responded, who received the lowest dose (2,500 U). All patients were asked to keep a voiding diary every 2 weeks postinjection and were noted to have an average of 5.27 fewer episodes of frequency per day after treatment. Since then, three further cases have been published with patients with NDO who were clinically suspected and electrophysiologically proven to have resistance to BTX-A, who were successfully treated with BTX-B (NEUROBLOC®) [73, 74]. A recent double-blind, controlled crossover trial in patients with IDO and NDO randomized patients to either 5,000 U of BTX-B or placebo [75]. Significant improvements were observed in average voided volume, frequency, incontinence episodes, and in quality of life using the KHQ, but the effects appeared to last for only 6 weeks. CISC was required in two patients. Other side effects included constipation ($n = 2$), dry mouth ($n = 2$), and general malaise was seen in one other patient. Although effective in treating symptoms, the effects appear to be too short-lived to merit use over BTX-A therapy. The use of BTX-B, in our opinion, should be reserved for those who fail treatment with or develop antibodies to BTX-A.

Techniques of Intradetrusor Administration of BTX

The original description of BTX-A injections for the treatment of NDO was through a collagen flexible needle using a rigid cystoscope [39]. Since then the technique has evolved, but the way in which the toxin is administered into the bladder has not been standardized, and indeed practice varies around the world. In the initial experience with BTX-A and NDO, the trigone was avoided on the assumption that paralyzing the trigonal muscle might induce

VUR. Since then there has been mounting evidence that BTX also may affect sensory nerves and that afferent mechanisms have an important role in the pathophysiology of DO [76]. Investigators in the United States have advocated injecting the trigone [56] based on the fact that this area of the bladder contains the highest density of nerve fibers, including afferent population. These authors did not formally assess patients for VUR but reported no episodes of symptomatic pyelonephritis in the treated patients. To resolve the issue as to which method is more efficacious in the treatment of DO, trials of trigonal versus nontrigonal injections of BTX are eagerly awaited.

An open label study using BTX-A for both NDO and IDO patients was begun in 2002 [61]. Initially BTX was injected using a rigid cystoscope under sedation. Thereafter, involved clinicians, led by Prokar Dasgupta at the National Hospital for Neurology and Neurosurgery, London (NHNN), began exploring an alternative method using a flexible cystoscope and an ultra-fine 4-mm flexible needle (Olympus, Keymed, UK) to perform injections. The objective was to ensure that the toxin could be delivered at an optimal depth into the submucosa or detrusor muscle, but not beyond. Experiments were carried out that involved injecting oranges under water using the ultra-fine needle, but it was soon realized that the needle was not steady enough to pierce the fruit's tegument. To overcome this difficulty a fine sheath (27 G) was introduced through the working channel of the cystoscope and the ultra-fine needle was passed through this sheath. The sheath not only provided the necessary stability to the needle resulting in excellent operator control and precision injection, but also provided protection to the flexible cystoscope in case of inadvertent puncture while feeding the needle down the channel. This was soon translated into clinical practice, and since has become known as the "Dasgupta technique," a minimally invasive daycase procedure performed under local anesthesia [77, 78].

Prophylactic antibiotics and 20 ml of 2% lignocaine intraurethral gel are administered prior to the procedure. The injections are evenly distributed over the dome, posterior, right, and left lateral walls of the bladder, avoiding the trigone (Fig. 20.4 and 20.5). The technique has obvious benefits in terms of cost and ease of administration, particularly in those with

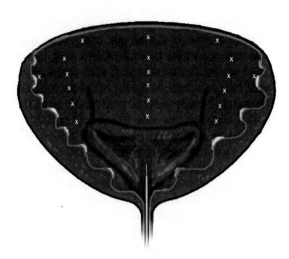

FIG. 20.4. Dasgupta technique: mapping of BTX injections

advanced neurological disease or significant comorbidity who are not fit for general or spinal anesthesia. In addition, the needle length is such that injection beyond the bladder is unlikely. Furthermore as an ultra-fine needle is used, the chance of backflow of the toxin after removal of the needle is reduced. These two important considerations may challenge the practice of using a longer and wider collagen needle with a rigid cystoscope, as traditionally employed in mainland Europe and the United States.

The "Dasgupta technique" is quick; the procedure taking on average 20 min to perform and also is well tolerated [61]. Patients who have a good response to treatment are willing to undergo repeat injections when their symptoms recur, which provides the most robust evidence to the technique's popularity. In the very few patients who tolerated the procedure poorly, instillation of 40 ml of 2% lignocaine for 30 min prior to injections eased the discomfort and made subsequent injections easily tolerable.

This minimally invasive technique has been adopted by some clinicians in the United States to treat patients with refractory OAB using 100 U of BTX-A [79]. Ten injections are utilized and injected submucosally into the bladder base and trigone only. In their series of ten patients similar efficacy was reproduced compared with their older rigid cystoscopic technique involving 30 injection sites. The added benefit appears to be that no patient developed urinary retention or an elevated

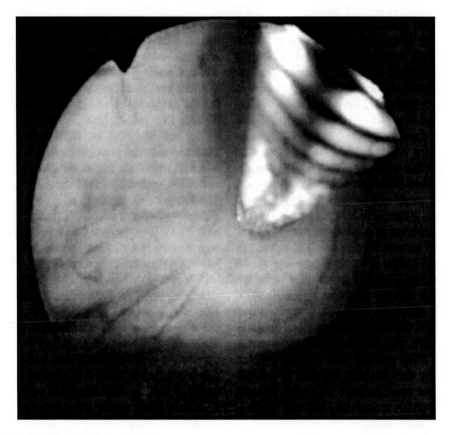

FIG. 20.5. Suburothelial injection of BTX

PVR with the use of a reduced dose of BTX-A and this modified technique.

It has been suggested that clinicians using the technique either for the first few injections or for teaching or demonstration purposes might add a dye to the reconstituted BTX such as indigo carmine [80] or methylene blue, to help identify injected areas and facilitate placement of further injections. Caution should be taken while doing this as redox reagents like methylene blue can detoxify BTX by photo-oxidation.

As there are no standardized guidelines or outcome measures of what constitutes "success" and "failure" with this form of therapy, evaluating which of the currently used techniques is superior is difficult. Further trials and perhaps head-to-head comparisons of rigid versus flexible cystoscopic techniques with the same outcomes being measured will establish whether the technique of administration has a role in efficacy of treatment. Certainly injecting the trigone in a systematic way will not be easily achieved using

a flexible cystoscope. It is reassuring that the results obtained using the flexible technique are comparable to and in some cases surpass those published globally using rigid cystoscopy.

Side Effects of BTX

Side effects of BTX are rare especially when considering its urological uses. Localized injection into the detrusor muscle may be associated rarely with an allergic reaction to the toxin or transient flu-like symptoms. Depending on the technique employed it is possible for patients to develop hematuria which in some cases may need admission and irrigation to resolve [49]. On the whole the injection technique is well tolerated even under local anesthetic with discomfort scores using a verbal 11-point Box Scale being 3.3±0.3 and 3.2±0.4 for patients with NDO and IDO, respectively [61]. Doses used in the intradetrusor injection of BTX are well below (one thousandth) the presumed fatal dose in a 70-kg man [81] and as the injection is localized, minute quantities only reach the systemic circulation. However, cases of generalized muscle weakness and prolonged paralysis in upper or lower limbs have been reported following BTX injection into the detrusor muscle [47–49, 82]. Some authors have speculated that the cumulative dose may have been too high or injection might have taken place in a thin-walled bladder where perivesical diffusion of the toxin took place, although this could not be proven. Another possibility is that systemic effects may be related to volume administered as opposed to dose.

Perhaps of greatest concern to patients is the theoretical possibility of hypocontractility of the detrusor resulting in voiding dysfunction with high PVRs or frank urinary retention following BTX injections. If this were to occur, patients would need to perform CISC until the effects of the toxin began to subside. This may not be of consequence to the many NDO patients who already perform CISC to empty their bladders but may be a major undertaking for some patients with IDO. Patients must have the ability to perform CISC and be counseled appropriately prior to the treatment.

While using BTX-A (MYOBLOC®) at a dose of 15,000 U, two patients experienced dry mouth and generalized malaise in a recent dose escalation study, and hence the authors have recommended that doses above this should be avoided [72]. At lower doses similar effects have been reported as well as constipation [75].

BTX treatment is to be avoided in any patient with preexisting neuromuscular conditions such as myasthenia gravis or Eaton-Lambert syndrome. Aminoglycosides such as gentamycin, commonly used by urologists, may potentiate neuromuscular weakness caused by BTX [83], and therefore these antibiotics also should be avoided in patients undergoing treatment. In certain clinical situations, repeat injections of BTX-A can cause an immune response with the build up of tolerance to its effects [84], although this happens in <5% of cases. The uses of other serotypes therefore are being investigated as an alternative therapy to type A toxin. BTX-C is thought to give a long-lasting paralysis similar to A [85], whereas the VAMP-associated toxins (B, D, F) are felt to have shorter duration of action [86]. When comparing serotypes of the toxin in a rat bladder model using fatigue stimulation, BTX-D was shown to elicit a more rapid response and a greater maximal inhibitory effect at 1 hour compared with type A [87].

Many urologists have expressed concern regarding the long-term effects of this form of treatment. To date two studies have reported on the repeatability and longevity of BTX treatment in both adult and pediatric populations [47, 70]. Additional concerns regarding histological change and long-term fibrosis recently have been addressed [88, 89]. Hafekamp et al. reported on a lack of structural changes before and after BTX injections in patients with NDO [90]. Contrary to reports with striated muscle very little axonal sprouting was observed following treatment. Comperat et al., when assessing bladder tissue at cystectomy in those who had previously received BTX injections within the last year with a control group, showed no difference in inflammation and edema [88]. Interestingly, those who had received BTX had less fibrosis of the bladder wall than those who had not, although this was based on their own grading scale using a cutoff of 20% ie, mild fibrosis if occupying <20% of muscle fibers and/or submucosa and important fibrosis if >20%.

Summary

In summary, BTX therapy appears to be a very attractive pharmacological agent to treat patients with DO resistant to anticholinergics and patients with symptoms of OAB. Recent evidence from randomized, controlled trials suggests that it is an effective treatment in both NDO and IDO. BTX-B is probably best reserved for those in whom treatment has failed with BTX-A. Whether other botulinum toxins will be come available for clinical use is not yet clear. Certainly further studies are needed to decide what is the optimum dose (currently being 300 U for NDO and between 100 and 200 U for IDO), for patients receiving BOTOX®. For those using DYSPORT® for NDO there is perhaps a consensus emerging that 750 U may be the optimum dose. Dose escalation studies currently are underway for patients with IDO and will help clarify the optimum dose in this setting, although the authors of this chapter believe that the dose will depend on certain patient factors such as severity of DO and that not one dose will "fix all," so to speak. The way in which the toxin is administered into the bladder has not been standardized, and indeed practice varies around the world. Whether the technique of administration has a role in efficacy of treatment also is uncertain. Further study with regard to distribution, depth, and volume of injection are necessary. The majority of side effects are minor and are related to infection, hematuria, and impaired contractility of the detrusor, resulting in high PVR. Careful counseling is mandatory in this context and patients' should be both physically able and willing to perform CISC prior to commencing treatment. This is particularly important for those with IDO. OAB is a chronic, debilitating condition that puts a huge strain on health resources worldwide. BTX is emerging as a useful therapeutic option in treating these patients, filling the void between anticholinergics and surgery. It is truly remarkable how one of the most poisonous substances known to mankind has been incorporated into the urologist's armory in treating such patients.

References

1. Arnon SS, Schechter R, Inglesby TV, et al. Botulinum toxin as a biological weapon: Medical and public health management. JAMA 2001; 285(8):1059–1070.
2. Gill DM. Bacterial toxins: A table of lethal amounts. Microbiol Rev 1982; 46(1):86–94.
3. Simpson LL. Molecular pharmacology of botulinum toxin and tetanus toxin. Annu Rev Pharmacol Toxicol 1986; 26:427–453.
4. Harper M, Fowler CJ, Dasgupta P. Botulinum toxin and its applications in the lower urinary tract. BJU Int 2004; 93(6):702–706.
5. Angaut-Petit D, Molgo J, Comella JX, et al. Terminal sprouting in mouse neuromuscular junctions poisoned with botulinum type A toxin: Morphological and electrophysiological features. Neuroscience 1990; 37(3):799–808.
6. Meunier FA, Schiavo G, Molgo J. Botulinum neurotoxins: From paralysis to recovery of functional neuromuscular transmission. J Physiol Paris 2002; 96(1–2):105–113.
7. de PA, Meunier FA, Molgo J, et al. Functional repair of motor endplates after botulinum neurotoxin type A poisoning: Biphasic switch of synaptic activity between nerve sprouts and their parent terminals. Proc Natl Acad Sci USA 1999; 96(6):3200–3205.
8. Naumann M, Jost WH, Toyka KV. Botulinum toxin in the treatment of neurological disorders of the autonomic nervous system. Arch Neurol 1999; 56(8):914–916.
9. de PA, Ashton AC, Foran P, et al. Botulinum A like type B and tetanus toxins fulfils criteria for being a zinc-dependent protease. J Neurochem 1993; 61(6):2338–2341.
10. Schiavo G, Papini E, Genna G, Montecucco C. An intact interchain disulfide bond is required for the neurotoxicity of tetanus toxin. Infect Immun 1990; 58(12):4136–4141.
11. Herreros J, Lalli G, Montecucco G, Schiavo G. Pathophysiological properties of clostridial neurotoxins. In: The comprehensive sourcebook of bacterial protein toxins. Academic Press, London, 2006.
12. Schiavo G, Matteoli M, Montecucco C. Neurotoxins affecting neuroexocytosis. Physiol Rev 2000; 80(2):717–766.
13. Carpenter FG. Motor responses of the urinary bladder and skeletal muscle in botulinum intoxicated rats. J Physiol 1967; 188(1):1–11.
14. Smith CP, Franks ME, McNeil BK, et al. Effect of botulinum toxin A on the autonomic nervous system of the rat lower urinary tract. J Urol 2003; 169(5):1896–1900.
15. Burnstock G. Purinergic nerves. Pharmacol Rev 1972; 24(3):509–581.
16. Mackenzie I, Burnstock G, Dolly JO. The effects of purified botulinum neurotoxin type A on cholinergic, adrenergic and non-adrenergic, atropine-resistant autonomic neuromuscular transmission. Neuroscience 1982; 7(4):997–1006.
17. Bayliss M, Wu C, Newgreen D, et al. A quantitative study of atropine-resistant contractile responses in human detrusor smooth muscle, from stable, unstable and obstructed bladders. J Urol 1999; 162(5):1833–1839.
18. O'Reilly BA, Kosaka AH, Knight GF, et al. P2X receptors and their role in female idiopathic detrusor instability. J Urol 2002; 167(1):157–164.
19. Mackenzie I, Burnstock G, Dolly JO. The effects of purified botulinum neurotoxin type A on cholinergic, adrenergic and non-adrenergic, atropine-resistant autonomic neuromuscular transmission. Neuroscience 1982; 7(4):997–1006.
20. Smith CP, Franks ME, McNeil BK, et al. Effect of botulinum toxin A on the autonomic nervous system of the rat lower urinary tract. J Urol 2003; 169(5):1896–1900.
21. Mackenzie I, Burnstock G, Dolly JO. The effects of purified botulinum neurotoxin type A on cholinergic, adrenergic and non-adrenergic, atropine-resistant autonomic neuromuscular transmission. Neuroscience 1982; 7(4):997–1006.

22. Smith CP, Franks ME, McNeil BK, et al. Effect of botulinum toxin A on the autonomic nervous system of the rat lower urinary tract. J Urol 2003; 169(5):1896–1900.

23. Apostolidis A, Dasgupta P, Fowler CJ. Proposed mechanism for the efficacy of injected botulinum toxin in the treatment of human detrusor overactivity. Eur Urol 2006; 49(4):644–650.

24. Smet PJ, Moore KH, Jonavicius J. Distribution and colocalization of calcitonin gene-related peptide, tachykinins, and vasoactive intestinal peptide in normal and idiopathic unstable human urinary bladder. Lab Invest 1997; 77(1):37–49.

25. Khera M, Somogyi GT, Kiss S, et al. Botulinum toxin A inhibits ATP release from bladder urothelium after chronic spinal cord injury. Neurochem Int 2004; 45(7):987–993.

26. Rapp DE, Turk KW, Bales GT, Cook SP. Botulinum toxin type A inhibits calcitonin gene-related peptide release from isolated rat bladder. J Urol 2006; 175(3 Pt 1):1138–1142.

27. Chuang YC, Yoshimura N, Huang CC, et al. Intravesical botulinum toxin A administration produces analgesia against acetic acid induced bladder pain responses in rats. J Urol 2004; 172(4 Pt 1):1529–1532.

28. Atiemo H, Wynes J, Chuo J, et al. Effect of botulinum toxin on detrusor overactivity induced by intravesical adenosine triphosphate and capsaicin in a rat model. Urology 2005; 65(3):622–626.

29. Apostolidis A, Dasgupta P, Fowler CJ. Proposed mechanism for the efficacy of injected botulinum toxin in the treatment of human detrusor overactivity. Eur Urol 2006; 49(4):644–650.

30. Apostolidis A, Popat R, Yiangou Y, et al. Decreased sensory receptors P2X3 and TRPV1 in suburothelial nerve fibers following intradetrusor injections of botulinum toxin for human detrusor overactivity. J Urol 2005; 174(3):977–982.

31. Welch MJ, Purkiss JR, Foster KA. Sensitivity of embryonic rat dorsal root ganglia neurons to *Clostridium botulinum* neurotoxins. Toxicon 2000; 38(2):245–258.

32. Purkiss JR, Welch MJ, Doward S, et al. A method for the measurement of [3H]-glutamate release from cultured dorsal root ganglion neurons. Biochem Soc Trans 1998; 26(2):S108.

33. Cui M, Khanijou S, Rubino J, Aoki KR. Subcutaneous administration of botulinum toxin A reduces formalin-induced pain. Pain 2004; 107(1–2):125–133.

34. Aoki KR. Review of a proposed mechanism for the antinociceptive action of botulinum toxin type A. Neurotoxicology 2005; 26(5):785–793.

35. Jankovic J, Schwartz K. Botulinum toxin injections for cervical dystonia. Neurology 1990; 40(2):277–280.

36. Leippold T, Reitz A, Schurch B. Botulinum toxin as a new therapy option for voiding disorders: Current state of the art. Eur Urol 2003; 44(2):165–174.

37. Smith CP, Chancellor MB. Emerging role of botulinum toxin in the management of voiding dysfunction. J Urol 2004; 171(6 Pt 1):2128–2137.

38. Sahai A, Khan M, Fowler CJ, Dasgupta P. Botulinum toxin for the treatment of lower urinary tract symptoms: A review. Neurourol Urodyn 2005; 24(1):2–12.

39. Schurch B, Stohrer M, Kramer G, et al. Botulinum-A toxin for treating detrusor hyperreflexia in spinal cord injured patients: A new alternative to anticholinergic drugs? Preliminary results. J Urol 2000; 164(3 Pt 1):692–697.

40. Kessler TM, Danuser H, Schumacher M, et al. Botulinum A toxin injections into the detrusor: An effective treatment in idiopathic and neurogenic detrusor overactivity? Neurourol Urodyn 2005; 24(3):231–236.

41. Bagi P, Biering-Sorensen F. Botulinum toxin A for treatment of neurogenic detrusor overactivity and incontinence in patients with spinal cord lesions. Scand J Urol Nephrol 2004; 38(6):495–498.

42. Hajebrahimi S, Altaweel W, Cadoret J, et al. Efficacy of botulinum-A toxin in adults with neurogenic overactive bladder: Initial results. Can J Urol 2005; 12(1):2543–2546.

43. Schulte-Baukloh H, Schobert J, Stolze T, et al. Efficacy of botulinum-A toxin bladder injections for the treatment of neurogenic detrusor overactivity in multiple sclerosis patients: An objective and subjective analysis. Neurourol Urodyn 2006; 25(2):110–115.

44. Klaphajone J, Kitisomprayoonkul W, Sriplakit S. Botulinum toxin type A injections for treating neurogenic detrusor overactivity combined with low-compliance bladder in patients with spinal cord lesions. Arch Phys Med Rehabil 2005; 86(11):2114–2118.

45. Reitz A, Stohrer M, Kramer G, et al. European experience of 200 cases treated with botulinum-A toxin injections into the detrusor muscle for urinary incontinence due to neurogenic detrusor overactivity. Eur Urol 2004; 45(4):510–515.

46. Kuo HC. Therapeutic effects of suburothelial injection of botulinum A toxin for neurogenic detrusor overactivity due to chronic cerebrovascular accident and spinal cord lesions. Urology 2006; 67(2):232–236.

47. Grosse J, Kramer G, Stohrer M. Success of repeat detrusor injections of botulinum A toxin in patients with severe neurogenic detrusor overactivity and incontinence. Eur Urol 2005; 47(5):653–659.

48. Patki PS, Hamid R, Arumugam K, et al. Botulinum toxin-type A in the treatment of drug-resistant neurogenic detrusor overactivity secondary to traumatic spinal cord injury. BJU Int 2006; 98(1):77–82.

49. Ruffion A, Capelle O, Paparel P, et al. What is the optimum dose of type A botulinum toxin for treating neurogenic bladder overactivity? BJU Int 2006; 97(5):1030–1034.

50. Schurch B, de SM, Denys P, et al. Botulinum toxin type A is a safe and effective treatment for neurogenic urinary incontinence: Results of a single treatment, randomized, placebo controlled 6-month study. J Urol 2005; 174(1):196–200.

51. Szallasi A, Blumberg PM. Vanilloid receptors: New insights enhance potential as a therapeutic target. Pain 1996; 68(2–3):195–208.

52. Chancellor MB, de Groat WC. Intravesical capsaicin and resiniferatoxin therapy: Spicing up the ways to treat the overactive bladder. J Urol 1999; 162(1):3–11.

53. Fowler CJ, Jewkes D, McDonald WI, et al. Intravesical capsaicin for neurogenic bladder dysfunction. Lancet 1992; 339(8803):1239.

54. Giannantoni A, Di Stasi SM, Stephen RL, et al. Intravesical resiniferatoxin versus botulinum-A toxin injections for neurogenic detrusor overactivity: A prospective randomized study. J Urol 2004; 172(1):240–243.

55. Rapp DE, Lucioni A, Katz EE, et al. Use of botulinum-A toxin for the treatment of refractory overactive bladder symptoms: An initial experience. Urology 2004; 63(6):1071–1075.

56. Smith CP, Nishiguchi J, O'Leary M, et al. Single-institution experience in 110 patients with botulinum toxin A injection into bladder or urethra. Urology 2005; 65(1):37–41.

57. Kuo HC. Clinical effects of suburothelial injection of botulinum A toxin on patients with nonneurogenic detrusor overactivity refractory to anticholinergics. Urology 2005; 66(1):94–98.

58. Werner M, Schmid DM, Schussler B. Efficacy of botulinum-A toxin in the treatment of detrusor overactivity incontinence: A prospective nonrandomized study. Am J Obstet Gynecol 2005; 192(5):1735–1740.

59. Flynn MK, Webster GD, Amundsen CL. The effect of botulinum-A toxin on patients with severe urge urinary incontinence. J Urol 2004; 172(6 Pt 1):2316–2320.

60. Kuo HC. Urodynamic evidence of effectiveness of botulinum A toxin injection in treatment of detrusor overactivity refractory to anticholinergic agents. Urology 2004; 63(5):868–872.

61. Popat R, Apostolidis A, Kalsi V, et al. A comparison between the response of patients with idiopathic detrusor overactivity and neurogenic detrusor overactivity to the first intradetrusor injection of botulinum-A toxin. J Urol 2005; 174(3):984–989.

62. Kalsi V, Apostolidis A, Popat R, et al. Quality of life changes in patients with neurogenic versus idiopathic detrusor overactivity after intradetrusor injections of botulinum neurotoxin type A and correlations with lower urinary tract symptoms and urodynamic changes. Eur Urol 2006; 49(3):528–535.

63. Schulte-Baukloh H, Weiss C, Stolze T, et al. Botulinum-A toxin detrusor and sphincter injection in treatment of overactive bladder syndrome: Objective outcome and patient satisfaction. Eur Urol 2005; 48(6):984–990.

64. Schmid DM, Sauermann P, Werner M, et al. Experience with 100 cases treated with botulinum-A toxin injections in the detrusor muscle for idiopathic overactive bladder syndrome refractory to anticholinergics. J Urol 2006; 176(1):177–185.

65. Sahai A, Khan MS, Dasgupta P. Efficacy of botulinum toxin-A for treating idiopathic detrusor overactivity: Results from a single center, randomized, double-blind, placebo controlled trial. J Urol 2007; 177(6):2231–2236.

66. Schulte-Baukloh H, Michael T, Schobert J, et al. Efficacy of botulinum-A toxin in children with detrusor hyperreflexia due to myelomeningocele: Preliminary results. Urology 2002; 59(3):325–327.

67. Riccabona M, Koen M, Schindler M, et al. Botulinum-A toxin injection into the detrusor: A safe alternative in the treatment of children with myelomeningocele with detrusor hyperreflexia. J Urol 2004; 171(2 Pt 1):845–848.

68. Altaweel W, Jednack R, Bilodeau C, Corcos J. Repeated intradetrusor botulinum toxin type A in children with neurogenic bladder due to myelomeningocele. J Urol 2006; 175(3 Pt 1):1102–1105.

69. Hoebeke P, De CK, Vande WJ, et al. The effect of botulinum-A toxin in incontinent children with therapy resistant overactive detrusor. J Urol 2006; 176(1):328–330.

70. Schulte-Baukloh H, Knispel HH, Stolze T, et al. Repeated botulinum-A toxin injections in treatment of children with neurogenic detrusor overactivity. Urology 2005; 66(4):865–870.

71. Dykstra DD, Pryor J, Goldish G. Use of botulinum toxin type B for the treatment of detrusor hyperreflexia in a patient with multiple sclerosis: A case report. Arch Phys Med Rehabil 2003; 84(9):1399–1400.

72. Dykstra D, Enriquez A, Valley M. Treatment of overactive bladder with botulinum toxin type B: A pilot study. Int Urogynecol J Pelvic Floor Dysfunct 2003; 14(6):424–426.

73. Pistolesi D, Selli C, Rossi B, Stampacchia G. Botulinum toxin type B for type A resistant bladder spasticity. J Urol 2004; 171(2 Pt 1):802–803.

74. Reitz A, Schurch B. Botulinum toxin type B injection for management of type A resistant neurogenic detrusor overactivity. J Urol 2004; 171(2 Pt 1):804–805.

75. Ghei M, Maraj BH, Miller R, et al. Effects of botulinum toxin B on refractory detrusor overactivity: A randomized, double-blind, placebo controlled, crossover trial. J Urol 2005; 174(5):1873–1877.

76. Apostolidis A, Dasgupta P, Fowler CJ. Proposed mechanism for the efficacy of injected botulinum toxin in the treatment of human detrusor overactivity. Eur Urol 2006; 49(4):644–650.

77. Harper M, Popat RB, Dasgupta R, et al. A minimally invasive technique for outpatient local anaesthetic administration of intradetrusor botulinum toxin in intractable detrusor overactivity. BJU Int 2003; 92(3):325–326.

78. Sahai A, Kalsi V, Khan MS, Fowler CJ. Techniques for the intradetrusor administration of botulinum toxin. BJU Int 2006; 97(4):675–678.

79. Smith CP, Chancellor MB. Simplified bladder botulinum-toxin delivery technique using flexible cystoscope and 10 sites of injection. J Endourol 2005; 19(7):880–882.

80. Schulte-Baukloh H, Knispel HH. A minimally invasive technique for outpatient local anaesthetic administration of intradetrusor botulinum toxin in intractable detrusor overactivity. BJU Int 2005; 95(3):454.

81. Scott AB, Suzuki D. Systemic toxicity of botulinum toxin by intramuscular injection in the monkey. Mov Disord 1988; 3(4):333–335.

82. Wyndaele JJ, Van Dromme SA. Muscular weakness as side effect of botulinum toxin injection for neurogenic detrusor overactivity. Spinal Cord 2002; 40(11):599–600.

83. Santos JI, Swensen P, Glasgow LA. Potentiation of *Clostridium botulinum* toxin aminoglycoside antibiotics: Clinical and laboratory observations. Pediatrics 1981; 68(1):50–54.

84. Pellizzari R, Rossetto O, Schiavo G, Montecucco C. Tetanus and botulinum neurotoxins: Mechanism of action and therapeutic uses. Philos Trans R Soc Lond B Biol Sci 1999; 354(1381):259–268.

85. Eleopra R, Tugnoli V, Rossetto O, et al. Botulinum neurotoxin serotype C: A novel effective botulinum toxin therapy in human. Neurosci Lett 1997; 224(2):91–94.

86. Meunier FA, Schiavo G, Molgo J. Botulinum neurotoxins: From paralysis to recovery of functional neuromuscular transmission. J Physiol Paris 2002; 96(1–2):105–113.

87. Smith CP, Boone TB, de Groat WC, et al. Effect of stimulation intensity and botulinum toxin isoform on rat bladder strip contractions. Brain Res Bull 2003; 61(2):165–171.

88. Comperat E, Reitz A, Delcourt A, et al. Histologic features in the urinary bladder wall affected from neurogenic overactivity – a comparison of inflammation, oedema and fibrosis with and without injection of botulinum toxin type A. Eur Urol 2006; 50:1058–1064.

89. Haferkamp A, Schurch B, Reitz A, et al. Lack of ultrastructural detrusor changes following endoscopic injection of botulinum toxin type A in overactive neurogenic bladder. Eur Urol 2004; 46(6):784–791.

90. Haferkamp A, Schurch B, Reitz A, et al. Lack of ultrastructural detrusor changes following endoscopic injection of botulinum toxin type A in overactive neurogenic bladder. Eur Urol 2004; 46(6):784–791.

Part V
Management of Pelvic Organ Prolapse

Chapter 21
Conservative Management of Pelvic Organ Prolapse: Biofeedback and Pessaries

Jill Maura Rabin

Pelvic organ prolapse is a complex, multifactorial, and dynamic condition. First and foremost, women presenting with disorders of the pelvic floor should have all presenting symptoms (relating to the gastrointestinal and genitourinary systems) thoroughly evaluated prior to the initiation of a treatment plan in order to identify all dysfunctions present. It is difficult to define the prevalence of pelvic organ prolapse because there is no clear distinction between normal and abnormal pelvic organ mobility [1]. Milder forms of prolapse are often asymptomatic [2] and a large proportion of women with symptomatic prolapse do not seek medical help [3]. Taking this into consideration, it is evident that pelvic organ prolapse is a common problem affecting 10–30% of the adult female population, predominately affecting middle-aged and elderly women [4].

Although surgical management of pelvic organ prolapse often is needed and is widely available, many women in this age group may suffer from severe medical comorbidities and other circumstances that may prevent them from having surgery, including patient choice. It is important therefore for gynecologists to continue to be skilled in the assessment and conservative management of pelvic organ prolapse.

The purpose of this chapter is to provide a comprehensive review of the conservative management of pelvic organ prolapse. Covered areas include symptoms, goals, and paradigms of treatment; current role of pessaries (including indications, insertion techniques, complications, contraindications, and factors affecting successful fitting); behavioral methods, biofeedback, and functional electrical stimulation (FES).

Goals and Paradigm of Treatment

Our treatment paradigm must be guided primarily by the extent to which the condition affects the patient's quality of life. This may be done either formally with quality of life questionnaires or may be incorporated into the overall health assessment (both verbal and written) or by the "Bother Index," scored from 1 to 10. Treatment options must be matched to the patient's specific situation, life-tyle, desires, wishes, and medical comorbidities. For example, some women do not want to use pessaries regularly, but may find these devices helpful and acceptable as a means to prevent further prolapse during exercise. It is of paramount importance to keep in mind our goals for each individual patient. We must keep abreast of the latest alternative, conservative approaches in the management of pelvic organ prolapse in order to be able to offer our patients a full spectrum of therapies for their conditions. Not only are these therapies and the surgical approach not mutually exclusive, they also may be synergistic in maximizing pelvic floor strength, increasing the durability of the surgical repair over time, and making it less likely for her to develop a recurrent problem. Some patients will not be surgical candidates due to medical comorbidities. In these cases, conservative management may prove to be invaluable.

Some women simply will not desire surgery, and we have a fundamental obligation as physicians to respect our patient's decisions and offer them non-surgical therapeutic options.

This chapter offers a spectrum of options with which to treat our patients. A treatment plan may dynamically change over time according to each individual patient's situation, anatomy, and degree of prolapse, as well as her desire and wishes for her individual treatment paradigm in the context of her life. By viewing the panoply of available options, we may better serve our patients not only in the short-term, but in formulating an effective dynamic long-term treatment and management paradigm and plan.

Pessaries: An Overview

Introduction

The pessary is a device or appliance of varied form introduced into the vagina in order to support the uterus, correct any malposition or displacement, and may be used to prevent conception as well as considered to be a medicated vaginal suppository [5]. Etymologically speaking, the word *pessary* has developed from the latin word "pessarium," as well as from the Greek word "pessos" meaning an oval stone. This is of historic interest since many of the original pessaries had at their core either a stone or other rounded object and then were wrapped or coated with various organic or inorganic material. The purpose of this section of the chapter is to provide the practitioner with a practical guide regarding pessary selection and use in the conservative management of pelvic organ prolapse for each individual woman.

Historical Perspective

Pessaries have enjoyed a long, rich, and colorful history dating back to biblical times. The oldest known reported use of the pessary was described by Hippocrates and later Soranus and Diocles, who used half of a pomegranate soaked in vinegar. Many naturally occurring substances such as other fruits and vegetables, cotton, bronze, and cork were used to construct a pessary of either the supportive or flap type and space-filling type. Often times

these were coated with various drugs, oil, butter, or wax in order to enhance the therapeutic use, enhance ease of insertion, and reduce disintegration or rotting. The bowl pessary was composed of linen held in place with a t-binder was composed of the Middle Ages by Trotula. In 1559, Casper Stromayr utilized a sponge that was tightly rolled and bound with string, then dipped in wax and covered with butter or oil. Hendrik Van Roonhuyse described a cork that was dipped in wax in 1663 in his operative gynecology textbook, which was the first of its kind [6]. Over 200 pessaries had already been created when Hugh Lenox Hodge created the contemporary lever pessary. The vulcanization of rubber by Goodyear in 1763 allowed the introduction of the rubber pessary, supplanting some of the early organic pessaries, adding to the overall attraction of this already popular mechanical device. Plastics were introduced in the 1950s, making pessaries more comfortable; subsequently, silicone-based products were added to the armamentarium of flexible, soft, and inert materials that serve as the basis of pessaries today. In the early 1900s, pessaries enjoyed their widest appeal; this declined with the introduction of asepsis and anesthesia, which allowed for the more widespread and safe use of surgical correction for pelvic organ prolapse. Nevertheless, there are over 20 types of pessaries in use today, available in a variety of sizes, and they are of ever-softer and flexible silicone. Having said this, the ideal pessary remains to be developed. Vaginal space not only is three-dimensional, but is a dynamic space that changes not only over time but with patient activity level, as well as with patient age and comorbidities. Therefore, it is essential that we think creatively about the future of pessaries. The development of such a device that is dynamic, in addition to being supportive and space-filling, must be given serious consideration.

Role of Pessaries and Indications for Their Use

Pessaries are most commonly used to relieve the symptoms associated with prolapse and are considered part of the initial treatment of primary or recurrent prolapse. Pessaries are invaluable devices prescribed by from 87 to 98% of gynecologists recently surveyed [7]. The role of this supportive device is both diagnostic as well as therapeutic and may be considered either short-term, long-term, or may change dynamically with a specific patient's individual situation. Therapeutically, pessaries may be used to relieve symptoms of primary prolapse or recurring prolapse including symptoms of backache, pelvic pressure, or various urinary symptoms including urgency. A properly fitted pessary may stabilize the urethrovesical junction. Urodynamic studies indicate that there is no increase in rectal, bladder, urethral, or detrusor pressure after pessary placement, despite an increase in urethral closure pressure. Thus, in most cases obstructed voiding or stress incontinence should not result from a properly fitted pessary [8]. Therapeutically pessaries can be enormously helpful both physically and emotionally for women with exteriorized prolapse including atrophic, cracked, dry, and ulcerated vaginal skin. Not only will a minimum of 2 months of topical estrogen cream and a subsequent placement of a good fitting pessary keep this bulge in situ, improving the patient's comfort level, but will allow for an improvement in the local environment including improvement in vascularity, decrease in air drying, and friction. One study examined the question of whether or not pessaries prevented the progression of pelvic organ prolapse. In fact, their data suggested there may be a therapeutic effect associated with the use a supportive pessary [9]. A special role for the pessary was proposed by Nygaard for use during physical activity, sports, and exercise when urinary incontinence is common even in young nulliparus women [10]. Patients reporting symptom relief with pessary placement may desire a more permanent approach to their situation such as surgery. Pessaries are especially useful in these cases, for example, in patients with recurrent prolapse who require some time with the pessary in order to recover physically, emotionally, and financially. This also is particularly helpful in patients who desire to wait a period of time prior to having surgery because of their individual situation, be it professional (a teacher who may have the entire summer for vacation may plan her prolapse surgery in these months), the caregiver of a sick husband or partner who may need to postpone definitive corrective to a more appropriate time, or the "snow bird." Typically, younger patients who benefit from symptomatic relief of their prolapse

will continue to wear a pessary until such time as they have completed their child-bearing.

The decision of whether or not to pursue surgical repair or to continue with long-term pessary management is an individual decision, and yet must be looked upon as a dynamic one, with the individual women along with her health care team. In summary, there have been no studies conducted to date to allow a physician to know in advance which patients are likely to accept and continue using the pessary. It is for this reason that all patients with symptomatic prolapse should be offered conservative management of their pelvic organ prolapse using pessaries.

Pessary Choice

Most pessaries today are either made of inert plastic or silicone, with the large majority composed of the latter. These pessaries last longer than the rubber types and have the advantage of not absorbing secretions and odors. Additionally, silicone pessaries also may be autoclaved and have a longer shelf-life than the other available materials. Borrowing one of the tenets of the principles of pelvic surgery, the least dangerous and least invasive procedure for the patient should be chosen as the first choice. Similarly, in choosing a pessary, the least invasive device should be chosen for the patient provided it reduces the prolapse, holds the pelvic organs in place, causes the least number and severity of localized symptoms, requires the least care and fewest changes possible without an increase in the symptoms, and additionally remains in place.

Although much has been written on the nature of pessary choice and fitting, this is as much an art as a science. The ultimate goal is to of fit the patient with the largest possible pessary that does not cause discomfort. There are two basic tenets of pessary choice [11, 12]. The first is the introitus, whether or not it is well-supported or relaxed. Second is the degree of pelvic organ prolapse including specific vaginal wall defects and overall pelvic muscle strength.

Stage 1 to 2 symptomatic pelvic organ prolapse generally is managed with a supportive pessary such as a ring or a donut pessary, which is generally gentler and less invasive than some of the other types of pessaries. Stage 3 to 4 pelvic organ prolapse usually requires a space-filling pessary such as a Cube or a Gellhorn.

One of the major areas in which experience of the provider comes into play in the art and science of fitting a pessary is the realization that there are two components in describing and in managing women with symptomatic prolapse in regard to the pelvic outlet (Fig. 21.1). It is helpful to regard the outlet as a three-dimensional structure with two important components, the first being the vagina. A vagina that is nonfunneled and cylinder-shaped will admit two or three fingers. Second, the perineal body will be intact, thick, and long. Although it has been said many times that the fitting of pessaries requires trial and error and that this is largely a function of individual physician experience and training, the greatest determinant of successful pessary choice and fitting remains the realization of the dual component of the three-dimensionally supported introitus/vaginal outlet.

All pessaries sit similarly in the vagina in an oblique position, lodged behind the pubic symphysis and extending to or near the levator plate fascia (toward the sacral promontory). In other words, pessaries basically sit in what we call the obstetric conjugate (anteroposterior diameter of the midplane of the bony pelvis). Pessaries that are supportive will rely on an intact vaginal outlet in order to stay properly positioned in the vagina as referenced above. Women will not be able to retain these pessaries in the face of a funneled vagina with a relaxed vaginal outlet, especially in cases of increased vaginal pressure occurring with defecation, for example. Pessaries that have the additional feature of a suction mechanism such as the Gellhorn or Cube type are able to reduce pelvic organ prolapse and remain in place because they function not only as a space-filling pessary but have the additional feature of this suction support. Nevertheless, some of the most challenging situations of pessary fitting remain this latter example of a relaxed vaginal outlet/deficient perineum and a long, funneled vagina.

One small prospective study investigated the risk associated with an unsuccessful pessary fitting trial in women with symptomatic pelvic organ prolapse and concluded that a short vaginal length and a wide vaginal introitus were risk factors for unsuccessful pessary fitting, and that Gellhorn pessaries more often are needed with stage 4 prolapse [14]. The use of a double pessary in grade 4 uterine and vaginal prolapse was proposed by one group who concluded that the placement of two pessaries often will be successful in women with long-standing

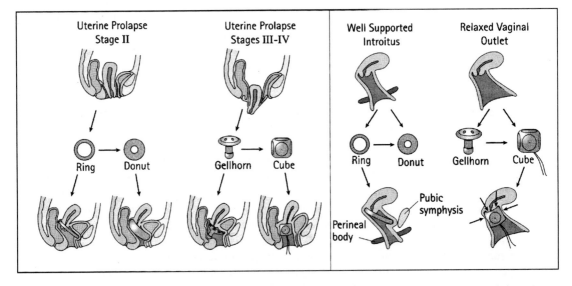

FIG. 21.1. The two determinants of pessary choice (from [13], with permission). The two factors determining pessary choice are the degree of pelvic organ prolapse (left) and the integrity of the pelvic outlet (right). Lesser degrees of pelvic organ prolapse usually are managed quite adequately with the less invasive, gentler ring or donut pessary. More severe or exteriorized lesions, however, may require the Gellhorn or Cube device

grade 4 prolapse who were unable to retain a single pessary [15]. Additionally, we have patented a pessary for treating vaginal prolapse that is dynamically conformable, provides support where it is most needed, and is coated with an antibacterial soft gel that reduces discharge, odor, and infection. Clinical trials are currently in progress [16].

Fitting and Insertion Techniques

After discussing the use of the pessary with the patient, we encourage her and instruct her in self-removal, cleaning, and reinsertion. This allows her to have more control over her pelvic organ prolapse and its management in private. She may take it out at night and reinsert it in the morning in order to minimize vaginal discharge, odor, as well as discoloration of the pessary. She thus may utilize the pessary when and if she decides to use it, for instance, during specific exercises or on certain days rather than other days when her schedule dictates greater degrees of intra-abdominal pressure increase and activity. Erosions and vaginitis may be best minimized. These are two of most common complications of pessary use. Finally, she will be in control and in charge of the management of her pelvic organ prolapse, thus making frequent visits to the physician for cleaning and management of the pessary unnecessary. Visits would be scheduled at appropriate intervals to check fit as well as checking for erosions and lesions and additionally for routine gynecological care (Table 21.1).

There is very little scientific information regarding the fitting of a pessary. It is important to discuss the use of a pessary in great detail with the patient. In particular, instructing her how to prevent expulsion during urination and defecation is very helpful, since many elderly women experience constipation. If a pessary fits properly, it either will not be visible or will barely appear on Valsalva maneuver in the lithotomy position with the labia separated. A device that is too small will fall out and a device that is too large may not fit properly in the obstetric conjugate and will cause additional discomfort and pressure, to say nothing of interference with micturition and defecation. It is helpful to teach the patient to palpate the pessary and hold it in place during Valsalva maneuver. Alternatively, squeezing the labia together effectively closes the vaginal outlet.

TABLE 21.1. Step-by-step pessary-fitting technique.

Discussion of pessary use with patient
Instruct patient to empty bladder and bowels
Vaginal examination for staging of the pelvic organ prolapse
Reduction of prolapse using Trendelenberg position and steady gentle pressure if pelvic organ prolapse is exteriorized
Approximate size estimation of pessary
Lubricate pessary: water soluble/estrogen cream/ Metronidazole vaginal /Trimosan
Reduction of diameter and or size of device as small as possible
Place widest diameter in the anterior posterior direction
Instruct patient in pelvic floor relaxation techniques
Placement of pessary, gently using a two-handed technique
Check placement of pessary in posterior fornix and behind pubic symphysis (obstetric conjugate placement)
Fitting of device that can be worn comfortably

In addition to instructing the patient on insertion, it is important to go through the steps verbally prior to initiating the fitting procedure. The patient is asked to empty her bladder. A pelvic examination is performed in order to assess the pelvis, the degree and type of prolapse, the vaginal length, perineum, and introitus. A type of pessary is chosen and a size estimate is made. Once the pessary type is chosen it is important to lubricate the tissues prior to reducing any prolapse present with a water-soluble lubricant or estrogen cream. It is important additionally to lubricate the particular pessary to be used and to reduce its diameter to a minimum prior to insertion. The pessary will sit with its widest diameter in an anteroposterior orientation and in the obstetric conjugate as previously mentioned. It is important to have the patient relax her pelvic floor prior to insertion of the pessary and place it during the patient's inhalation. A two-handed technique is performed whereby the pessary is reduced to its smallest diameter and held in the practitioner's dominant hand. The thumb and fingers are used to squeeze the pessary. The index finger of the nondominant hand is used to assist the patient in relaxing her introitus. The pessary is guided into the posterior fornix and the distal edge behind the pubic symphysis. Some pessary types, such as a ring pessary, need to be rotated 90°. Following this the patient must perform a Valsalva movement and the fit must be assessed. The pessary in situ must have a fingertip width's room between the perimeter of the pessary and the vaginal walls. The largest possible device must be fit, provided it is comfortable. If the patient notes expulsion during her activities in the office, a larger or different pessary should be tried. If she notes pressure or discomfort in the pelvis, a smaller or different pessary should be fitted. The patient is instructed to report any difficulty with defecation or urination. A test fit protocol is then conducted (Table 21.2).

It is important to spend considerable time with the patient in the examination room (either the physician, nurse, or nurse practitioner) asking the patient to ambulate, as well as sit, to perform the Valsalva maneuver, and to attempt to void prior to leaving the office. Further, instructions should be given to the patient in terms of self-management or at least to her caregiver. Ideally, the pessary should be removed every night, washed with soap and water, and reinserted in the morning. Many patients prefer to perform this exercise weekly, while others prefer to leave it in place for 6–8 weeks at time. If the latter scenario is the case, the patient must return at regular intervals, depending on the individual patient from 1 to 6 months, with the average being 2–3 months.

We keep a current list of patients using pessaries in order to ensure that each patient using a pessary is followed regularly at intervals determined by both the physician and patient. This will reduce complications associated with pessary use that will be elaborated on in a subsequent section.

While vaginal discharge is associated with long-term pessary use, with regular follow-up the discharge should not be excessive. This being stated, if the patient notes an excessive, foul-smelling, or bloody vaginal discharge, she should report to the office immediately.

Successful pessary fitting is one where the pessary is not expelled with Valsalva maneuver or cough, and where the patient is comfortable without pressure or pain symptoms as well as not being aware of the pessary in situ with ambulation, sitting, voiding, or defecation.

Care of the Pessary

Follow-up intervals for patients vary on whether they are self-inserting and removing, or if it is being performed by the practitioner (Table 21.3). The time interval also varies with the type of pessary. For example, a Gelhorn pessary or Cube may require more frequent physician and/or patient cleaning. Topical creams should be used and they may be in the form of water-soluble gels, such as KY jelly or estrogen cream, Metronidazole vaginal gel, or Trimosan. It is helpful when the patient presents for device check to compose a 50:50 mixture of peroxide and saline and to swab

TABLE 21.2. Testing the fit of the pessary.

Ask the patient to walk for a minimum of 15–20 min in the exam room and not to sit, to attempt position

If discomfort, pressure, or expulsion: instruct the patient on self-management

If expulsion of the pessary is noted: a larger or different pessary must be tried

If the patient experiences significant discomfort or pressure: a smaller or different pessary should be tried

The patient is asked to report any pelvic pressure or discomfort, a slow stream or pressured defecation, or an inability to urinate or defecate immediately

Patient is asked to return within 1 week to check pessary placement, size, and type

Check once again after 1 month if 1 week visit was successful

Ask the patient to make an appointment to return within 3 months if she is not self-managing, or within 6 months if she is pursuing self-management

TABLE 21.3. Pessary care.

Self-insertion or removal follow-up every 6 months (follow-up varies with pessary type)

Estrogen cream, Metronidazole gel, Trimosan, (follow-up intervals varies with pessary type)

Solution is mixed one half peroxide, one half sterile water and vagina is swabbed out with single-use swab prior to device removal

Lubricate fingers of glove and remove device

Device is washed and inspected

Vagina is swabbed with the peroxide, sterile water mixture; any bleeding is noted

Vagina is carefully inspected for any erosions, ulcers, or lesions and if found these are addressed (including biopsy if necessary)

Mild vaginitis: vagina is irrigated and painted with Betadine; with severe vaginitis the pessary is discontinued temporarily and any erosions or ulcerations are addressed

If pessary is to be replaced, lubricate pessary well with estrogen cream, Metronidazole gel, or Trimosan before it is replaced (as in this table above)

the vagina with a large swab soaked in the mixture. This helps reduce any odor from vaginal discharge. The gloved hand is then lubricated and one or two fingers are used to remove the pessary. It is helpful on removal to also use the two-handed technique in order to more adequately control the pessary emerging from the vagina. Any bleeding is noted. The pessary is examined for wear and tear. Similarly the vagina is examined for any erosion, ulceration, or necrosis and these are noted in the chart. The patient is questioned as to the ease of her urination and defecation, and if urinary retention is suspected, postvoid residual via ultrasound or catheterization should be performed prior to pessary removal. The urine may be sent for culture and sensitivity, especially if the patient is symptomatic. If mild vaginitis is found, the vagina may be irrigated and swabbed with betadine. The follow-up interval in this case may need to be sooner. If severe vaginitis, erosions, or ulcerations are identified, the pessary is not reinserted at this visit. Once it is cleaned, it is returned to the patient. She is asked to return within a 1- to 2-week interval after utilizing one of the topical creams as mentioned above to assist in the healing process. Usage of low-dose estrogen cream (1/2–1 g two nights per week) is recommended by many practitioners and does not result in significant systemic absorption.

Many patients prefer to remove the device each night, or at least once a week, to leave it out overnight or several days, and to douche, swab the vagina, and clean their own pessary, and reinsert it. Once it is established that the patient is able to do this, a follow-up of every 3–6 months is acceptable. One study specifically studied women who self-managed their pessaries, and the author found good acceptance, with very little in the way of complications, and these were actually minor [17]. A new pessary should be substituted if inspection reveals either physical defects or cracking, or other signs of wear and tear. Discoloration does not require replacement. However, severe discoloration may indicate breakdown of the silicone and substitution may be prudent.

Types of Pessaries

See Table 21.4

The Ring Pessary With and Without Support

There are two types of ring pessaries available: the open ring or the ring with a supportive membrane (Fig. 21.2). These pessaries are among the simplest to use requiring less frequent visits, allow for easy self-insertion, removal, and permit coitus. The ring with supportive membrane is utilized in patients with procidentia who otherwise may experience organ prolapse through an open ring. The ring pessaries themselves are considered the least invasive and are associated with the lowest incidence of heavy vaginal discharge. They actually are very similar in appearance to the contraceptive diaphragm and are available in sizes 0–13. The most common sizes utilized are sizes 3–5. These are most effective for women with mild to moderate pelvic organ prolapse. This particular pessary does require an intact vaginal outlet. The ring with support is especially useful for women with an accompanying cystocele. The pessary is folded in half and inserted in a controlled manner, and also folded for removal. This particular type of pesary is turned 90 degrees following insertion due to its uni-directional bend which assists in limiting expulsion, and similarly turned prior to removal. The patient can assist with removal of the pessary by bearing down as the pessary is removed, and this will also assist in folding the ring which will decrease its diameter and facilitate removal. The Shaatz is a supportive pessary also used for mild to moderate uterine and vaginal prolapse in patients requiring a slightly greater degree of support than those utilizing the ring pessary. It fits between the levator muscles and ultimately into the obstetric conjugate. Insertion and removal is similar to the ring pessary with the exception that it may be folded in half at any point along the circumference.

The incontinence dish and the incontinence dish with support are used in cases of mild pelvic organ prolapse including mild cystocele. Sizing is similar to the ring and Shaatz pessaries and are most commonly used in sizes 3–5. The knob is intended to be positioned at the urethrovesical junction, as these pessaries are indicated in cases of mild stress incontinence and most notably may be used during exercise. Insertion and removal is similar to the ring pessary described above.

TABLE 21.4. Incontinence dish and incontinence dish with support.

Pessary	Type	Size	Mechanism of action	Indications	Require intact vaginal outlet	Pros	Cons	Follow-up	Comments
Schaatz	Support	3–5	Fits obliquely between pubic symphysis and sacral promontory (obstetric conjugate)	Mild pelvic organ prolapse with or without cystocele	Yes	Easy insertion, removal and self-care, coitus possible, may be used for exercise-specific stress incontinence/leakage. Vaginitis, none to mild	Less effective for severe pelvic organ prolapse	Initially after 3 months, then q3–6 months	More effective with node (if present) anterior near urethrovesical junction. May cause vaginal and rectal discomfort with rotation of node
Donut	Space filling	2½–3 in.	Fills vaginal vault occluding facing prolapse	Moderate to severe uterine or vaginal vault prolapse. Mild genuine stress urinary incontinence	Yes	For moderate to severe uterine or vaginal vault prolapse	Coitus not possible, vaginitis frequent, frequent removal necessary	Monthly for 3 months then q3 months	Deflation prior to insertion, reinflation after insertion, deflation prior to removal facilitates insertion and removal
Inflato-ball	Space filling	Medium and large	Fills vaginal vault repositions pelvic organ prolapse cephalad and occludes upper vagina	Moderate to severe uterine and vaginal prolapse	No	Self-insertion and removal. None to mild vaginitis	May be Difficult to retain		Must not be used with patient latex allergy
Gehrung	Support	3–5	Supports cystocele by directing pressure via double arch against anterior vaginal wall with legs of pessary directed posteriorly, supporting rectocele by double arch sitting against rectocele and posterior vaginal wall with its legs directed anteriorly	Cystocele or rectocele	No	Isolated cystocele or rectocele, ease of self-insertion or removal, coitus possible	Mild to moderate vaginitis	Monthly for the first 3 months, then every 2–3 months	Designed specifically for cystocele or rectocele

Gelhorn	Space filling	The dish portion has a shallow cup oriented cephalad against the cervix or vaginal vault reducing prolapse in a cephalad manner, the stem sits in the vagina directed toward the introitus or posterior fourchette, suction	1–5 (3–5 most common)	Moderate to severe pelvic organ prolapse	No	Excellent choice for moderate to severe pelvic organ prolapse	Insertion and removal may be difficult, severe vaginal discharge or vaginitis may develop, coitus not possible, more frequent patient visits for cleaning and management ___ may be required	Initially 1–2 weeks and then 1–3 months	Assure patient compliance, removal may be difficult (use of single-tooth tenaculum or ring forceps in nondominant hand may assist with traction on stem, dominant index finger breaks suction between vagina and dish prior to removal portion)
Cube	Space filling	Severe pelvic organ prolapse	0–7 (2–4 most common)	Severe pelvic organ prolapse	No	For severe pelvic organ prolapse	Heavy vaginitis and discharge, vaginal ulcerations, frequent removals, coitus not possible	Every 1–2 weeks, subsequently every 4 weeks	Cutting holes between surfaces will decrease the hypoxic environment and allow vaginal discharge to escape. Newer models have incorporated this feature. May cause severe vaginal ulcerations in diabetes and patients should be monitored carefully.

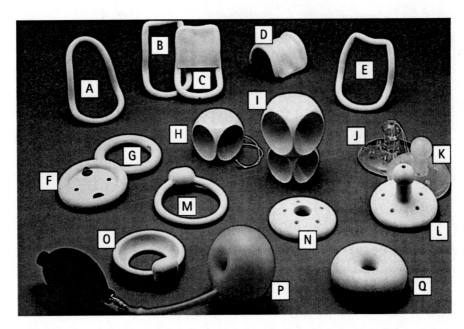

FIG. 21.2. Currently available vaginal pessaries (Cooper Surgical, with permission). (**a**) Smith (silicone, folding), (**b**) Hodge without support (silicone, folding), (**c**) Hodge with support (silicone, folding), (**d**) Gehrung with support (silicone, folding), (**e**) Risser (silicone, folding), (**f**) ring with support (silicone, folding), (**g**) ring without support (silicone, folding), (**h**) Cube (silicone, flexible), (**i**) Tandem-Cube (silicone, flexible), (**j**) rigid Gelhorn (acrylic, multiple drain), (**k**) 95% rigid Gelhorn (silicone, multiple drain), (**l**) flexible Gelhorn (silicone, multiple drain), (**m**) ring incontinence (silicone), (**n**) Shaatz (silicone, folding), (**o**) incontinence dish (silicone, folding), (**p**) inflatoball (latex), and (**q**) donut (silicone)

The donut pessary is considered the pessary of choice if a person is unable to successfully retain the ring pessary and those mentioned previously. It is very popular for moderate to severe pelvic organ prolapse and is considered a space-filling pessary by supporting the prolapse by filling the vaginal vault. It does require an intact vaginal outlet. Follow-up is monthly for the first several months and every 1–3 months thereafter. Once the proper size has been chosen, the pessary is folded in half and lubricated. In order to decrease the diameter further, some have suggested removing the air within the pessary utilizing a 20 cc syringe and 18–21 gauge needle (Fig. 21.3). The plunger of the syringe is removed, the needle is inserted into the inflated pessary, and the pessary is compressed allowing the air to go through the barrel of the syringe. The pessary is then squeezed in half to its minimum diameter and is inserted with the widest part of the donut entering the vagina using a two-handed technique as referenced above and guiding the leading edge into the posterior fornix

(Fig. 21.4). Following this maneuver, the index finger of the nondominant hand is placed into the vagina and into the donut's hole, pulling the distal edge into the introitus a bit so that a portion of the

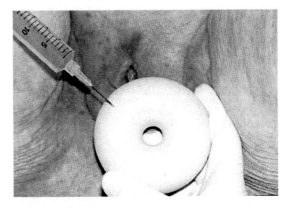

FIG. 21.3. Donut pessary (from [67], with permission). After approximating the most appropriate size, the air is removed via a 21-gauge needle and 20-cc syringe. With the plunger out, the pessary is compressed and after maximizing deflation, the needle is removed

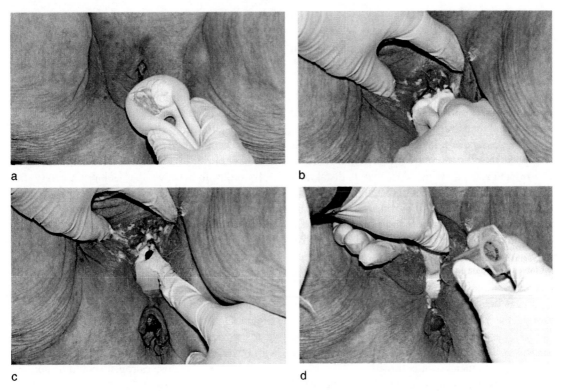

FIG. 21.4. Insertion of donut pessary. (from [67], with permission). (**a**) The deflated donut occupies less space. (**b**) When lubricated, the donut is very easily inserted through the separated labia. (**c**) Once the widest part of the donut enters the vagina through the introitus, it tends to slip away from the physician's grasp. (**d**) It is held near the introitus with an index finger in the donut's hole so that the needle and syringe without plunger can again be inserted through the silicone wall and the pessary reinflated by equilibrating with room atmosphere. The needle is removed and the pessary slides apically

pessary is visible. The needle and the syringe once again can be inserted into the pessary without the plunger and reinflated, allowing the donut pessary to receive room atmospheric pressure. The pessary then is guided cephalad with the distal end positioned behind the pubic symphysis as far as possible. Removal is facilitated by drawing the pessary down with the examiner's index finger in order that a portion of the pessary is visible at the introitus. A 20-cc syringe with 18–21 gauge needle with the plunger in can be used to withdraw 40–60 cc of air. The pessary then is removed gently.

The inflatoball is similar to the donut in that it is a space-occupying pessary used most often to manage moderate to severe uterine and/or vaginal vault prolapse. It is made of latex and should be used with caution unless absence of latex allergy can be confirmed. The inflatoball is similar in its shape and mechanism of action as compared with the donut. It was designed for self-care and can be inflated with air once it is placed in the patient's vagina. It is necessary to remove, cleanse the pessary and vagina, and reinsert the pessary two to three times per week since it is composed of latex and may absorb odors. The pessary is inserted in an oblique angle by the patient with the labia separated, placed high in the vagina, and then inflated by the patient with the specifically designed top, which is then removed after inflation. It remains inflated because of the small bead located inside a Y connector. Once inflated the bead is placed above the branch point of the Y connector and therefore remains inflated. For deflation, the patient moves the bead into one of the shorter arms of the Y thus deflating the pessary, It is then easily removed by the patient.

The Gehrung pessary is a shapable pessary specifically designed for a cystocele, but also may be used for a rectocele. For cystocele it is situated with the convex surface against the anterior vaginal wall. Its legs are directed posteriorly toward the posterior fornix on the patient's left and right. This pessary requires an intact vaginal outlet. Visits are monthly and then every 1–2 months thereafter. The Gehrung pessary is folded in half for insertion. It is slipped into the vagina with its convex surface upward and rotated 90° in order that its distal arch is situated transversely behind the pubic symphysis and the proximal arch will sit transversely high in the vagina in the uppermost limit of the cystocele or slightly higher. To replace rectocele, the above maneuver is repeated with the convexity directed downward and the double arches supporting the rectocele. Removal is facilitated by insertion of the dominant index finger into the vagina and gently turning the pessary as it is drawn down toward the introitus. Patients may assist with a Valsalva maneuver. The Gehrung pessary will automatically decrease its diameter as it is turned.

The Gelhorn pessary is available in either rigid acrylic or rigid or flexible silicone but often is used in its flexible silicone form. It is an extremely effective pessary for patients with moderate to severe prolapse and complete procidentia and does not require an intact vaginal outlet. It is one of the strongest available pessaries not only because of its size and shape but also because of its partial suction effect. Insertion and removal may be difficult, and thus care is typically performed by the practitioner. In order to minimize the vaginal discharge, which may be moderate to severe, patients may elect to douche two to three times per week with either water and vinegar solution or Povidone–Iodine as referenced above. Patients experience the greatest success with Gelhorn pessary if there is a somewhat intact perineal body present. In order to insert the Gelhorn pessary, the device is inserted with lubricant liberally applied. There are two methods of insertion (Fig. 21.5). Small Gelhorn pessaries from the size of 1½–2¼ in. can be inserted directly with the dish portion parallel to the anterior posterior diameter of the introitus directing the leading edge of the dish into the posterior fornix with the following edge directed under the pubic symphysis and the knob rotated perpendicular to the introitus. The knob can be adjusted in order that the flat portion or dish reaches the highest point against the cervix or the upper vagina. Alternatively and most notably, with the Gelhorn of larger size (from 2¼ to 3½ in.) a two-handed technique is adopted. The dish is folded in half between the thumb and forefinger to its minimum diameter. Every attempt is made to control the pessary during insertion. It is prudent to allow the patient a short period of time to become used to the sensation of the pessary placement prior to adjustment with the stem.

In order to remove the Gelhorn pessary the thumb and forefinger of the nondominant hand may be used while the patient is bearing down in order to grasp the stem. Alternatively, a single-tooth tenaculum or ring forceps can be applied to the stem and gentle traction applied in a downward fashion (Fig. 21.6). The index finger of the dominant hand can be used to break the suction by interposing the finger between the dish and the vagina. Once the suction is broken, the examiner's hands work synchronously to gently guide the pessary out of the vagina. If erosions or ulcerations are noted, topical low-dose estrogen should be applied at regular intervals and the pessary should be replaced only when complete healing is noted. This may take from 1 to 4 weeks or longer depending on the patient's situation. In diabetics, development of these erosions may occur with greater regularity and healing may be delayed.

The Cube pessary is very useful in cases of moderate to severe prolapse and generally is used when the above pessaries have not produced a satisfactory result. It is a soft, self-positioning pessary with six suction cups, one present on each side of the cube. It is usually associated with a high-risk of vaginal ulcerations and necrosis most notably in patients who are diabetic and/or atrophic. In these patients it must be used with great caution and as a last resort; use may be facilitated by creating small holes cut between the cups in order to let air get into this otherwise hypoxic environment. The pessary is inserted by compressing it into its smallest diameter and moved into the uppermost portion of the vagina against the cervix and/or vaginal vault by steady pressure. In order to remove the pessary, the labia are separated; the string is grasped, suction is broken, and all available sides are gently grasped, pulled down, and out of the vagina maintaining gentle traction on the string.

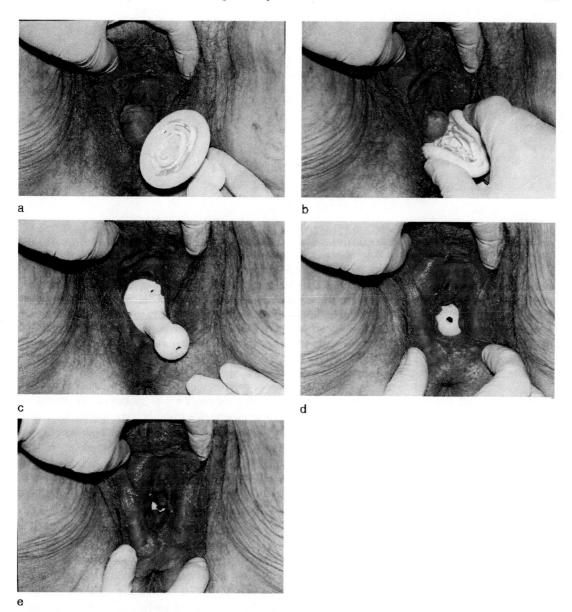

FIG. 21.5. Insertion of a Gelhorn pessary (from [67], with permission). (**a**) Metronidazole gel is copiously applied with Gelhorn and Cube pessaries to counteract anaerobic growth in the hypoxic environment above the Gellhorn dish or cube cup. Small Gelhorns like the one pictured (2¼ in.) can be inserted directly with the dish parallel to the anteroposterior diameter of the introitus, inserting the side of the dish first. (**b**) Alternatively, and particularly with larger Gelhorns, the dish can be pinched or folded to compress its size and inserted obliquely through the vulva held open with the contralateral hand. (**c**) Once the dish is in the vagina, it will spontaneously and easily turn into the proper axis. It should sit obliquely with the dish positioned under the vaginal apex and the horn pointing toward the perineum. (**d**) After giving the patient a chance to relax, the pessary is pushed up into the vaginal apex. (**e**) A properly positioned Gelhorn pessary has its presenting horn pointing down toward the perineum and just barely visible with the vulva held apart and the patient performing a Valsalva maneuver

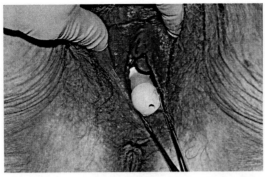
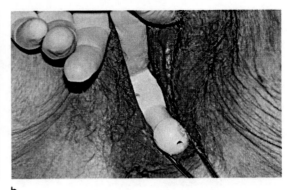

a   b

FIG. 21.6. Removal of a Gelhorn pessary (from [13], with permission). (**a**) Removal is facilitated by finding the distal horn with the fingers and grasping it with a single-toothed tenaculum. (**b**) Gentle traction on the tenaculum posteriorly will allow an intravaginal index finger of the other hand to slip above the dish and break the suction. Once the suction is broken, the two hands working together will gently guide the Gelhorn pessary down through the vagina and out with the dish in the anteroposterior diameter. After removing a Gelhorn or a Cube pessary, a careful observation of the vaginal walls, using a speculum, should be done to look for lacerations, erosions, or ulcerations. Significant foreign body-related lesions warrant a temporary moratorium from pessary use until topical estrogen-mediated healing occurs. Vaginal discharge can occur with any pessary and is sometimes quite copious and purulent with the Cube and Gelhorn types. After pessary removal and inspection, the vagina can be painted with procto-swabs soaked in povidone–iodine

In addition to all of the above, a Tandem-Cube is used for patients with moderate to severe pelvic organ prolapse, in particular, uterine procidentia, when a single Cube provides inadequate support. All of the above caveats should be noted.

Lever pessaries such as Smith, Risser, and Hodge are all variations of a design by Hodge developed to correct a retroverted uterus by displacing the cervix posteriorly. Currently, their main indication is for the management of stress urinary incontinence as they support the urethrovesical junction. Since these types generally are not used in cases of pelvic organ prolapse, they will not be covered further in this chapter

Complications with and Contraindications to Pessary Use

A noncompliant patient is an absolute contraindication to continue pessary use. Patients satisfied with their pessaries continue to use them for several years. As these women (not infrequently elderly woman) continue the aging process, their situation is a dynamic one and they change medically and/or psychosocially. Many may develop diabetes, making more frequent visits to the office necessary in order to check for erosion and ulceration. A patient no longer may be able to easily come to the office, often relying on family and friends, and therefore may not be able to keep her appointments for pessary follow-up. Similarly along these lines, a patient's mental status may change. She no longer may be able to perform self-care or douche as frequently or follow-up at the office every several months. This increases the propensity toward an increase in vaginal discharge. The neglected pessary may become trapped in the vagina under a dense vaginal scar or cicatrix [18]. This would necessitate surgical removal of the pessary. The Gelhorn pessary is most often associated with serious complications when neglected which include severe ulcerations, necrosis, and migration of the pessary into the bowel, bladder, or abdominal cavity. It can become densely adherent to other pelvic structures and eventuate into a situation that is extremely difficult to treat. These case reports have been associated with other pessaries as well. Applying estrogen cream to an impacted pessary may generally assist in its removal. Migration into bowel and bladder as mentioned above is rare, as is fistula formation, but these have been noted in the literature [19–24] (Fig. 21.7).

The most common complication of pessary use is irritation of the vaginal mucosa with accompanying

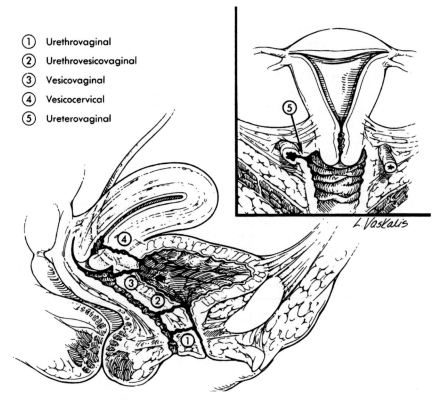

① Urethrovaginal
② Urethrovesicovaginal
③ Vesicovaginal
④ Vesicocervical
⑤ Ureterovaginal

L. Vaskalis

FIG. 21.7. "Fistulas associated with pessary use" (from [25], with permission)

discharge, odor, ulceration and bleeding, and necrosis. These are minimized with careful attention to pessary care as previously mentioned. In the face of erosions and ulcerations, pessary use should be temporarily discontinued. Low-dose vaginal cream two to three times per week can be used to assist in the healing process and may be continued as part of pessary care including lubrication subsequent to healing of the ulcerated areas. Recurrent erosions may be avoided by changing either the style or size of pessary. If the current erosions continue to develop, pessary use should be discontinued for longer periods or even permanently. All suspicious lesions should be biopsied to rule-out neoplastic process. Cervical and vaginal carcinomas associated with pessary use have been reported, but are rare [26].

Despite the above, there are almost no contraindications to pessary use other than the noncompliant patient. With careful attention to patient selection and meticulous follow-up care, the vaginal supportive pessary serves both the practitioner and patient well and serves an extremely valuable clinical function.

Successful Long-Term Pessary Use and Patient Satisfaction

The ring pessary seems to be used most often due to its ease of use both for patients and physicians. Complications are rare and minor complications are generally easily dealt with [27, 28]. One study cited a high success rate of 82% among pessary users with a satisfaction rate of approximately 70% in patients using a ring pessary. This study did not distinguish patients with a successful pessary fitting and those who no longer use the pessary [29].

Hopefully future studies will answer such questions such as: which specific pessary is most suitable for specific pelvic organ prolapse types and whether or not pelvic floor physical therapy will enhance the patient's ability to retain an intravaginal pessary. These are but some of the questions that remain to be answered. One study from Holland concluded that most patients using the pessary for vaginal prolapse opted for continuation of this therapy [30]. Interestingly and similarly a recent study found that pessaries also can have a therapeutic effect. In 21% of patients, an improvement of the prolapse was found and in no women was a worsening of their prolapse found [31]. Interestingly, although pessary use is quite common and has remained so over the past several decades, there has not been a full evaluation of their efficacy in comparison to other modes of treatment such as pelvic floor muscle exercise (PFME) or surgery. Pessaries have stood the test of time and it is important to incorporate them into gynecologists' practices. This is a safe and useful alternative for conditions that are seen by gynecologists every day. Most notably and stated by Novak, as he concluded a discussion of pessaries by quoting Bantock who wrote, "I am not aware that there is on record a single case in which a woman has lost her life for the use, or even the abuse, of the vaginal pessary." Unfortunately, the outcomes associated with pelvic surgery are not always as clear-cut or safe [32, 33].

Behavioral Treatments in the Management of Pelvic Organ Prolapse

Prevention is the first step when employing behavioral therapies for pelvic organ prolapse. There currently is no vigorous evidence from randomized controlled trials regarding the use of conservative interventions for the management of pelvic organ prolapse. Nevertheless, lifestyle interventions including weight loss, smoking cessation, and reducing activities that exacerbate the prolapse, such as lifting and coughing, as well as improving bowel habits, may ameliorate the symptoms of pelvic organ prolapse. A program of pelvic floor muscle education and exercise instituted prior to the development of prolapse may prove effective in the long-run for our generations of young women. Appropriate abdominal and pelvic floor muscle control during all activities of daily living, including elimination of bladder and bowel, are essential components of treatment. Parents can teach their young children that urinary and defecatory functions are controlled by pelvic floor muscles, and

that control of these muscles brings regular and complete emptying of the bowel and bladder. Young women engaging in competitive sporting activities, most notably high impact sports such as soccer, basketball, and gymnastics should be taught pelvic floor muscle education and exercise including bracing of the core trunk musculature and pelvic floor prior to impact.

Once the diagnosis of pelvic organ prolapse has been made, behavioral therapies may be initiated. The essential components of behavioral therapies are patient education regarding bowel and bladder training, pelvic floor muscle rehabilitation including PFME, vaginal weight-training, biofeedback therapy (alone or in combination with PFME), and pelvic floor electrical stimulation.

Behavioral therapies in the management of pelvic organ prolapse serve two major roles. First and foremost, the behavioral therapies serve as an initial treatment point for the patient and her physician and one that may be revisited and reformatted through the patient's life regarding her particular subsequent lifestyle choices. Second, one of the cornerstones of the behavioral therapies is patient education over the course of her lifetime. Thus the conversation may be continued between the patient and her physician when additional behavioral and other therapies are developed. Behavioral therapies have large potential benefits and are associated with very little, if any, risk. They are also ideal therapies for the elderly patient, where the risk of medication side effects, as well as surgical complications, can be substantial. The behavioral therapies may prove to be most effective in motivated patients with pelvic organ prolapse with or without urinary or fecal incontinence.

Pelvic Floor Muscle Exercise

PFME is considered the cornerstone of all pelvic floor muscle rehabilitation programs in the conservative management of pelvic organ prolapse. In one extensive review of the literature regarding the utilization of pelvic muscle exercises, it was suggested by the authors that, "regular exercises of the pelvic floor should be as much a part of the preventative health-care routine of women as annual Pap smears, and monthly breast self-examination" [34]. The principle of restoring the function of the segregated group of muscles with specific program, method, or aid of reeducation was taken from the orthopedic, neuromuscular, plastic surgery, and physical medicine and rehabilitation literature noted in the gynecological arena, a method of rehabilitation by Arnold Kegel in his original article published in 1948. His work in World War II on muscle function and recovery concluded that, "in the preservation or restoration of muscular function, nothing is more fundamental than the frequent repetition of correctly guided exercises" instituted by the patient's own efforts [35]. Although his original exercise regimen was developed for recovery in the postpartum period, he widened the potential net of usefulness for patients when they would come for a period of what he called "active exercise" in order to prevent pelvic organ prolapse, as well as to provide an improvement in surgical outcome after pelvic floor reconstructive surgery. Coordination of the pelvic floor muscle contractions is the first step in the pelvic floor muscle education training program process. A multidisciplinary approach often is very helpful including the physician, nurse practitioner, and ultimately a physical therapist, especially if the patient is going to continue on her particular program for the long term. Since patients do have to be shown how to do a pelvic floor muscle contraction, a mirror may be helpful in order to actually observe the contraction. This allows the patient to see her pelvic floor elevation. Placing a tampon in the vagina, or the examiner's middle and index finger, or alternatively placing a lubricated cotton swab in the urethra may be able to help the patient actually see her pelvic floor elevation, while observing the perineum using a mirror. Physical examination may allow the physician to evaluate the patient's baseline ability to contract her pelvic floor. With the initial pelvic floor contraction and proper pelvic floor elevation, the patient will observe a slight disappearance of the end of the tampon, near the insertion of the tampon string. The examiner will feel and the patient will observe a pulling upward on his or her fingers and an elevation of the pelvic floor. Valsalva maneuver performed subsequent to this, will allow the patient to visualize the different between a pelvic floor contraction and a Valsalva maneuver. She will be able to see how the Valsalva maneuver and subsequently coughing produced descent of the perineum and urethra. Anatomic models may be utilized, as well as pictorial repre-

sentations of the muscles of the pelvic floor. Only one fifth to one third of women who believe they perform Kegel exercises (pelvic floor contractions) correctly actually exhibit the correct technique. Most women have to be shown how to do these exercises correctly in the stepwise fashion [36]. After this initial stage of observation and palpation of the initial pelvic floor contraction by the physician and patient, the second phase of the pelvic floor muscle education program is initiated. This second stage is a strengthening phase, during which time the patient attempts pelvic floor contractions repeatedly and rapidly, counting how many times she can do this without losing her coordination, quickly and for 1 s each. This "flick contraction" exercise can be performed by contracting and relaxing the levator ani as tightly as possible for 1 s. This exercise helps to augment the fast-twitch fibers (anaerobic-glycolytic), which are the type II muscle fibers (largest diameter). They are the fibers responsible for fast, forceful contractions activated as a short-term response to increased abdominal pressure. The third and next stage is determination and strengthening of the ability of the patient to contract her pelvic floor after a brief rest and hold this contraction for at least 6 s, subsequently resting the pelvic floor for 10–12 s. This exercise will enable the patient to sustain her pelvic floor tone over longer periods of time and mainly are governed by the slow-twitch fibers that are aerobic-oxidative, (smaller diameter), and will enable to patient to develop her baseline pelvic floor strength over the long haul. Additionally, recruitment takes place of the fast-twitch fibers by fast contractions in order to develop strength as well as slow-twitch fibers by slow contractions, as mentioned above, in order to increase long-term endurance [37]. After a strengthening program has been devised the fourth and final step of the pelvic floor muscle education program is the phase where the patient is sent home to practice the program and gradually increase her ability to contract her pelvic floor with exercises referenced above. This particular phase of the program will be most successful if a trained physical therapist, nurse, or nurse practitioner follows the patient on a regular basis and tracks her progress with frequent office visits as determined by the patient, the physician, and the physical therapist as appropriate. It is most important that women be taught to contract their pelvic floor muscles before any rise of intra-abdominal pressure such as lifting, coughing, sports, or any other anticipated increase in intra-abdominal pressure. This is also termed "pelvic bracing" and is believed to help augment the success of pelvic floor muscle education programs for pelvic organ prolapse. Cammu et al. reported that the majority of patients who respond successfully to pelvic floor muscle education programs (physiotherapy programs) remain satisfied after 10 years or more [38]. There are various protocols with PFME currently available. The number of contractions range from 100 per day to Kegel's original dissertation recommending 300 contractions per day [35]. Burgio et al. recommended 45 exercises daily divided into three sessions of 15 exercises each and then increasing the length of the sustained contraction. The use of vaginal cones may serve as adjunctive therapy to any pelvic floor muscle education program in order to augment and enhance the patient's overall long-term muscle strength. These were developed by Plevnik in order to improve pelvic floor muscle strength. These range in weight approximately 5–100 g, and are of equal shape and volume as well as appearance. The patient is asked to introduce the vaginal cone and to attempt to retain it intravaginally by contracting her muscles while ambulating for a period of 15–30 min, once to twice a day. This provides feedback to the patient to maintain pelvic floor contractions and increase hypertrophy and augment her slow-twitch fibers responsible for this baseline pelvic floor contraction. The patient begins with the lowest weight she can easily retain and is instructed to progress to the next heaviest weight after approximately 1 month of twice daily use without this initial weight falling out vaginally for 30 consecutive days. The patient is then instructed to progress to the next heaviest weight until she is able to maintain the heaviest weight intravaginally twice daily, for 30 min, for a period of 30 days. She may continue utilizing the weights once to twice per day for up to 30 min. Peattie et al. studied 39 premenopausal women and found that after 1 month of use, 70% of patients were either improved or cured.

Recently, a new intravaginal device designed to allow PFME to treat advanced degrees of vaginal prolapse by acting as a space-occupying sphere above the levators muscles has become available (Fig. 21.8). The Colpexin sphere (Adamed, New Jersey, USA) is placed into the vaginal canal, above

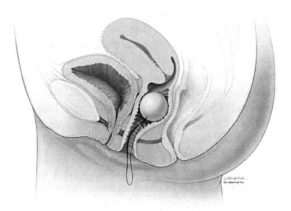

Fig. 21.8. Colpexin sphere in place, elevating the prolapsed genital tissues above the levator muscles while the patient performs pelvic floor exercises

the levator plate, thus reducing any significant prolapse, and allowing Kegel exercises to help provide support to the prolapsed tissues. Over time, the levator muscles hypertrophy and the size of the levator hiatus decreases, leading to improved pelvic floor support. Additional benefits include reduction of urinary incontinence episodes with the device in place [39].

The Role of Biofeedback

Biofeedback is a training technique as well as a process and is defined in the behavioral medicine literature as "a process in which a person learns to reliably influence physiological responses of two kinds: either responses which are not under voluntary control or responses which are ordinarily easily regulated but for which regulation has broken down due to trauma or disease" [40]. It also is a training technique "soundly based on the principles of human behavior and learning, and supported by considerable evidence derived from years of experimental investigation" [41]. Biofeedback is used in conjunction with many of the techniques and therapies previously mentioned in this chapter as part of a pelvic floor muscle training program.

Biofeedback is provided to the patients with a visual display such as light, a computerized graphic display, or by means of an auditory signal (Fig. 21.9). Vaginal or rectal probes are easy to use and comfortable for patients during insertion and removal, and

FIG. 21.9. Biofeedback instruments for home use (used with permission of Marks LE, OTR and Freedman M, PT, BCIA-PMDB)

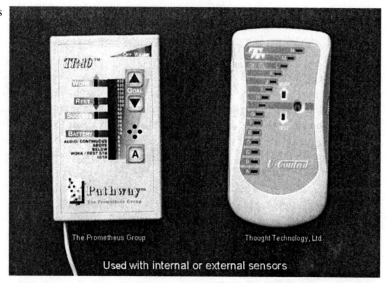

also may afford the patient control over her pelvic floor muscle biofeedback program. During the initial phase of vaginal EMG it may be useful for an additional surface electrodes to be placed on accessory muscles (usually abdominal wall sensors) in order to teach the patient to accurately isolate a pelvic floor muscle contraction. Biofeedback therapy needs to elicit low pelvic floor muscle resting tension prior to and following an exercise session. Patients are instructed to selectively contract and relax their pelvic floor musculature without increasing their intra-abdominal pressure.

Home training programs then may be subsequently developed on an individual basis for patients presenting with pelvic organ prolapse either with or without stress or urge incontinence. EMG electrodes embedded in vaginal or rectal probes are easily utilized by patients in a home setting. This affords the patient privacy as well as ease and comfort of use.

Biofeedback when utilized as a component of a pelvic floor exercise program ensures that exercises of the pelvic floor are being performed properly. Patients may do very well with biofeedback as part of an integrated PFME program; this may prove to be synergistic, in regard to the patient's ultimate outcome and satisfaction with her treatment. Randomized controlled trials are needed to determine whether the increase in pelvic floor muscle strength associated with biofeedback training

programs actually result in a clinically significant reduction in pelvic organ prolapse in the short- as well as the long-term period. Having said this, biofeedback is easily incorporated into any PFME program and generally is well accepted by patients, in particular because this gives the patient a sense of control over her body and bodily functions. Knowledge about anatomy and physiology may aid the patient by gaining knowledge and thereby gaining power over her own condition and may have a positive effect on her ultimate outcome.

Functional Electrical Stimulation

Functional electrical stimulation (FES) was first utilized in 1963 by Caldwell for correction of urinary and fecal incontinence. Since that time electrical stimulation has proved to be a valuable adjunct to biofeedback and additionally as a standalone method in the armamentarium of conservative alternative approaches for the management of pelvic organ prolapse and additionally to treat stress and urge incontinence [42]. As with the conservative approaches previously mentioned, electrical stimulation allows the patient to learn how to strengthen as well as more properly utilize her pelvic floor muscles either alone or in combination with biofeedback therapy. FES in conjunction with biofeedback therapy can enable the patient to sense her pelvic floor muscles as they contract and ultimately to be able to contract them and perform these exercises with or without biofeedback, without the assistance of a pelvic floor contraction created by electrical stimulation per se. Therefore electrical stimulation of the pelvic floor can help elicit a reflex contraction of the pelvic musculature, especially during activities such as lifting, laughing, and coughing. A low-mid frequency current (50 Hz) is utilized in order to stimulate a contraction of the levator ani muscles. It is quite bearable to the patient. Lower frequencies (10–25 Hz) are useful to reduce bladder overactivity.

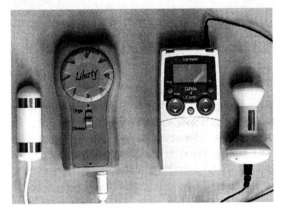

Fig. 21.10. Electrical stimulation units (used with permission of Marks LE, OTR and Freedman M, PT, BCIA-PMDB)

FES is particularly useful for patients who do not have adequate awareness of their pelvic floor musculature and who may be unable to isolate a pelvic floor contraction. Electrical stimulation in these cases may help the patient properly identify the location of the pelvic floor muscles while providing proprioception as well as assisting the patient in performing the contraction.

Pelvic floor exercises alone have been demonstrated to improve pelvic floor muscle strength, thus reducing prolapse and additionally assisting in the reduction of incontinence [42]. Adding to basic PFME programs, biofeedback with or without electrical stimulation has been proven to be not only comfortable for the patient, but without significant side effects and quite synergistic in regard to reeducation of the pelvic floor muscles (Figs. 21.10 and 21.11).

The principle of electrical stimulation per se is based on restoring normal, physiological reflex mechanisms in abnormal muscles and nerves [43]. Electrophysiological data suggest that a partial denervation occurs along with weakening of the pelvic floor musculature during childbirth. There additionally is a loss of levator ani muscle tone. FES promotes tissue growth and potentially nerve regeneration. Therefore reinnervation of the pelvic floor may occur through the judicious use of electrical stimulation with persistent biofeedback therapy or electrical stimulation alone.

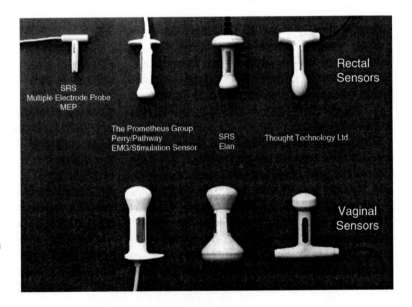

Fig. 21.11. Vaginal and rectal sensors for biofeedback and electrical stimulation (used with permission of Marks LE, OTR and Freedman M, PT, BCIA-PMDB)

Vaginal muscle strength increased significantly over that of control subjects who utilized the SHAM device for investigating transvaginal pelvic floor electrical stimulation for genuine stress incontinence [44]. Electrical stimulation has been shown to be effective in patients who initially are unable to perform a pelvic floor muscle contraction or to identify the correct muscles to contract. Thus pelvic floor muscle education is provided through initial stimulatory and then subsequently voluntary pelvic floor muscle contractions [45].

Contraindications to electrical stimulation are fairly few: patients who utilize on-demand high pacemakers, patients who are pregnant, patients with postvoid urine residuals >100 ml, and patients with urethral obstruction, bleeding (sessions must not be held during menstruation), and urinary pelvic or vaginal infections.

Electrical stimulation is a valuable and effective therapeutic tool, in particular in patients who are unable to identify and contract the correct pelvic floor muscles initially. Biofeedback-triggered electrical stimulation may actually be more effective than either treatment alone, and additionally has the attraction of reducing the lag time to evident treatment response [46]. Finally, as with other conservative methods for the reduction of pelvic organ prolapse, patient motivation and commitment of the therapist and patient are crucial elements for successful therapeutic outcome. On average these therapies require approximately 2 months of an intensive program in order begin to see therapeutic results. Additionally, in most cases, these programs must be continued for the duration of the patient's lifetime if improvement or cure is to be maintained. Finally, improvement in a patient's overall pelvic health is enormous. The results, in many cases, are rewarding for both patient and therapist.

Conclusions

The decision to elect conservative treatment modalities for pelvic organ prolapse involves a time commitment on the part of both the physician and the patient. All treatment options must be considered carefully in the context of the individual patient's life and health. There must be a willingness to accept the possibility of the delayed results that may be associated with conservative treatments. These therapies should be considered for any patient who is deemed to be high-risk due to medical comorbidities, patients who do not desire surgery or who do desire repeat surgery, patients who are not yet completed with their childbearing, patients who are exceptionally motivated, and patients who are agreeable to periodically reevaluating their unique situations as they change dynamically over time. Finally, in patients who elect to use pessaries, physicians must be extremely cognizant of the importance of regular routine pessary care and vigilant in their follow-up, which must be meticulous due to the potential for complication. Although rare, complications due to the "forgotten pessary" must be avoided at all costs.

Future areas of research must focus on comparing and evaluating various conservative therapies in the management of pelvic organ prolapse. We must systematically examine which patients would benefit most from these therapies including pessaries, as well as what specific type of conservative therapies should be used and under what circumstances.

Acknowledgments. Marilyn Freedman, Physical Therapist, for her editorial assistance, support, and friendship. Elise Stettner, Physical Therapist, for her support and her technical expertise. Susan Gimmi, for her manuscript preparation skills. Sigrid Anderson, for typing of the manuscript. Dennis Skahill and Adam Cooper, NSLIJHS, for their assistance with figures and photos. Debbie Rand, Chief of Library Services, LIJMC. Shfra Atik, Senior Librarian, LIJMC. Rita Feigenberg, Librarian, LIJMC. Norma Frankel, Librarian, LIJMC. Carlos Arguelles, Librarian, LIJMC. And to my family, especially Aaron and Bobbie, for their love and encouragement.

References

1. Swift S, Theofrastous JP. Aetiology and classification of pelvic organ prolapse. In: Cardozo L, Staskin D, eds. Female urology and urogynecology. London: Isis Medical Media; 2001:576–585.
2. Samuelsson EC, Arne Victor FT, Tibblin G, Svardsudd KF. Signs of genital prolapse in a Swedish population of women 20 to 59 years of age and possible related factors. Am J Obstet Gynecol 1999; 180:299–305.
3. Karram M, Portur R. Pathophysiology, diagnosis and management of rectoceles. In: Cardozo L.

Staskin D, eds. Female urology and urogynaecology. London: Isis Medical Media; 2001:616–625.

4. Olsen AL, Smith VJ, Bergstrom JO, et al. Epidemiology of surgically managed pelvic organ prolapse and urinary incontinence. Obstet Gynecol 1997; 89:501–506.

5. Stedman, TL. Stedman's medical dictionary. Baltimore, MD: Williams and Wilkins, 1976:1062.

6. Miller, DS. Contemporary use of the pessary. In: Gynecology and obstetrics, Vol. 1. Sciarra JJ, ed. Philadelphia: Lippincott; 1995:1–12.

7. Cundiff GW, Weidner AC, Visco AG, et al. A survey of pessary use by members of the American Urogynecologic Society. Obstet Gynecol 2000; 95:931–935.

8. Niemiec TR. Adequate follow-up "essential" after placement of pessary. Obstet Gynecol News 1989; 24:1.

9. Handa VL, Jones M. Do pessaries prevent the progression of pelvic organ prolapse? Int Urogynecol J 2002; 13(6):349–352.

10. Nygaard IE, Zinsmeister AR. Treatment of exercise incontinence with a vaginal pessary: A preliminary study. Int Urogynecol J 1993; 4:133–137.

11. Trowbridge ER, Fenner DE. Conservative management of pelvic organ prolapse. Clin Obstet Gynecol 2005; 48(3):668–681.

12. Young SB. Nonsurgical management of prolapse. In: Atlas of clinical gynecology, Vol. 5. Thomas Benson J, ed. Philadelphia: McGraw-Hill; 1999:8.1–8.13.

13. Stenchever MA, Benson JT. Atlas of clinical gynecology, vol. V, Urogynecology and reconstructive pelvic surgery. 2000; Philadelphia: Current Medicine.

14. Clemons JL. Aguilar VC, Tillinghast TA. et al. Risk factors associated with an unsuccessful pessary fitting trial in women with pelvic organ prolapse. Am J Obstet Gynecol 2004; 90(2):345–350.

15. Myers DL, LaSala CA, Murphy JA. Double pessary use in grade 4 uterine and vaginal prolapse. Obstet Gynecol 1998; 91:1019–1020.

16. Rabin JM, et al. Gelift: patent #5,894,842. April 20, 1999.

17. Kunczicky V, Uhl-Steidl M, Pontpasch H. Safety and acceptance of self-application of the pubic and uretheral ring pessaries. Gynakol Geburtshilf Rundschr 1998; 38:242–246.

18. Poma PA. Management of incarcerated vaginal pessaries. J Am Geriatr Soc 1981; 29:325–327.

19. Goldstein I, Wise GJ, Tancer ML. A vesicovaginal fistula and intravesical foreign body. A rare case of the neglected pessary. Am J Obstet Gynecol 1990; 163(2):589–591.

20. Grody MH, Nyirjesy P, Chatwani A. Intravesical foreign body and vesicovaginal fistula: A rare complication of a neglected pessary. Int Urogynecol J Pelvic Floor Dysfunct 1999; 10(6):407–408.

21. Sivasuriya M. Cervical entrapment of a polyethylene vaginal ring pessary a clinical curiosity. Aust M Z J Obstet Gynecol 1987; 27:168–169.

22. Ott R. Richte H, Behr J, Scheele J. Small bowel prolapse and incarceration caused by a vaginal ring pessary. Br J Surg 1993; 80:1157.

23. Roberge RJ, Keller C, Garfinkel M. Vaginal pessary induced mechanical bowel obstruction. J Emerg Med 2001; 20:367–370.

24. Meinhardt W, Schuitemaker MW, Smeets NJ, Venema PL. Bilateral hydronephrosis with urosepsis due to neglected pessary. Case report. Scand J Urol Nephrol 1993; 27:419–420.

25. Nichols DH, Randall CL. Vaginal surgery, 4th ed. 1996; Lippincott: Williams & Wilkins.

26. Schraub S, Sun, XS, Maingon P, et al. Cervical and vaginal cancer associated with pessary use. Cancer 1982; 69:2505–2509.

27. Pott-Grinstein E, Newcomer JR. Gynecologists' patterns of prescribing pessaries. J Reprod Med 2001; 46(3):205–208.

28. Sulak PJ, Kuehl TJ, Shull BL. Vaginal pessaries and their use in pelvic relaxation. J Reprod Med 1993; 38(12):919–923.

29. Bai SW, Yoon SB, Kwon JY, et al. A survey of the characteristics and satisfaction degree of the patients using a pessary. Int Urogynecol J 2005; 16:182–186.

30. Clemons JL, Aguilar VC, Sokol ER, et al. Patient characteristics that are associated with continued pessary use versus surgery after 1 year. Am J Obstet Gynecol 2004; 191:159–164.

31. Morgan-Jahanshir L, Shott S, Fenner DE. Factors affecting patients' ability to retain a pessary. AM Urogyn Society, 19th Annual Scientific Meeting. Washington, DC; November 1998.

32. Novak E. The vaginal pessary: Its indications and limitations. JAMA 1923; 80:1294–1298.

33. Bantock GG. In defense of the pessary. J Obstet Gynecol Br Emp 1905; 7:17–29.

34. Wall LL, Davidson TG. The role of muscular re-education by physical therapy in the treatment of genuine stress urinary incontinence. Obstet Gynecol Surg 1992, 47:322–331.

35. Kegel A. A progressive resistance exercise in the functional restoration of the perineal muscles. Am J Obstet Gynecol 1948; 56:238–246.

36. Bo K, Larsen S, Oseid S, et al. Knowledge about and ability to correct pelvic floor muscle exercises in women with urinary incontinence. Neurol Urodyn 1998; 7:261–262.

37. Samples JT, Dougerthy MC, Abrams RM, Batich CD. The dynamic characteristics of the circumvaginal muscles. JOGNN 1988; 17(3):194–201.

38. Cammu H, Van Nylen M, Amy J. A ten-year follow-up after Kegel pelvic floor muscle exercises for genuine stress incontinence. BJU Int 2000; 85:655–658.

39. Lukban JC, Aguirre OA, Davila GW, Sand. Safety and effectiveness of Colpexin Sphere in the treatment of pelvic organ prolapse. Int Urogynecol J Pelvic Floor Dysfunct. 2006 Sep;17(5):449–54. Epub 2005 Nov 19.

40. Feuerstein M, Labbe EE, Kuczmierczyk AR. Health psychology: A psychobiological perspective. 1986; New York: Plenum Press.

41. Burgio KL. Urinary incontinence; non-surgical therapies: Biofeedback therapy. In: Benson JT, ed. Female pelvic floor disorders. New York: WW Norton Company; 1992:210–218.

42. Caldwell KPS. The electrical control of sphincter incontinence. Lancet 1963; 2:174–175.

43. Fall M, Erlandson BE, Carlsson CA, Lindstrom S. The effect of intravaginal electrical stimulation on the feline urethra and urinary bladder: neuronal mechanisms. Scand J Urol Nephrol Suppl 1977; 44:19–30.

44. Sand PK, Richardson DA, Staskin VR, et al. Pelvic floor electrical stimulation in the treatment of genuine stress incontinence: A multicenter, placebo-controlled trial. Gen Obstet Gynecol 1995; 173(1):72–79.

45. Bo K. Effect of electrical stimulation on stress and urge urinary incontinence. Clinical outcome and practical recommendations based on randomized controlled trials. Acta Obstet Gynecol Scand 1998; 77(Suppl 168):3–11.

46. Yamanishi T, Yasuda K. Electrical stimulation for stress incontinence. Int Urogynecol J 1998; 9: 281–290.

Chapter 22
Surgery for Pelvic Organ Prolapse: An Historical Review

Baharak Amir and Alfred E. Bent

What drugs will not cure, the knife will; what the knife will not cure, the cautery will; what the cautery will not cure must be considered incurable.

Hippocrates

In reviewing the history regarding surgery for pelvic organ prolapse, it becomes apparent that although the evolution of medicine is amazing, there is a constant yet dynamic ebb and flow of conflicting theory and evidence. The literature regarding the history of gynecologic surgery is a testament to the fast pace of advancement yet a controversy to what is currently practiced. Richard H. Meade says of the task of writing the history of surgery – "the task is undertaken with due humility" [1]. His words resound clearly when discussing the history and evolution of current gynecologic surgery and in particular pelvic floor surgery.

It appears that our first understanding and knowledge of pelvic organ prolapse comes from the ancient Egyptians [1]. In the Kahun papyrus of Egypt, dating to 2000 BC, and in the Ebers papyrus, some 500 years later, there are medical records referring to pelvic organ prolapse [2]. Little else is known of how ancient civilizations treated this female condition. It has been suggested that astringent solutions such as vinegar and pessaries molded from beeswax or round fruit such as pomegranates were used in ancient Egypt for reducing prolapse, with the earliest description of a pessary being provided by Hippocrates. A device made of bronze, believed to be a pessary, was found in the ruins of Pompeii [3].

Hippocrates was also the first to provide advice for the treatment of pelvic organ prolapse that was considered irreducible by traditional methods. This has become known as *hippocratic succussion* (Fig. 22.1). As depicted in this illustration, the patient was bound by her feet and hung upside-down along a ladderlike frame. Held in this position for several minutes, the frame was moved up and down behind the patient, causing her to shake. The upside-down position, gravity, and shaking were thought to help reduce the prolapse [2].

In 1910, Henry Wellcome, a British collector of medical artifacts and instruments, found an incised stone tablet in the Temple at Rom-Ourbos near the city of Cairo. The temple, built by Ptolemy VII (181–146 BC), depicts a number of surgical instruments that are thought to be obstetric and gynecologic [3]. This would suggest that there may have been more than conservative treatment available for pelvic organ prolapse over 2000 years ago.

Soranus of Ephesus, a physician of the Greco-Roman Era, considered to be the authority of gynecology in antiquity, is purported to have been the first to propose and perform excision of the gangrenous prolapsed uterus (98–138 AD) [2]. Many authors have suggested that although no reports exist for the actual performance of a hysterectomy before the sixteenth century, this procedure is mentioned in several ancient records, such as those of Aretaeus of Cappodocia, between the second and third centuries AD and again by Paulus Aegina, in the seventh century AD [3].

Fig. 22.1. Hippocratic succussion (from
[2], original picture from Appolonius
of Kitium, Appolonius of Kitium.
Illustrieter Kommentar zu der hippok-
ratischen Schrift hEP APqPWN (Peri
Arthron), V.H. Schone (Ed.). Teubner,
Leipzig, 1896)

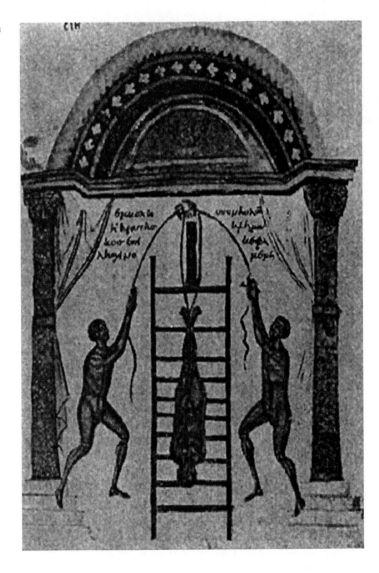

The first official record of a uterus being excised was written by anatomist and surgeon Berengaria da Carpi of Bologna. He witnessed his father excise a prolapsed and gangrenous uterus vaginally from a woman in the early 1500s [1]. It is believed that this patient did in fact live for many more years but was unable to enjoy intimate relations with her husband [3]. Berengaria da Carpi also performed the surgery himself once and subsequently assisted a colleague with another. He describes his technique for vaginal hysterectomy as consisting of ligating the prolapsed uterus with thick twine. This twine was tightened progressively to the point of severing the organ. [3]. Celebrated French surgeon,

Ambroise Paré (1509–1590), also provided similar details of his approach for the removal of a gangrenous prolapsed uterus [3].

Prior to the sixteenth century, limited knowledge of anatomy and physiology restricted appropriate management for female pelvic organ prolapse. Changing views of science, less hindered by religion, led to cadaveric dissections and those who provided accounts and teaching of what lay within the human body. Although Leonardo Da Vinci (1452–1519) provided many beautiful illustrations including those of female pelvic anatomy (Fig. 22.2), few in his time were privy to his work. It was Andreas Vesalius (1514–1564) who revolu-

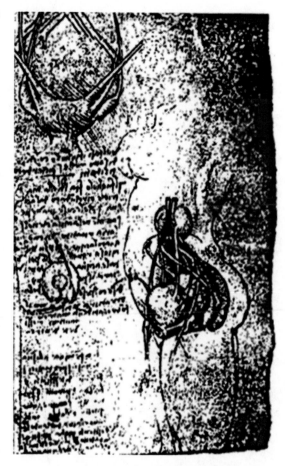

FIG. 22.2. The female organs of generation by Leonardo da vinci (from [4])

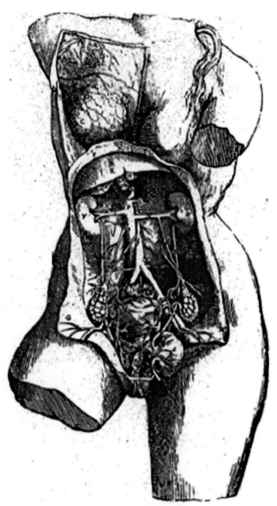

FIG. 22.3. The female pelvic organs as illustrated by Vesalius (from [4] Original from *De humani corporsis fabrica*, 1543)

tionized our understanding of the human female pelvis by providing the first accurate description of the female genital tract through cadaveric dissection. His teachings and descriptions became the foundation for anatomy and physiology of the female pelvis (Fig. 22.3). Shortly thereafter, the engravings of Johannes Scultetus (1595–1645) in his *Armementarium Chirurgicum*, provide the first illustrations in step-by-step account of pelvic surgery (Fig. 22.4a, b). In this body of work is found the first known illustration of procidentia [2].

During the seventeenth century, uterine prolapse became better described and classified. Among other gynecologic subjects in his book, the physician James Cooke (1614–1688) also describes *procidentia uteri* [3]. In the latter part of the century, there appeared to be significant debate regarding the appropriate measures to be taken with a prolapsed uterus. Namely, many experts did not favor surgical therapy and believed that all uteri could be reduced even if temporarily with conservative methods such as pessaries (Fig. 22.5a, b).

It was during the eighteenth century that other aspects of vaginal prolapse were first characterized. Perineal and vaginal hernias were first described by French physician Jean Mèry in 1713 [2]. The famous Scottish obstetrician William Smellie also provided case reports of the same in 1731. During the middle of the eighteenth century, an interest in relaxation of the vaginal walls, particularly

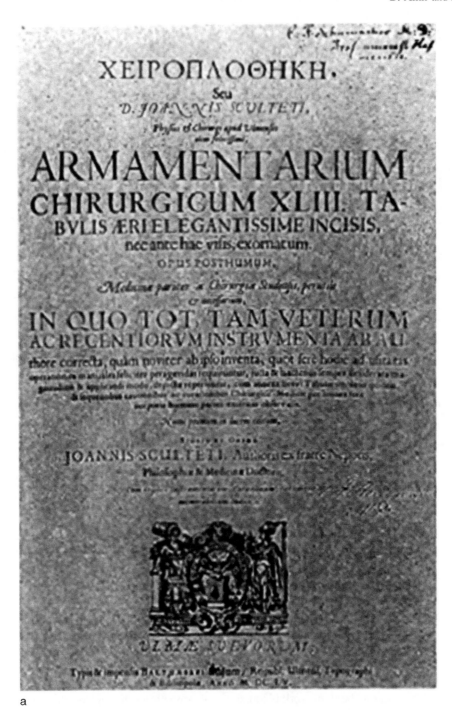

a

FIG. 22.4. (**a**) 1655 edition of Aramentarium Chirurgicum by Johann Schultes (Scultetus) and selected illustrations (from [4]). (**b**) 1655 edition of Aramentarium Chirurgicum by Johann Schultes (Scultetus) and selected illustrations (from [4])

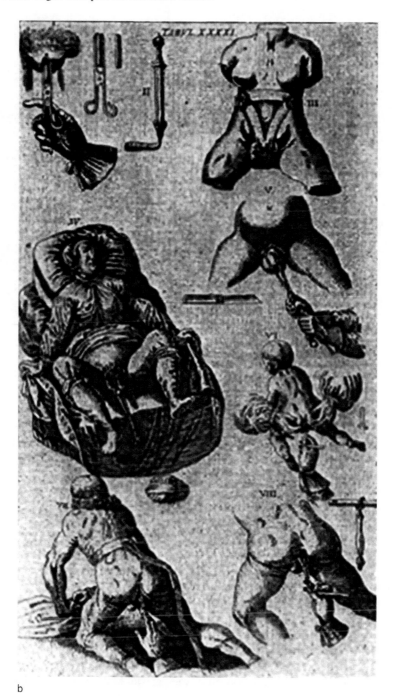

b

Fɪɢ. 22.4. (continued)

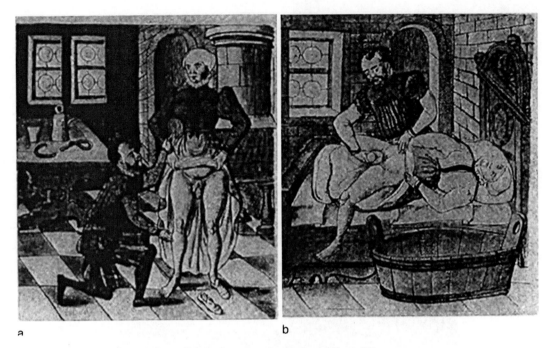

a   b

FIG. 22.5. (**a, b**) The examination and reinsertion of uterine prolapse (from [4])

cystocele and rectocele, which were termed hernias of the bladder and rectum, began with René-Jacques-Croissant de Garengoet (1688–1759). He was the first to describe using a vaginal speculum to conduct his examination of the vagina and differentiate areas of pelvic relaxation [5].

Although much changed regarding our understanding of medicine by the valuable contributions of those mentioned and many more to human physiology and anatomy, much remained unchanged with regard to gynecologic therapy. Prior to the nineteenth century, treatment for female conditions such as menorrhagia, pelvic organ prolapse, and vaginal fistulae were primarily conservative in nature. The most popular treatment for pelvic organ prolapse remained the vaginal pessary. Many of these pessaries were quite elaborate in design with straps and belts to keep them in place. During the nineteenth century and in particular after the understanding and development of antiseptic technique, surgical therapy gained favor. The eighteenth century also saw the establishment of the anatomic classification of pelvic organ prolapse that we still use today.

The first vaginal hysterectomy specifically for pelvic organ prolapse is believed to have been performed by American Civil War surgeon Samuel Choppin in 1861, in New Orleans. His patient is said to have survived and later presented before a medical class with her uterus held in her hand as proof of her survival after the procedure [2]. Other surgeons such as James Blundell in Great Britain in 1829, and J.C. Warren in the United States that same year had each performed vaginal hysterectomy on a prolapsed uterus for removal of a cancerous cervix [2].

By the end of the nineteenth century, vaginal hysterectomy became a primary operative procedure for pelvic organ prolapse. Indeed, Parisian physician Pierre Delbet, in 1896, described his modification of the vaginal hysterectomy for pelvic organ prolapse that he called "colpocystopexie," whereby he supported the superior aspect of the vaginal wall to the round ligaments [2].

The first successful abdominal hysterectomy was performed by Walter Burnham in 1853 [6]. Burnham was a prominent Massachusetts surgeon and professor who had begun an exploratory laparotomy on a female patient with a pelvic mass when during the surgery she vomited and pushed out an enlarged uterus. He could not reinsert the uterus and had no choice but to remove it. His patient survived this procedure and Burnham went on to perform 15 abdominal hysterectomies, thus introducing another means of removing the uterus.

J. Marion Sims, well known for his contributions toward repair of vesicovaginal fistulae, was the first to describe the vaginal repair for a cystocele. In 1866, Sims described the denudation of an elliptical segment of the anterior vaginal wall followed by primary closure of this incision [7]. Many of the procedures aimed to correct pelvic organ prolapse, involved this denudation of the vaginal mucosa. In 1877, French surgeon, Leon Le Fort's procedure involved denudation of the entire vaginal wall for total vaginal occlusion [2].

During the twentieth century more modifications for surgical repair of pelvic organ prolapse occurred. Abdominal approaches evolved to correct prolapse such as D.T. Gilliam's uterine suspension in 1900 [8], and the Manchester approach for conserving the uterus by cervical amputation with anterior and posterior repairs. Fothergill proposed suturing the cardinal ligaments to the anterior aspect of the cervix, and hence evolved the procedure known today as the Manchester–Fothergill operation [2].

Howard Atwood Kelly, known as the father of modern gynecology, arrived at Johns Hopkins University in 1888, where he became the first professor of Gynecology with special interest in the area of urogynecology. His many contributions include the initiation of organized training in the area of gynecologic and urologic surgery. It was in 1918 that urology developed as a separate specialty following Kelly's pioneering work in cystoscopy [9]. His other contributions include the development of specific surgical tools such as the Kelly clamp, which is still indispensable in vaginal and abdominal hysterectomies, and two gynecologic textbooks with extensive illustrations (Fig. 22.6) by famous Johns Hopkins' medical illustrator, Max Brödel [10, 11].

In 1914, Kelly and his colleague W.M. Dumm were the first to publish their modified technique for cystocele repair with periurethral plication meant also to treat stress urinary incontinence [12]. Their technique is still practiced by many surgeons today. Many more modifications of Kelly and Dumm's method ensued, mostly involving ways to reinforce surgical technique to prevent the high recurrence rate of cystocele and cure stress urinary

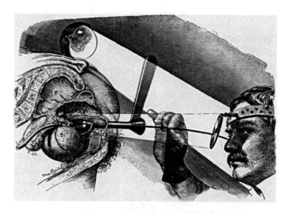

FIG. 22.6. Max Brodel's illustration of Kelly performing cystoscopy and catheterization of the left ureter (from [11])

incontinence. In 1936, W.T. Kennedy modified Kelly's plication technique and advocated its use for the management of urinary incontinence at the time of hysterectomy [2].

As a result of the work of esteemed surgeons such as Mayo, Heaney, Richardson, Pratt, Te Linde, and others, vaginal hysterectomy with colporrhaphy became the most popular surgery for uterovaginal prolapse in North America [13].

With better understanding of female surgical anatomy, the concept of central and lateral defects to the anterior vaginal wall developed. George R. White first described what he believed to be the reason for the consistent failure to provide a permanent cure for a cystocele [14]. In 1909, he described reattachment of the vaginal sulci to the "white line of pelvic fascia" or the *arcus tendineous fascia*, and thus corrected what we now understand as a paravaginal or lateral defect. Although he clearly described his vaginal technique and reported excellent cure rates, it was not until A. Cullen Richardson described four distinct defects in the anterior vaginal wall support from his cadaveric dissections (Fig. 22.7a, b) and devised an abdominal approach to correcting the anterior vaginal wall defect, that the term "paravaginal defect" was coined and this procedure gained favor [15].

Repair of posterior vaginal defects gained momentum during the past century. Prior to the twentieth century there is a paucity of information regarding the surgical management of such defects as rectoceles. R.J.C de Garengoet was the first to describe an enterocele in 1736. He coined the term *enterocele*

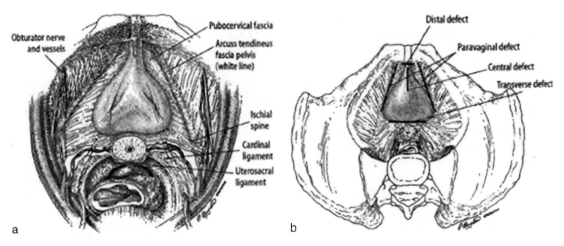

FIG. 22.7. (**a, b**) A.C. Richardson's illustration of endopelvic fascia and locations of anterior vaginal wall support defects (from [15])

vaginale and created a specific pessary for this condition [5]. Thereafter, anatomist Edward Sandifort in 1777, through cadaveric dissection, described a condition he called "intestinovaginal hernia" or perhaps what we now know as rectocele–enterocele [3]. The reason for so little historical literature on the management of rectoceles is likely that women during the nineteenth and early twentieth century were less inclined than modern women to complain of such concerns as fecal incontinence and needing to manually reduce posterior vaginal defects to have bowel movements.

As with cystocele and uterine prolapse, prior to the twentieth century, management for rectoceles appears to have been primarily conservative. In 1867, however, Simon of Heidelberg may be considered the first to have described the technique for repairing posterior vaginal wall defects and originated the term posterior "colporrhaphy" [16, 17]. His technique attempted to reduce rectoceles and uterovaginal prolapse by plication of the levator ani muscles and the inferior aspect of the vagina [16, 18]. Hegar in 1870 went on to introduce his method of posterior repair by creating a tight introital ring [16]. One hundred years later, in 1970, A. Cullen Richardson described five sites along the rectovaginal fascia that could be broken and produce defects, and as with his correction for anterior vaginal wall defects he advocated a site-specific method for the repair of a rectocele [15].

With many more independent surgeons communicating with one another and sharing theories, tools, and techniques many of the relatively simple surgeries for prolapse have evolved and matured to what are now known. In 1942, H.S. Heaney provided his experience after performing hundreds of vaginal hysterectomies for pelvic organ prolapse, wherein he clearly described his successful technique for the procedure [19]. In 1957, M.L. McCall published his culdoplasty technique for repairing an enterocele [20].

With many more hysterectomies being performed in the middle of the preceding century, a new concern in the form of vaginal vault prolapse developed. Now investigators were introducing techniques for diagnosis, treatment, and prevention of vault prolapse. E.H. Richardson in 1937 with the Spalding–Richardson composite operation [21] and McCall with the posterior culdoplasty provided efforts to prevent this complication of hysterectomy. In 1962, Lash and Levin suggested a radiological technique for the diagnosis of vaginal vault prolapse [22].

Now experts describe apical vaginal prolapse and specialized surgeries such as sacrospinous colpopexy, which have been introduced by Amreich, Richter, Nichols, and Randall [23]. Sacrospinous vaginal vault fixation was first developed by German surgeons Amreich and Richter. This procedure is still performed extensively in Europe and is called the

Amreich–Richter procedure. Nichols, who learned the procedure from Amreich, later performed and published information regarding this procedure with colleague Randall, in the United States.

The abdominal counterpart for vaginal vault prolapse, the sacrocolpopexy, was first described by Parsons and Ulfelder, and has become another popular method for the correction of vaginal vault prolapse [24]. Indeed, following publication of results from the first large series by W.H. Addison and colleagues, it is now considered the gold standard for restoration of the vaginal vault [25].

Today there are numerous variations for vaginal vault repairs including techniques involving suspensions to the iliococcygeus fascia [26] and uterosacral ligaments [27]. All of these procedures for vaginal vault prolapse are well described in the literature, with many surgeons favoring one over another in different circumstances and ongoing debate regarding the best approach to take.

Also along with advanced technology has come the use of adjuvant graft material to reinforce repairs, whether the repair is done abdominally or vaginally. In 1964, W.H. Ferguson was the first to describe the use of Marlex mesh as part of the repair for vaginal vault prolapse [28]. Traditionally, very few biomaterials and synthetic materials were used in vaginal surgery. In a resurgence of performing vaginal operations that are more durable, these materials increasingly have been utilized. There is a growing market for such materials as is generally the case with new technology, yet there is no conclusive evidence supporting the use of either synthetic or biological graft materials in vaginal reconstructive surgery. Despite this, there continues to be a steep evolution with regards to the quality of graft material. Today, the most common biomaterials in use are xenograft: porcine dermis, bovine pericardium, porcine small intestinal mucosa; allograft: cadaveric fascia and dermis; and autologous: harvested rectus fascia or fascia lata. The most common synthetic material used today for vaginal repairs and abdominal sacrocolpopexy continues to be polyprolpylene as a large-pore mesh.

Since the 1970s there also has been amazing growth in endoscopy and laparoscopy. For every surgery there are new minimally invasive techniques [29]. Many procedures such as hysterectomies [30], vault suspensions, and paravaginal repairs [31] can be performed laparoscopically. This has led to reduced morbidity and mortality and reduced hospital stay and an ever-expanding realm of new tools and techniques.

To describe the list of further developments over the course of the last two to three decades is a hefty task. It is sufficient to say that this aspect of medicine—the correction of pelvic floor disorders such as pelvic organ prolapse—remains dynamic and is constantly evolving to improve and provide justification for old techniques and also provide new methods.

In order to improve the communication between different investigators, systems for quantifying and standardizing the severity of pelvic organ prolapse were devised (Fig. 22.8). Methods that have been used to grade pelvic organ prolapse have included the Baden halfway system [32] and the International Continence Society (ICS) classification, which has adopted the Pelvic Organ Prolapse Quantification (POP-Q) system [33, 34].

With improved communication between independent medical investigators and advanced technology, growth in medical knowledge during the twentieth century can be simply described as exponential. Specialized fields such as urology and gynecology branched off and within them further subspecialties such as urogynecology and pelvic floor surgery have evolved. Each member of the medical scientific community now has his or her own unique area of medicine on which to concentrate all of their scientific efforts.

Thus the concept of evidence-based medicine has evolved. It now is simply not enough to theorize or describe exciting new tools and practices, but now you must prove efficacy and effectiveness under the ever-constant scrutiny of peer review.

In many respects, evidence-based medicine has become a standard of care, but it also evokes controversy, and at times confusion, particularly for surgical techniques that have been performed for many years but do not have sufficient evidence to justify their practice. There are multiple ways of correcting one aspect of a pelvic floor defect and the modern pelvic floor surgeon must decide which procedure, in what context, for each individual patient is necessary.

Also, in dividing medicine into smaller compartments, there is some overlap of care for such

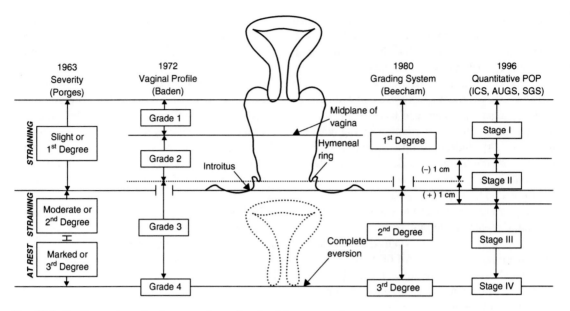

F_IG. 22.8. Grading systems for degree and severity of pelvic organ prolapse

things as the female pelvic floor. This of course can engender some degree of dispute among the different specialties, whether good or bad, to prove one more superior to deal with the issues at hand over the others. Wall and Delancey in 1991 illustrate this feud exceptionally well [35] . In modern medicine, however, the ideal approach toward management and treatment of a patient affected by a pelvic floor disorder such as pelvic organ prolapse is as a multidisciplinary team, including possibly a gynecologist, colorectal surgeon, neurologist, urologist, and a physiotherapist all working together toward this common goal.

References

1. Meade RH. An introduction to the history of general surgery. Philidelphia, Saunders, 1968.
2. Emge LA, Durfee RB. Pelvic organ prolapse: Four thousand years of treatment. Clin Obstet Gynecol 1966; 9(4):997–1032.
3. Ricci JV. The genealogy of gynaecology. History of the development of gynaecology throughout the ages, 2000 B.C.–1800 A.D. Philadelphia, The Blakiston Company, 1943.
4. Speert H. Iconographia gyniatrica: A pictorial history of gynaecology and obstetrics. Philadelphia, F.A. Davis Company, 1973.
5. Garengeot, René-Jacques Croissant de. Traité des operations de chirurgie. Seconde edition, revûe, corrigée & augmentée par l'auteur. Paris, chez Huart, 1740.
6. Benrubi GI. History of hysterectomy. J Fla Med Assoc 1988; 75:533542.
7. Drutz HP, Herschorn S, Diamant NE. Female pelvic medicine and reconstructive pelvic floor surgery. London, Springer, 2003.
8. Gilliam DT. Round ligament ventrosuspension of the uterus. Trans Am Assoc Obstet Gynecol 1901; 13:282.
9. Bent AE. Howard Atwood Kelly (1858–1943). Int Urogynecol J 1996; 7:48–61.
10. Kelly HA. Operative gynecology, Vol. 1, New York, D. Appleton, 1898.
11. Kelly HA, Burnham CF. Diseases of the kidneys, ureters and bladder. New York, D. Appleton, 1914.
12. Kelly HA, Dumm WM. Urinary incontinence in women without manifest injury to the bladder. Surg Gynecol Obstet 1914; 18:444.
13. Rock JA, Thompson JD. Te Linde's operative gynecology, 8th edn. Philadelphia, Lippincott-Raven Publishers, 1997.
14. White GR. Cystocele. A radical cure by suturing lateral sulci of the vagina to the white line of pelvic fascia. JAMA 1909; 80(21):1707–1710.
15. Richardson AC, Lyon JB, William NL. A new look at pelvic relaxation. Am J Obstet Gynecol 1976; 126:568–578.

16. Jeffcoat TNA. Posterior colpoperineorrhaphy. Am J Obstet Gynecol 1959; 77:490–502.
17. Kahn MA, Stanton SL. Techniques of rectocele repair and their effects on bowel function. Int Urogynecol J Pelvic Floor Dysfunct 1998; 9(1):37–47.
18. Bent AE, Ostergard DR, Cundiff GW, Swift SE. Ostergard's urogynecology and pelvic floor dysfunction. Philadelphia, Lippincott Williams & Wilkins, 2003.
19. Heaney HS. Technique of vaginal hysterectomy. Surg Clin North Am 1942; 22:76.
20. McCall ML. Posterior culdeplasty. Surgical correction of enterocele during vaginal hysterectomy: A preliminary report. Obstet Gynecol 1957; 10:595–602.
21. Richardson EH. An efficient composite operation for uterine prolapse and associated pathology. Am J Obstet Gynecol 1937; 34:814.
22. Lash AF, Levin B. Roentgenographic diagnosis of vaginal vault hernia. Obstet Gynecol 1962; 20:427–433.
23. Nichols DH, Randall CL. Vaginal surgery, 4th edn. Baltimore, Williams & Wilkins, 1996.
24. Parsons L, Ulfelder H. An atlas of pelvic operations, 2nd edn. Philadelphia, WB Saunders, 1968.
25. Addison WA, Livengood CH, Sutton GP, Parker RT. Abdominal sacral colpopexy with Mersilene mesh in the retroperitoneal position in the management of post-hysterectomy vaginal prolapse and enterocele. Am J Obstet Gynecol 1985; 153:140–146.
26. Meeks GR Washburne JF, McGehee RP, Wiser WL. Repair of vaginal vault prolapse by suspension of the vagina to iliococcygeus (pre-spinous) fascia. Am J Obstet Gynecol 1994; 171:1444–1452.
27. Shull BL, Bachofen C, Coates KW, Kuehl TJ. A transvaginal approach to repair of apical and other associated sites of pelvic organ prolapse with uterosacral ligaments. Am J Obstet Gynecol 2000; 1365–1374.
28. Ferguson WH. New functional repair of posthysterectomy vaginal vault prolapse with Marlex mesh. Am Surg 1964; 30:227–230
29. Litynski GS. Endoscopic surgery: The history, the pioneers. World J Surg 1999; 23:745–753.
30. Reich H. Laparoscopic hysterectomy. Surg Laparosc Endosc 1992; 2(1):85–88.
31. Ross JW. Laparoscopic approach for severe pelvic vault prolapse. J Am Assoc Gynecol Laparosc 1996; 3(4 Suppl):S43.
32. Baden WF, Walker TA. Genesis of the vaginal profile: A correlated classification of vaginal relaxation. Clin Obstet Gynecol 1972; 15(4):1048–1054.
33. Hall AF, Theofrastous JP, Cundiff GW, et-al.. Interobserver and intraobserver reliability of the proposed International Continence Society, Society of Gynecologic Surgeons, and the American Urogynecologic Society Pelvic Organ Prolapse Classification System. Am J Obstet Gynecol 1996; 175:1467–1470.
34. Bump RC, Mattiasson A, Bo K, et-al.. The standardization of terminology of female pelvic organ prolapse and pelvic floor dysfunction. Am J Obstet Gynecol 1996; 175:10–17.
35. Wall LL, Delancey JOL. The politics of prolapse: A revisionist approach to disorders of the pelvic floor in women. Perspec Biol Med 1991; 34:486–496.

Chapter 23
Biomaterials: Natural and Synthetic Grafts

Kaytan V. Amrute and Gopal H. Badlani

Introduction

Traditional methods of treatment for pelvic organ prolapse (POP) and stress incontinence have varied over time. From the ancient use of pomegranates as pessaries to the modern use of synthetic pessaries, or surgical techniques utilizing native tissue, these treatment modalities may not provide durable results. Cystoceles conventionally are repaired by anterior colporrhaphy, but recurrence in up to 40% of patients is reported [1]. Data from a large managed care population in Oregon estimate the lifetime risk for a woman to undergo surgery for POP or incontinence by age 80 is 11.1%, with reoperation occurring in 29.2% of cases [2].

As POP affects up to half of all women over age 50, population projections of women aged 65 and over are estimated to double to 35 million by 2030 [3, 4]. With approximately one third of patients undergoing reoperation and the eventual rise in incidence, surgical repair techniques need to evolve to meet these challenges. Along with restoration of anatomy and preservation of sexual function, repair techniques need to incorporate durability as a goal for success. Biomaterials assist in the attainment of these goals; use of biomaterials will not, of course, replace sound surgical practice, but may augment it for long-term efficacy.

Biomaterial refers to any biocompatible substance that integrates into host tissue during treatment and, in the case of grafts, can be natural or synthetic. Biological grafts are further divided into autologous grafts (patient's native tissue), allografts

(cadaveric tissue), and xenografts (animal tissue). Synthetic grafts are either absorbable, nonabsorbable, or a combination of the two. Synthetic grafts also are identified by woven structure (monofilament vs. multifilament) and pore size (macroporous vs. microporous or both). Selection of biomaterial is dependent on the inherent characteristics of the graft, individualized patient need, and surgeon preference. Biomaterial use, however, is not free from controversy. Potential complications such as erosion and infection are present and limited data exist for long-term outcomes [5]. Comprehension of biomaterial qualities and indications, though, will undoubtedly limit these complications and maximize efficacy.

Use of Biomaterials: A Biochemical and Genetic Raison d'Être

Alterations of Collagen Metabolism: Hernia Investigations

Some of the notable risk factors for prolapse include increasing age, menopausal status, high parity, and history of hysterectomy [6]. Other proposed causes of prolapse include denervation or direct injury of the pelvic floor musculature. A common link between these factors is the disruption of normal endopelvic fascia and ligamentary support; integrity of the muscles and connective tissue of the pelvic floor is the key for continence and pelvic organ support. Alterations of collagen and elastin metabolism have been suggested as another underlying mechanism of pelvic organ support loss and incontinence: previous research on individuals with connective tissue disorders or with hernias demonstrates credence to this premise.

It is well recognized that persons with connective tissue disorders such as Ehlers–Danlos and Marfans syndrome have a higher rate of urinary incontinence and pelvic prolapse. Initial studies conducted in a female population with Ehlers–Danlos diagnosis showed a 20% higher incidence of stress urinary incontinence than those without any known connective tissue disorder [7]. Likewise, Carley et al. confirmed these data in a population of women afflicted with either Ehlers–Danlos or Marfans syndrome. A comparison between these two groups demonstrated a higher rate of prolapse in those with Ehlers–Danlos [8].

In normal individuals, collagen is made up of mainly type I and type III collagen, in a 4:1 ratio [9]. Types I and III collagen are produced primarily by connective tissue fibroblasts and enable flexibility and tensile strength. Stability of the collagen fibers is a result of cross-linking between proline and hydroxyproline amino acids within collagen. Elastin, another component of connective tissue, facilitates compliance and stretching [10]. Hernia patients demonstrate a different fibroblast phenotype, and consequently, produce abnormal collagen systemically [9, 11].

Individuals with hernias have an overexpression of type III collagen, leading to abnormal cross-linking with type I collagen and, ultimately, production of tenuous fibers [11]. Klinge et al. [12] demonstrated a significant decrease in collagen type I/III ratio in the skin of patients with indirect or direct hernia compared to controls. The authors concluded that hernias could be isolated manifestations of a systemic problem of collagen metabolism and this could delineate the high recurrence rates with repeated suture repair. Enhanced elastolytic activity and decreased antiprotease action has been illustrated as well [13]. Matrix metalloproteinases (MMP) are proteases involved in collagen degradation and remodeling and are regulated by tissue inhibitors of metalloproteinases (TIMP). A certain type of MMP, MMP-2, was noted to be significantly overactive in the fibroblasts of the tranversalis fascia in patients with direct inguinal hernia [14].

Other factors, such as aging or smoking, may contribute to the formation of hernias. Nicotine has an inhibitory effect on fibroblasts and decreased oxygen levels obviate normal collagen metabolism [9]. Muscle wasting, inherent changes in connective tissue, and increased MMP activity may possibly explain the effects of the aging process on hernia formation. These comorbidities along with others, such as obesity and genetic predispositions, may be additive and lead to symptomatic hernia formation [9].

Parallels to Pelvic Prolapse and Incontinence

Research findings of abnormal collagen metabolism in patients with inguinal hernias have been applied to those with pelvic support loss and incontinence. Jackson et al. [15] compared the vaginal–epithelial tissue of premenopausal women with genitourinary prolapse to a control group. Significant reduction of total collagen content and solubility was associated with the afflicted group, attributable to increased collagenolytic activity. Chen et al. [16] noted increased collagen degradation in the vaginal wall tissue of women with stress incontinence or severe prolapse, demonstrated by an increase in the expression of mRNA of MMP-1 ($P = 0.05$) and in MMP-1/TIMP-1 ratio ($P = 0.04$) compared to controls. Vaginal connective tissue in individuals with prolapse also demonstrates an increased expression of collagen type III fibers [17]. Gabriel et al. recently performed a histological and immunohistochemical comparison of uterosacral ligaments of patients with and without prolapse [18]. While there was no difference between collagen type I and smooth muscle content between the two groups, the prolapse group had a significantly higher expression of collagen type III ($P < 0.001$).

As with individuals with hernias, a systemic process of abnormal collagen metabolism may exist. Collagen content in nonsupportive tissue such as the uterine cervix in women with prolapse is significantly lower compared to a control group [19]. Ulmsten et al. demonstrated that the skin and ligamentum rotundum of women with stress incontinence had 25–40% less hydroxyproline than that of unaffected women in a similar age group, indicating lower collagen content [20]. Concentration of helical peptide $\alpha 1$ (I) 620–633, a urinary collagen degradation product, is significantly higher in patients with stress incontinence compared to those without stress incontinence [21]. Histopathological differences of skin and endopelvic fascia biopsies in stress-incontinent women and unaffected women show reduced collagen content in the incontinent group [22]. Elastin metabolism also may be affected as significantly decreased levels of α-1 antitrypsin mRNA, a serine protease inhibitor, were noted in women with stress incontinence and/or prolapse [23]. Elevated elastase activity is evident in plasma of patients with stress incontinence and provides further evidence of systemic process [24].

Genetic predisposition plays a significant role in laxity of the pelvic floor as well. Bladder neck and urethral hypermobility is partly determined genetically, as demonstrated in a translabial ultrasound study with nulligravid twin sister pairs with approximately 59% of bladder neck descent variance due to genetic factors [25]. Bushbaum et al. [26] quantitatively compared the degree of prolapse using the pelvic organ prolapse quantification (POP-Q) exam in 101 pairs of nulliparous and their parous postmenopausal sisters. While a majority of patients had no significant prolapse, a high concordance in prolapse stage was evident among sister pairs. In discordant sister pairs, ie, prolapse in one sister greater than two or more stages of prolapse compared to the other, the parous sister demonstrated advanced stages of prolapse in more than 80% of the cases [26]. A recent case series reported on ten patients with early-onset prolapse (average age 37 years old) and family history of prolapse [27]. Genetic analysis on this small population of patients revealed an autosomal inheritance pattern with incomplete penetrance, with both maternal and paternal transmissions. Furthermore, the relative risk of prolapse to the siblings of the affected patients was five times greater than the risk for the general population [27]. A genome-wide linkage scan performed on one family with a generational history of prolapse suggests a polymorphic variant in the promoter of laminin gammal (LAMC 1) gene in vaginal tissue may increase the susceptibility of early-onset POP [28].

Clinical Translation

Abnormal collagen and elastin metabolism, together with inciting factors such as childbirth, may lead to symptomatic pelvic floor defects and incontinence. After repair of such defects, failure of surgical therapy and recurrence of prolapse may be explicated by this biochemical phenomenon. As certain patients may have a genetic predisposition, use of biomaterial grafts may offer a solution to recurrence of pelvic support loss.

The "Ideal" Biomaterial and Host Remodeling

Biomaterial Paradigm

The ideal biomaterial should represent the following characteristics: inert, sterile, noncarcinogenic, noninflammatory, nonimmunogenic, mechanically durable, ability to withstand modification or enzymatic degradation by host tissue, inexpensive, accessible, convenient, and easy to use. Current biomaterials do not meet all of these criteria, but come close to this paradigm [29]. Ultimately, selection of graft material is tailored according to patient need and surgeon preference. The requirements for the mechanical properties of grafts used in pelvic prolapse have not yet been defined and insights have been extrapolated from abdominal hernia repair [9]. Synthetic mesh implants used in hernia repairs have a minimum tensile strength that far exceeds the increased intra-abdominal pressures noted during Valsalva maneuvers. "Dry" laboratory conditions demonstrate that most meshes are stronger than what is physiologically required. Consequently, implants with lesser tensile strength or more elasticity may result in better clinical outcomes [9].

Host Response of Remodeling

Although biomaterials strive to be biologically inert and nonimmunogenic, all invariably cause a foreign body response, with the synthetic grafts inducing a more vigorous response compared to natural grafts [9]. Initially, after implantation, the host reacts to the injury and covers the material with a biofilm. Low-molecular-weight proteins, such as albumin, and later more complex proteins such as fibrinogen, immunoglobulins, extracellular matrix proteins are incorporated onto the graft. If bacteria are present, alterations in the biofilm may occur to cause future clinical consequences, such as erosion. The biofilm becomes immunogenic through structural changes

Stage 1: (first 7 days): intense inflammation with capillary proliferation, granular tissue, and giant cell

Stage 2: (after 14 days): granular tissue remains with more giant cells

Stage 3: (after 28 days): the acute inflammation has disappeared and number of histiocytes and giant cells has increased

Stage 4: presence of giant cells on the external cells on the external surface of the implant with dense fibrous tissue

FIG. 23.1. Host remodeling: initial histological reaction. Adapted from [30]

of the adsorbed proteins, thereby triggering a typical acute inflammatory response, involving the complement system, binding of antibodies, and blood clotting and fibrinolysis activation [9].

A chronic inflammatory reaction then ensues: formation of granulation tissue with fibroblasts, macrophages, and ultimately foreign body giant cells (see Fig. 23.1 [30]). Neovascularization also occurs followed by fibrosis. Macrophages, differentiated from extravascular monocytes, are the critical cell type in the clinical response of the biological acceptance or rejection of the graft. Roles include interaction with lymphocytes and production of mediators that induce protein synthesis and cell proliferation, ie, fibroblasts [9]. Fibroblasts eventually predominate as capillaries and inflammatory decrease in number. Consequently, collagen and other matrix proteins are deposited, resulting in fibrous tissue formation.

The host response of fibrosis and scarring eventually should engender a successful clinical outcome. Yet, the remodeling process itself can be responsible for failure of graft material and recurrence of symptoms. The inflammatory reaction, requisite for fibrosis, may cause some adverse effects such as erosion, adhesion formation, and graft shrinkage. Another consideration is the deposition of abnormal collagen, as the process occurs in an individual with inherent defective collagen production and metabolism [9]. Ideally, biological acceptance of the graft should demonstrate little inflammatory response with early infiltration of fibroblasts [30].

Natural Biomaterials

Biological grafts may be harvested from a patient's own fascia (autologous graft), from cadaveric tissue (allograft), or from animal tissue (xenografts). Each in

TABLE 23.1. Indications for biological grafts.

- Poor vaginal healing
- Pelvic bone trauma
- History of pelvic radiation
- Urethral reconstruction
- Known allergic reaction to synthetic biomaterial
- Surgeon preference

turn have particular strengths and may be used when synthetic grafts are contraindicated (see Table 23.1). Advantages include in vivo tissue remodeling, histological similarity, and reduced erosion rates. Potential shortcomings are limited supply, cost, unpredictable host tissue integration, inconsistent strength, lack of long-term data, and possible infectivity with allografts and xenografts [31].

Autologous Biomaterial

Autologous grafts traditionally are harvested from two sites: rectus abdominis fascia or tensor fascia lata. Due to size restrictions, autologous grafts are used mainly in sling procedures and rarely in POP repair. Alridge first described the use of bilateral strips of rectus fascia, passed through the rectus muscles, and ligated together posterior to the urethra [32]. Beck et al. [33] reported the use of fascia lata as a suburethral sling for recurrent stress incontinence treatment. Current surgical techniques are described in detail elsewhere in this book.

The rectus abdominis fascia is obtained usually through a Pfannenstiel incision, and unlike the fascia lata harvest, repositioning of the patient is not required. Transmission of infectious agents is minimal. While the harvest may be straightforward, potential complications include a limited length of fascia obtained, increased morbidity secondary to incision pain or wound infection, risk of future abdominal hernia, and added procedure and recovery times. Previous surgery or radiation therapy at the harvest site also may preclude the acquirement of good tissue of sufficient length and quality.

Recent studies on rectus fascia have demonstrated high success rates with minimal complications. Morgan et al. [34] reported on 247 women with type II or III stress incontinence treated with pubovaginal slings, composed of rectus fascia. At a mean follow-up of 51 months, continence rates were 88% overall, 91% for type II and 84% for type III. Secondary procedures, consisting of transurethral collagen injections or repeat slings, were performed in 14 patients. A complication rate of 4% was noted and included pelvic hematoma, incisional hernia, deep venous thrombosis, and pulmonary embolus. However, no erosions or extrusions were evident [34]. Another retrospective study showed a 92% overall success rate with a minimum of 1 year follow-up (median 3.1 years, range 1–15) in 251 patients; permanent urinary retention occurred in only four patients, while de novo urge incontinence occurred in 3% of patients and persistent urge incontinence in 23% [35].

Tensor fascia lata may offer several advantages over rectus fascia. Fascia lata, with dimensions of approximately 20 × 2 cm, is obtained laterally from the upper thigh from the ileotibial band, with the aid of a device such as the Masson fascial stripper (Marina Masson Fasicalata Stripper, Marina Medical, Hollywood, Florida, USA) or the Crawford fascia stripper (Bausch & Lomb Storz Instrument Company, San Dimas, CA, USA) (see Fig. 23.2). Fascia lata has greater tensile strength than rectus fascia [36]. Concerns of length, history of previous abdominal surgery, and future complication of abdominal hernia are irrelevant. Disadvantages include increased operating time, repositioning of the patient, and possible cosmetic issues. Potential complications include acute hematoma, seroma requiring serial aspiration or drainage, prolonged postoperative pain, muscle herniation, and infection.

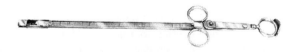

FIG. 23.2. Crawford fascia stripper

Success rates with autologous fascia lata grafts by and large have been similar to rectus fascia. In 170 patients, Beck et al. demonstrated a 92% success rate with minimal de novo urgency rates and no erosions [37]. Another retrospective review, supplemented by the urogential distress inventory (UDI)-6 questionnaire with a mean follow-up period of 4.4 years, demonstrated 85% of 100 patients reported being dry or improved and 93% being pain-free at the harvest site by the seventh day postoperatively. No infections at the harvest site or lower extremity thrombotic events were noted [38]. The same authors also retrospectively evaluated use of fascia lata in abdominal sacrocolpopexy in ten patients and noted POP-Q stage II or lower in all patients with a follow-up range of 19 to 42 months [39].

Allograft Biomaterial

As with autologous grafts, cadaveric grafts are associated with a low risk of infectivity and erosion. Use of allografts also confers the advantages of absence of donor site morbidity, shorter operating times, more rapid recovery time, and similar efficacy to autologous grafts [40]. Furthermore, size restrictions are not applicable; in addition to use in pubovaginal slings, allografts may be used in other reconstructive procedures, such as abdominal sacrocolpopexy or anterior colporrhaphies. Processing techniques, however, potentially may compromise biomechanical properties of cadaveric fascia, thereby contributing to an unpredictable resorption and integration process [40].

Donor cadaveric grafts, usually harvested from the tensor fascia lata, undergo several processing techniques to decrease infectivity and antigenicity, thereby reducing a host immune response. Donors usually are screened first with a thorough medical and social history and serological testing for HIV, Hep B, Hep C, and HTLV-1. After completion of the screening process, harvest of tissue then should occur under strict aseptic conditions. Removal of infectious and antigenic material varies according to manufacturer [40]. Tissue processing of cadaveric fascia may include freeze-drying, after a wash to remove various bacterial, viral, and fungal organisms. Suspend Tutoplast® by Coloplast (Marietta, GA, USA) undergoes a multistep solvent dehydration method with various organic solvents which has the added benefit of eliminating prions, the agent responsible for Creutzfeldt–Jakob disease. Suspend Tutoplast® also is further sterilized with gamma-irradiation to decrease infection transmission risk [40].

Although infectivity and antigenicity is lessened, allograft quality may be affected by the various processing methods. Lemer et al. [41] noted a significantly lower tensile strength and stiffness in freeze-dried fascia compared to autologous grafts and solvent-dehydrated cadaveric fascia. Independent of freeze-drying, incomplete rehydration of allograft of less than 1 h also can affect quality. This may trap water between collagen fibers as they expand, thereby creating a decrease in structural integrity [40]. While irradiation at high levels (over 30 kGy) may be virucidal, damage to the tertiary structure of collagen can occur and affect the tensile strength and graft stiffness. To preserve collagen structure and achieve sterility, along with other processing methods, cadaveric fascia usually is exposed to 20–25 kGy of radiation. In addition, donor factors may play a role in graft quality. Instead of well-developed, well-nourished, athletic individuals, allograft donors usually consist of an elderly population that may be sedentary, malnourished, and have age-related attenuated fascia [40].

Clinically, tissue-processing techniques and donor factors may explicate the reduced functional outcomes of allografts noted in pubovaginal sling surgery. Success rates of cadaveric fascia used for midurethral slings range from 65 to 98% [42]. McBride et al. performed a retrospective comparison of autologous slings against Suspend Tutoplast®, the solvent-dehydrated and gamma-radiated cadaveric fascia [43]. Overall, 92.3% of the autologous patients ($n = 39$) and 90.5% of the allograft patients ($n = 32$) reported subjective stress continence at 24 months. No differences were noted in subjective quality-of-life measures, maximum urethral closure pressures, and bladder neck mobility. However, 41.7% of allograft patients demonstrated urodynamic stress incontinence compared to 0% of autologous patients ($P = 0.007$) [43].

Poor outcomes also were noted in a recent study of 303 patients with a median overall follow-up time of 5.6 years comparing autologous rectus fascia ($n = 153$) to freeze-dried cadaveric fascia ($n = 150$) [44]. Recurrent stress incontinence symptoms (39.6% vs. 28.3%, $P = 0.04$) and reoperation (12.7% vs. 3.3%, $P = 0.003$) occurred more in the cadaveric versus the autologous group, respectively. Adjusting for differences in follow-up time, the cadaveric group revealed higher rates of incontinence (16 vs. 5 per 100 women-years, $P < 0.0001$) and higher rates of reoperation (4 vs. 1 per 100 women-years, $P < 0.0003$) [44]. FitzGerald et al. performed a histopathological analysis of retrieved freeze-dried, irradiated graft material on 7 of 12 patients who underwent reoperation for recurrence of prolapse or stress incontinence symptoms [45]. The results revealed that most of the graft remnants demonstrated areas of disorganized remodeling patterns and graft degeneration. Unpredictable host integration of the allograft may be related to several factors such as rate of tissue remodeling, antigenicity of the graft material, and high levels of stress placed on the graft during remodeling [45].

For use in prolapse surgery, Culligan and colleagues performed a randomized controlled trial in 100 patients who underwent abdominal sacrocolpopexy, where 54 patients received polypropylene mesh and 46 Suspend Tutoplast® [46]. Objective anatomic failure was defined as POP-Q stage 2 or more at any time during the follow-up period. At 1-year follow-up, a significant difference in objective cure rates was noted: 91% in the mesh group and 68% in the solvent dehydrated, gamma-radiated fascia group ($P = 0.007$) [46]. A prospective randomized trial of 154 patients by Gandhi et al. compared standard anterior colporrhaphy with or without solvent-dehydrated graft [47]. Sixteen women in the graft group (21%; $n = 76$) and 23 in the control group (29%; $n = 78$) experienced recurrent anterior vaginal wall prolapse ($P = 0.229$). While the difference was not statistically significant, the authors concluded use of cadaveric fascia will not decrease prolapse recurrence rates.

In brief, data suggest autologous grafts may be superior to allografts in clinical results of pubovaginal sling procedures. If cadaveric fascia is considered for use, solvent dehydration processing appears to be superior to freeze-dried methods. Unpredictable host remodeling of the allografts after placement possibly explains the difference in clinical outcomes [40].

Xenograft Biomaterial

Xenografts are derived from other species, mainly porcine or bovine sources, and act as acellular collagen-based scaffolds. Collagen sources include porcine small intestine submucosa, porcine dermis, fetal bovine skin, and bovine pericardium. Production is governed strictly by Food and Drug Administration (FDA) guidelines, which encompass information of the animal herd, vaccination status, feed source, and bovine spongiform encephalopathy clearance. Furthermore, the collagen-based implants can be cross-linked or not; cross-linking between the collagen fibrils protects against host collagenase degradation, rendering the implant relatively nonabsorbable [9].

Pelvicol® (Bard Urological Division, Covington, GA, USA) is a porcine dermal collagen implant composed of a flexible sheet of fibrous, acellular collagen and elastin fibers cross-linked by hexamethylene-di-isocyanate (HMDI). The implant also is terminally sterilized by gamma irradiation. In addition to providing stability against enzymatic degradation, HMDI cross-linking also may cause less of an immune response. However, a host cytotoxic effect may not be completely absent [48]. In a rat model comparing the inflammatory responses of Pelvicol® with Prolene synthetic graft, a lesser inflammatory response was demonstrated in the former group, where decreased granulocytes and macrophages were noted [49]. Pelvicol® induced a slower, but more orderly collagen deposition paralleling the surface of the implant and fewer adhesions were apparent. In lieu of tissue ingrowth, encapsulation occurred, thereby challenging mechanical strength and causing possible seroma formation [49]. To promote tissue infiltration and vascularization, a porous version of Pelvicol® is available (Pelvisoft®, Bard Urological Division, Covington, GA, USA).

Gandhi et al. [50], performing a retrospective histological study on cross-linked porcine dermis in 7 of 12 patients who underwent reoperation secondary to pubovaginal sling complications, showed variable tissue reaction. In patients who were reoperated for urinary retention at a time period of 6–42 weeks later, explanted specimens showed a trend toward graft preservation, with minimal tissue ingrowth and remodeling. In two patients who reoperated for stress incontinence recurrence,

with a longer time frame from initial surgery, the grafts appeared to be replaced with dense fibroconnective tissue and moderate neovascularization without any inflammatory response [50]. Although histological comparison was not performed with biopsies from successful operations and the sample size is small, the study raises questions concerning predictability of host tissue reaction to cross-linked porcine dermis. The cross-linking process may prevent cellular infiltration by the host, consequently affecting the remodeling process and eventually leading to graft failure.

Wheeler et al. [51] analyzed outcomes of use of cross-linked porcine dermis in 36 women who underwent high vaginal uterosacral suspension and cystocele repair. Dissection in the anterior compartment was performed laterally for exposure of sufficient paravaginal tissue capable of graft attachment. Postoperatively, with a median follow-up time of 17 months, significant improvement was demonstrated in mean scores of the Incontinence Impact Questionnaires-7 (IIQ-7) and Urogential Distress Inventory-6 (UDI-6) ($P < 0.01$). Overall postoperative mean POP-Q measurements also showed significant improvement, but approximately 50% of patients had a stage II or greater anterior compartment prolapse; 28.6% of patients had point Ba beyond the hymen. Complications included graft resorption in one patient and reoperation in a total of four patients. Although the study was not a randomized, controlled trial and graft attachment was not as far lateral as to the arcus tendineous, use of porcine dermis did not produce any significant advantages [51].

Gomelsky and colleagues recently retrospectively evaluated the incidence of vaginal extrusion and management in 270 women who underwent pubovaginal sling placement or prolapse repair with Pelvicol® over a 5-year period [52]. Nineteen women (7%) had complete or partial vaginal extrusion. Of the 13 patients who underwent pubovaginal sling surgery, 11 patients healed by re-epitheliazation and two required operative debridement. Two of the six patients who underwent prolapse repair required reoperation for extensive extrusion and had reoccurrence of prolapse while the remaining patients healed with minimal incisional separations. Statistical analysis revealed that vaginal extrusion was significantly associated with concomitant urethral diverticulectomy and pubovaginal sling surgery [52].

Non-cross-linked porcine dermis (InteXen™ and InteXen LP™, American Medical Systems, Minnetonka, MN, USA) was introduced to address the limitations of the cross-linked dermis. It is an acellular material that should minimize risk of rejection and decrease inflammatory response. The lack of cross-linked collagen fibrils theoretically should facilitate host tissue integration. InteXen LP differs from InteXen in that it is not irradiated but terminally sterilized by ethylene oxide then lyophilized. A histological comparison of three implanted porcine dermis biomaterials (InteXen, InteXen LP, and Pelvisoft) was reported using Sprague-Dawley male rat models [48]. At day 84, the endpoint of the study, InteXen LP had significantly more vascularization ($P<0.03$) and the most even distribution of cellular infiltration within the material. A higher capillary count and cellular infiltration was noted in the pores of Pelvisoft compared to within the graft material. Pelvisoft and InteXen LP had a higher degree of surface area persistence, or material integrity, at the end of the study period. Also, at day 84, tensile strength was similar in all groups as well as fibroblast count. In this model, non-cross-linked porcine dermis and porous cross-linked dermis seem to facilitate vascularization and remodeling [48].

Gomelsky et al. [53] retrospectively reviewed outcomes in 70 women who underwent repair of high-grade cystocele with porcine dermis graft interposition with InteXen. The graft was secured to three points on the arcus tendineous bilaterally with delayed absorbable suture after proper dissection. Concomitant repairs of stress incontinence and prolapse occurred in 65 patients (with pubovaginal sling) and 50 patients (iliococcygeous vault suspension), respectively. After 24 months of follow-up, 59 (91%) of patients were dry while 10 (14%) patients had recurrent prolapse: one with vaginal vault prolapse (POP-Q value of $C = -2$) repaired with abdominal sacrocolpopexy, six with grade II asymptomatic cystocele (Ba = 0), and three with grade III (Ba = + 2) cystocele who elected no surgical intervention [53].

Porcine small intestinal submucosa (SIS) (Surgisis®, Cook Medical, Bloomington, IN, USA), is composed of non-cross-linked collagen processed such that immunogenic cells are removed while the complex extracellular matrix and natural growth factors are left intact. It is obtained from the tunica submucosa of the small intestine and is the layer of connective tissue arrange immediately under the mucosa layer. SIS contains collagen types I, III, and V and growth factors TGF-b and FGF-2 and exists as vacuum-pressed or freeze-dried two-, four-, and eight-layer implants [9]. Acting as a biological scaffold, SIS is usually degraded in 4–12 weeks by an active remodeling process that replaces the graft gradually by host connective tissue. Specifically, SIS enables the ingrowth of fibroblasts, rapid angiogenesis, differentiation of myofibroblasts, and resurfacing of epithelial cells [9, 54]. Weidemann and Otto [55] in their series of 15 patients performed a histopathological analysis of SIS graft in three patients who underwent reoperation for failed pubovaginal sling procedures after a mean of 12.7 months. The biopsies revealed minimal focal residue and absence of a foreign body or chronic inflammatory reaction. Compared to other biomaterials, SIS produces the highest stimulus for the formation of collagen fibers surrounding the graft [56].

Clinically, SIS has demonstrated good short-term results in some studies. In one series of 152 pubovaginal sling patients, a 93% cure rate for stress incontinence was noted at 4 years, but 50.7% of patients showed urge incontinence [57]. A more recent retrospective study of 34 patients showed 27 (79%) cured of stress incontinence at 2-year follow-up. One patient developed de novo urgency while three patients (9%) developed suprapubic inflammation at 10, 21, and 45 days after surgery, resolved with antibiotics. No prolonged urinary retention, erosions, or other complications were noted [58]. Ho et al. also noted in six of ten patients receiving eight-ply SIS pubovaginal slings symptomatic postoperative inflammation. Pain and induration at the abdominal incision site occurred in this series 10–39 days after surgery and all patients were treated conservatively, with an exception of one patient who required abscess drainage [59]. For prolapse repair, a case-control study of 14 patients undergoing traditional anterior repair and 14 patients with SIS graft anterior repair demonstrated significant improvements in quality-of-life parameters such as role and physical limitations at 6-month follow-up in the latter group [60]. SIS graft repair improved all POP-Q measurements

TABLE 23.2. Amid classification and types of synthetic mesh.

Type	Pore size and filament number	Material (trade names)
1	Macroporous[a], Monofilament	Polypropylene (Prolene, Marlex, Atrium), Polypropylene/Polyglactin 910 (Vypro I and II), Polyglactin 910 (Vicryl)
2	Microporous[a], Multifilament	Expanded Polytetrafluoroethylene (PTFE) (Gore-tex)
3	Macroporous/Microporous, Multifilament	Polytetrafluoroethylene (PTFE) (Teflon), Polyethylene tetraphthalate (Mersilene), Braided polypropylene (Surgipro)
4	Submicronic[b], Monofilament	Polypropylene sheet (Cellgard)

[a]Macroporous: defined as >75 mm, Microporous ≤75 mm
[b]<1 mm, not used in pelvic reconstructive surgery

significantly except for total vaginal length. At 2-year follow-up, no significant difference was noted in quality-of-issues or POP severity between both groups; in terms of long-term efficacy, the initial greater improvement of POP-Q measurements in the SIS graft group was not evident [60].

Synthetic Biomaterials

Classification and Host Remodeling

Synthetic grafts are classified according several parameters; mainly pore size, nature of fiber filaments, and durability. Other important characteristics include flexibility and mechanical strength. Amid [61] established a classification system for synthetic grafts used in abdominal herniorrhaphy based on pore size and fiber type (see Table 23.2). Synthetic mesh is usually created from knitted single-fiber filaments (monofilament) or braided with monofilament yarns into multifilament fibers and the tensile strength will vary with fiber type, the weight-to-area ratio, and the weave [62]. The fibers may be absorbable or nonabsorbable material, or a combination of both. Flexibility is determined by the individual stiffness of its yarns, the knitting procedure, the pore size, and the amount of material per unit of surface. Multifilament implants generally are more supple [9].

Pore size is the diameter of the open spaces while interstitial distance is measured between the fibers (see Fig. 23.3). Greater flexibility is noted in grafts with a larger pore size, while grafts that are more interlooped have smaller pores and a higher degree of stiffness [9]. Pore size and interstitial distance

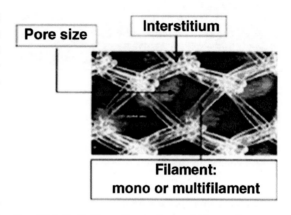

FIG. 23.3. Definition of terms for synthetic mesh

also are the most important characteristics that determine whether host inflammatory cells, fibroblasts, and collagen can infiltrate the mesh structure [62]. Pore size >75 mm, defined as macroporous, enable rapid ingrowth of fibroblasts and capillaries necessary to integrate the implant with native tissue. Interstices, in multifilament implants, are smaller than the actual pores and increase the contact surface with the host tissue. Although better integration occurs, a stronger inflammatory reaction can result. Yet, there seems to be an absolute lower limit for filament size: when filament size is less than 4/0, a constant granulomatous reaction was demonstrated irrespective of the fiber type or number of filaments [63].

Pore sizes or interstices of less than 10 mm hypothetically allow passage of bacteria (2 mm or less) but not leukocytes (9–15 mm) and macrophages (16–20 mm) (see Fig. 23.4). These cell

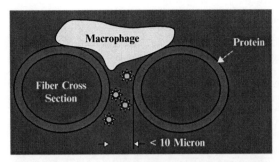

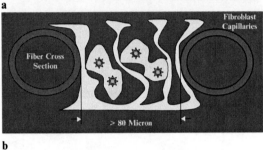

FIG. 23.4. (**a**) Small pore sizes (<10 mm) enable the passage of bacteria and block the components for tissue ingrowth, such as macrophages and fibroblasts while, (**b**) larger pore sizes (>75 mm) allow for the remodeling process and neovascularization to occur

populations are necessary for clearance of infection and play a vital role in the remodeling process [9]. Peak ingrowth occurs at a pore size approximately at 400–500 mm. Large pores limit the remodeling process to the perifilament region, as the pores are occupied by adipose cells [63]. A mesh with smaller pores (<50 mm) or a solid product will be encapsulated or induce an increased foreign body reaction, consequently filling the pores by bridging from one filament to another [9]. Bobyn et al. [64] reported that the best mechanical anchorage occurs when the pore size was between 50 and 200 mm with an average of 90 mm. Furthermore, elasticity in the range of 20–35% has been reported to match the compliance of the surrounding tissues to avoid both extrusion and patient discomfort [65].

Types of Synthetic Mesh

A variety of synthetic mesh is available for use, differing in porosity, fiber materials, weight, stiffness, and resistance to degradation. Polypropylene is commonly used as a nonabsorbable, type 1 macroporous, monofilament mesh and available

in different weaves and weights. Examples of heavier mesh are Prolene (85 g m^{-2}) and Marlex (95 g m^{-2}), while Gynemesh PS (43 g m^{-2}) is significantly lighter (see Fig. 23.5). An example of an absorbable product is polyglactin 910 (Vicryl, Ethicon, Summerville, NJ, USA) while Vypro I and II are examples of combination absorbable and nonabsorbable mesh (50% polyglactin 910/50% polypropylene).

Julian [66] first described the use of synthetic mesh in anterior vaginal colporrhaphy in a prospective randomized study of 24 patients. Marlex (CR Bard, Branston, RI, USA), a type 1 monofilament polypropylene mesh, was placed proximally to the vaginal apex and laterally to the levator fascia in 12 patients after routine colporrhaphy. At 24 months' follow-up, the success rate in the Marlex group was 100% compared to 66% in the control group undergoing colporrhaphy alone. However, a high rate of erosion was noted in four patients (25%) [66]. Flood et al. [67] retrospectively analyzed 142 patients who similarly underwent anterior repair with Marlex augmentation. In this series, the success rate, defined as prolapse less than grade 1, was 100% with no mesh-related complications.

Short-term efficacy of polyglactin 910 has been evaluated in two randomized controlled trials. In one, 114 patients with stage 2 or 3 cystoceles were randomly allocated into three groups: standard anterior repair, standard plus polyglactin 910 mesh, and ultralateral anterior repair [68]. At the median follow-up time of 23.3 months, 83 patients were available for evaluation: success rates (defined stage 0 or stage 1 at points Aa and Ba) were noted in 10 of 33 (30%) in the standard group, 11 of 26 (42%) in the standard and mesh group, and 11 of 24 (46%) in the ultralateral group. The results were not statistically significant, and as such the addition of polyglactin did not seem to improve surgical outcome [68]. Sand et al. [69] prospectively randomized 161 patients in need of anterior and posterior colporrhaphy into a control group of standard repair ($n = 80$) and a group with mesh augmentation ($n = 80$). Of those available for follow-up ($n = 143$), at 1 year, 43% (30/70) of the control group and 25% (18/73) with polyglactin 910 mesh had recurrent cystoceles beyond the midvaginal plane ($P = 0.02$). Recurrent cystoceles to the hymenal ring occurred in eight patients (11.4%) in the control group and in two patients (2.7%) with mesh

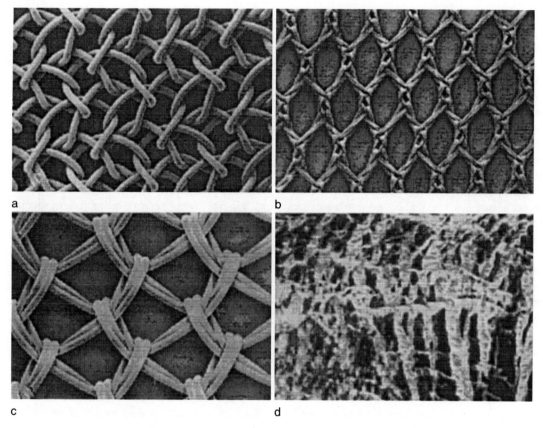

FIG. 23.5. Examples of synthetic mesh knits and weaves. (**a**) Marlex, (**b**) Mersilene, (**c**) Prolene, (**d**) Gore-tex

($P = 0.04$). No recurrent rectoceles to the hymenal ring occurred in either groups [69].

Great efficacy may be achieved with use of polypropylene mesh along with a higher risk of erosion. Compared to other materials, polypropylene induces a far less intense inflammatory reaction [56]. Using a lightweight polypropylene mesh (Gynemesh; Gynecare, Johnson & Johnson, NJ, USA), de Tayrac et al. [70] performed transvaginal repair of the anterior compartment with mesh augmentation in 87 consecutive cases. The polypropylene mesh was placed in a tension-free fashion from the retropubic space to the inferior portion of the bladder. Cure in this series was defined according to the POP-Q staging system with point Ba in stage 0 (optimal) or stage 1 (satisfactory). At the median follow-up time of 24.3 months, 91.6% (77/84 patients) were cured, 5.9% patients had asymptomatic stage 2 anterior vaginal wall prolapse, and

2.4% had recurrent stage 3 prolapse. Mesh erosion was noted in 8.3% of patients, and four patients required reoperation for partial excision. De novo dyspareunia was noted in 16.7% of 30 sexually active patients and de novo urgency was noted in 6.8% of patients [70].

Synthetic biomaterials can be fashioned according to specific patient anatomical defects and pelvic dimensions. A soft polypropylene 5 × 5 cm circular mesh is used in a new transvaginal technique described by Rodriguez and colleagues [71]. After placement of a distal urethral sling and vaginal dissection, the mesh is situated to correct the central and lateral defects of high grade cystoceles (POP-Q stages 3 and 4); points of attachment include the obturator fascia laterally, the bladder neck distally, and sacrouterine/cardinal ligament complex proximally. In 98 patients who had the procedure, with minimum 1-year follow-up, post-operative POP-Q scores showed 85% of patients with stage 0–1, 13% with stage 2, and 2% with stage 3 anterior vaginal wall prolapse. De novo urge and stress incontinence were seen in three and three patients, respectively. No erosions were reported [71].

At our institution, a 6- × 8-cm polypropylene mesh is specially fashioned into an "H" shape and fixed to four points in a tension-free manner to repair anterior compartment defects and provide vaginal vault support. After proper vaginal dissection, the anterior arms of the mesh are passed retropubically to provide midurethral and bladder neck support, the middle portion addresses anterior vaginal wall defects, and the posterior arms aid in vaginal vault suspension via bilateral sacrospinous ligament fixation. A retrospective analysis on 96 patients with Baden-Walker stage 3 or 4 who had the procedure from January 2000 to June 2005 recently was performed [72]. Seventy-six patients (79%) were available with a mean follow-up time of 31 months. Four patients (5.2%) reported recurrence of prolapse. Sixty-eight patients (89%) were completely dry or almost dry, defined as an occasional leak. For those with preoperative incontinence ($n = 36$), average pad use per day decreased significantly from 2.1 ± 0.4 to 0.8 ± 0.2 ($P < 0.005$) postoperatively. Twelve patients (15.7%) reported of de novo urgency. Other complications included vaginal erosions in two patients (2.1%), urinary retention secondary to obstruction in one patient (1.1%), palpable vaginal suture in one patient (1.1%), and recurrent stress incontinence in two patients (2.1%). Among those who were sexually active ($n = 21$), 90.4% denied any dyspareunia and patient satisfaction overall was high [72].

Diagnosis and Management of Erosion and Extrusion

Inherent risks to the use of biomaterials are the complications of erosion and extrusion. Although not universally applied as of yet, newer studies are differentiating the inherently similar two terms: "erosion" generally is defined as the presence of graft material in the lumen of the urinary tract, while "extrusion" is defined as the presence of exposed graft in the vagina [73]. Erosion and extrusion rates mainly are extrapolated from pubovaginal sling or abdominal sacrocolpopexy procedures;

limited data exist for the newer synthetic graft kits used in pelvic reconstructive surgery.

The first reported incidence of vaginal extrusion from sling placement ranged from 0.3 to 23%, with decreased rates with the use of biological grafts [74]. More recently, reported extrusion rates range from 0.4 to 4.8% for TVT (Gynecare, Johnson & Johnson, NJ, USA), 1–10.5% for SPARC (American Medical Systems, Minnetonka, MN, USA), and 0–6.7% for MONARC (American Medical Systems, Minnetonka, MN, USA) [75–79]. Several theories have been postulated as to etiology, ranging from operative techniques to specific properties of the sling material to patient characteristics (see Table 23.3). Although type II and III meshes are multifilamentous and may allow bacteria to pass through, the small pore size (<10 mm) may not allow the passage of macrophages and leukocytes, important for the remodeling process (see above). Type IV mesh rarely is used in pelvic reconstructive surgery secondary to the small pore size as well. Operative techniques such as inadequate plane of dissection, poor tissue irrigation, excessive tension, and bacterial infection secondary to draining hematoma or nonsterile mesh are other factors. Finally, patient comorbidities such as diabetes or menopausal status and early resumption of sexual activity may play a role [73, 80].

Patient presentation ranges from asymptomatic to a variety of symptoms such as vaginal discharge, vaginal or groin pain, dyspareunia, de novo urgency, stress incontinence, hematuria, recurrent urinary tract infection, obstruction, or partner discomfort during intercourse. Careful pelvic examination

TABLE 23.3. Possible etiologies for erosion/extrusion.

- Implant characteristics
  - Small pore size, poor elasticity, basic tissue compatibility
- Operative technique
  - Plane too close to urethra, inadequate vaginal tissue coverage, excessive tension, rolled edges of mesh
- Unrecognized complications
  - Urethral/ bladder injury, poor vaginal tissue vascularity, bacterial infection, hematoma formation and drainage, placement of nonsterile mesh
- Patient factors
  - Uncontrolled diabetes mellitus, tobacco use, prior history of pelvic irradiation, vaginal estrogen status, repeat procedures, early resumption of sexual intercourse

may reveal granuloma formation, anterior vaginal tenderness, eroded tape, or suture. An examination under anesthesia may be requisite to evaluate the full extent of extrusion. Cystourethroscopy is also of paramount importance to exclude bladder/urtheral erosion, particularly if the patient presents with irritative or obstructive symptoms, hematuria, de novo urgency, recurrent urinary tract infections, or bladder stones. Pelvic magnetic resonance imaging (MRI) may be needed when clinical signs of pelvic or perineal abscess are noted [80].

Management depends on type of material, presence of infection, size, and location [73]. Vaginal extrusion of type I polypropylene mesh can be managed conservatively: if less than 1–2 cm in size, use of local estrogen replacement therapy, antibiotics if infection is present, and abstinence from sexual intercourse is recommended. If the vaginal mucosa fails to re-epithelialize after 6–8 weeks, transvaginal excision of exposed mesh with debridement and reapproximation of surrounding tissue is performed. Persistent infection or failure to heal mandates complete mesh excision. Vaginal extrusion of types II, III, and IV require complete excision, since these are prone to higher infection rates and poor healing [73].

Erosion into the urethra or bladder mandates complete mesh excision, regardless of mesh type. Bladder erosion is rare and traditionally has been excised using a transvesical approach [73]. Cystoscopic removal has been described but maximal removal of exposed mesh is required to avoid further erosion and continual symptoms. For urethral erosions, Clemens et al. [74] recommends removal of all synthetic material (sutures and sling), since a distinct plane of scar and old synthetic material usually is present and can be removed in a piecemeal fashion. The synthetic material in that review was a bovine collagen-injected polyester sling (Protogen, Boston Scientific, Natick, Massachusetts, USA) which has been removed from the market. If a defect in the urethra is identified, it should be closed; if not visualized, prolonged urethral catheterization (2 weeks) should result in closure, followed by a pullout cystourethrogram at time of catheter removal. In a study of 57 patients who underwent urethrolysis for urtheral obstruction after pubovaginal sling placement, nine patients were identified with erosion [81]. Three patients with synthetic mesh underwent removal of whole sling, multilayer closure of urtheral defect, and use of Martius flap, if necessary. The remaining patients, with allografts or autologous graft, underwent sling incision and multilayer closure of the defect. At mean follow-up of 30 months, there was no recurrence of urethral erosions or fistulas in either group, while two patients had persistent stress incontinence, two with urge incontinence, and one with urinary retention [81].

Conclusions

Because a high rate of recurrence of prolapse exists, traditional methods of repair may need augmentation with the use of biomaterials. Certain patient populations may need biomaterials due a variety of risk and host factors, such as abnormal collagen metabolism. However, choice of biomaterial depends on several factors, ie, surgeon preference, patient need, and inherent characteristics of the graft. Several key points should be kept in consideration [82]:

- Graft integration into host tissue is vital for successful outcomes. Collagen ingrowth and neovascularization should occur without the occurrence of infection or significant inflammatory reaction. Poorly integrated grafts include synthetic micorporous grafts and xenografts treated with chemical cross-linking. As such, these types of grafts may become encapsulated, leading to hardening or shrinkage. Clinical manifestations then may include recurrence of prolapse, dyspareunia, or alteration of normal anatomy. Examples of well-integrated biomaterials are non-cross-linked biological grafts, and in terms of synthetics, low-weight, large-pore, monofilament mesh with an elasticity between 20 and 35%. A possible disadvantage of non-cross-linked grafts is rapid host degradation before proper integration, leading to failure in a small percentage of patients. Processing methods such as freeze-drying also may compromise biological graft quality.
- More randomized trials are needed: abdominal sacrocolpopexy and pubovaginal slings are the only procedures where prospective randomized trials and clinical outcomes have demonstrated the need for graft material and the greater efficacy of synthetics compared to biological material. Currently, published data on graft material are lim-

ited and do not completely delineate indications and contraindications for graft use. Long-term efficacy data of synthetic mesh for pelvic prolapse repair isarelacking. Future clinical research must involve standardized outcomes, including pre- and postoperative POP-Q evaluations and use of validated questionnaires for quality-of-life issues, sexual function, and incontinence.

- With lack of evidence-based medicine, use of biomaterials needs to be judicious and individualized. Complications of biomaterials such as erosion and dyspareunia, especially with synthetic grafts, can alter patient lifestyle and may present as clinical challenges. Ultimately, the goals of surgical restoration must include patient satisfaction.

References

1. Weber AM, Walters MD, Piedmonte MR, et al. Anterior colporrhaphy: A randomized trial of three surgical techniques. Am J Obstet Gynecol 2001; 185: 1299–1306.
2. Olsen AL, Smith VJ, Bergstrom JO, et al. Epidemiology of surgically managed pelvic organ prolapse and urinary incontinence. Obstet Gynecol 1997; 89: 501–506.
3. Samuelsson EC, Arne Victor FT, Tibblin G, et al. Signs of genital prolapse in a Swedish population of women 20 to 59 years of age and possible related factors. Am J Obstet Gynecol 1999; 180:299–305.
5. Davila GW, Drutz H, Deprest J. Clinical implications of the biology of grafts: Conclusions of the 2005 IUGA grafts roundtable. Int Urogynecol J Pelvic Floor Dysfunct 2006; 17(Suppl 7):S51–55.
6. Weber AM, Richter HE. Pelvic organ prolapse. Obstet Gynecol 2005; 106: 615–634.
7. McIntosh LJ, Mallett VT, Frahm JD, et al. Gynecologic disorders in women with Ehlers–Danlos syndrome. J Soc Gynecol Investig 1995; 2:559–564.
8. Carley ME, Schaffer J. Urinary incontinence and pelvic organ prolapse in women with Marfan or Ehlers–Danlos syndrome. Am J Obstet Gynecol 2000;182: 1021–1023.
9. Deprest J, Zheng F, Konstantinovic M, et al. The biology behind fascial defects and the use of implants in pelvic organ prolapse repair. Int Urogynecol J Pelvic Floor Dysfunct 2006; 17(Suppl 7):S16–25.
10. Karlovsky ME, Thakre AA, Rastinehad A, et al. Biomaterials for pelvic floor reconstruction. Urology 2005; 66: 469–475.
11. Wagh PV, Read RC. Collagen deficiency in rectus sheath of patients with inguinal herniation. Proc Soc Exp Biol Med 1971; 137: 382–384.
12. Klinge U, Zheng H, Si ZY, et al. Expression of the extracellular matrix proteins of collagen I, collagen III, fibronectin, and matrix metalloproteinases 1 and 13 in the skin of patients with inguinal hernia. Eur Surg Res 1999; 31:480–490.
13. Cannon DJ, Read RC. Metastatic emphysema: A mechanism for acquiring inguinal herniation. Ann Surg 1981; 194: 270–278.
14. Bellón JM, Bajo A, Ga-Honduvilla N, et al. Fibroblasts from the transversalis fascia of young patients with direct inguinal hernias show constitutive MMP-2 overexpression. Ann Surg 2001; 233: 287–291.
15. Jackson SR, Avery NC, Tarlton JF. Changes in metabolism of collagen in genitourinary prolapse. Lancet 1996; 347: 1658–1651.
16. Chen B, Wen Y, Li H, Polan ML. Collagen metabolism and turnover in women with stress urinary incontinence and pelvic prolapse. Int Urogynecol J Pelvic Floor Dysfunct 2002; 13:80–87.
17. Moalli PA, Shand SH, Zyczynski HM, et al. Remodeling of vaginal connective tissue in patients with prolapse. Obstet Gynecol 2005; 106: 953–963.
18. Gabriel B, Denschlag D, Gobel H, et al. Uterosacral ligament in postmenopausal women with or without pelvic organ prolapse. Int Urogynecol J Pelvic Floor Dysfunct 2005; 16: 475–479.
19. Wong MY, Harmanli, OH, Agar M, et al. Collagen content of nonsupport tissue in pelvic organ prolapse and stress urinary incontinence. Am J Obstet Gynecol. 2003; 189: 1597–1599.
20. Ulmsten U, Ekman G, Giertz G, et al. Different biochemical composition of connective tissue in continent and stress incontinent women. Acta Obstet Gynecol Scand 1987; 66: 455–457.
21. Kushner L, Mathrubutham M, Burney T, et al. Excretion of collagen derived peptides is increased in women with stress urinary incontinence. Neurourol Urodyn 2004; 23: 198–203.
22. Chen Y, DeSautel, M, Anderson, A, et al. Collagen synthesis is not altered in women with stress urinary incontinence. Neurourol Urodyn 2004; 23: 367–373.
23. Chen B, Wen Y, Polan ML. Elastolytic activity in women with stress urinary incontinence and pelvic organ prolapse. Neurourol Urodyn 2004; 23:119–126.
24. Shah DK, Kushner, L, Rao, SK, et al. Elastase activity in plasma: Screening tool for stress urinary incontinence. Abstract presented at AUA Meeting, Orlando, FL, 2002.
25. Dietz HP, Hansell NK, Grace ME, et al. Bladder neck mobility is a heritable trait. BJOG 2005; 112: 334–339.
26. Buchsbaum GM Duecy EE, Kerr LA, et al. Pelvic organ prolapse in nulliparous women and their

parous sisters. Obstet Gynecol 2006; 108(6): 1388–1393

27. Jack GS, Nikolova G, Vilain E, et al. Familial transmission of genitovaginal prolapse. Int Urogynecol J Pelvic Floor Dysfunct 2006; 17(5): 498–501.

28. Nikolova G, Lee H, Berkovitz S, et al. Sequence variant in the laminin gamma 1 (LAMC1) gene associated with familial pelvic organ prolapse. Hum Genet 2007; 120(6): 847–856.

29. Karlovsky ME, Kushner L, Badlani GH. Synthetic biomaterials for pelvic floor reconstruction. Curr Urol Rep 2005; 6:376–384.

30. Birch C. The use of prosthetics in pelvic reconstructive surgery. Best Pract Res Clin Obstet Gynaecol 2005; 19:979–991.

31. Silva WA, Karram MM. Scientific basis of use of grafts during vaginal reconstructive procedures. Curr Opin Obstet Gynecol 2005; 17: 519–529.

32. Alridge AH. Transplantation of fascia for relief of urinary stress incontinence. Am J Obstet Gynecol 1942; 44: 398–411.

33. Beck RP, Grove D, Arnusch, D, et al. Recurrent urinary stress incontinence treated by the fascia lata sling procedure. Am J Obstet Gynecol 1974; 120:613–621.

34. Morgan TO, Westney OL, McGuire EJ. Pubovaginal sling: 4-Year outcome analysis and quality of life assessment. J Urol 2000; 163: 1845–1848.

35. Chaikin DC, Rosenthal J, Blaivas JG. Pubovaginal fascial sling for all types of stress urinary incontinence: Long-term analysis. J Urol 1998; 160: 1312–1316.

36. Haab F, Zimmern,PE, Leach GE. Diagnosis and treatment of intrisinic sphincter deficiency in females. AUA Update Series. Lesoon 35, Vol. XV. American Urological Association: Baltimore, MD, 1996:282–287.

37. Beck RP, McCormick S, Nordstrom L. The fascia lata sling procedure for treating genuine stress incontinence of urine. Obstet Gynecol 1988; 72:699–703.

38. Latini JM, Luxx MM, Kreder KJ. Efficacy and morbidity of autologous fascia lata sling cystourethropexy. J Urol 2004; 171: 1180–1184.

39. Latini JM, Brown JA, Kreder KJ. Abdominal sacral colpopexy using autologous fascia lata. J Urol 2004; 171: 1176–1179.

40. Moalli PA. Cadaveric fascia lata. Int Urogynecol J 2006; 17:S48–50.

41. Lemer ML, Chaikin DC, Blaivas JG. Tissue strength analysis of autologous and cadaveric allografts for the pubovaginal sling. Neurourol Urodyn 1999; 18:497–503.

42. Kobashi KC, Hsaio KC, Grovier FE. Suitability of different sling materials for the treatment of female stress urinary incontinence. Nat Clin Pract Urol 2005; 2: 84–91.

43. McBride AW, Ellerkmann RM, Bent AE, et al. Comparsion of long-term outcomes of autologous fascia lata slings with Suspend Tutoplast fascia lata allograft slings for stress incontinence. Am J Obstet Gynecol 2005; 192:1677–1681.

44. Howden NS, Zyczynski HM, Moalli PA, et al. Comparison of autologous rectus fascia and cadaveric fascia in pubovaginal sling continence outcomes. Am J Obstet Gynecol 2006; 194:1444–1449.

45. FitzGerald MP, Mollenhauer J, Bitterman P, et al. Functional failure of fascia lata allografts. Am J Obstet Gynecol 1999; 181:1339–1346.

46. Culligan, PJ, Blackwell L, Goldsmith LJ, et al. A randomized controlled trial comparing fascia lata and synthetic mesh for sacral colpopexy. Obstet Gynecol 2005; 106: 9–37.

47. Gandhi S, Goldberg RP, Kwon C, et al. A prospective randomized trial using solvent dehydrated fascia lata for the prevention of recurrent anterior vaginal wall prolapse. Am J Obstet Gynecol 2005; 192: 1649–1654.

48. Winter JC. InteXen tissue processing and laboratory study. Int Urogynecol J 2006; 17:S34–38.

49. Zheng F, Lin Y, Verbeken E, et al. Host response after reconstruction of abdominal wall defects with porcine dermal collagen in a rat model. J Obstet Gynecol 2004; 191(6):1961–1970.

50. Gandhi S, Kubba L, Abramov Y, et al. Histopathologic changes of porcine dermis xenografts for transvaginal suburethral slings. Am J Obstet Gynecol 2005; 192:1643–1648.

51. Wheeler TL 2nd, Richter HE, Duke AG, et al. Outcomes with porcine graft placement in the anterior vaginal compartment in patients who undergo high vaginal uterosacral suspension and cystocele repair. Am J Obstet Gynecol 2006; 194(5): 1486–1491.

52. Gomelsky A, Haverkorn RM, Simoneaux WJ, et al. Incidence and management of vaginal extrusion of acellular porcine dermis after incontinence and prolapse surgery. Int Urogynecol J Pelvic Floor Dysfunct 2007; 18: 1337–1341.

53. Gomelsky A, Rudy DC, Dmochowski RR. Porcine dermis interposition graft for repair of high-grade anterior compartment defects with or without concomitant pelvic organ prolapse procedures. Urol 2004; 171(4): 1581–1584.

54. Hiles M, Hodde J. Tissue engineering a clinically useful extracellular matrix biomaterial. Int Urogynecol J 2006; 17:S39–43.

55. Wiedemann A, Otto M. Small intestine submucosa for pubourethral sling suspension for the treatment of stress incontinence: First histopathological results in humans. J Urol 2004; 172(1):215–218.

56. Thiel M, Rodrigues PPC, Riccetto LZ, et al. A stereological analysis of fibrosis and inflammatory reaction induced by four different synthetic slings. BJU Int 2005; 95: 833–837.

57. Rutner AB, Levine SR, Schmaelzle JF. Processed porcine small intestine submucosa as a graft material for pubovaginal slings: Durability and results. Urology 2003; 62:805–809.

58. Jones JS, Rackley RR, Berglund R, et al. Porcine small intestinal submucosa as a percutaneous mid-urethral sling: 2-Year results. BJU Int 2005; 96: 103–106.

59. Ho KL, Witte MN, Bird ET. 8-Ply small intestinal submucosa tension-free sling: Spectrum of postoperative inflammation. J Urol 2004; 171:268–271.

60. Chaliha C, Khalid U, Campagna L, et al. SIS graft for anterior vaginal wall prolapse repair – a case-controlled study. Int Urogynecol J Pelvic Floor Dysfunct 2006; 17(5): 492–497.

61. Amid P. Classification of biomaterials and their relative complications in an abdominal wall hernia surgery. Hernia 1997; 1: 15–21.

62. Dwyer PL. Evolution of biological and synthetic grafts in reconstructive pelvic surgery. Int Urogynecol J Pelvic Floor Dysfunct 2006; 17 (Supple 7): S10–15.

63. Klinge U, Losterhalfe B, Birkenhaure V, et al. Impact of polymer pore size on the interface scar formation in a rat model. J Surg Res 2002; 103:208–214.

64. Bobyn JD, Wilson GJ, Macgregor DC, et al. Effect of pore size on the peel strength of attachment of fibrous tissue to porous-surfaced implants. Biomed Mater Res 1982; 16:517–584.

65. Barbolt TA. Biology of polypropylene/polyglactin 910 grafts. Int Urogynecol J Pelvic Floor Dysfunct 2006; 17 (Supple 7):S26–30.

66. Julian TM. The efficacy of Marlex mesh in the repair of severe recurrent vaginal prolapse of the anterior mid vaginal wall. Am J Obstet Gynecol 1996; 175: 1472–1475.

67. Flood CG, Drutz HP, Waja L. Anterior colporrhaphy reinforced with Marlex mesh for the treatment of cystoceles. Int J Urogynecol 1998; 9: 200–204.

68. Weber AM, Walters MD, Piedmonte MR, et al. Anterior colporrhaphy: A randomized trial of three surgical techniques. Am J Obstet Gynecol 2001; 185: 1299–1304.

69. Sand PK, Koduri S, Lobel RW, et al. Prospective randomized trial of polyglactin 910 mesh to prevent recurrence of cystoceles and rectoceles. Am J Obstet Gynecol 2001; 184:1357–1362.

70. de Tayrac R, Gervaise A, Chauveaud A, et al. Tension-free polypropylene mesh for vaginal repair of anterior vaginal wall prolapse. J Reprod Med 2005; 50(2):75–80.

71. Rodriguez LV, Bukkapatnam R, Shah SM, et al. Transvaginal paravaginal repair of high-grade cystocele central and lateral defects with concominant suburethral sling: Report of early results, outcomes, and patient satisfaction with a new technique. Urology 2005; 66 (Suppl 5A):57–65.

72. Amrute KV, Eisenberg ER, Rastinehad AR, et al. Analysis of outcomes of single polypropylene mesh in total pelvic floor reconstruction. Neurourol Urodyn 2007; 26(1):53–58.

73. Nazemi TM, Kobashi KC. Complications of grafts used in female pelvic floor reconstruction: Mesh erosion and extrusion. Ind J Urol 2007; 23(2):153–160.

74. Clemens JQ, DeLancey JO, Faerber GJ, et al. Urinary tract erosions after synthetic pubovaginal slings: Diagnosis and management strategy. Urol 2000; 56:589–595.

75. Abouassaly R, Steinberg JR, Lemieux M, et al. Complications of tension-free vaginal tape: A multi-institutional review. BJU Int 2004; 94:110–113.

76. Huang KH, Kung FT, Liang HM, et al. Management of polypropylene mesh erosion after intravaginal midurethral sling operation for female stress urinary incontinence. Int Urogynecol J Pelvic Floor Dysfunct 2005; 16:437–440.

77. Lord HE, Finn JC, Tsokos N, et al. A randomized controlled equivalence trial of short-term complications and efficacy of tension-free vaginal tape and suprapubic urethral support sling for treating stress incontinence. BJU Int 2006; 98:367–376.

78. Yamada BS, Govier FE, Stefanovic KB, et al. High rate of vaginal erosions associated with mentor ObTape. J Urol 2006; 176:651–654.

79. But I. Vaginal wall erosion after transobturator tape procedure. Int Urogynecol J Pelvic Floor Dysfunct 2005; 16:506–508.

81. Amundsen CL, Flynn BJ, Webster GD. Urethral erosion after synthetic and nonsynthetic pubovaginal slings: Differences in management and continence outcome. J Urol 2003; 170: 134–137.

82. Davila GW, Drutz H, Deprest J. Clinical implications of the biology of grafts: Conclusions of the 2005 IUGA Grafts Roundtable. Int Urogynecol J 2006; 17 (Suppl 7):51–53.

Chapter 24
Pelvic Reconstructive Surgery: Vaginal Approach

Daniel Biller and G. Willy Davila

Introduction

The goals for surgical correction of pelvic support defects include normalizing support of all anatomic compartments, alleviating clinical symptoms, and optimizing sexual, bowel, and bladder function. Care must be taken to restore normal anatomy and function to all compartments, without precipitating new support or functional problems. A thorough evaluation of the apical, anterior, and posterior compartments as described in previous chapters is necessary prior to surgical correction.

The importance of an accurate pelvic exam cannot be overemphasized. In addition to assessing the degree and type of prolapse present, it is important to perform the vaginal examination with a surgical planning point of view, especially if the patient is considering surgical therapy. The presence of any fascial tears or defects usually can be predicted during careful vaginal examination, since they are visualized as areas of sudden change in vaginal wall thickness or rugations. By the end of the pelvic examination, the surgeon should have developed a surgical plan for repair of the prolapse. Urodynamic assessment will help determine the type of a concomitant anti-incontinence procedure to be performed, if necessary.

The choice of surgical approach should be based on what is best for the patient's individual variables [1]. The greatest advantage of the vaginal approach is that all compartment defects (resulting in apical prolapse, cystocele, rectocele, enterocele, and perineal body defects) may be repaired concomitantly, frequently through the same incision. The following factors are particularly important when planning a surgical approach for vaginal prolapse:

1. Importance of sexual function. If the patient reports that vaginal sexual function is of great importance to her (age may be an unrelated issue here), a sacrocolpopexy may be considered primarily.
2. Vaginal length. If the vaginal apex (dimples) reaches the ischial spines with ease, the patient will do well with a vaginal procedure, while those whose apex does not reach the ischial spines may be better served by an abdominal procedure or an obliterative procedure, if appropriate.
3. Previous reconstructive procedures. The degree of existent scarring and fibrosis must be kept in mind, as the area around the sacral promontory or sacrospinous ligaments may be difficult or risky to reach. This is especially important in this age of commonplace graft use.
4. Presence of large paravaginal defects. Although paravaginal defect repairs can be performed vaginally, they can be technically difficult and their long-term outcomes have not been reported. Thus, an abdominal paravaginal approach or a grafted repair may be preferable if significant paravaginal defects are present.
5. Medical comorbidities. In the face of a medically delicate or advanced-age patient, a vaginal, often obliterative, procedure under regional anesthesia is preferable.

6. Tissue quality and presence of large fascial defects. Tissue quality usually will improve with preoperative local estrogen therapy, but large fascial defects adjacent to the cuff may require graft reinforcement, which can be accomplished during surgical repair.

7. Associated colorectal problems. The frequent coexistence of colorectal dysfunction in women with vaginal prolapse requires that these problems be kept in mind during surgical planning. As such, a woman with extensive rectal prolapse may best undergo a concomitant rectopexy and sacrocolpopexy or a perineal proctosigmoidectomy and vaginal-approach vaginal repair.

Optimizing Surgical Outcomes

The success rate of any surgical procedure is in great part based on appropriate patient preparation. A clear understanding of the present anatomic defects and voiding dysfunction as diagnosed by urodynamics will help identify the most appropriate procedures to be performed. Tissue preparation with low-dose estrogen cream (ie, 1 gm two nights per week) is crucial for most postmenopausal women. Medical clearance should be obtained and perioperative safety is optimized by appropriate DVT prophylaxis (SC Heparin or pneumatic compression device per surgeon's preference), and prophylactic antibiotics. Postoperatively, vaginal packing is placed for 24 h to prevent stress on suture lines secondary to coughing or vomiting. For 6 weeks postoperatively, patients are instructed to lift no more than 5 pounds or exert themselves to any significant degree. Estrogen cream is restarted and the patient is instructed to perform Kegel exercises as a part of her daily routine after the 6-week postoperative visit.

Vaginal Apical Suspension

The vaginal approaches to surgical repair of apical prolapse include McCall–Mayo culdoplasty, uterosacral ligament suspension, iliococcygeal suspension, sacrospinous ligament fixation, and the new grafted "minimally invasive" vault procedures.

McCall–Mayo Suldoplasty

The technique of plicating the uterosacral ligaments in the midline while reefing the peritoneum in the cul-de-sac combined with a posterior culdoplasty was introduced by McCall in 1957 [2]. The importance of this technique for prevention of posthysterectomy vaginal vault prolapse cannot be overemphasized, especially in cases where vaginal hysterectomy is performed for pre-existing vaginal vault prolapse. The goal is the restoration of the integrity and attachment of the apical endopelvic fascia to the cardinal–uterosacral ligament complex at the apex.

Nonabsorbable sutures incorporate both uterosacral ligaments, intervening cul-de-sac peritoneum, and full thickness apical vaginal wall (Fig. 24.1). Multiple sutures may be required if extensive prolapse is present. As a general rule, the uppermost suture is placed on the uterosacral ligaments a distance from the cuff equal to the amount of vault prolapse that is present (ie, POP-Q: TVL minus point D, or C if uterus is absent).

Care must be taken not to injure or kink the ureters when placing the suture through the uterosacral ligaments, since the ureters lay 1–2 cm lateral at the level of the cervix. We recommend cytoscopy with visualization of ureteral patency following the procedure. Reported success rates are high, but objective long-term data are limited. Most pelvic surgeons would recommend that a

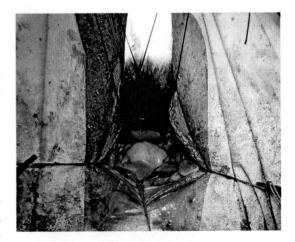

FIG. 24.1. McCall culdoplasty with placement of permanent sutures through the uterosacral ligaments, cul-de-sac peritoneum and full thickness vaginal wall

McCall culdoplasty be performed whenever a vaginal hysterectomy is performed, especially for uterine prolapse.

Uterosacral Ligament Suspension

Excellent anatomic outcomes have been described with reattachment of the uterosacral ligaments to the vaginal apex, similar to the McCall technique (Table 24.1). The physiological nature of this technique makes it very attractive. This technique involves opening the vaginal wall from the anterior to the posterior over the apical defect and identifying the pubocervical fascia, rectovaginal fascia, and uterosacral ligaments. One permanent 1–0 suture and one delayed absorbable 1–0 suture are placed in the posterior-medial aspect of each uterosacral ligament 1–2 cm proximal and medial to each ischial spine. One arm of each permanent suture then is placed through the pubocervical and rectovaginal fascia, and one arm of each delayed absorbable suture is placed in a similar fashion but also incorporates the vaginal epithelium. After all additional defects are repaired, the sutures are tied, suspending the vault.

Potential pitfalls include ureteral injury and difficulty identifying the uterosacral ligaments in cases of extensive prolapse secondary to redundant peritoneum and preexisting weak and attenuated ligaments. Reported ureteral injury rates range from 0 to 11% [3–8]. Therefore, cystoscopy to confirm ureteral patency is essential.

Success rates range from 82 to 96% over a follow up of 6 months to 3 years. The largest study was performed by Shull et al., who reported on 289 patients undergoing uterosacral ligament suspension [3]. Eighty-seven percent (251/289) had no postoperative support defects at any site. Karram et al. recently reported 5-year outcome data on 72 patients, who underwent high uterosacral vaginal vault suspension. Concomitant procedures included vaginal hysterectomy (37.5%), posterior colporrhaphy (87.5%), anterior colporrhaphy (58.3%), and suburethral sling (31.9%). Failure was defined as symptomatic recurrent prolapse of stage 2 or greater in one or more segments, and was reported in 11 of 72 patients (15.3%), specifically apical recurrent prolapse of stage 2 or greater in 2 of 72 patients (2.8%). The authors concluded this procedure seemed to be durable for repair of vaginal enterocele and vault prolapse [4].

It must be emphasized that uterosacral ligament vault suspension at a time of vaginal hysterectomy (when the ligaments are readily identifiable) is vastly different from the procedure when performed for posthysterectomy vault prolapse. Higher success rates and decreased morbidity are likely associated with the greater ease at identifying the ligaments at their attachment site to the uterus.

Iliococcygeus Suspension

Originally described by Inmon in 1963, elevation of the vaginal apex to the iliococcygeus muscles along the lateral pelvic sidewall is a safe and simple procedure [9]. It can be performed without a vaginal incision by placing a monofilament permanent suture (ie, polypropylene) full thickness through the apical vaginal wall into the muscle and fascia unilaterally or bilaterally in nonsexually active women where a suture knot in the vagina will not be problematic. It thus is useful in elderly patients where complete restoration of vaginal anatomy is not necessary or as a salvage operation

TABLE 24.1. Uterosacral ligament suspension results.

	Patients	Follow-up mean months (range)	Number cured (rate)	Ureteral injury number (%)
Silva et al. [4]	72	5.1 (3.5–7.1)[a]	61/72 (84%)	5 (2.4)
Amundsen et al. [5]	33	28 (6–43)	27/33 (82%)	NR[b]
Shull et al. [3]	289	48	251/289 (87%)	1 (1)
Barber et al. [6]	46	15.5 median (3.5–40.8)	90% (symptoms)	5 (11)
Jenkins [7]	50	33 (6–48)	48/50 (96%)	0 (0%)

[a]Years
[b]Not reported

TABLE 24.2. Sacrospinous ligament fixation.

Investigator	Duration of follow-up	No. available for follow-up	No. cured (rate)
Richter/Albright, 1981	1–10 years	81	37 (70%)
Nichols, 1982	≥2 years	163	158 (97%)
Morley and DeLancey, 1988	1 year 11 months	92	75 (82%)
Kettel and Herbertson, 1989		31	25 (81%)
Shull, 1992	2–3 years	81	53 (65%)

Adapted from [18]

for someone with suboptimal vault support and good distal vaginal anatomy, such as after a unilateral sacrospinous fixation.

It also can be performed in an open fashion following a posterior vaginal wall dissection and entering the pararectal space. The sutures are placed into the fascia overlying the iliococcygeus muscle, anterior to the ischial spine inferior to the arcus tendineus fascia pelvis, and incorporated into the pubocervical fascia anteriorly and the rectovaginal fascia posteriorly.

Shull reported a 95% cure rate of the apical compartment with a follow-up of 6 weeks to 5 years of 42 women. He did, however, note a 14% occurrence rate of prolapse at other sites [10]. Other long-term data for this procedure are scant.

Sacrospinous Ligament Fixation

Fixation of the apex to the sacrospinous ligaments is likely the most common currently performed apical suspension procedure from the vaginal approach. It was first described by Sederl in 1958 and has undergone multiple modifications [11]. Indications for this procedure are correction of complete procidentia, posthysterectomy vault prolapse, and vaginal enterocele [12–17].

The sacrospinous ligaments are identified after entering the pararectal space through a posterior vaginal wall dissection, and two nonabsorbable sutures are placed *through* the ligament, rather than around it, as the pudendal neurovascular bundle passes behind the ligament. The first suture is placed 2 cm medial to the ischial spine and the second 1 cm medial to the first. Each suture is then secured to the underside of the vaginal apex, short and long term results are overall acceptable (Table

24.2). Surgical approach will be based on the proper identification of these support defects.

Although most surgeons perform the procedure unilaterally, on the right side, as originally described by right-handed surgeons, a bilateral procedure results in more physiological suspension of the apex (Fig. 24.2). It does not appear that reinforcement of the apex with a graft improves surgical outcome, as we noted in a retrospective review.

Overall, transvaginal vault suspension is associated with excellent results. Improvements still can be made in long-term cure of subsequent anterior compartment prolapse and associated morbidity [18].

Anterior Wall Repairs

Anterior wall prolapse remains the most challenging aspect of vaginal prolapse repair. Despite advancements in surgical technique, recurrence rates after a traditional repair remain quite high (40–60%). Anatomic concepts have guided surgeons through a progression from central fascial plication (for a midline fascial stretching defect), to paravaginal detachment correction (for separation of the vaginal sidewall sulcus from the arcus tendineus fascia pelvis along the lateral pelvic sidewall), to identification and correction of specific fascial tears (for site-specific hernia-type tears) without a significant reduction in recurrence rates when analyzed on a long-term basis. It is likely that most patients have a combination of fascial stretch defects, apical paravaginal separation, and site-specific fascial tears. Thus, one technique may not be sufficient for a satisfactory repair in a given patient.

FIG. 24.2. Bilateral sacrospinous fixation is a more physiologic approach than the unilateral approach, a graft does not appear to improve outcomes

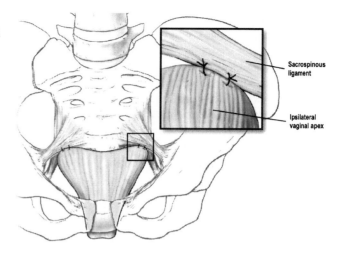

Sacrospinous ligament

Ipsilateral vaginal apex

Anterior Colporrhaphy

The anterior colporrhaphy was popularized by Howard Kelly in 1912, and is a commonly used technique for transvaginal correction of anterior vaginal prolapse secondary to midline support defects. A midline incision is made in the vaginal epithelium from the bladder neck to approximately 2 cm from the uterine cervix or vaginal cuff. Sharp and blunt dissection then is performed bilaterally to separate the vaginal epithelium from the vaginal muscularis (fascia) to the lateral sulcus. After completing the dissection, the pubocervical fascia is plicated in the midline in one or more layers with interrupted stitches of delayed absorbable or permanent suture, thereby repairing the central defect and elevating the bladder base and anterior vagina toward the apex. The fascia then must be incorporated into the cervix (nonhysterectomized patient) or the cardinal–uterosacral ligament complex (hysterectomized patient) at the apex (Fig. 24.3). Apical support must be addressed to ensure durability of the repair, especially when anterior enterocele is present. Concomitant anti-incontinence procedures may be done through the same incision or a different incision depending on surgeon preference. Excess vaginal epithelium trimmed with care taken not to excise too much vaginal wall to avoid stricture formation. The incision is then closed with a 2–0 absorbable suture. Cystoscopy is then should be performed to ensure bladder and ureteral integrity. A vaginal pack is placed for postoperative hemostasis.

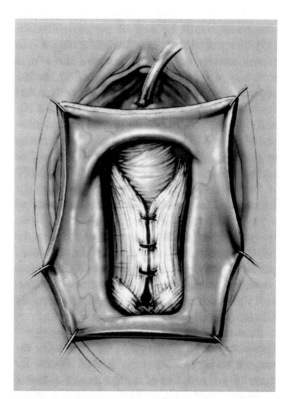

FIG. 24.3. An anterior colporrhaphy must include placation of healthy fascia in the midline and reattachment to the vaginal cuff/cervix to achieve a satisfactory result

Reported failure rates range from 0 to 60% for traditional anterior colporrhaphy for the treatment of anterior compartment prolapse [19–22]. Degree of lateral dissection may be important in achieving an improved result, since a wide dissection to the lateral vaginal sulcus was reported to be superior to a limited anterior wall dissection [23]. Many studies focus on prolapse of the anterior compartment after sacrospinous fixation and/or in conjunction with Kelly plication for stress urinary incontinence, which may not fully evaluate the effectiveness of a midline plication procedure. Graft usage as reinforcement or as primary repair has been studied and success rates range from 75 to 100%.

Paravaginal Defect Repair

In 1909, White described the paravaginal repair as an anatomic correction of cystoceles [24]. Richardson, in 1976, reintroduced the concept of repairing anterior compartment prolapse with the site-specific repair by way of paravaginal repair [25]. The goal of the paravaginal defect repair is to correct anterior vaginal wall prolapse that results from loss of lateral support by reattaching the lateral vaginal sulcus and the associated pubocervical fascia to its normal lateral attachment site. The lateral vagina attaches to the levator ani muscle bilaterally along a line from the anterior pubic ramus to the ischial spine known as the "white line" or arcus tendineus fasciae pelvis (ATFP). The ATFP is formed from a condensation of the obturator internus and levator ani fascia and is composed of organized fibrous collagen connective tissue. When the pubocervical fascia separates laterally from the ATFP, a paravaginal defect results. As mentioned previously this defect is identified on careful vaginal physical examination and most commonly presents as a right-sided unilateral defect, although certainly bilateral defects and left-sided defects occur.

Paravaginal defect repair using the transvaginal approach can be challenging, but it enables the surgeon to repair concurrent central defects for those women with loss of midline as well as lateral anterior vaginal support. Initial dissection of the pubocervical fascia from the vaginal epithelium is identical to colporrhaphy. Entrance is gained into the paravaginal space as the fascia is separated to the lateral vaginal sulcus and urogenital diaphragm. Once a paravaginal defect is identified, the normal site of lateral attachment of the vagina should be clearly visualized. A Briesky-Navratil retractor then can be used to retract the bladder medially, exposing the levator ani muscle and the course of the ATFP from the ischial spine to the inferior aspect of the pubic ramus. Four to six interrupted nonabsorbable sutures are placed through the ATFP and the aponeurosis of the levator ani muscle from the level of the ischial spine to the pubic symphysis at 1-cm intervals. Each suture then is placed through the lateral edge of the detached pubocervical fascia at its corresponding level along the lateral vaginal wall sulcus and tied. The vaginal epithelium then is trimmed and closed. Cystoscopy is performed to confirm ureteral patency and absence of intravesical sutures.

Results of the vaginal paravaginal repair for cystocele have ranged from 67 to 100% [26–29]. Shull reported a 93% success rate of less than grade 2 recurrent prolapse (to the hymen) with follow up of 1.6 years in 56 patients who underwent vaginal paravaginal repair [26]. Elkins reported a 92% (23/25) cure rate [27], and Young et al. reported a 98% objective cure rate in 55 patients followed for 1 year. However, 22 patients had recurrent midline cystocele and 21 major complications occurred with a 16% rate of transfusion [28]. Karram reported a 97% cure rate in 35 patients with mean follow-up of 20.2 months. He did note, however, recurrent enterocele in 20% (seven patients) and recurrent rectocele in 14% (five patients). Serious complications did occur including retropubic hematoma, abscess, and ureteral obstruction [29]. To date there are no randomized controlled studies on vaginal paravaginal repair.

Posterior Compartment Reconstruction

Herniation of the rectum or posterior vaginal wall into the vaginal canal resulting in a vaginal bulge is commonly termed a "rectocele." Symptoms consist of perineal and vaginal pressure, obstructive defecation, constipation, and the need to splint or digitally reduce the vagina in order to defecate. Defects in the integrity and attachments of the posterior vaginal wall and rectovaginal septum may result in posterior wall defects.

The normal posterior vaginal wall is lined by squamous epithelium overlying the lamina propria, which is a layer of loose connective tissue and a fibromuscular layer referred to as the rectovaginal fascia. Defects in this support structure result in posterior wall defects. When the defect occurs superiorly as a tear off the apex or cervix, traditional anatomic concepts term it an "enterocele." Tears from the perineal body are thought to result in rectocele and perineocele. Recent anatomic studies have shown that many rectoceles actually are due to an apical fascial separation which can readily be identified when the dissection is carried up to the vaginal apex (Fig. 24.4b). A rectocele typically develops at or below the levator plate along the vertical vagina as an attenuation of the perineal body integrity (Fig. 24.4a)

Transvaginal repair of posterior wall prolapse allows for correction of vaginal as well as rectal symptomatic dysfunction. Posterior colporrhaphy in conjunction with perineoplasty is commonly performed to address a rectocele or relaxed perineum and widened genital hia-

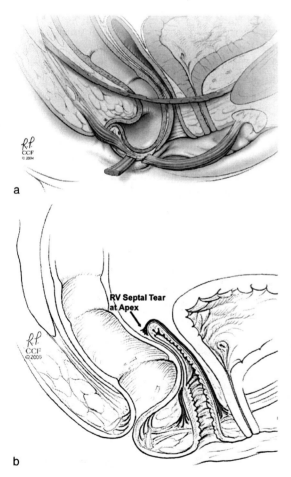

a

b

FIG. 24.4. (a) A rectocele develops as an anterior weakness of the perineal body, and (b) is frequently associated with a fascial separation from the vaginal apex or cervix

tus. A midline incision then is made along the length of the vagina to the superior edge of the rectocele. Dissection then is carried laterally to the lateral vaginal sulcus to separate the posterior vaginal epithelium from the underlying rectovaginal fascia. If an apical fascial separation is noted, the fascial edges should be reattached to the apex–cervix prior to repairing the lower vagina. The rectovaginal fascia overlying the levator ani muscles is plicated with interrupted delayed absorbable sutures. In the presence of a large rectocele, multiple suture layers may be necessary. Concomitant perineoplasty is performed by plicating the bulbocavernosus and transverse perineii muscles. This reinforces the perineal body and provides enhanced support to the anterior rectal wall–corrected rectocele.

Discrete site-specific repair has been popularized secondary to the high rate of dyspareunia after posterior colporrhaphy likely secondary to plication of the levator ani muscles [30–32]. The intent of the site-specific repair of rectoceles is to identify the fascial tears and reapproximate the edges with interrupted absorbable sutures. Further discussion of posterior compartment repair and results are discussed in Chap. 27.

Mesh and Grafts in Vaginal Surgery

Adopting the principles of hernia repair by general surgeons, reconstructive pelvic surgeons have begun adopting reinforcement of transvaginal repairs with synthetic and biological prostheses. Synthetic mesh such as polypropylene (PP) has been demonstrated to be useful for anti-incontinence surgery (slings) and abdominal sacrocolpopexy (ASC) for repair of vaginal vault prolapse. Although high success rates have been reported for ASC, erosion of the mesh and infection have been reported [33]. As such, only monofilament, macroporous (PP type 1) mesh should be used in order to minimize the risk of erosion. Biological grafts used in reconstructive surgery include autologous grafts (from another body part, ie, fascia lata) and allografts including cadaveric fascia lata, rectus sheath, and dermal grafts. Xenograft materials used include porcine dermis, bovine pericardium, and small intestinal mucosa. There are scant long-term outcome data on these materials in the literature. Although grafts appear to improve short-term success rates, lack of long-term data leads to concerns of regarding graft exposure/erosion, long-term integrity, and consequences especially in sexually active women.

Grafted Apical Procedures

Minimally invasive techniques for apical suspension have relied on placement of synthetic tapes from the apex to strong pelvic structures. Introduced as the infracoccygeal sacropexy, the posterior intravaginal slingplasty (posterior IVS, Tyco/US Surgical, Norwak, CT, USA) was the initial apical suspension "kit" procedure [34]. Concerns regarding resultant vaginal length and healing abnormalities due to the multifilament nature of the tape used led to its poor acceptance. However, the concept of placing a tape to provide apical support was attractive to many, and the approach was modified to allow placement of the tape from ischial spine to ischial spine in an analogous position to endogenous cardinal ligaments in order to restore apical support. Entry into the pararectal space, as for sacrospinous fixation, is needed, and the needle tunneler device is used to appropriately place the tape. Early results were quite promising with apical support restoration resulting in over 90% of patients and vaginal lengths of approximately 8 cm [35, 36].

Vaginal Wall Graft Use

Drutz reported on 142 women who underwent anterior colporrhaphy reinforced with Marlex mesh with mean follow-up of 3.2 years. Symptomatic recurrence was reported at 5.7%, and objective recurrence greater than stage II (descent less than halfway to hymen) was not detected (0 of 142). Mesh erosion was observed in 3 (2.1%) [37].

Sand reported on 132 women undergoing either standard rectocele repair or repair plus reinforce-ment with polyglactin mesh (absorbable). He found no difference in recurrence rates. However, placing a piece of polyglactin 910 mesh within the suture line of an anterior colporrhaphy was demonstrated to reduce recurrence rates in a prospective, randomized design [38].

Even fewer studies demonstrate the use of a biological graft to enhance longevity of a repair. Porcine dermis implantation improved the outcome of anterior colporrhaphy results in a 1-year follow-up study [39]. Using bovine pericardium, we demonstrated an improvement in outcomes over a standard plication cystocele repair, which became apparent after 6 months [40]. A summary of findings is found in Table 24.3.

No definitive study has yet been performed to demonstrate the benefit of a graft for anterior or posterior wall repairs. Until the literature provides more conclusive evidence, surgeons must weigh the potential benefit of reduced prolapse recurrence rates versus the risk of vaginal wall erosion (synthetic grafts), premature graft breakdown (non-cross-linked biological grafts) and graft encapsulation and distortion/hardening (cross-linked biological grafts) when deciding whether to use an implanted graft.

Prolapse Repair Kits

The growing awareness of prolapse as a surgically treatable condition has led to an increased volume of reconstructive procedures. As a natural consequence of increased surgical volume, surgeons have teamed up with surgical device companies to produce standardized, mesh-based surgical kits to simplify the treatment of genital prolapse. This process followed in the footsteps of midurethral slings for stress incontinence, such as TVT, which revolutionized urogynecologic surgery. However,

TABLE 24.3. Review of prosthetic surgical grafts in the management of cystoceles.

Author	Type of mesh	No. of patients	Duration of follow-up	Success rate cystocele (%)
Julian	Marlex, Control	12, 12	2 years, 2 years	100, 66
Flood	Marlex	142	3.2 years	100
Sand	Polyglactin, AC (no mesh)	73, 70	1 year, 1 year	75, 57
Weber	Polyglactin, AC (no mesh)	26, 57	23 months, 23 months	42, 37
Gomelsky [39]	Porcine dermis	70	2 years	91
Guerette [40]	Bovine pericardium (no graft)	47, 47	1 year	83

Adapted from: Table 2 of [44]

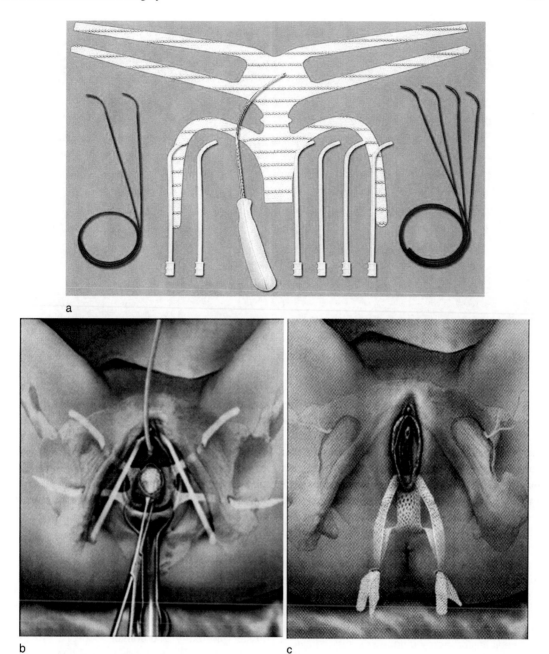

FIG. 24.5. Kits currently available for comprehensive prolapse repair include: (**a**) Prolift, (**b**) Avaulta anterior, (**c**) Avaulta posterior, (**d**) Apogee, and (**e**) Perigee

much controversy has resulted due to the lack of sufficient long-term data prior to commercialization to satisfy more conservative surgeons.

Currently available commercial prolapse repair kits include Prolift (Gynecare/Ethicon) for comprehensive repairs, Avaulta (Bard) in anterior and pos- terior versions, and Apogee and Perigee (American Medical Systems) for apical–posterior and anterior wall repairs (Fig. 24.5). Apogee and Perigee are available in PP synthetic and biological graft for- mulations, while Prolift and Avaulta are available only in synthetic PP versions.

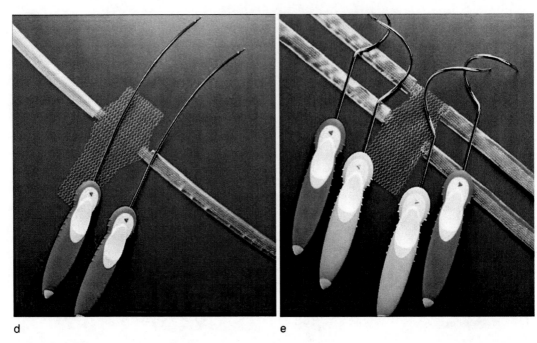

d   e

Fig. 24.5. (continued)

Available data to date on the use of the new kits are limited to short- and medium-term single- or multicenter case series. The largest use case series has been collected by a group of seven French surgeons reporting on a series of over 600 patients undergoing Prolift procedures of a period of over 5 years. Their sequential reports of outcomes have been invaluable in guiding pelvic surgeons in the use of grafts in the pelvis. They have reported a prolapse recurrence rate of 6.3% [41]. Most importantly, they have shed light on means of minimizing the risk of mesh erosions: appropriate tissue preparation preoperatively, subfascial tissue dissection, minimizing of mucosal trimming prior to vaginal wall closure, and avoiding performance of vaginal hysterectomy if not medically indicated. They clearly demonstrated that avoidance of a "T" incision along the anterior apical vagina reduced the rate of erosion from 16 to 5%. Uterine preservation also greatly reduces operative time and provides a strong structure (the cervix) to attach the mesh to apically. American surgeons also have demonstrated promising outcomes with the same technique [42].

Early outcomes demonstrated that apical support requires a synthetic graft rather than a degradable biological graft, as has been found with sacrocol-

popexy. Thus, current Apogee kits have a synthetic apical tape to recreate cardinal ligaments. Repair of the posterior and anterior vaginal walls with a synthetic or biological graft demonstrated restoration of normal anatomy with 1-year follow-up in 100% of anterior wall repair kits, 91.2% of posterior–apical repair kits, and 95.5% when a combination of both is used [43].

Summary

Advancements in the vaginal repair of genital prolapse have been aimed at achieving similar results to the abdominal approach, without the associated higher morbidity and longer recovery. All compartments can be addressed simultaneously, and selective use of grafts may enhance longevity and optimize operation room time utilization.

References

1. Biller DH, Davila GW. Vaginal vault prolapse: Identification and surgical options. Clev Clin J Med 2005;72:S12–S19.
2. McCall ML. Posterior culdoplasty: Surgical correction of enterocele during vaginal hysterectomy. A preliminary report. Obstet Gynecol 1957;10:595–602.

3. Shull BL, Bachofen C, et al. A transvaginal approach to repair of apical and other associated sites of pelvic organ prolapse with uterosacral ligaments. Am J Obstet Gynecol 2000;183:1365–1373.

4. Silva WA, Pauls RN, Segal JL, et al. Uterosacral ligament vault suspension: Five year outcomes. Obstet Gynecol 2006;108 (2):255–263.

5. Amundsen CL, Flynn BJ, Webster GD. Anatomical correction of vaginal vault prolapse by uterosacral ligament fixation in women who also require a pubovaginal sling. J Urol 2003;169:1770–1774.

6. Barber MD, Visco AG, et al. Bilateral uterosacral ligament vaginal vault suspension with site specific endopelvic fascia defect repair for treatment of pelvic organ prolapse. Am J Obstet Gynecol 2000;183:1402–1411.

7. Jenkins VR II. Uterosacral ligament fixation for vaginal vault suspension in uterine and vaginal vault prolapse. Am J Obstet Gynecol 1997;177:1337–1343.

8. Aronson MP, Aronson PK, Howard AE, et al. Low risk of ureteral obstruction with "deep" (dorsal/posterior) uterosacral ligament suture placement for transvaginal apical suspension. Am J Obstet Gynecol 2005;192:1530–1536.

9. Inmon WB. Pelvic relaxation and repair including prolapse of vagina following hysterectomy. South Med J. 1963;56:577–582.

10. Shull BL, Capen CV, Riggs MW, Kuehl TJ. Bilateral attachment of the vaginal cuff to iliococcygeus fascia: An effective method of cuff suspension. Am J Obstet Gynecol 1993;168(6):1669–1677.

11. Sederl J. Zur operation des prolpases der blind endigenden sheiden. Geburtshilfe Frauenheilkd 1958;18:824–828.

12. Richter K, Albright W. Long term results following fixation of the vagina on the sacrospinous ligament by the vaginal route. Am J Obstet Gynecol 1981;141:811–816.

13. Kettel LM, Herbertson RM. An anatomic evaluation of the sacrospinous ligament colpopexy. Surg Gynecol Obstet 1989:1–45.

14. Morley G, DeLancey JO. Sacrospinous ligament fixation for eversion of the vagina. Am J Obstet Gynecol 1988;158:872.

15. Randall C, Nichols D. Surgical treatment of vaginal inversion. Obstet Gynecol 1971;38:327–332.

16. Nichols D. Sacrospinous fixation for massive eversion of the vagina. Am J Obstet Gynecol 1982;142:901–904.

17. Shull BL, Capen CV, et al. Preoperative and postoperative analysis of site-specific pelvic support defects in 81 women treated with sacrospinous ligament suspension and pelvic reconstruction. Am J Obstet Gynecol 1992;166:1764–1771.

18. Sze EH, Karram MM. Transvaginal repair of vault prolapse: A review. Obstet Gynecol 1997;89:466–475.

19. Porges RF, Smilen SW. Long term analysis of the surgical management of pelvic support defects. Am J Obstet Gynecol 1994;171:1518–1526.

20. Stanton SL, Hilton P, Norton C, Cardozo L. Clinical and urodynamics effects of anterior colporrhaphy and vaginal hysterectomy for prolapse with and without incontinence. Br J Obstet Gynaecol 1982;89:459–463.

21. Walter S, Olesen KP, Hald T, et al. Urodynamic evaluation after vaginal repair and colposuspension. Br J Urol 1982;54:377–380.

22. Weber AM, Walters MD. Anterior vaginal prolapse: Review of anatomy and techniques for surgical repair. Obstet Gynecol 1997;89(2):311–318.

23. Weber AM, Walters MD, Piedmonte MR. Anterior colporraphy: A randomized trial of three surgical techniques. Am J Obstet Gynecol 2001;185:1299–1306.

24. White GR. Cystocele: A radical cure by suturing lateral sulci of vagina to white line of pelvic fascia. JAMA 1909;853:1707–1710.

25. Richardson AC, Lyon JB, Williams NL. A new look at pelvic relaxation. Am J Obstet Gynecol 1976;126:568–573.

26. Shull BL, Benn SJ, Kuehl TJ. Surgical management of prolpase of the anterior vaginal segment: An analysis of support defects, operative morbidity, and anatomic outcome. Am J Obstet Gynecol 1994;171(6):1429–1439.

27. Elkins TE, Chesson RR, Videla F. Transvaginal paravaginal repair: A useful adjunctive procedure in pelvic relaxation surgery. J Pelvic Surg 2000;6:11–15.

28. Young SB, Daman JJ, Bony LG. Vaginal paravaginal repair: One-year outcomes. Am J Obstet Gynecol 2001;185(6):1360–1366.

29. Mallipeddi PK, Steele AC, Kohli N, Karram MM. Anatomic and functional outcome of vaginal paravaginal repair in correction of anterior vaginal wall prolapse. Int Urogynecol J 2001;12:83–88.

30. Mellgren A, Anzen B, Nilsson BY, et al. Results of rectocele repair: A prospective study. Dis Colon Rectum 1995;38:7–13.

31. Francis W, Jeffcoate T. Dyspareunia following vaginal operations. J Obstet Gynecol Br Comnwlth 1961;68:1–10.

32. Kahn M, Stanton S. Posterior colporrhaphy: Its effects on bowel and sexual function. Br J Gynecol 1997;104:82–86.

33. Iglesia CB, Fenner DE, Brubaker L. The use of mesh in gynecologic surgery. Int Urogynecol J 1997;8:105–115.

34. Vardy MD, Brodman M, et al. Anterior IVS tunneller device for stress incontinence and posterior IVS tunneller for apical vault prolapse—A 2 year prospective multicenter study. Int Urogynecol J 2006;17(S3):S400 (abstract).

35. Davila G. Restoration of vaginal apical and posterior wall support with the Apogee system. J Minim Invasive Gynecol 2005;12(5):S42 (abstract).

36. Biller DH, Jean-Michel M, Davila GW. Apical prolapse repair using the Apogee system. Int Urogynecol J 2007;18(Suppl):S41 (abstract).

37. Flood CG, Drutz HP, Waja L. Anterior colporraphy reinforced with Marlex mesh for the treatment of cystocele. Int Urogynecol J 1998;9:200–204.

38. Sand PK, Koduri S, Lobel RW. Prospective randomized trial of polyglactin 910 mesh to prevent recurrences of cystoceles and rectoceles. Am J Obstet Gynecol 2001;184:1357–1364.

39. Gomelsky A, Rudy DC, Dmochowski RR. Porcine dermis interposition graft for repair of high anterior compartment defects with or without concurrent pelvic organ prolapse procedures. J Urol 2004;171:1581.

40. Guerette N, Aguirre O, VanDrie D, et al. Multi-center randomized prospective trial comparing anterior colporrhaphy alone to bovine pericardium collagen matrix graft reinforced anterior colporrhaphy: 12-Month analysis. Int Urogynecol J 2006;17(Suppl 3):S384–S385.

41. Collinet P, Bilot F, Debodinance P, et al. Transvaginal mesh technique for pelvic organ prolpase repair: Mesh exposure management and risk factors. Int Urogynecol J 2006;17(4):315–320.

42. Miller DP, Lucente V, Robinson D, Babin E. Prospective clinical assessment of the total vaginal mesh (TVM) technique for treatment of pelvic organ prolapse: 6 and 12 month results. Int Urogynecol J 2006; 17(S3):S402 (abstract).

43. Davila GW, Flaherty JF, Lukban JC, et al. Retrospective analysis of efficacy and safety of Perigee™ and Apogee™ in patients undergoing repair for pelvic organ prolapse. J Min Invast Surg 2006;13(5 Suppl):S27.

44. Maher C, Baessler K. Surgical management of anterior vaginal wall prolapse: an evidence based literature review. Int Urogynecol J 2006;17:195–201.

Chapter 25
Pelvic Reconstruction: Abdominal Approach

Lawrence R. Lind and Harvey A. Winkler

Surgical repair of pelvic organ prolapse can be accomplished via a laparoscopic approach, abdominal approach, vaginal approach, robotically, or a combination of routes. In some instances, medical necessity requires a patient to have a laparotomy for nonreconstructive indications, and in such instances it makes sense to take advantage of the abdominal incision which provides generous access to pelvic support structures and good availability of anchoring sites to accomplish the desired reconstructive surgery. In other instances, surgeons choose an abdominal approach because data have shown excellent, long-lasting results through the abdominal approach and because the surgeon believes that the patient's severity of prolapse and/or the life expectancy of the patient mandates the more invasive abdominal approach in order to obtain lasting results [1].

The main objectives of pelvic reconstructive surgery are the restoration of normal vaginal anatomy, relief of symptoms presumed to be caused by abnormal pelvic floor anatomy, restoration or maintenance of normal bladder and bowel function, and restoration and/or maintenance of normal sexual function. Abdominal repairs for pelvic reconstructive surgery include paravaginal repair for cystocele, methods for vaginal apex suspension (ligament suspensions of the vaginal apex, and abdominal sacral colpopexy (ASC). Pelvic cul-de-sac closure techniques also are used for prevention or treatment of enterocele. With some modifications, the ASC also can be used to repair a wide spectrum of defects including cystocele, rectocele, as well as vaginal apex prolapse. Each of the procedures performed through an abdominal approach can be accomplished via a laparoscopic approach; however, technical skills to accomplish these procedures are advanced, and in general, only surgeons with advanced laparoscopic skills and previous experience with open reconstructive surgeries can execute laparoscopic repairs with safety and efficacy.

Abdominal Sacral Colpopexy

ASC is performed primarily for advanced prolapse of the vaginal apex. With modifications, it also can be very effective for anterior and posterior vaginal wall relaxation. This procedure is appealing to many surgeons because it repairs defects in multiple compartments with a single procedure; there is a large body of data supporting the long-term efficacy of the procedure [1–4]. In performing an ASC, graft material (either synthetic or biological) is attached to the vaginal apex. Depending on the individual anatomy, the graft may be extended to varying lengths along the anterior and posterior vaginal walls to correct additional defects. The other end of the graft is attached to the longitudinal ligament overlying the sacrum just distal to the sacral promontory. The anatomic goals of ASC include restoring normal midline vaginal position, correction of vaginal apex prolapse, and correction of high cystocele and rectocele.

Pelvic Anatomy in Consideration of Abdominal Sacral Suspension

Figure 25.1 demonstrates a lateral view of advanced vaginal vault prolapse. The surgical principles of ASC are based on repairing the deficient support tissues that allow this level of herniation. The fascial planes and support structures of the anterior vaginal wall and vaginal apex are demonstrated in Figs. 25.2 and 25.3. Note the pubocervical fascia between the bladder and the vagina and the rectovaginal fascia between the vagina and the rectum converge at the level of the cervix to form a pericervical ring. The supporting fascia is then in continu-

ity with the uterosacral ligaments providing natural attachment of the vaginal walls to the sacrum. In an ASC, mesh is typically configured to run in the same plane as the pubocervical fascia, rectovaginal fascia, or both; to recreate a strong suspension for the vaginal walls, bladder, and rectum, and uterus (if retained).

The selection of materials (biological vs. synthetic) is subject to much debate. There have been studies documenting disappointing results with donor fascia [5]. A few prospective studies comparing the various graft materials currently available reveal improved outcomes when using permanent synthetic polypropylene graft materials.

Surgical Technique

ASC can be performed in a patient with a previous hysterectomy, at time of total abdominal hysterectomy, or in conjunction with a supracervical hysterectomy. A few studies have demonstrated that the risk of mesh erosion into the vagina is significantly increased by the presence of the vaginal cuff incision required to complete a total abdominal hysterectomy [6]. In an attempt to reduce the risk of erosions, therefore, increasing numbers of supracervical hysterectomies are performed at the time of ASC. This trend mandates increased attention to screening a patient's risk factors for subsequent cervical malignancy and creates surgical challenges if a trachelectomy is required subsequent to an ASC.

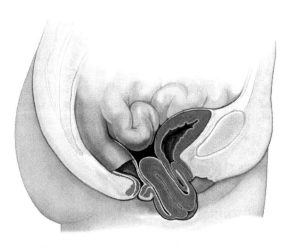

FIG. 25.1. A lateral view of the pelvis demonstrates advanced pelvic organ prolapse

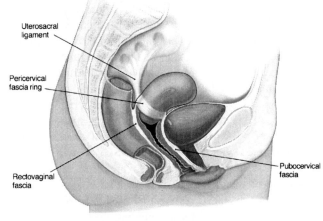

FIG. 25.2. A lateral view of the pelvis demonstrates the support structures of the vaginal vault and gynecologic organs. Note the pubocervical and rectovaginal fascias fusing at the level of the pericervical ring. These fibers are then in continuity with the uterosacral ligaments which provide proximal attachment to the sacrum

FIG. 25.3. An oblique view of the pelvis demonstrates the pubocervical fascia fibers traversing laterally to their insertion point at the arcus tendineus fascia pelvis or "white line." This view also demonstrates the concept of the fusion of the fascias at the pericervical ring and the continuity of those fibers with the uterosacral ligaments

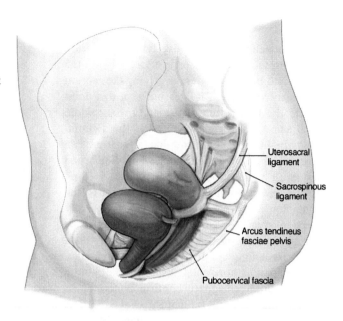

Uterosacral ligament

Sacrospinous ligament

Arcus tendineus fasciae pelvis

Pubocervical fascia

There are many variations in technique; however, a few general principles are followed by the majority of experienced surgeons. A broad surface area of attachment to the vagina allows enhanced correction of anatomic defects. Volume of material is concerning for erosion; however, a focal or "pinpoint" attachment site is felt to be more vulnerable to failure and erosions. Attachment of graft to both the anterior and posterior vaginal walls and respective fascias allows symmetric elevation of the apex as well as allowing customized correction of the anterior and posterior defects.

There is no comparative scientific evidence to guide the choice of permanent versus absorbable sutures to attach to the vaginal apex to the mesh. We have observed that erosions (our own and those referred to us) almost always have a permanent surgical knot at the center focus of the erosion. Mesh configurations have taken a trend toward having wider pores; theoretically to allow for rapid ingrowth, to permit macrophage entry, and to decrease the total mass of foreign material. At any point on the mesh where a permanent suture has been attached, the mesh no longer retains the wide pore configuration at that site. Instead, it represents permanent synthetic mesh material gathered into a central location at the base of three to five knots. For these reasons, we use delayed absorbable

monofilament suture for attachment of the mesh to the vagina.

Surgical Steps

After the abdomen is entered, nonreconstructive surgery is performed first. The bladder is dissected down off of the anterior vaginal wall and the rectosigmoid reflection off of the posterior vaginal wall. The patient typically is in low adjustable stirrups in the supine position, allowing both abdominal and vaginal access to the vagina. An EEA sizer is used to distend the vaginal apex and assists in creating countertraction during dissection (Fig. 25.4). The end point for dissection is based on preoperative examination, extent of prolapse, and operative assessment. We typically end our dissection when a clamp placed at the distal limit of the dissection is able to pull the vaginal wall to a horizontal plane (based on the sensations of a vaginal examining hand).

Figure 25.5a–c demonstrate mesh configurations customized for three different patients: the first with somewhat pure, symmetric vaginal apex prolapse; the second with a dominant cystocele; and the third with dominant posterior vaginal relaxation. Multiple delayed absorbable sutures are used to attach the mesh to the vaginal walls and fascia.

Sacral Dissection

The peritoneum is entered overlying the sacrum
and the presacral fatty tissue is dissected until the
sacrum and fine vasculature overlying the sacrum
are clearly visualized. It is essential at this point
to note the bifurcation of the aorta, the middle
sacral vessels, the right ureter, and the sigmoid
colon. Failure to complete this dissection can
result in passing of sutures somewhat blindly and
may result in catastrophic sacral venous bleeding
[7]. The exact point of attachment distal to the
promontory is not critical. Surgeons typically
select an area in the midline that appears to be
the safest based on the location of small veins.
Three ascending sutures, typically permanent,
are placed in a horizontal fashion. Each suture
is tested with tension to confirm a good pass
through the supportive ligament (Fig. 25.6). A
vaginal examining hand is used to judge the elevation of the anterior wall, posterior wall, and vaginal
apex. The goal is replacement to normal position
without additional tension. One must avoid the
temptation to pull the repair tight since experience
has demonstrated that pain, erosions, and possible
urinary incontinence are potential complications.

There are different configurations of the mesh
used for ASC including one piece of mesh, two
pieces of mesh, or one piece of mesh that is folded
over the anterior and the posterior vaginal walls.
It is our preference to use two separate pieces
of mesh. This allows the support of the anterior
vaginal wall and posterior vaginal wall to be

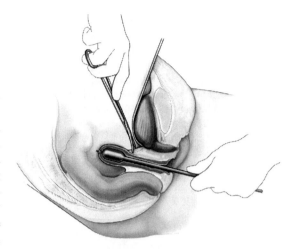

FIG. 25.4. Abdominal sacral colpopexy: An EEA sizer
is placed in the vagina to allow surgical countertraction
while dissecting the bladder reflection off the anterior
vaginal wall in preparation for graft placement

customized based on the patient's pre-operative
anatomy. After tension adjustment of each mesh,
the sacral promontory sutures are passed through
the mesh at the appropriate location and tied down.
A final result in a patient who retained the cervix
is demonstrated in Fig. 25.7. Peritoneum is used to
cover as much of the mesh as is possible. There is
no agreement as to whether or not the mesh should
be fully covered in a retroperitoneal position.
Advocates of covering the mesh completely suggest that there is a decreased chance of adhesion
formation and bowel obstruction.

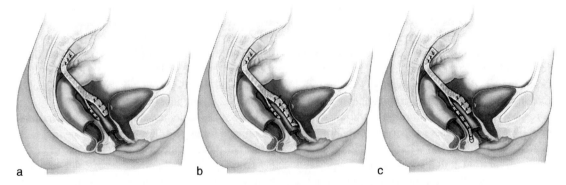

FIG. 25.5. Three variations of abdominal sacral colpopexy: (**a**) symmetric anterior and posterior defect support, (**b**)
apical support and dominant anterior vaginal support with elongated anterior mesh segment, and (**c**) apical support
and dominant posterior vaginal support with elongated posterior mesh segment

Closure of the Cul-de-Sac

Surgeon preference and operative findings guide decisions regarding whether or not the cul-de-sac should be closed posterior to the mesh. The goal of this maneuver is to obliterate the anatomic deep cul-de-sac, preventing enterocele and avoiding bowel entrapment posterior to the mesh [3, 8]. Figure 25.8 shows the hollow cul-de-sac and the vulnerable entrapment space behind the mesh and Fig. 25.9 demonstrates bowel that has moved into this space. There is no consensus regarding closure of this space and there are a variety of methods incorporated to obliterate the space.

A more radical modification of the ASC has been described to treat patients with vaginal vault prolapse combined with full-length posterior vaginal wall relaxation including perineal mobility. The "abdominal sacral colpoperineorrhaphy" incorporates a mesh that runs the full distance of the posterior vaginal wall and retrieval of such mesh via a posterior vaginal wall incision to enable suturing of the mesh at the level of the perineum (Fig. 25.5c) [9].

Concomitant Procedures

The goal of all pelvic reconstructive surgery is to restore normal anatomy of all surgical compartments, anterior, apical and posterior. Some surgeons feel that the length of mesh applied to the anterior and posterior vaginal walls can alleviate most anterior and posterior defects, while others are of the opinion that a dedicated paravaginal cystocele repair is required for significant anterior vaginal relaxation. Training and experience dictate which methods are necessary for each individual patient. If the posterior mesh is not extended enough to correct a sizeable rectocele, then a dedicated vaginal rectocele repair is indicated.

There are data indicating that a reasonable number of patients who were continent before an ASC may become incontinent after the procedure [10]. There also are randomized, prospective data indicating that a Burch bladder suspension at the time of ASC significantly reduces the chances of urinary incontinence after the procedure [10]. Based on this study, many (but not all) surgeons feel that a Burch procedure should be performed with all ASC regardless of preoperative incontinence testing results.

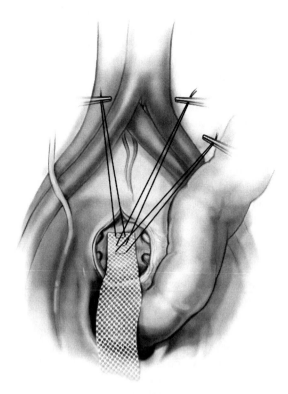

FIG. 25.6. Abdominal sacral colpopexy. Placement of sacral sutures into the longitudinal ligament distal to the sacral promontory

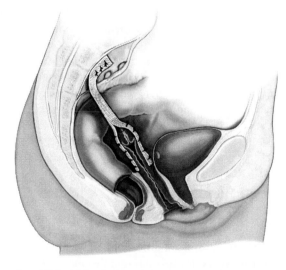

FIG. 25.7. Abdominal sacral colpopexy. A completed repair in a patient following supracervical hysterectomy

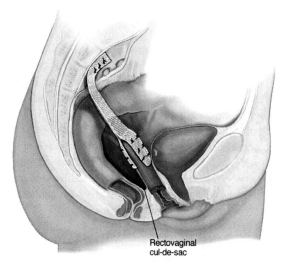

Rectovaginal
cul-de-sac

FIG. 25.8. Abdominal sacral colpopexy. The posterior cul-de-sac is a potential anatomic site for enterocele formation or bowel entrapment

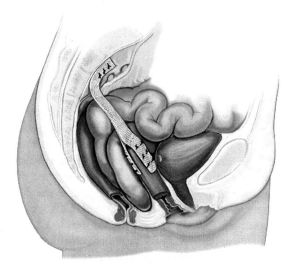

FIG. 25.9. Abdominal sacral colpopexy. Artistic representation of small bowel which has moved posterior to the graft representing the potential for bowel obstruction

Efficacy of Abdominal Sacral Colpopexy

Success rates as defined by absence of recurrent prolapse tend to be between 85 and 100% for ASC, with most success rates 90% or higher [1, 9, 11–14]. The tools used to measure objective and subjective results vary between studies; however, what is compelling is the consistent good

efficacy in most studies. There are only a few randomized trials that compare ASC to vaginal methods. Benson and Lucente found a higher success rate for the abdominal group as compared to the sacrospinous vaginal group to such an extent that the study was terminated early [15]. Lowe and Wang compared unilateral sacrospinous suspension to ASC and found optimal effectiveness in 80% of women in the vaginal group and in 94% of the abdominal group [16]. Maher and others did a similar comparison; however, they found no statistical difference between the groups, but the trend once again was favoring better results with the abdominal approach [17].

Complications

The most concerning complications of ASC include bleeding, bowel injury, bowel obstruction, bladder injury, dyspareunia, and infection or erosion of the graft material. Fortunately, most of these complications occur in 5% or less of cases [1]. In general the rate of mesh erosion varies between 0 and 5.5%, with an average of 3.4% [1, 18–26]. There are no comparative data to definitively prove one mesh material causes less erosion than another. The intuitive thought that a biological mesh might cause less erosion than a synthetic mesh has not been proven and some studies have created concern regarding the long-term reliability of the biological materials.

ASC is an excellent option for advanced pelvic prolapse, has stood the test of time, and is supported extensively in the literature. While this abdominal procedure is the most invasive method for repair of pelvic floor defects, long-lasting results and the ability to correct multiple anatomic defects with one procedure have made it one of the more common and desirable procedures used to treat advanced pelvic prolapse.

Ligament Suspensions of the Vaginal Apex and Closure of the Cul-de-Sac

There are several modifications of vaginal apex suspensions performed through the abdomen that use one or more existing pelvic ligaments to suspend the vaginal apex. The advantages of "autologous" procedures include elimination of a foreign body (graft), elimination of the sacral dissection required for ASC, and time efficiency. The uterosacral and cardinal ligaments are most commonly used for this purpose. Some surgeons use only one pair of ligaments while others use both pairs. In general, it is felt that ligament suspensions may not have as reliable long-term success compared to the ASC; however, randomized comparative objective data do not exist to definitively quantify an advantage. Decisions for ligament procedures versus ASC are based on surgeon preference, severity of prolapse, life expectancy of the patient, and anticipated patient activity level. Some surgeons use these techniques for prevention of prolapse at the conclusion of an abdominal hysterectomy to prevent prolapse at a later time, while other surgeons use these techniques to directly treat vaginal apex prolapse.

Uterosacral Ligament Vaginal Apex Suspension

After removal of the uterus, the uterosacral ligaments are placed on traction to allow tracking of the ligament several centimeters cephalad from the distal attachment point to the uterus. As the strength of the ligament is variable at its distal limit it is essential to track it back to a point where good strong support fibers can be palpated. As shown in Fig. 25.10, the uterosacral ligament on each side is encircled and pierced. The suture then passes through the vaginal cuff on each side. The tied sutures bring the vaginal apex to the supporting ligaments as shown in Fig. 25.11. In some variations of technique, the pair of ligaments are pulled toward the midline incorporating the anterior rectal serosa and the posterior of the vaginal wall (Fig. 25.12a, b). In all of these techniques, identification of the ureters is essential to avoid inadvertent suturing or kinking of the ureters, which are in close proximity to the uterosacral ligaments.

Prevention of Enterocele Formation

In conjunction with vaginal apex suspensions and in cases with isolated enteroceles, the deep cul-de-sac can be obliterated to prevent abdominal contents from herniating between the vagina and rectum. While surgeons differ in their understanding of enteroceles, there is agreement that bowel contents herniating into the deep cul-de-sac can cause signifi-

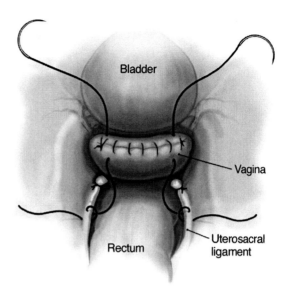

FIG. 25.10. Ipsilateral suspension of the vaginal apex to the uterosacral ligaments: Sutures are passed through the uterosacral ligament on each side and then through the vaginal apex

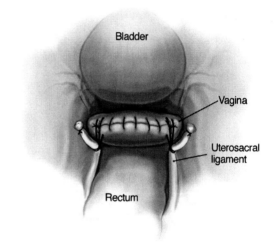

FIG. 25.11. Ipsilateral suspension of the vaginal apex to the uterosacral ligments: The vaginal vault is pulled up to the strong supporting uterosacral ligaments. Note that the distal limits of the uterosacral ligaments which have been tied after the hysterectomy are not the final attachment points. A position proximal to the previous uterine attachment point is selected to obtain a strong portion of the ligament

cant clinical symptoms. Therefore, addressing this potential hernia site is an important component of comprehensive pelvic reconstructive surgery.

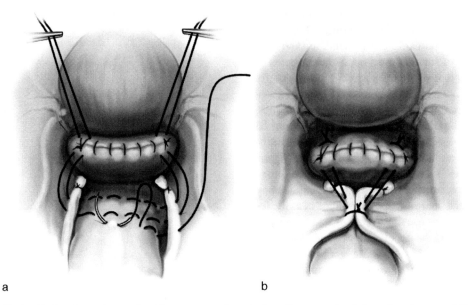

a   b

FIG. 25.12. (**a, b**) An alternative method for uterosacral vaginal vault suspension brings the uterosacral ligaments toward the midline and incorporates the anterior rectal serosa to close the cul-de-sac and support the vaginal apex in one maneuver

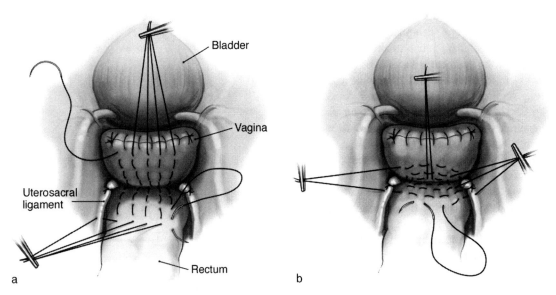

FIG. 25.13. Two variations in technique for closure of the cul-de-sac. Both techniques incorporate the uterosacral ligaments, rectal serosa, posterior vaginal wall, and peritoneum of the deep cul-de-sac: (**a**) demonstrates sutures placed in a vertical orientation and (**b**) demonstrates sutures placed in concentric circles

One technique for cul-de-sac closure incorporates sutures that run anterior to posterior along the posterior vaginal wall, along the peritoneum of the deep cul-de-sac, then along the anterior serosa of the rectum (Fig. 25.13a). An alternative method runs concentric circles of suture through the uterosacral ligaments and (in a superficial plane) through the vaginal and rectal walls (Fig. 25.13b).

Paravaginal Repair

The concept that cystoceles may result from the separation of the pubocervical fascia from its lateral attachment to the pelvic sidewall has been considered as early as 1909 [27]. In the 1960s, Burch developed one of the most popular procedures for urinary incontinence [28]. While searching for the ideal anchoring point for his paraurethral sutures (for what would become the "Burch urethropexy"), he originally chose the lateral pelvic sidewall for his first few patients. He eventually favored Cooper's ligament as an attachment point, but the lateral pelvic sidewall was considered initially.

Most of the anatomic dissections for paravaginal defects and the subsequent translation into an established procedure for paravaginal repair of cystocele are credited to Cullen Richardson. After he observed the anterior–lateral vaginal sulcus evert in a patient with a cystocele (with Valsalva), he began several years of cadaver dissections and formally brought paravaginal repair into the reconstructive armamentarium of pelvic surgeons [29, 30]. More recent clinical studies have supported the effectiveness of this procedure for repair of cystocele [31]. While some have advocated this repair for stress incontinence, the preponderance of data relating to this procedure support its use for cystocele repair and not for urinary incontinence.

In order to select proper patients for paravaginal cystocele repair, the distinction between "midline" cystoceles and "lateral detachment" cystoceles must be established preoperatively. A lateral detachment cystocele is suggested by asymmetric eversion of the anterior vaginal wall with straining and resolution of the cystocele with support of the anterior lateral vaginal sulci. This can be accomplished in an office assessment with ring forceps. Classic teaching was that all cystoceles were the result of midline weakening or stretching of support tissues. Standard repair was an anterior repair that brought lateral tissues across the midline to elevate the bladder in the midline. Richardson's cadaver dissections and clinical experience suggested that the majority of cystoceles were the result of lateral defects. Intact paravaginal fascia is demonstrated in Fig. 25.14a, a unilateral left paravaginal defect in Fig. 25.14b, and a bilateral defect in Fig. 25.14c. The fascia defect allows movement of the anterior

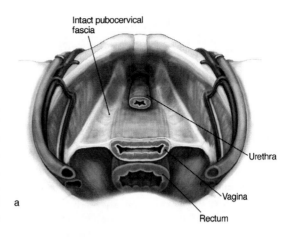

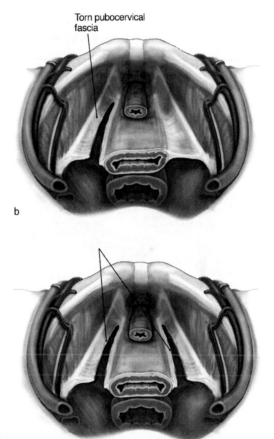

Fig. 25.14. Paravaginal fascia support and paravaginal defects: (**a**) demonstrates intact pubocervical fascia, (**b**) depicts a left-sided paravaginal defect, and (**c**) depicts bilateral paravaginal defects (courtesy of Boston Scientific Corp, Massachussetts)

vaginal wall and bladder toward the vaginal outlet, resulting in a clinical cystocele.

Surgical Technique: Abdominal Paravaginal Repair

A Pfannensteil incision is made and any necessary intraperitoneal procedures are performed first. If there is no requirement for surgery within the peritoneum, then this procedure is performed without entering the peritoneum. The retropubic space is developed with blunt dissection between the bladder and the superior pubic ramus. The nondominant hand is placed in the vagina and one or two fingers are used to explore the lateral vaginal sulci. The goal is to attach the anterior lateral vaginal wall to its original anatomic support site—

the arcus tendineus *fascia* pelvis—or "white line." The white line runs from the posterior–inferior edge of the pubic symphysis to the ischial spine. This linear density should be palpated and visualized before placing sutures. If a Burch procedure is necessary for stress incontinence, typically the Burch sutures are placed first and paravaginal sutures continue along the lateral vaginal wall about a centimeter apart starting a centimeter or two above the higher pair of Burch sutures. Figure 25.15a, b demonstrate the placement of the vaginal (pubocervical) sutures and the lateral "white line" sutures. A unilateral paravaginal repair is demonstrated in Fig. 25.16a and a bilateral repair in Fig. 25.16b. A Burch suspension and bilateral paravaginal repair is demonstrated in Fig. 25.16c. If a Burch is not indicated, the paravaginal repair

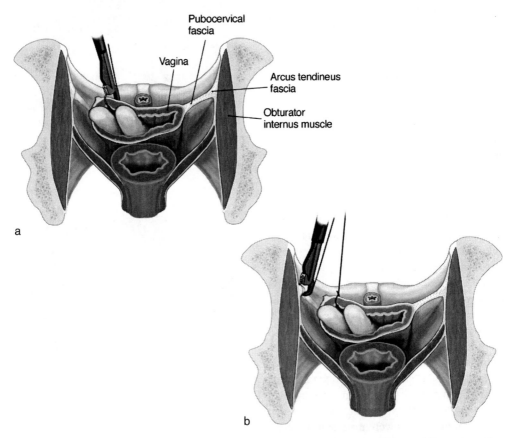

FIG. 25.15. Paravaginal repair: (**a**) The surgeon's nondominant hand is within the vagina guiding suture placement into the anterior lateral vaginal wall incorporating the pubocervical fascia and the anterior lateral vaginal wall. (**b**) Placement of the suture through the arcus tendineus fascia pelvis (*white line*) (courtesy of Boston Scientific Corp., Massachusets)

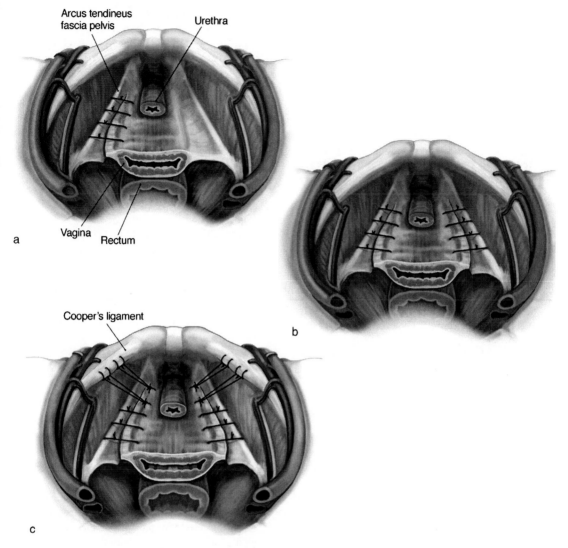

FIG. 25.16. Three variations of completed paravaginal repairs: (**a**) unilateral left paravaginal repair, (**b**) bilateral paravaginal repair, and (**c**) bilateral paravaginal repair with concomitant Burch procedure

typically starts lower with the first two vaginal sutures very similar in location to those that would have been used for a Burch procedure. The only difference on the distal sutures is that they are attached laterally to the white line rather than to Cooper's ligament. The highest stitch is about 1 cm in front of the ischial spine. Each suture is placed first through the anterior lateral vaginal wall and overlying fascia, then through the corresponding (slightly cephalad) location on the white line. Cystoscopy is recommended. Most surgeons prefer permanent suture. Some surgeons advocate bilateral repairs on all patients regardless of preoperative findings while others feel that if a defect is purely unilateral that a unilateral repair is indicated.

Conclusion

Abdominal repairs for female pelvic organ prolapse have a variety of techniques. Selection of techniques is guided by surgeon experience and patient characteristics. The popularity of the ASC is due to excellent long-term results. Abdominal repairs include suspension of the vaginal apex, cystocele repair, high rectocele repair, and prevention of enterocele.

References

1. Nygaard IE, McCreery R, Brubaker L, et al. Abdominal sacrocolpopexy: A comprehensive review. Obstet Gynecol (United States) 2004;104(4):805–823.
2. Addison WA, Livengood CH III, Sutton GP, Parker RT. Abdominal sacral colpopexy with Mersilene mesh in the retroperitoneal position in the management of posthysterectomy vaginal vault prolapse and enterocele. Am J Obstet Gynecol 1985;153: 140–146.
3. Addison WA, Gundiff GW, Bump RC, Harris RI. Sacral colpopexy is the preferred treatment for vaginal vault prolapse. J Gynecol Technol 1996;2: 69–74.
4. Hendee AE, Berry CM. Abdominal sacropexy for vaginal vault prolapse. Clin Obstet Gynecol 1981;24:1217–1226.
5. FitzGerald MP, Mollenhauer J, Bitterman P, Brubaker L. Functional failure of fascia lata allografts. Am J Obstet Gynecol 1999;1339–1346.
6. Bensinger G, Lind L, Lesser M, et al. Abdominal sacral suspensions: Analysis of complications using permanent mesh. Am J Obstet Gynecol 2005;193:2094–2098.
7. Sutton GP, Addison WA, Livengood CH III, Hammond CB. Life-threatening hemorrhage complicating sacral colpopexy. Am J Obstet Gynecol 1981;140:836–837.
8. Addison WA, Timmons MC, Wall LI, Livengood CH III. Failed abdominal sacral colpopexy: Observations and recommendations. Obstet Gynecol 1989;74:480–483.
9. Cundiff GW, Harris RL, Coates K, et al. Abdominal sacral colpoperineopexy: A new approach for correction of posterior compartment defects and perineal descent associated with vaginal vault prolapse. Am J Obstet Gynecol 1997;177:1345–1355.
10. Brubacker L, Cundiff GW, Fine P, et-al. Abdominal sacrocolpopexy with Burch colposuspension to reduce urinary stress incontinence. N Engl J Med 2006; 354(15):1557–1566.
11. Arthure HG, Savage D. Uterine prolapse and prolapse of the vaginal vault treated by sacral hysteropexy. J. Obstet Gynaecol Br Emp 1957;64:355–360.
12. Lane FE. Repair of posthysterectomy vaginal vault prolapse. Obstet Gynecol 1962;20:72–77.
13. Birnbaum SJ. Rational therapy for the prolapsed vagina. Am J Obstet Gynecol 1973;115:411419.
14. Culligan PJ, Murphy M, Blackwell L, et al. Long-term success of abdominal sacral colpopexy using synthetic mesh. Am J Obstet Gynecol 2002;187:1473–80; discussion 14811482.
15. Benson JT, Lucente V, McClellan E. Vaginal versus abdominal reconstructive surgery for the treatment of pelvic support defects: A prospective randomized study with long-term outcome evaluation. Am J Obstet Gynecol 1996;175:14181422.
16. Lo T-S, Wang AC. Abdominal colposacropexy and sacrospinous ligament suspension for severe uterovaginal prolapse: A comparison. J Gynecol Surg 1998;14:5964.
17. Maher CF, Qatawneh AM, Dwyer PL, et al. Abdominal sacrocolpopexy or vaginal sacrospinous colpopexy for vaginal vault prolapse: A prospective randomized study. Am J Obstet Gynecol 2004;190:20–26.
18. Cundiff GW, Addison WA. Management of pelvic organ prolapse. Obstet Gynecol Clin North Am 1998;25:907921.
19. Visco AG, Weidner AC, Barber MD, et al. Vaginal mesh erosion after abdominalsacral colpopexy. Am J Obsete Gynecol, 2001;184:297–302
20. Pilsgaard K, Mouritsen L. Follow-up after repair of vaginal vault prolaspse with abdominal colposacropexy. Acta Obstet Gynecol Scand 1999;78: 66–70.
21. Brizzolara S, Pillai-Allen A. Risk of mesh erosion with sacral colpoexy and concurrent hysterectomy. Obstet Gynecol 2003;102:301–310.
22. Virtanen H, Hirvonen T, Makinen J, Kiihloma P. Outcome of thirty patients who underwent repair of posthysterectomy prolapse of the vaginal vault with abdominal sacral colpopexy. J Am Coll Surg 1994;178:283–287.
23. Baker KR, Beresford JM, Campbell C. Colposacropexy with Prolene mesh. Surg Gynecol Obstet 1990;170:51–54.
24. Scettini M, Fortunato P, Gallucci M. Abdominal sacral colpopexy with Prolene mesh. Int Urogynecol J Pelvic Floor Dysfunct 1999;10:295–299.
25. Diana M, Zoppe C, Mastrangeli B. Treatment of vaginal vault prolapse with abdominal sacral colpopexy using Prolene mesh. Am J Surg 2000;179:126–128.
26. Van Lindert AC, Groenendijk AG, Scholten PC, Heintz AP. Surgical support and the suspension of genital prolapse, including preservation of the uterus, using Gore-Tex soft patch (a preliminary report). Eur J Obstet Gynecol Reprod Biol 1993;50:133–139.
27. White GR. Cystocele, a radical cure by suturing lateral sulci of vagina to white line of pelvic fascia. J Am Med Assoc 1909;53:1707–1711.

28. Burch JC. Urethrovaginal fixation to Cooper's ligament for the correction of stress incontinence, cystocele, recotcele, and prolapse. Am J Obstet Gynecol 1961;82:281–290.

29. Richardon AC.Paravaginal repair. In: Glenn Hurt W, ed. Urogynecologic surgery. Gaithersburg: Aspen Publication, 1992:73–80.

30. Richardson AC, Lyon JB, Williams NL. A new look at pelvic relaxation. Am J Obstet Gynecol 1976;65:586.

31. Shull BL, Baden WF. A six year experience with paravaginal defect repair for stress urinary incontinence. Am J Obstet Gynecol. 198;160:1432–1436.

Chapter 26
Laparoscopic Sacrocolpopexy: Indications, Technique and Results

Jens J. Rassweiler, Ali S. Goezen, Walter Scheitlin, Christian Stock, and Dogu Teber

Introduction

The introduction of the pelvic lymph node dissection by Schuessler in 1991 represented a milestone for urological laparoscopy [1]. Within the last 15 years, this minimally invasive technique experienced an enormous technical development. Initially, urological laparoscopy was limited by technical problems such as subtle hemostasis or the difficulties with endoscopic suturing [2]. However, following the successful introduction of laparoscopic radical prostatectomy by Gaston, Guillonneau, and Vallancien in 1999, a significant increase of interest was observed [3–5]. In 2001, Binder and Kramer performed the first robot-assisted laparoscopic radical prostatectomy using the da Vinci device [6]. However, in 2003, Menon and Ahlering showed the easy transfer of robotic-assisted from open radical prostatectomy, which thereafter revolutionized the management of localized prostate cancer in the United States [7, 8]. In 2007, almost 60% of all radical prostatectomies are performed with the da Vinci system. Interestingly, all these developments based on extensive experience with laparoscopic sacrocolpopexy by Gaston [5].

The technique of sacral fixation of the vagina for correction of genital prolapse (promontofixation) was first described in the year 1889, respectively, 1892, by Freund and Zweifel using a transperitoneal as well as a transvaginal approach [9], but it was Ameilen Hugier who in 1957 presented a more detailed description of open sacral colpopexy [10]. Miller described in 1927 a transvaginal colpopexy

to the sacrospinal ligaments [11], which was further modified by various authors including Richter and Albrich [12].

Scali in 1974 proposed the suspension by placement of prosthetic slings between the vagina and the bladder, which was anchored to the sacral promontory [13]. In the early 1990s, the gynecologists Dorsey and Nezhat described a laparoscopic sacropexy [14, 15]. In contrast to the technique of laparoscopic bladder neck suspension or colposuspension, which has not been performed frequently after its introduction due to worse results, respectively, recent less invasive techniques such as tension-free vaginal tape (TVT) or (TOT) [16, 17], laparoscopic sacrocolpopexy is used increasingly for pelvic floor repair [10, 18–22]. In 2004, Di Marco reported the successful use of the da Vinci robot for a robotic-assisted laparoscopic sacrocolpopexy for the treatment of vaginal vault prolapse [23] followed by others [24].

In this chapter, we want to outline the indications and technical approach of laparoscopic sacrocolpopexy together with an analysis of results reported by other authors, particularly in comparison to new techniques, such as tension-free vaginal mesh (TVM) for repair of pelvic organ prolapse (POP).

Indication

POP affects millions of women around the world. American data suggest that 10% of all women need surgery for prolapse or stress incontinence, with

30% of those patients requiring repeated surgical repair for recurrent prolapse [25]. These figures are predicted to rise by 45% in the next 30 years due to the increased life expectancy of women in the Western world and increasing prevalence of pelvic floor dysfunction with age [26].

Genital prolapse can involve the anterior vaginal wall, the apical vagina, the posterior vaginal wall, or a combination of these sites [27]. It can be classified as anterior if it compromises cystocele with or without urethral hypermobility; posterior, when rectal herniation occurs; and apical if it involves an enterocele, uterine, or vault prolapse [28]. This is further defined by the degree of descent through the introitus in the DeLancey classification utilizing four grades [29].

There are a variety of symptoms, affecting the pelvic floor, the lower urinary tract, as well as producing bowel or sexual dysfunction. The optimal treatment depends on several issues, such as patient's general health status, symptoms, quality of life impairment, and prolapse type and grade. There is a large number of open, vaginal, laparoscopic and robot-assisted laparoscopic techniques described

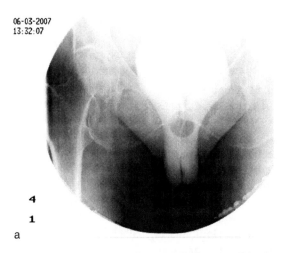

a

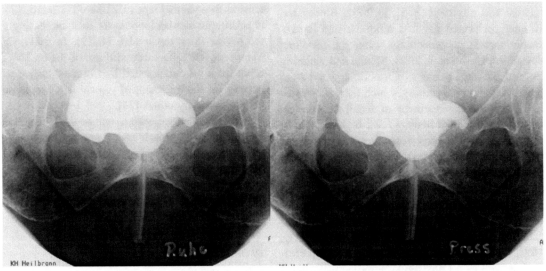

b

Fig. 26.1. Cystogram before and after laparoscopic sacrocolpopexy: (**a**) massive vaginal vault prolapse and (**b**) complete correction of POP after laparoscopic sacrocolpopexy with and without Valsalva (Ruhe and Press)

in the literature [27, 29–32]. Their common goal is to restore the vagina and descended pelvic organs to their correct anatomical position in order to improve or relieve symptoms and restore their normal physiological function [27, 30–32].

Diagnostic Work-Up

The preoperative workup involves a detailed urogynecologic history and physical examination to determine the type and degree of genital prolapse as well as to determine the presence of any concurrent stress urinary incontinence. The latter must be further assessed by performing the Bonney and Ulmsten maneuver or even by a urodynamic study. Urine analysis, Pap smear, and pelvic ultrasound must be performed routinely in order to exclude malignancy or large uterine volume (ie, indication for a simultaneous hysterectomy). For a better classification of the degree of the pelvic prolapse, all patients should have a cystogram with and without Valsalva maneuver (Fig. 26.1). In case of a enterocele, real-time dynamic MRI studies might be helpful (Fig. 26.2). All patients with a posterior prolapse require a gastroenterological consultation. All patients with concomitant anal incontinence are

presented to the surgical department of our certified continence center.

Technique

Trocar Placement

Based on adequate preoperative diagnosis, the procedure can be performed also with an intact uterus. Prior to the operation, we place a Foley catheter under sterile conditions.

In a 30° Trendelenburg and lithotomy position, a transperitoneal access is performed (Verress-needle, 15 mm Hg max. pressure of CO_2) using five trocars:

- 3 × 10 mm (telescope, midright port for suturing (Fig. 26.3) and introduction of the meshes, midleft port for dissecting tools and retracting peanut holder)
- 2 × 5 mm (left and right lateral port)

Optionally, the camera can be moved by use of the AESOP 3000 robot (Intuitive Surgical, Menlo Park, USA). The procedure is performed by one surgeon on the left side of the patient and two assistants, one of them sitting between the patient's legs to manipulate the surgical blade retractor, which

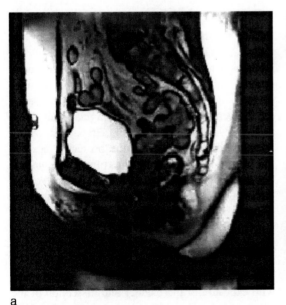
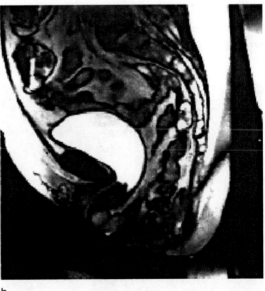

a   b

FIG. 26.2. Dynamic MRI imaging of severe enterocele following hysterectomy: (**a**) without Valsvalva: normal position of the bladder and bowel and (**b**) with Valsalva: massive vaginal vault prolapse with enterocele

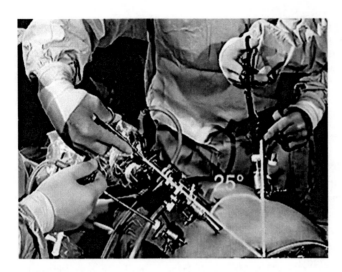

FIG. 26.3. Arrangement of trocars for laparoscopic sacrocolpopexy. The midright port is used for suturing to provide an adequate angle between the instruments (i.e., >25°)

is introduced into the vagina at the beginning of the operation. We are using only bipolar coagulation during the entire procedure. Once all trocars are placed, the uterus (if present) is fixed to the abdominal wall with a 0-Prolene-suture on a straight needle passed through the skin (Fig. 26.4).

Surgical Principle

The transperitoneal laparoscopic sacrocolpopexy is based on the anterior and posterior fixation of the vaginal wall to the sacral promontory using nonresorbable meshes (ie, polypropylene, polytetrafluorethylene, polyester single side covered silicone)

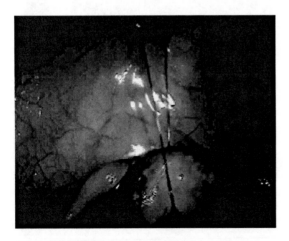

FIG. 26.4. Fixation of the uterus by a transcutaneous stay suture with straight needle (Prolene 2/0)

(Fig. 26.5a). The two meshes are fashioned from two 6 × 11 cm sheets (ie, Prolene-mesh, Ethicon, Norderstedt, Germany), measuring 11 cm in length and tapering from a width of 5 cm at the vaginal end to 3 cm at the sacral end (Fig. 26.5b). If indicated, simultaneous (prophylactic) correction of associated urinary stress continence can be accomplished using either a TVT or a laparoscopic Burch procedure using three suspension sutures on either side.

Posterior Dissection

Pulling on the transcutaneous stay suture of the uterus provides an excellent exposure of the Douglas pouch (Fig. 26.4). We now incise the peritoneum horizontally at the line between the uterosacral ligaments to enter the rectovaginal space for dissection of the posterior vaginal wall down to both levator ani muscles (Fig. 26.6a). Following adequate dissection we fix the posterior mesh to the vaginal wall either by interrupted or continuous sutures (2/0 prolene, 15 cm). A broad fixation including lateral parts of the levator ani muscle is of upmost importance (Fig. 26.6b).

Anterior Dissection

This step includes the opening of the Retzius space with exposure of the bladder and dissection of the anterior vaginal wall by adequate exposure of the intervesicovaginal space (Fig. 26.7a). If the uterus is present, a window through the broad ligament

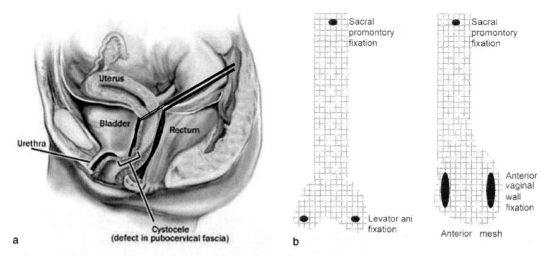

FIG. 26.5. Principle of sacral colpopexy. (**a**) Placement of two meshes sutured to the anterior and posterior vaginal anchored to the sacral promontory. (**b**) Tapering of the two meshes (modified from Rozet et al. [13])

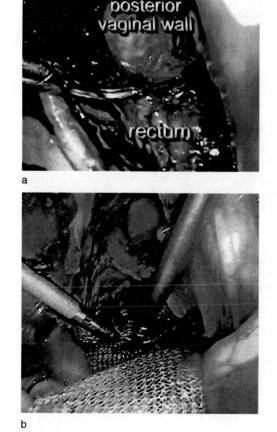

FIG. 26.6. Posterior dissection between vagina and rectum. (**a**) Endoscopic view at the end of dissection. (**b**) Fixation of the mesh to the levator ani muscle on the right side

on the right side must be created (Fig. 26.7c). For this purpose, the uterine stay suture is released. Subsequently, we introduce the anterior mesh and fix it to the anterior vaginal wall using either interrupted of continues sutures (2/0 prolene; 15 cm) (Fig. 26.7b).

Presacral Dissection and Sacropexy

Finally, we expose the sacral promontory medial to the sigmoid following transsection of the uterosacral ligaments and suture both meshes to the periosteum using two interrupted sutures (2/0 prolene 12 cm). We start with the posterior mesh. During the fixation, the vagina is pushed cranially by use of the retractor blade and the knot is secured by the assistant (Fig. 26.8). If the mesh is too long, we trim it endoscopically. The anterior mesh is put through the window of the broad ligament (Figs. 26.7c and 26.8b). Finally, the peritoneum is closed over both meshes by use of continuous 2—0 –Vicryl sutures (Fig. 26.9).

Incontinence Procedure

In case of a pronounced cystocele (anterior prolapse), we prefer to perform a Burch colposuspension using three suspension sutures (1/0 Ethibond) on either side. All other cases with verified stress incontinence are treated by a transvaginal TVT placed under laparoscopic control.

Results

Operating room times range between 97 and 276 min with a conversion rate to open surgery between 2 and 7%. Postoperative complications in experienced centers vary between 6 and 16%, including bowel lesions, mesh infections, spondylicitis, and vaginal erosions. The overall success rates depend on definition and technical considerations (ie, anterior mesh vs. anterior plus posterior mesh) and range between 66 and 94%. Compared to recently published open transabdominal [30, 33, 34] and transvaginal series [33, 35], these results are comparable (Table 26.1)

Discussion

Sacral colpopexy is the most commonly performed abdominal procedure to restore support to the vaginal apex [36, 37]. It has several advantages when approaching the complex problem of vaginal

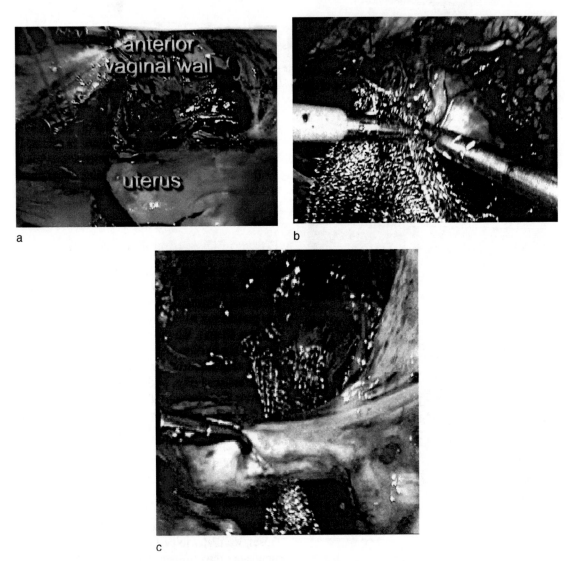

a   b

c

FIG. 26.7. Anterior dissection between vagina and bladder distal to the uterus. (a) Endoscopic view at the end of dissection. (b) Endoscopic suturing to fix the anterior mesh at the vaginal wall. (c) Transposition of the mesh through the window created at the right broad ligament

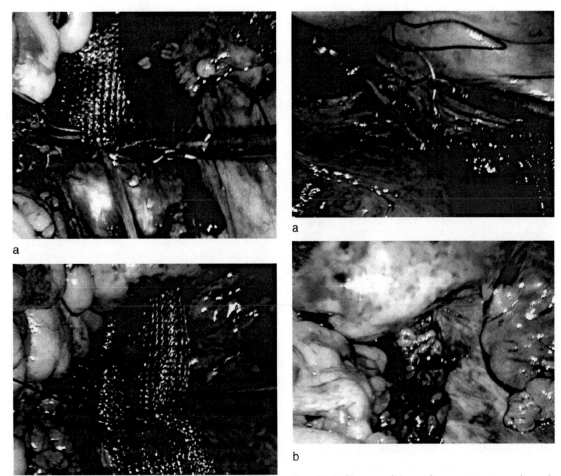

FIG. 26.8. Promontofixation. (**a**) Endoscopic suturing of the posterior mesh to the sacral promotory. The assistant pulls on the mesh to provide a tension-free knotting. (**b**) Fixation of the anterior mesh which was guided through the window at the right broad ligament

FIG. 26.9. Closure of the peritoneum to retroperitonealize both meshed. (**a**) Starting the suture anteriorly. (**b**) Final view at the sacral promontory with complete closure of the peritoneum

vault prolapse, namely, consistent anatomy, the most definitive enterocele repair, and culdeplasty. This procedure maintains a functional vagina and restores maximal vaginal length by securing the vaginal apex to the periosteum of the sacrum. Sacrospinous fixation is the most commonly performed transvaginal suspension procedure [12, 35, 38]. Its advantages include achieving a functional vagina, avoiding the morbidity of an abdominal incision and the ability to repair coexisting anterior and posterior compartment defects using a single surgical site. Because the technique displaces the vaginal axis posteriorly, it leads to the development of new anterior compartment defects. Other reported complications include intraoperative hemorrhage due to pudendal artery laceration, vaginal shortening, sexual dysfunction, pudendal nerve injury, and postoperative pain.

In this scenario, the laparoscopic sacrocolpopexy may combine the advantages of both traditional techniques offering excellent anatomical correction with minimal invasiveness and morbidtity. However, there are several issues to be taken into consideration.

TABLE 26.1. Results of laparoscopic and robotic-assisted sacrocolpopexy compared to open series.

Author	N	OR-time (min.)	Conversion (%)	Complication (%)	Success rate (%)	Fixation
Laparosocpic						
Cosson[19] 2002	83	276 (120–360)	7	16	94	ant + post
Antiphon[22] 2004	108	261 (120–450)	3	6	84	ant + post
					66	anterior
Rozet[13] 2005	363	97 (45–156)	2	9	94	ant + post
Rassweiler + 2008	21	216 (157–263)	–	8	92	ant + post
Robot-assisted						
Di Marco[23] 2004	30	186 (120–241)	3	7	95	ant + post
Abdominal						
Ng[36] 2004*	113	133 (32–227)	n.a.	11	96	ant + post
Limb[30] 2005	61	260 (135–420)	n.a.	4	91	ant + post
Blanchard[37] 2006	40	162 (90–270)	n.a.	20	80	anterior
Transvaginal						
Lantzsch[38] 2001	200	n.a.	n.a.	16	87	posterior
Ng[36] 2004*	64	78 (28–156)	n.a.	11	80	posterior

+ present study; * comparative study; n.a. = not applicable

Definition of Success

Blanchard et al. emphasized the varying definition of success following correction of pelvic organ prolapse studies [34]. Many investigators define success as the absence of recurrent vault prolapse, but the incidence of site-specific pelvic organ defects after sacrocolpopexy has not been clearly reported. However, it always has to be taken into consideration which type of defect exists and whether the patients had undergone only an anterior repair [22].

Important Technical Issues

There is still a controversy as to whether an anterior and posterior mesh repair should be performed routinely during laparoscopic and open sacrocolpopexy. Antiphon et al. clearly demonstrated a significantly lower posterior compartment failure rate (5.9% vs. 31.3%) following a double, anterior, and posterior, mesh [22]. However, it also increased the postoperative complication rate (ie, constipation rate 75% vs. 31%). In accordance with the huge experience of Rozet and colleagues [13], we prefer the systematic placement of two prosthetic meshes, which directly impacts on a lower rectocele relapse (only 4%). Moreover, one should take into consideration that laparoscopic sacrcocolpopexy mainly

is indicated in case of severe pelvic organ prolapse in patients predisposed to develop recurrencies in untreated compartments of the pelvic floor.

Another issue might be the type of mesh used [20]. Based on long-term experiences with bladder neck suspension, transvaginal sling procedures, and laparoscopic hernia repair, we prefer the use of polypropylene, which provides larger pore and interstices size (type 1 synthetic graft). In our hands, the risk of erosion is minimal. However, the retroperitonealization of the implant is mandatory to avoid any bowel lesion (Fig. 26.9).

Comparison with Other Techniques

To our knowledge, there is only a single study [39] comparing laparoscopic transabdominal sacropexy with either open abdominal approach, but none comparing it to the vaginal approach or even those using the new total mesh techniques. Paraiso et al. found 50 min longer operative time for laparoscopic sacrocolpopexy (269 vs. 281 min), but a significantly shorter hospital stay (1.8 vs. 4.0 days), with similar complication and success rates [39].

However, there are studies showing better cure rates (ie, 95.6% vs. 79.7%) when comparing open abdominal sacrocolpopexy with vaginal sacrospinous ligament fixation [33] (Table 26.1). In this study, however, the postoperative morbidity was high after the transabdominal approach, including pyrexia (52% vs. 28%) and hematuria (25% vs. 4%). One may argue that such complications could be significantly diminished by the laparoscopic approach without deterioration of the success rates.

Until now, there have been no peer-reviewed studies published comparing the new total vaginal mesh techniques with other established procedures. Novara et al. [37] recently analyzed the data regarding such minimally invasive total prosthetic implant techniques in the literature (i.e., Prolift, Apogee, Perigee) and emphasizing the relatively high rate of mesh erosion (max 12%), mesh shrinkage (max 17%), and de novo voiding symptoms (max 12%).

Advantages of Laparoscopic Prolapse Repair

There are several newer treatments in addition to the classic abdominal sacrocolpopexy and vaginal sacrospinous ligament fixation in the management of severe uterovaginal or vault prolapses, including less invasive methods such as laparoscopic pelvic floor repair [31, 32]. The laparoscopic route offers superior vision and less traumatic access compared with the traditional techniques. This could be translated into a better assessment, more precise and correct anatomical repair, the use of strong and acceptable material as a substitute for weak tissues, faster recovery, and excellent anatomical and functional results.

Problems of Laparoscopic Technique

There is no doubt that the laparoscopic approach requires a high degree of skill and expertise based on a specialized training. The learning curve takes a longer time and as a result not every surgeon may achieve competence in this methods [39, 40]. On the other hand, urologists focusing on laparoscopic or robotic-assisted techniques are well trained with endoscopic dissection and suturing techniques based on their daily practice. There already are well-established training programs [41–43]. Such trained surgeons have to be only instructed in the assessment of the specific pathologies of vaginal vault prolapse. This is underlined by our own experience: despite significantly fewer numbers

of cases, our operative time and follow-up results do not differ from other experienced groups (Table 26.1). We therefore would like to motivate urological laparoscopists to include this procedure in their list of indications.

Perspectives

Despite a significant number of patients who already have undergone laparoscopic sacrocolpopexy, there are no phase III trials comparing the approach with the traditional open techniques or with the newer total vaginal mesh techniques. Such studies should be realized by high-volume centers or as a multi-institutional trial to really define the role of the procedure. Based on a significant experience with pelvic laparoscopy and pelvic floor reconstruction, we believe that laparoscopic placement of two meshes (anterior and posterior) together with an anti-incontinence procedure if indicated represents a highly effective technique with minimal morbidity for the patients. Other options seem to work, too, but are associated with a higher complication rate (ie, erosion of TVM tchniques), higher morbidity (ie, open abdominal sacral colpopexy), or lower success rates (ie, transvaginal sacrofixation). Finally, as we already experienced with the example of radical prostatectomy, the use of the da Vinci robot may further allow the technique to result in a significant increase of laparoscopic sacrocolpopexy [23, 24, 44].

References

1. Schuessler WW, Vancaille RG, Reich H, Griffith DP. Transperitoneal endosurgical lymphadenectomy in patients with localized prostate cancer. J Urol 1991; 145:988–991.
2. Rassweiler J, Janetschek G, Griffith DP. Laparoscopic surgery in urology. Thieme Stuttgart, New York 1996.
3. Guillonneau B, Cathelineau X, Barret E, et-al.. Laparoscopic radical prostatectomy: Technical and early oncological assessment of 40 operations. Eur Urol 1999; 36:14–20.
4. De la Rosette JJMCH, Abbou CC, et-al.. Laparoscopic radical prostatectomy: A European virus with global potential. Arch Esp Urol 2002; 55:603–609.
5. Rassweiler J, Hruza M, Teber D, Su L-M. Laparoscopic and robotic assisted radical prostatectomy—critical analysis of the results. Eur Urol 2006; 49:612–624.

6. Binder J, Kramer W. Robotically assisted laparoscopic radical prostatectomy. BJU Int 2001; 87:408–410.

7. Menon M, Shrisvastava A, Tewari A, et-al.. Laparoscopic and robot assisted radical prostatectomy: Establishment of a structured program and preliminary analysis of outcomes. J Urol 2002; 168:945–949.

8. Ahlering TE, Skarecky D, Lee D, Clayman RV. Successful transfer of open surgical skills to a laparoscopic environment using a robotic interface: Initial experience with laparoscopic radical prostatectomy. J Urol 2003; 170:1738–1741.

9. Zweifel P. Vorlesungen über klinische Gynäkologie, Hirschwald, Berlin, 1892.

10. Hugier A. Sacral colpopexy. Gynecol Obstetrique 1957; 56:114–117.

11. Miller NF. A new method of correcting complete inversion of the vagina with or without complete prolapse, two cases. Surg Gynecol Obstet 1927; 44:550–554.

12. Richter K, Albrich W. Long-term results following fixation of the vagina on the sacrospinal ligament by the vaginal route. Am J Obstet Gynecol 1981; 141:811–816.

13. Rozet F, Mandron E, Arroyo C, et-al.. Laparoscopic sacral colpopexy approach for genito-urinary prolapse: Experience with 363 cases. Eur Urol 2005; 47:230–236.

14. Dorsey JH, Cundiff G. Laparosopic procedures for incontinence and prolapse. Curr Opin Obst Gynecol 1994; 6:223–231.

15. Nezhat CH, Nezhat C, Nezhat F. Laparoscopic sacral colpopexy for vaginal vault prolapse. Obstet Gynecol 1994; 84:885–888.

16. Rassweiler J, Frede T, Seemann O, Jaeger T. Laparoscopic colposuspension with the Burch technique—fact or fiction. Urologe B 2000; 40:330–332(Engl. Abstract).

17. El-Toukhy, Davies AE. The efficacy of laparoscopic mesh colposuspension: Results of a prospective controlled. BJU Int 2001; 88: 361–366.

18. Paraiso MFR, Falcone T, Walters MD. Laparoscopic surgery for enterocele, vaginal apex prolapse and rectocele. Int Urogynecol J 1999; 10:223–229.

19. Cosson M, Rajabally R, Bogaert E, et-al.. Laparoscopic sacrocolpopexy, hysterectomy, and Burch colposuspension: Feasibility and short-term complications of 77 procedures. 2002; JSLS 6:115–119.

20. Deval B, Haab F. What's new in prolapse surgery? Curr Opin Urol 2003; 13:315–323.

21. Sundaram CP, Ramakrishna V, Landman J, Klutke CG. Laparosopic sacrocolpopexy for correction of vaginal vault prolapse. J Endourol 2004; 18:620–624.

22. Antiphon P, Elard S, Benyoussef A, et-al.. Laparoscopic promontory sacral colpopexy: Is the posterior, recto-vaginal mesh mandatory? Eur Urol 2004; 45:655–661.

23. Di Marco DS, Chow GK, Gettman MT, Elliott DS. Robotic-assisted laparoscopic sacrocolpopexy for treatment of vaginl vault prolapse. Urology 2004; 63:373–376.

24. Daneshgari F, Paraiso MF, Kaouk J, et-al.. Robotic and laparoscopic female pelvic floor reconstrction. BJU Int 2006; 98(Suppl 1):62–68.

25. Boyles S, Weber A, Meyn L. Procedures for pelvic organ prolapse in the United States. Am J Obstet Gynecol1997; 186:712–716.

26. Luber KM, Boero S, Choe JY.The demographics of pelvic floor disorders: Current observations and futures perspectives. Curr Opin Urol 2005; 15:256–262.

27. Novara G, Galfano A, Secco S, et-al.. Prolapse surgery: An update. Curr Opin Urol 2007; 17:237–241.

28. Baden WF, Walker TA. Genesis of the vaginal profile: A correlated classification of vaginal relaxation. Clin Obstet Gynecol 1972; 15:1048–1054.

29. DeLancey JOL. Anatomic aspects of vaginal eversion after hysterectomy. Am J Obstet Gynecol 1992; 166:1717–1728.

30. Limb J, Wood K, Weinberger M, et-al.. Sacral colpopexy using mersilene mesh in the treatment of vaginal vault prolapse. World J Urol 2005; 23:55–60.

31. Palma P, Riccetto C, Dambros M, Rodrigues Netto N. New trends in the transobturator management of cystoceles. BJU Int 2006; 97:201–210.

32. Reisenauer C, Kirschniak A, Drews U, Wallwiener D. Anatomical conditions for pelvic floor reconstruction with polypropylene implant and its application for the treatment of vaginal prolapse. Eur J Obstet Gynecol Reprod Biol 2007; 131(2):214–225.

33. Ng CCM, Han WHC. Comparison of effectiveness of vaginal abdominal routes in treating severe uterovaginal or vault prolapse. Singapore Med J 2004; 45:475–481.

34. Blanchard KA, Vanlangendonck R, Winters JC. Recurrent pelvic floor defects after abdominal sacral colpopexy. J Urol 2006; 175:1010–1013.

35. Lantzsch T, Goepel C, Wolters M, Koelbl H, Methfessel. Sacrospinous ligament fixation for vaginal vault prolapse. Arch Gynecol Obstet 2001; 265:21–25.

36. Wattiez A, Canis M, Mage G, et-al.. Promontofixation for the treatment of prolapse. Urol Clin N Am 2001;28:151–157

37. Novara G, Artibani W. Surgery for pelvic organ prolapse: current status and future perspectives. Curr Opin Urol 2005; 15:256–262.

38. Flynn BJ, Webster G. Surgical management of the apical vaginal defect. Curr Opin Urol 2002; 12:353–358.

39. Paraiso MF, Walters M, Rackley R, et-al.. Laparoscopic and abdominal sacropexies. A comparative cohort study. Am J Obstet Gynecol 2005; 192:1752–1758.

40. Ross JW, Preston M. Laparoscopic sacrocolpopexy for severe vaginal vault prolapse: Five year outcome. J Minim Invasive Gynecol 2005; 12: 221–226.

41. Teber D, Dekel Y, Frede T, et-al.. The Heilbronn laparoscopic training programm for laparoscopic suturing: Concept and validation. J Endourol 2005; 19: 230–238

42. Frede T, Erdogru T, Zukosky D, et-al.. Comparison of training modalities for performing laparoscopic radical prostatectomy: Experience with 1,000 patients. J Urol 2005; 174:673–678

43. Stolzenburg J, Schwaibold H, Bhanot SM, et-al.. Modular surgical training for endoscopic extraperitoneal radical prostatectomy. BJU Int 2005;96: 1022–1027.

44. Nezhat C, Saberi NS, Shahmohamady B, Nezhat F. Robotic-assisted laparoscopy in gynecological surgery. JSLS 2006; 10:317–320

Chapter 27
Posterior Compartment Repair and Fecal Incontinence

Gil Levy and Brooke H. Gurland

Introduction

Women with lower urinary tract symptoms and pelvic organ prolapse frequently report coexistent problems with the posterior pelvic compartment. This may include fecal urgency or incontinence, constipation, rectal pain syndromes, and rectal prolapse. Functional bowel disorders are the most understudied of all pelvic floor disorders. Little evidence exists regarding accepted definitions, treatments, and the relationship between anatomical findings and function [1]. We believe that understanding the complexity of the relationship between the pelvic floor organs, support system, and rectal function requires a multidisciplinary approach that addresses the posterior compartment as a functional unit in the pelvic floor.

This chapter will encompass the most common functional bowel disorders, the challenges involved in evaluating patients with posterior compartment disorders, and the relevant surgical anatomy and physiology. Furthermore, we will provide a multidisciplinary approach to the evaluation of patients with bowel symptoms, the use of anorectal testing, and the various treatment concepts for posterior compartment disorders.

Posterior Compartment Dysfunction: Definitions and Challenges

The prevalence of functional bowel disorders in patients with urinary incontinence and pelvic organ prolapse using standardized definitions (Table 27.1) is reported as 19% of patients with fecal incontinence and 36% with constipation [2]. Patients with constipation are further categorized into 19% of patients with outlet constipation, 5% functional constipation, 5–7% irritable bowel syndrome (IBS) and its subtypes, and 25% of patients with anorectal pain disorders. Rectal prolapse is reported in only 2% of the population; however, concomitant pelvic floor disorders have been reported in 8–27% of these patients [3, 4]. Case-control studies reveal that patients with rectal prolapse undergo genital prolapse surgery more frequently and at a significantly younger age than age-matched controls [5].

Fecal incontinence is thought to coexist with urinary incontinence and pelvic organ prolapse as a result of direct sphincter trauma or neuropathic injuries from vaginal deliveries [6]. In otherwise healthy younger women, obstetric anal sphincter injury is the principal causative factor in the development of fecal incontinence [7]. In women over the age of 65 years old fecal incontinence is significantly associated with chronic health conditions, liquid stool consistency, and bowel surgery [8].

Outlet type constipation is most common in women with pelvic organ prolapse as a result of the loss of pelvic floor support. Childbirth, hysterectomy, and chronic straining can damage the pelvic diaphragm and rectal vaginal supports, resulting in abnormal perineal descent of the distal rectum, sigmoid colon, or small bowel causing obstructive symptoms.

Rectal pain syndromes are the least well understood. Proctalgia fugax and levator spasm may occur in patients with prolapse, a result of stretching of the pelvic floor supports or muscular spasm.

Rectal prolapse is associated with chronic straining and a loss of fixation of the rectal attachments. Fecal incontinence is reported in 50–70% of these patients [9, 10]. Possible etiologies include stretching of the anal muscles, inhibition of the internal anal sphincter due to rectal reflexes, impairment of rectal sensation, or denervation of the pelvic floor muscles. Outlet constipation is reported in 72% of patients with rectal prolapse due to a mechanical-like obstruction [11].

Surgical repair of prolapse is based on the premise that correction of anatomical defects will improve symptoms. Thus, it is important to understand which symptoms are directly related to pelvic organ prolapse and which symptoms are associated with other disorders. Weber et al. reports 79.7% of women with posterior vaginal wall prolapse had one or more bowel complaints, but the authors could not correlate the bowel symptoms to the degree of posterior vaginal wall prolapse [12]. Several other studies report similar findings with the exception of a significant correlation between perineal descent and outlet constipation [13, 14]. Furthermore, da Silva et al. reveals that bowel symptoms correlate with abnormal anal physiology testing and primary anorectal pathology, but symptoms do not correlate with advanced posterior vaginal wall prolapse [15].

The literature that discusses surgical treatment can be difficult to interpret because of the use of broad, nonstandardized definitions and paucity of adequate outcome tools to evaluate function. The ROME II criteria (Table 27.1) are a set of criteria agreed upon by gastroenterologists and colorectal surgeons to describe functional bowel disorders, but these definitions and their relationships have not been validated in patients with prolapse or incontinence.

The Pelvic Organ Quantification Score (POP-Q), which is the accepted tool to evaluate pelvic organ prolapse, does not correlate with radiological findings [16, 17]. Its posterior compartment measuring points do not allow the determination among rectocele, sigmoidocele, enterocele, or intussusception during physical examination. Although defecography will differentiate these findings and is considered the "gold standard" to evaluate evacuation disorders, there is no consensus in the gynecology literature to its recommended use [18].

These are some of the challenges confronting physicians who are managing patients with posterior compartment dysfunction. We will begin this chapter by highlighting the surgical anatomy and physiology of the posterior compartment, which is essential in approaching patients with these disorders.

Anatomy and Physiology

The posterior pelvic compartment has the following borders: (1) posterior: the anterior surface of the sacrum and the levator muscles; (2) anterior: the posterior vaginal wall and the posterior vaginal fornix; (3) inferior: the perineum, anal muscles, and perineal body; and (4) superior: the peritoneal reflection and pouch of Douglas. The compartment contains the rectum and anus (Fig. 27.1).

Sacrum

The sacrum and coccyx comprise the posterior border of this compartment. These structures are covered by a thick layer of fascia, known as Waldeyer's fascia, which fuses with the fascia propria of the rectum above the anorectal ring. A lack of fixation of the fascial support of the rectum against the sacrum can lead to internal rectal prolapse, intussusception, and ultimately full thickness rectal prolapse. The coccyx, ischial spine, and sacrospinous ligaments can be palpated during clinical examination or accessed through

TABLE 27.1. Definitions of common posterior compartment terminology.

Fecal urgency is a symptom rather than a condition and is defined as "the patient's statement of the overwhelming desire to defecate accompanied by fear of leakage of bowel contents"

Fecal incontinence is defined as recurring episodes of involuntary loss of gas, solid, or liquid stool that are a social or hygienic problem. The time frame and the character of loss should be specified

Functional constipation/ROME II criteria[a]

The presence of at least 12 weeks (which do not need to be consecutive) in the previous year of two or more of the following symptoms:

• <3 Bowel movements (BMs) per week
• Hard or lumpy stools for more than 25% of BMs
• Straining with defecation for more than 25% of BMs
• A sensation of incomplete evacuation for more than 25% of BMs
• The use of manual maneuvers to assist defecation for more than 25% of BMs

Outlet constipation is a subtype of functional constipation. Patients also must report one of the following: a sensation that stool cannot be passed, a need to press on the perineum to complete the bowel movement, or difficulty relaxing and allowing the stool to come out

Dyssnergia constipation involves similar symptoms as above with EMG evidence of nonrelaxing puborectalis

Irritable bowel syndrome/ROME II criteriaa

The presence of at least 12 weeks (which do not need to be consecutive) in the previous year, of two or more of the following symptoms:

• Intermittent loose stools or constipation
• Abdominal pain or cramping
• Pain relieved with defecation

Rectal pain syndromes/ROME II criteriaa

Proctalgia fugax is defined as having more than 1 episode of aching pain or pressure in the anal canal over the last year that lasts for seconds to minutes and disappears completely

Levator ani syndrome includes the same pain which can last more than 20min up to several days or longer and has occurred frequently or continuously over the last 3 months

Rectal prolapse is a true intussusception of the rectum with protrusion of the full thickness of the rectum through the anal opening

[a]Source: Thompson WG, Longstreth G, Drossman DA, Heaton K, Irvine EJ, Muller-Lissner S. Functional bowel disorders and functional abdominal pain, pages 351–432. Whitehead WE, Wald A, Diamant NE, Enck P, Pemberton JH, Rao SSC. Functional disorders of the anus and rectum, pages 483–532. In: Drossman DA, Corazziari E, Talley NJ, Thompson WG, Whitehead WE, eds. ROME II The functional gastrointestinal disorders, diagnosis, pathophysiology and treatment: A multinational consensus. 2nd edn. Allen Press, Lawrence, KS

the pararectal space during surgical dissection. The sacrospinous ligament originates on the ischial spine and inserts onto the sacrum. The sacral plexus lies immediately next to the sacrospinous ligament on its cephalic border and passes through the greater sciatic foramen. Just before its exit, the plexus gives off the pudendal nerve, which, with its accompanying vessels, passes posterior to the sacrospinous ligament at its attachment to the ischial spine. Entrapment of these nerve fibers can cause gluteal pain. The levator ani muscles, iliococcygeus, and pubococcygeus arise from the ischial spine and pubic bone, respectively, and insert on S3, S4, and the coccyx and anococcygeal ligament. The puborectalis muscle is the most

medial portion of the levator muscle. The levator ani is supplied by S4 root on the pelvic surface and by the perineal branch of the pudendal nerve on its inner surface. The genital hiatus allows for passage of the lower rectum, vagina, and urethra.

Posterior Vaginal Wall

The rectovaginal septum is an elastic fibromuscular tissue layer that invests the posterior vaginal wall and is covered by mucosa up to the level of the cervix [19]. Superiorly, it is an extension of the endopelvic fascia and attaches to the cervix and the cardinal uterosacral complex, which supports the vaginal apex. Laterally, it attaches to the

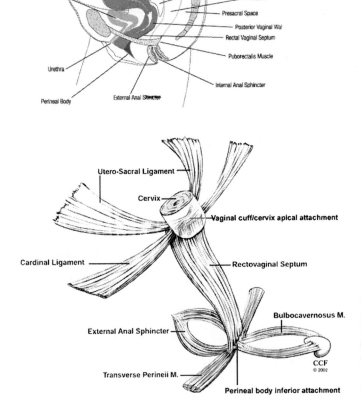

FIG. 27.1. Anatomical structures of the pelvic compartments

FIG. 27.2. Anatomical relationship of the perineal body and the rectovaginal septum (reprinted with permission from Cleveland Clinic Foundation: Pollack J, Davila GW. Rectocele Repair: The Gynecologic Approach. Clinics in Colon and Rectal Surg 2003; 16:61–69)

pelvic sidewalls and fuses with the aponeurosis of the levator ani muscle along a line referred to as the arcus-tendineus-fascia-rectovaginalis [20]. The rectovaginal septum fuses with the perineal body at its inferior portion.

Proximal injuries to the rectovaginal septum will permit the peritoneum to come into direct contact with the vaginal epithelium, resulting in small bowel or sigmoid protrusion, enterocele or sigmoidocele, respectively. Defects that are more distal will lead to bulging of the rectum into the posterior vaginal wall causing rectocele (Fig.27.2). The site-specific surgical repair of rectocele and enterocele is geared toward identifying and repairing defects in the rectovaginal septum [21].

Perineal Body

The perineal body is a pyramidal structure located between the vaginal introitus and anus with its base along the perineum. It is an attachment of the inferior central tendon, bulbocavernosus, transverse perineii muscles, and external sphincter muscles (Fig. 27.2). The perineal body also is connected to the rectovaginal septum, causing the retraction of the intergluteal cleavage. This cleavage disappears when the attachment of the perineal body is injured, causing perineal descent. Detachments of the rectal vaginal fascia from the perineal body can lead to distal rectocele in patients with normal posterior vaginal wall support. Richardson reported this as a "perineal rectocele" and a possible etiology for persistent difficult rectal evacuation in patients who underwent rectocele repair [21].

Pouch of Douglas

The peritoneal pocket located between the vaginal apex and the rectum is called the cul-de sac or pouch of Douglas. This space can be stretched deep in between the vagina and rectum allowing the peritoneum, small bowel, or redundant sigmoid colon to interpose those structures, causing peritoneocele, enterocele, or sigmoidocele.

Anal Sphincter Muscles/Anal Canal

The external anal sphincter (EAS) is fused to the perineal body anteriorly and is attached to the coccyx posteriorly by the anoccygeal ligament. The EAS is an elliptical cylinder of striated muscle that surrounds an inner tube of smooth muscle, the internal sphincter muscle (IAS), but ends slightly distal to it. The deepest part of the EAS is intimately related to, but embryologically distinct from, the puborectalis muscle. The puborectalis muscle is a U-shaped strong loop of striated muscle, which slings the anorectum junction to the back of the pubis, maintaining an acute anorectal angle [22]. The inferior rectal branch of the pudendal nerve innervates the EAS.

The IAS represents the distal 2.5- to 4-cm long condensation of the inner circular layer of the rectum. The anal opening or lower-most edge of the anus, also known as the anal verge, is closed at rest due to tonic circumferential contractions of the sphincters and the anal cushions. As a smooth muscle, the IAS is at a state of constant contraction due to intrinsic myogenic and extrinsic autonomic properties and represents a natural barrier to the involuntary loss of stool. The IAS is responsible for 50–85% of the resting tone, the EAS accounts for 25–30%, and the remaining 15% is attributed to expansion of the anal cushions [23, 24].

The surgical anal canal extends from the sulcus between the IAS and EAS for approximately 4cm to the anorectal ring. The anorectal ring, the upper end of the puborectalis muscle and IAS, is an easily recognizable boundary of the anal canal on physical examination. Vaginal delivery, perineal laceration, and instrumental deliveries can lead to anal sphincter injury and fecal incontinence.

Rectum

The rectum is a 12- to –15-cm long segment of large intestine that occupies the sacral concavity and ends 2–3cm inferior to the tip of the coccyx. At the tip of the coccyx, the rectum ungulates backward, passing through the levators and becomes the anal canal. The rectum is a very compliant organ that accommodates stool contents and acts as a reservoir so that defecation can be delayed.

Defecation

Regulated bowel habits rely on the interaction of complex neurological and muscular features under the influence of the central nervous system. Stool consistency, intestinal motility, delivery of stool to the rectum, rectal capacity and compliance, anorectal sensation, integrity of the anal sphincter mechanism, neurological function of the pelvic floor muscles and nerves all contribute to "normal" bowel activity.

The sigmoid colon fills the rectum and triggers defecation. Rectal distention is interpreted as a desire to defecate. Following the rectal fill, the IAS relaxes by opening the upper anal canal and allowing sampling of contents. The EAS contraction reflex maintains continence during this phase. If the call to stool is answered, then sitting or squatting positions are assumed and increased abdominal pressure and rectal contractions squeezes the part of the rectum that lies above the pelvic diaphragm. The EAS and puborectalis relax and the anorectal angle becomes more obtuse and defecation occurs. If defecation is to be deferred, conscious contraction of the EAS occurs with rectal compliance and contractions of the puborectalis pull the distal vagina and anorectal junction toward the pubic symphysis, creating a near 90 angle, anorectal angle, which facilitates fecal continence. In diarrheal states high volumes of liquid stool empty rapidly into the rectum, overwhelming the sphincter mechanism, leading to fecal urgency and incontinence.Disorders that relate to poor rectal compliance or loss of rectal reservoir can result in fecal urgency or incontinence. Sensory neuropathy (diabetes) or altered mental status (stroke or dementia) may selectively reduce conscious sensation and awareness of rectal fullness. In these patients relaxation occurs before the sensation of rectal distention, which results in fecal impaction and overflow incontinence. Anal sphincter injuries can result in the inability to maintain adequate resting and squeeze pressures and a noncompliant rectum.

For patients with motility disorders, markedly delayed intestinal transit may result in nonfilling of the sigmoid colon, thus delaying the defecation process. Patients with outlet-type constipation can have nonrelaxation of the puborectalsis (anismus). Thus, the anorectal angle remains abnormally contracted at the time of defecation.

Furthermore, chronic straining can lead to stretching of the pudendal nerves and denervation of the external sphincter muscle and fecal incontinence. Denervation of the pelvic diaphragm results in opening of the genital hiatus and laxity of the endopelvic fascia, which then is prone to attenuation and tearing. In this pathological state of excessive perineal descent, the pelvic organs are allowed to pass through the genital hiatus.

Patient Evaluation

Medical Intake

Women with posterior compartment prolapse may complain of urinary dysfunction, bowel disorders, or hernia-like symptoms. Urinary urgency, frequency, and incontinence frequently are identified concomitantly with posterior compartment disorders and are discussed in detail in prior chapters. In order to create a systematic evaluation of posterior compartment complaints we grouped the symptoms into two categories: (1) bowel complaints including fecal incontinence, constipation, rectal pain, and rectal prolapse; and (2) vaginal complaints including vaginal pressure, a feeling of a bulge, visible prolapse, vaginal pain or bleeding,, and sexually related symptoms.

When evaluating patients with bowel disorders the consistency and frequency of bowel movements and the use of enemas and laxatives needs to be documented. The inability to control gas, liquid, or solid stool and the frequency of loss are reported as well as the presence of passive, urgent, or mixed incontinence. Passive loss of stool, without the patient knowing until the accident has occurred, implies that there is a rectal

sensory deficit. Urgency incontinence implies that the patient has the sensation to move her bowels but cannot control the movement. This may occur with chronic diarrheal states, irritable bowel, or anal sphincter injuries. Soiling, a streak of stool on the underwear, may be related to liquid stool consistency or seepage of stool from fecal impaction and overflow incontinence. A number of fecal incontinence scoring systems have been proposed and validated to assist in clinical decision-making. We use the Wexner fecal incontinence score (FICS) to evaluate the degree of fecal incontinence (Table 27.2). Prior validations report a FICS 9 correlate with significant fecal incontinence [25].

To evaluate patients with complaints of constipation we use the ROME II criteria (Table 27.1). Patients with rectal pain are asked to describe the quality and duration of their symptoms and its association with bowel movements. Prolapse of tissue from the anus, the presence of rectal bleeding, and the quantity and frequency of blood loss are documented.

Underlying medical and surgical conditions and medications, which may alter bowel habits, need be investigated. Patients who fit the criteria for IBS should be referred for the appropriate workup (Table 27.1). The risk of malignancy also should be considered, specifically where there has been a change in bowel habits or bleeding, and appropriate evaluation with colonoscopy initiated. The conditions associated with fecal incontinence are summarized in Table 27.3. Medical conditions associated with constipation are reported in Table 27.4. Outlet obstruction constipation can be further categorized by the mechanism of action (Table 27.5). Patients with internal intussusception or full thickness rectal prolapse also may complain of fecal urgency or incontinence, mucus discharge or soiling, outlet constipation, rectal pressure, rectal bleeding, or pain. Rectal bleeding may be associated with internal intussusception, full thickness rectal prolapse, and solitary rectal ulcer syndrome.

The common vaginal symptoms associated with posterior compartment disorders include feeling of a bulge, heaviness, or pain. Pain can be reported as pelvic, abdominal, lower back, or perineal. In cases of advanced genital prolapse the patient may describe visible prolapse of the vagina.

Symptoms may relate to sexual dysfunction and include dyspareunia or decreased sensation.

TABLE 27.2. Wexner fecal incontinence.

	Solid stool	Liquid stool	Gas	Wears pad	Lifestyle change
Frequency of accidents					
Never	0	0	0	0	0
Rarely <1 month	1	1	1	1	1
Sometimes <1/week, >1/month	2	2	2	2	2
Usually >1/week	3	3	3	3	3
Always >1/day	4	4	4	4	4

Score (0 = perfect continence and 20 = complete incontinence)
Source: Jorge J, Wexner S. Ethiology and management of fecal incontinence. Dis Colon Rectum 1993; 36:77–97

TABLE 27.3. Etiologies of fecal incontinence.

I Altered stool consistency — diarrheal states
A. Irritable bowel syndrome
B. Inflammatory bowel disease
C. Infectious diarrhea
D. Laxative abuse

II Inadequate reservoir capacity or compliance
A. Inflammatory bowel disease
B. Surgical removal of the rectum
C. Collagen vascular disease

III Inadequate rectal sensation
A. Neurological conditions
i. Dementia/cerebrovascular accident
ii. Multiple sclerosis
B. Central nervous system injuries or neoplasms
C. Sensory neuropathy
i. Diabetes
D. Overflow incontinence
i. Fecal impaction
ii. Psychotropic drugs

IV Abnormal sphincter mechanism or pelvic floor
A. Anatomic sphincter defect
i. Traumatic
a. Obstetric injury
b. Anorectal surgery
B. Pelvic floor denervation
i. Pudendal neuropathy
ii. Chronic straining of stool
iii. Descending perineal syndrome
iv. Aging
v. Vaginal deliveries
vi. Rectal prolapse

TABLE 27.4. Conditions associated with constipation.

Organic disorders	Diabetes
	Amyloidosis
	Hypokalemia
	Hypocalcemia
	Hyperparathyroidism
	Parkinson's disease
	Cerebral vascular disease
	Autonomic neuropathy
Medications	Anticholinergics
	Opiates
	Antihypertensives

the severity of symptoms. We repeat the assessment following intervention to measure the success of treatment [26, 27].

Physical Examination

Perineal, vaginal, anal, and rectal evaluations are important components of the physical examination. Inspection may reveal previous scars and atrophic changes, dermatologic conditions, a gaping introitus or prior episiotomy scars. A short, distorted perineal body associated with the "dovetail sign" is suspicious of an anterior anal sphincter defect. A gaping patulous anus may indicate neurological injury or full thickness rectal prolapse. Palpation of the external genitalia can reveal localized tenderness and irritation. Neurological examination to sharp and soft stimuli and sensory, motoric, and reflex functions should be evaluated. The bulbocavernosus reflex or anal wink reflex refers to contractions of the external sphincter with gentle touching of the clitoris or anus. Flattening of the perineum during Valsalva beyond the ischial tuborosities is suggestive of excessive perineal descent and can be

Dyspareunia should be documented in various parts of penetration or intercourse positions. Lack of sensation needs to be differentiated from decreased libido and documented in the various parts of the sexual stages.

We use validated multicompartment scoring systems and quality of life questionnaires to address

TABLE 27.5. Etiologies of outlet type constipation.

Mechanism	
1. Impaired rectal sensation	1. Megarectum
2. Functional outlet obstruction	1. Inefficient inhibition of the IAS
	a. Hirschsprung's
	b. Chagas
	2. Inefficient relaxation of the pelvic floor muscles
	a. Anismus
	b. Spinal cord lesions
	c. Multiple sclerosis
3. Mechanical obstruction	1. Full thickness rectal prolapse
	2. Internal intussusception to the anal verge
	3. Large enterocele
4. Redirection of expulsion force	1. Rectocele
	2. Descending perineum syndrome
	3. Total rectal prolapse

TABLE 27.6. Physical examination findings.

Inspection
- Vaginal skin integrity
- Posterior vaginal wall descent
- Perineal body thickness and integrity
- Stool particles around the anus
- Anus closed or open (patulous)
- Scars or muscular defect
- Anal skin reflex to palpation (anal wink)
- Mucosal versus full thickness prolapse with Valsalva
- Perineal descent with Valsalva below the ischial tuborosities

Palpation
- Pain/tenderness at the introitus
- Vaginal/uterine prolapse
- Masses
- Resting pressures
- Squeeze pressure
- Sphincter defects
- Rectal content
- Relaxation of the puborectalis
- Tenderness over the levators
- Rectocele

Endoscopy
- Rectoanal intussusception
- Mucosal lining/colitis
- Malignancy

felt with the patient sitting on the examiner's hand palpating the perineum.

Internal vaginal examination may reveal tenderness over the levator muscles, which is suggestive of levator spasm as a possible etiology for pelvic pain and dyspareunia. During speculum examination atrophic changes and posterior vaginal wall support are reported. Evaluation of the posterior vaginal wall is routinely performed using single-blade speculum to retract the anterior wall and allow direct visualization of the posterior wall and fornix during rest and Valsalva maneuver. The Pelvic Organ Prolapse Quantification score (POP-Q) is used to report the degree of prolapse [16]. Bimanual vaginal and rectal examination may be performed in the standing position to elicit the maximal prolapse of the pelvic organs as they descend through the pouch of Douglas.

During anorectal examination, sphincter coordination is noted when patients are asked to squeeze, relax, and push. Valsalva maneuver usually is required to elicit full thickness rectal prolapse. Digital examination reveals resting and squeeze anal tone and a large rectocele or sphincter defect frequently may be palpated. If rectal prolapse is suspected, then we have the patient sit on the commode and attempt evacuation in order to visualize the rectal prolapse. Physical examination finding are summarized in Table 27.6.

Anoscopy is performed to evaluate patients for mucosal abnormalities and rectoanal intussusception. Colonoscopy is recommended to rule out anatomic lesions and inflammatory conditions.

Diagnostic Studies

Anorectal physiology permits objective measures of subjective functional colorectal problems and helps to distinguish between among pathophysiological mechanisms that would not otherwise be detected on clinical examination [28] (Table27.7).

Anorectal Manometry

Anorectal manometry measures intra-anal and intrarectal pressures at rest and during squeeze and Valsalva to measure internal and external sphincter function. We use a system that can accommodate both urodynamic and anorectal testing. A thin catheter with a balloon secured to the end is introduced into the anus and pressure measurements are reordered along the length of the anal canal (Fig. 27.3). There is a graduated increase in pressure

TABLE 27.7. Diagnostic studies.

Test	Purpose
Anorectal manometry	To measure resting and squeeze anal pressures
	Rectal sensation/compliance and RAIR
Electromyography	
Needle EMG	To measure sphincter injuries by assessing reinervation patterns
Surface EMG	To measure relaxation of the puborectalis
Pudendal nerve terminal latency studies	To measure the integrity of the pudendal nerve
Endorectal ultrasound	Anatomic mapping of the internal and external anal sphincter
Cinedefecography	To evaluate for incomplete or delayed rectal evacuation and possible etiologies: rectocele, intussusception, rectal prolapse, enterocele, perineal descent
MRI	Anatomic view of all pelvic floor compartments

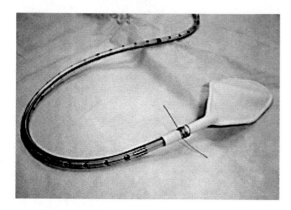

FIG. 27.3. Anal manometry catheter

proceeding distally and the highest resting pressures are generally recorded from 1 to 2cm from the anal verge. The mean anal canal resting pressure in healthy adults ranges from 40 to 60 (cm/H_2O) and is lower in elderly patients. During normal squeeze effort intra-anal pressures double or triple their baseline resting pressures (80 –180cm/H_2O) (Fig. 27.4) [29]. Low anal pressures are seen in patients with incontinence from anal sphincter

defects, neurogenic incontinence, rectal prolapse, and perineal descent.

The rectal anal inhibitory reflex (RAIR) and rectal sensation are measured by injecting air into an intrarectal balloon at the end of the catheter. Rectal distention causes reflex transient IAS relaxation and EAS contraction, thus permitting rectal sampling of fecal contents. Patients with Hirschsprungs and Chagas disease have an absent RAIR.

The first rectal sensation usually is between 10 and 20ml of air. As more air is introduced, the rectum distends and the patient reports the urge to move her bowels. Viscous and elastic properties intrinsic to the rectum allow it to maintain a low intraluminal pressure despite a large volume [30]. Through this mechanism of rectal compliance, stool contents can be accommodated so that defecation can be delayed. Low rectal compliance is identified in patients with inflammation to the rectum such as proctitis and inflammatory bowel disease and in patients with anal sphincter injuries. Some believe that the development and maintenance of a compliant rectum is related to a competent sphincter [31]. It is unclear whether poor rectal compliance is a cause or a consequence of fecal incontinence. High sensory thresholds have been associated with diabetes, peripheral neuropathy, perineal descent syndrome, fecal impaction, encopresis, spina bifida, and meningeocele and may be related to overflow fecal incontinence or difficult evacuation [32].

Neurological Studies: Electromyography/ Pudendal Nerve Latency

Electromyography (EMG) is used to investigate the electrical activity of the EAS and pelvic floor muscles. Concentric needle, monopolar, and single-fiber electrodes are techniques that require insertion of a needle into the EAS or puborectalis to measure motor unit potentials (MUP). Muscular defects can be demonstrated by assessing reinervation patterns.

Surface EMG using patch electrode on the external sphincter muscles or a sponge electrode in the anal canal is noninvasive and well tolerated by the patient. During squeezing, the amplitude of the MUP will increase, while pushing or simulated defecation appears very similar to the resting pattern. Nonrelaxation of the puborectalis can be diagnosed by an abnormal pattern during Valsalva (Fig. 27.5).

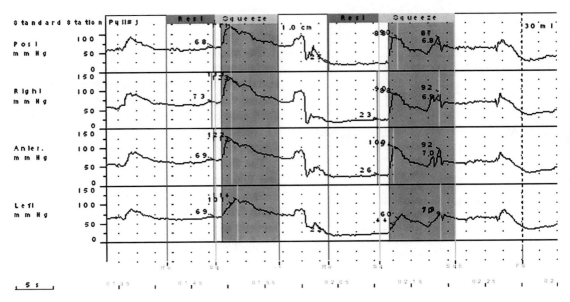

FIG. 27.4. Normal manometry measurements during rest and squeeze cycle

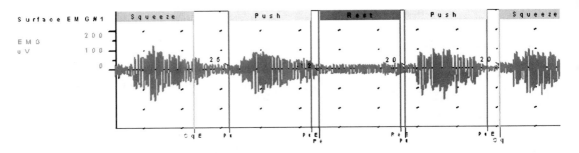

FIG. 27.5. EMG of the pelvic floor muscles demonstrating nonrelaxing puborectalis

Pudendal nerve terminal latencies (PNTML) are measured by stimulating the pudendal nerve intra-rectally with the St. Mark's electrode on a gloved finger to assess pudendal neuropathy. Prolongation of the PNTML indicates pathology to the pudendal nerve; however, the nature and the site of the lesion remain uncertain. Moreover, the conduction velocity of a nerve may have little bearing on its functional integrity. The prevalence of prolonged PNTML in patients presenting for anorectal physiology studies is reported at 20–28% with unilateral neuropathy and 11–12% with bilateral neuropathy [33, 34]. Bilateral, not unilateral pudendal neuropathy is associated with diminished sphincter function and higher incontinence scores. In some studies, pro-longed pudendal nerve latencies have been shown to be an important prognostic factor in patients undergoing anal sphincter repair [35]. Figure 27.6 demonstrates normal and abnormal PNTML.

Imaging Studies

Ultrasound

Anal endosonography requires an ultrasound scanner, a 360 endoprobe at 7 or 10mHz with a rigid cap for evaluation of the anal canal musculature (Fig. 27.7). The probe is moved in or out of the anal canal and images are taken at the upper, middle, and distal anal canal. At the upper anal canal the puborectalis is visualized as a hyperechoic U-shaped structure. At the middle anal canal the external and internal sphincter muscles form a complete ring and outer hyperechoic and inner

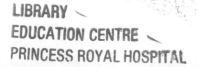

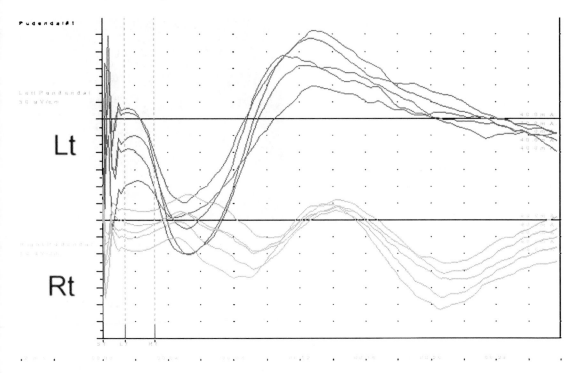

FIG. 27.6. Measurements of pudendal nerve latency (normal <2.2 ms). *Left* 2.1 ms, *Right* 3.1 ms. The *bottom curves* demonstrate slow conduction consistent with unilateral neuropathy

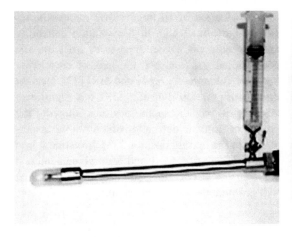

FIG. 27.7. Anal ultrasound probe

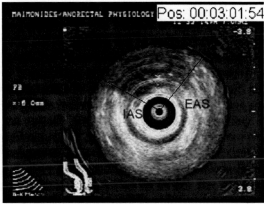

FIG. 27.8. Anal ultrasound demonstrating anterior anal sphincter defect

hypoechoic circles are visualized. At the distal anal canal only the subcutaneous EAS is visualized as a hyperechoic ring. Anal sphincter injuries are detected by a break in the muscular ring. Defects may be reported as EAS, IAS, or combined injuries (Fig. 27.8). Ultrasound measure-

ments of the perineal body increase the sensitivity of detecting anal sphincter injuries [36]. A finger is placed into the vaginal introitus at the level of the middle anal canal and the distance between the tip of the finger to the IAS is measured and perineal body measurements less than 10mm are suspicious for sphincter injuries [37]. Ultrasound measurements of perineal body do not correlate with POP-Q measurements [38].

In most practices, endoanal ultrasound has become the preferred modality for evaluation of sphincter defects. It provides an anatomic view but is not helpful in assessment of neuromuscular activity. Although needle EMG can be very uncomfortable for the patient, endoanal ultrasound and needle EMG may be complementary when the presence of a defect is uncertain.

Three-dimensional anorectal endosonography takes the data from a series of closely spaced two-dimensional images combined with a three-dimensional image. Improved visualization of the anal musculature is an exciting prospect. The clinical significance of this modality has yet to be proven.

Cinedefecography

Cinedefecography is a dynamic study that requires opacification of the pelvic floor structures with contrast and simulation of defecation [39]. It is performed on patients with difficult evacuation or selectively on patients with fecal incontinence to identify internal or full thickness rectal prolapse. Oral contrast is given to opacify the small bowel, liquid barium to opacify the sigmoid colon, and barium paste is inserted into the rectum and vagina. Opacification of the bladder or the peritoneum will enhance visualization of cystoceles and enteroceles. Cinedefecography is performed in the fluoroscopy suite with the aid of videorecording and freeze-framing with the patient sitting on a specialized water-filled commode. Images are taken at rest, squeeze, and pushing, and evacuation is recorded. We look for delayed or incomplete rectal emptying, changes in the anorectal angle, the presence and size of an anterior or posterior rectocele and evacuation of the rectocele, sigmoid or small bowel descent below the pubococcygeal line (sigmoidocele or enterocele, respectively), perineal descent, internal intussusception, and full thickness rectal prolapse (Fig. 27.9). Cinedefecography is able to identify pathology not visualized on clinical examination [17]. There is a 33% incidence of internal rectoanal intussusception in patients with clinical rectoceles and defecatory dysfunction [40]. Although internal prolapse is unlikely to progress into overt prolapse, it may contribute to the evacuation

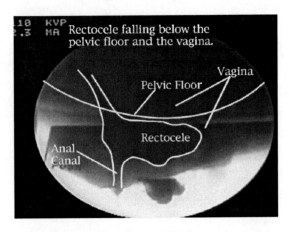

FIG. 27.9. Large rectocele marked on defecography (reprinted with permission Lahr, C. Why Can't I Go, Charleston: Sunburst Press, 2004)

symptoms. Furthermore, enterocele diagnosed by defecography is associated with a high likelihood of other pelvic floor findings [41] (Fig. 27.10).

Magnetic Resonance Imaging Systems

The development of fast sequence magnetic resonance imaging (MRI) provides a quick, efficient, detailed, and reproducible evaluation of pelvic organ prolapse and pelvic floor relaxation. Evaluation of all three pelvic compartments can be performed with high-resolution capability and no radiation. Disadvantages to MRI are the cost, supine position, and the lack of correlation between videoproctography and MRI [42]. Upright open-configuration dynamic MRI has significant advantages over the supine position, allowing the patient to simulate defecation and prolapse associated with the upright position [43]. Investment into open-configuration MRI and a combined interest between the pelvic floor surgeon and radiologist will promote the use of this exciting technology.

Treatment Concepts and Surgical Techniques

Surgical Treatment of Symptomatic Posterior Vaginal Wall Prolapse

The surgical treatment of symptomatic posterior wall prolapse is based on the concept that the restoration of anatomy will alleviate pelvic

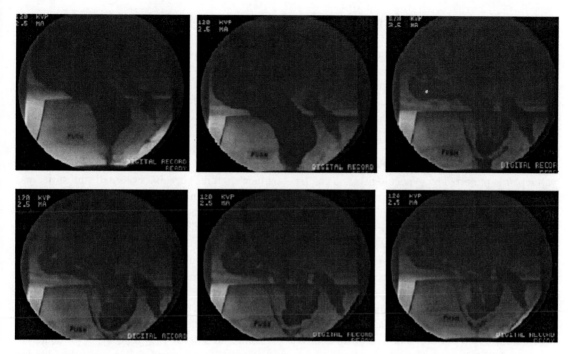

FIG. 27.10. Enterocele demonstrated during defacography. Series of frames prior and during valsalva maneuver demonstrating small bowel loop descent deep into the perineum (reprinted with permission Lahr, C. Why Can't I Go Charleston: Sunburst Press, 2004)

TABLE 27.8. NIH criteria for posterior compartment surgical outcome.

Optimal anatomical outcome	Cure	No prolapse of the posterior vagina is demonstrated	Stage 0 by ICS staging, with points Ap and Bp at −3cm
Satisfactory anatomical outcome	Improvement	Descent of the posterior vagina to within 1cm above the hymen	Stage 1 by ICS staging, with point Ap or Bp at −2cm
Unsatisfactory anatomical outcome	Persistence or recurrence, failed treatment	Descent of the posterior vagina to 1cm proximal to the hymen or lower, or no change or worsening from pretreatment stage	Stage 2 or worse by ICS staging, with points Ap or Bp at −1cm or lower, or no change or worsening from pretreatment position

floor symptoms. In order to compare the various surgical techniques discussed in the literature, success needs to be evaluated from anatomical and functional perspective. The National Institutes of Health have established criteria to evaluate anatomical repair of the posterior compartment (Table 27.8) using POP-Q scoring, but have failed to provide a validated and standardized tool to evaluate postoperative functional results and their effects on quality of life. Other difficulties in the analysis of the relevant surgical literature include:

1. Variability in inclusion and exclusion criteria
2. Multiple modifications of the surgical techniques
3. Short-term published follow-up
4. Lack of independent postoperative reviewers
5. Combination with other reconstructive procedures
6. Lack of validated symptom scales

The surgical approach for the treatment of posterior vaginal wall prolapse can be divided into transvaginal, transanal, transperineal, and abdominal, and open or laparoscopic procedures.

Independent of the surgical technique, chronic increased abdominal pressure can cause recurrence of the anatomical defect. High intraperitoneal pressure is associated with body mass index (BMI) >35; heavy smokers; chronic heavy lifters, such as nurses or impact sports players; and chronic constipation. Established risk assessment scales to improve success rate predictions of these high-risk patients do not exist.

The transvaginal approach to posterior vaginal wall repair is preferred by gynecologists and can be divided into four surgical techniques: (1) midline plication of the levator ani muscles [44]; (2) plication of the rectovaginal septum [45]; (3) site-specific repair of the discrete tears in the rectovaginal septum [46]; and (4) posterior colporrhaphy using graft material. Overall, all of these techniques provide adequate anatomic repair of the posterior vaginal wall, but they vary in regard to functional success and complications. Midline levator ani plication has been criticized due to reports of postoperative constipation and dyspareunia in 19–41% of patients [44, 47–49]. The midline plication of the rectovaginal fascia was reported to improve obstructed defecation in over 80% of patients [50, 51]. Patients who underwent the site-specific repair had a higher anatomical failure rate compared to those who underwent rectovaginal septum plication. However, patients who underwent site-specific repair denied significant dyspareunia, but they failed to document an improvement in fecal symptoms. The literature describing the use of graft material for posterior vaginal wall repair is limited to case series reports that lack level I evidence. Graft material initially was used to augment the site-specific repair using the graft as a buttress. As the techniques evolved, grafts were used to replace the rectovaginal septum with the assumption that the defect not only is a physical tear and/or detachment but is due to an intrinsic weakness of the tissue from decreased collagen quality secondary to genetic, hormonal, and aging factors. It was theorized that the grafts would provide scaffolding for regeneration of collagen. This premise was based on laboratory evidence of fibroblast migration into the biomaterial as early as a few weeks after surgery [52–55]. However, further studies failed to document histological evidence of an increased endogenous collagen production at the posterior compartment implant site 6 months after surgery [56].

There are many variations of graft materials and anchoring techniques. Both biological and synthetic graft materials have been used to repair posterior vaginal wall prolapse. The biological materials include allografts and xenografts. Allografts are harvested from cadaveric fascia or dermis. Chemical cross-linking of cadaveric products increases durability but also can result in an inflammatory reaction, fibrosis, or scar formation. However, allografts are at an extremely low risk for erosion. Xenografts include porcine dermis or small intestine and bovine pericardium. Xenografts also can be chemically cross-linked or minimally processed. The synthetic materials used are either absorbable (Polyglactine 910 = Vicryl) or permanent [polypropylene (Prolene), polytetrafluoroethylene (Gore-Tex), polyester fiber (Mersilene), or knitted polyesther (Dacron)]. The synthetic materials are fenestrated with holes of at least 100mm to allow fibroblasts migration and tissue regeneration.

Kohli and Miklos [57] reported 93% anatomic success rate, at 12-month follow-up, using porcine dermis as a buttress following site-specific posterior colporrhaphy. Altman et al. [58] reported 41% success rate using the same biomaterial anchored to the levator muscles, perineal body, and the upper rectovaginal septum without performing the site-specific repair. Furthermore, he reported a dramatic drop in success rate with long-term follow-up. Symptoms of incomplete emptying and a decreased need for hand-assisted defecation significantly improved, but overall the improvement was reported in less than 50% of patients.

There are few reports that describe the use of synthetic graft material for posterior vaginal wall repair. The synthetic grafts usually are anchored to strong anatomical structures such as the sacrospinous ligaments, arcus tendineous, obturator fascia, and muscle. An alternative to graft fixation was described by Petros, who introduced the concept of a neoligament as an anchoring technique using the IVS tunneler in an infracoccygeal approach [59].

Short-term follow-up for patients undergoing posterior repair with synthetic mesh reveals an anatomic success rate of 85% and a subjective cure rate of 60–80%. The main complications reported after synthetic graft use are postoperative dyspareunia and mesh erosion in 69 and 13%, respectively [60]. However, de Tayrac et al. reported their series of patients undergoing posterior colporraphy with synthetic graft material anchored to the sacrospinous ligaments and perineal body without site-specific repair [61]. He reported significant improvement in bowel symptoms and sexual function using validated questionnaires and quality of life tools.

The transanal or transperineal approaches are preferred by colorectal surgeons who have limited training operating on the vagina. The indications for surgery are complaints of difficult evacuation, manual digitation, rectocele >4cm, and residual contrast in the rectocele by defecography [62]. Evidence of nonrelaxing puborectalis is associated with poor functional results [63].

Most studies reveal improvement of rectal symptoms with transanal rectocele repair [64, 65]. However, there is level I evidence that transvaginal repair is superior to transanal because of better anatomic repair with equivalent functional results reporting cure rates approaching 75%, independent of the approach [66, 67].

The transperineal approach involves the same surgical techniques used in the transvaginal route except the approach to the surgical space is made through a perineal incision, avoiding incision of the vaginal mucosa [68]. Insertion of the mesh for the reconstruction of the rectovaginal septum through the perineum provides comparable success rates but lacks long-term follow-up [69]. The transperineal approach may be the preferred technique when rectocele repair is performed in combination with overlapping sphincteroplasty and perineoplasty.

Abdominal open or laparoscopic procedures usually are performed for a combination of apical and posterior wall prolapse and are based on the sacrocolpopexy techniques with the use of graft material. Lyons and Winer [70] report a laparoscopic approach using absorbable material with 80% resolution of prolapse symptoms and digital-assisted defecation at 1-year follow-up. Other authors have suggested additional modifications to the abdominal sacrocolpopexy by extension and fixation of the mesh down to the level of the levator ani or perineal body. In addition to correcting apical prolapse and posterior compartment defects, these procedures are designed to improve excessive perineal descent [71]. Fox and Stanton [72] reported 93% success rate using a Teflon mesh, but functional symptoms did not improve. On the other hand, Sullivan et al. describe their experience with a total Marlex pelvic mesh repair achieving excellent anatomical results and 75% improvement in bowel symptoms [73].

Classic teachings have included obliteration of the pouch of Douglas, enterocele repair, as an integral part to the success of apical and posterior compartment reconstruction. Procedures such as the Moschcowitz and Hallban culdoplasty involved obliteration of the cul-de-sac by approximating the peritoneum [74, 75]. The Mayo-modified McCall technique with reconstruction of level one support was reported to provide an anatomical success rates of 82% [76–78].However, it is impossible to analyze the contribution of the enterocele resection to the final anatomical or functional success, because enterocele repair usually performed in conjunction with other prolapse procedures. It is interesting to note that current surgical techniques using graft material for the repair of vaginal apex do not emphasize enterocele resection as a mandatory step to avoid recurrence.

Richardson proposed that an enterocele resulted from a defect in the integrity of the endopelvic fascia at the vaginal apex [79]. He described enterocele repair in combination with site-specific rectocele repair by reapproximation of the upper edge of the rectovaginal septum to the pubocervical fascial edge and uterosacral ligament. High anatomic success rates were reported using this site-specific approach but functional results were not discussed [80].

Treatment Options for Fecal Incontinence

The initial management of patients with fecal incontinence focuses on improving stool consistency and decreasing the overall number of bowel movements with a high-fiber diet, bulking agents, and constipating medications. Most medical therapies reported are geared toward the treatment of diarrhea rather than fecal incontinence and little evidence exists to guide the physician in the selection of drug therapies [81]. For patients with leakage of stool secondary to fecal impaction or decreased rectal sensation, fiber therapy, laxatives, and a daily enemas help to empty the rectal vault and minimize fecal accidents. Noninvasive modalities such as intra-anal and pelvic floor muscle strengthening exercises (biofeedback) for the treatment of fecal incontinence are reported to improve continence scores [82]. Due to a limited number of studies and methodological weaknesses, the Cochrane Incontinence Group Trials Register failed to identify a major difference in outcome between any method of biofeedback or exercises for fecal incontinence or an improvement compared to conservative measures [83]. We offer intra-anal biofeedback for fecal incontinence to patients with normal sphincter anatomy or to patients who refuse or are poor candidates for surgical repair.

Bulking agents injected into the anal sphincter such as those approved for use in patients with urinary stress incontinence also have been tried to treat passive fecal leakage for patients with normal sphincter anatomy or patients with isolated internal sphincter injuries. Different materials and injection techniques have been reported but are confined to small pilot studies and presently are not available for widespread use [84]. The SECCA procedure is an additional option for patients with normal sphincter anatomy and fecal incontinence. This involves radio frequency energy delivery into the anal canal and has been proven to be well tolerated and efficacious [85].

Anterior anal sphincter injuries frequently are identified in patients who complain of fecal incontinence in addition to other pelvic floor disorders such as urinary incontinence or advanced pelvic organ prolapse [86]. Surgical repair can be performed concomitantly with other pelvic floor procedures with good outcomes and cost effectiveness [87]. Furthermore, Steele et al. reports that patients who underwent anterior overlapping sphincter repair in conjunction with total pelvic floor repair had better functional results than patients with sphincteroplasty alone [88]. Other authors have not corroborated these findings. We offer these patients combined urinary, prolapse, and anorectal surgical procedures. The additional benefits to the patient include a single anesthesia and recovery time and overall decreased disability.

There are several techniques described for anal sphincteroplasty. Obstetricians most commonly perform apposition of the external anal sphincter with an end-to-end technique. Overlapping sphincteroplasty is preferred by colorectal surgeons for external or external and internal anal sphincter injuries. For immediate primary repair following obstetric injury overlap repair is associated with less fecal urgency and lower incontinence scores at 1 year compared to end-to-end approximation [89, 90]. Although fecal incontinence scores are improved following sphincteroplasty, complete continence is difficult to achieve and tends to deteriorate over time [91, 92]. Pudendal neuropathy has been implicated as a poor prognostic indicator in patients undergoing overlapping sphincter repair, but it is not a contraindication to surgery [35, 93].

Postanal repair involves posterior levatorplasty and is thought to improve continence by lengthening the anal canal and making the anorectal angle more acute. Postanal repair can be considered in patients without a sphincter defect and low resting pressures who failed or do not wish to undergo biofeedback. It also is an option for patients for whom overlapping sphincter repair has achieved anatomical but not functional improvement. Reports of poor long-term success rates and the introduction of newer, less invasive techniques have discouraged many surgeons from offering postanal repair [94].

Sacral nerve stimulation (SNS) is geared toward neuromodulation instead of anatomic repair. It has been proven beneficial for the treatment of voiding disorders, and European studies document up to 80% success rate using SNS in the treatment for patients with fecal incontinence, an intact sphincter, and normal sacral plexus [95–97]. The most common technique includes a two-phase procedure. An electrically stimulated spinal needle is placed percutaneously under fluoroscopic guidance in the S3 foramina. The electrode is connected to an external pulse generator for the testing period of 10–14 days and the patient is asked to complete a symptom diary. Patients that demonstrate at least 50% improvement are offered the second phase during which a permanent stimulator is implanted subcutaneously in the upper part of the gluteal area. SNS was thought to increase the anal canal closure pressure resulting from contraction of the puborectalis and sphincter muscles and transformation of fast twitch, fatigable muscle fibers (type 2) to slow twitch, fatigue-resistant fibers (type 1) [98]. However, changes in anal resting and squeeze pressure have not been consistently reported. Other authors propose that SNS improves rectal sensation and compliance, thus decreasing fecal urgency [99, 100].

Neosphincter procedures are an option for patients with congenital abnormalities, neurogenic incontinence, or those who have failed other repairs. These procedures control continence by mimicking the natural action of the sphincter muscles using a muscle interposition, dynamic graciloplasty, or an inflatable plastic cuff around the anus [artificial bowel sphincter (ABS)]. Controlled clinical trials reveal that either procedure improves continence or quality of life. However, adverse events such as infection, erosion, or ulceration are common [101–103]. The neurotransmitter used to stimulate the gracilis muscle is no longer available in the United States leaving the ABS as the procedure of choice for patients considering a neosphincter.

It is difficult to make comparisons among the procedures listed above. Presently, there are no randomized trials comparing the techniques, identifying one procedure as superior to another. Furthermore, for patients who have intractable fecal incontinence and who have failed other measures permanently, colostomy is a viable option.

Treatment of Outlet Type Constipation

The initial management of patients with complaints of constipation is to exclude organic and anatomic causes, colonic dysmotility, and extraintestinal processes. First-line therapies include bulking agents, laxatives, enemas, and enterokinetic agents. Increased dietary fiber (bulking agents) increases stool weight and frequency of defecation and decreases intestinal transit time in nonconstipated patients. Most symptoms associated with functional constipation can be improved by increasing dietary fiber to 20–30g per day. In some situations, increasing dietary fiber may make symptoms worse, resulting in cramping and flatulence.

Laxatives liquefy stool and increase the propulsive activity, thus overcoming abnormal expulsive forces. Osmotic laxatives include magnesium-containing products, polyethelyene glycol, and nonabsorbable sugars such as lactulose and sorbitol. Through different mechanisms these products increase intraluminal water content and promote bowel activity. Stimulant laxative—senna and bisacodyl—are metabolized by intestinal flora and then increased fluid and electrolyte accumulation in the distal ileum and colon. There are concerns that long-term use of stimulant laxatives harm the

colon and promote dependency and habituation. However, these products may be useful in patients with occasional constipation [104]. Enema use may consist of tap water, saline, or commercially available sodium phosphate combinations. These may be helpful in patients with diminished rectal sensation or megarectum.

Enterokinetic agents increase intestinal motility through various mechanisms. Presently, there are only two commercially available medications: tegaserod and lubiprostone. Tegaserod (Zelnorm) is a 5-hydroxytryptamine agonist that stimulates intestinal motility by facilitating enteric cholinergic transmission. It is FDA approved for women with constipation-predominant IBS and in some studies shows modest effectiveness for chronic constipation in men and women younger than 65 years old [105]. Lubiprostone, a selective type 2 chloride channel activator, accelerates small bowel and colonic transit by activating intestinal chloride channels and increases intestinal fluid secretion without altering serum electrolyte levels. It is approved for patients of all ages with chronic constipation. These medications are fairly new and trials are needed to assess their role in outlet type constipation.

Pelvic floor biofeedback aims at retraining the pelvic floor muscles to relax, strengthening, and sensory training. Uncontrolled studies suggest that approximately 70% of patients with pelvic floor dyssynergia type constipation (paradoxical contraction of the puborectalis) benefit from biofeedback to learn to effectively relax the pelvic floor during defecation [106]. A randomized, controlled trial of biofeedback compared to laxative treatment revealed that five biofeedback sessions are more effective than continuous polyethylene glycol for treating pelvic floor dyssynergia [107]. For patients with dyssynergia who fail conservative measures and biofeedback, there is anecdotal evidence that botulinum toxin injected intramuscularly into the puborectalis provides symptomatic relief [108].

Biofeedback and diet modification for patients with large rectoanal intussusception (occult rectal prolapse) reveal 30% improvement of evacuation symptoms with these noninvasive modalities [109]. Despite the low success rate, biofeedback frequently is offered as first-line therapy for patients with rectoanal intussusception because there is no consensus in the literature as to the benefit of surgical repair. Johnson et al. reports improvement of evacuation symptoms following rectopexy or sigmoid resection and rectopexy [110]. However, other authors report that abdominal rectopexy or mucosal resection are associated with high recurrence rate for constipation [111, 112].

Stapled transanal rectal resection (STARR) is a promising technique specifically for patients with outlet-type constipation and clinical findings of rectal intussusception, rectocele, and mucosal prolapse. STARR is based on the stapled hemorrhoidopexy procedure frequently used by colorectal surgeon for the treatment of hemorrhoids. It employs a double-stapled circumferential full thickness resection of the lower rectum using two proximate PPH-01 stapling guns (Ethicon Endosurgery, Ohio USA). The first staple line is placed anteriorly and reduces the intussusception and the bulging rectocele, correcting the anterior wall defect, and the second staple line is placed posteriorly and is aimed at correcting the intussusception.

Boccasanta et al. report a prospective multicenter trial of 90 patients who underwent the STARR with 100% improvement of constipation symptoms and no complaints of worsening fecal incontinence or dyspareunia. The outcome at 1 year was excellent in 53%, good in 37%, fairly good in 6%, and poor in 4% [113]. Renzi et al. report their results on 14 patients who underwent STARR and a successful outcome was achieved in 90% [114]. At this time there is only limited objective analysis available for the STARR. Contraindications to this procedure include full thickness rectal prolapse, enterocele at rest, the presence of mesh or foreign material adjacent to the rectum, anal incontinence, and proctitis [115].

Rectocele repair for symptomatic outlet-type constipation is discussed in detail earlier in this chapter with a mean improvement of difficult evacuation of 75–80% regardless of transanal or transvaginal techniques [66, 67]. At our institution rectocele repair is performed through the transvaginal route by the urogynecologist, but concomitant rectal pathologies are identified preoperatively and combined procedures are performed if needed.

Sacral nerve stimulation presently is under investigation for use in constipation. As a coincidental finding in patients undergoing sacral nerve stimulation for lower urinary tract dysfunction, many patients experienced an increase in bowel frequency and improved defecation. Ongoing trials suggest modest symptomatic improvement [116, 117].

Treatment of Rectal Prolapse and Combined Pelvic Organ Prolapse

Correction of rectal prolapse can be performed through a perineal, abdominal, or laparoscopic technique. Narrowing the anal canal with encircling devices, Thiersch wire, or its modifications can prevent the prolapse from emerging but does not repair the process and is reserved for patients whose comorbid status is too high for other options [118]. For elderly women, we prefer the perineal approach, while younger, healthier patients are offered abdominal and laparoscopic procedures. The perineal approach can be performed under regional anesthesia and is associated with minimal postoperative pain and avoids the complications and disabilities associated with abdominal surgery.

There are two widely used perineal procedures: mucosal resection (Delorme procedure) and perineal rectosigmoidectomy (Altemeier procedure). The Delorme procedure involves resection of the redundant rectal mucosa and plication of the muscular layer. Perineal rectosigmoidectomy entails full thickness rectal and sigmoid resection through a transanal approach. The addition of levatorplasty is associated with improved fecal continence. Agachan et al. compared the Delorme procedure, perineal rectosigmoidectomy, and perineal rectosigmoidectomy with levatorplasty and found recurrence rates of 38, 13, and 5%, respectively [119]. Postoperative continence was improved in all three procedures, but incontinence scores were lowest for patients who underwent perineal rectosigmoidectomy with levatorplasty. We prefer this procedure for elderly patients with extensive rectal prolapse. However, this is difficult to perform on patients with minimal prolapse or in those whose prolapse is not full thickness in its entire circumference and a modification of the Delorme procedure is offered [120].

Overall, recurrence rates are the lowest with an abdominal procedure at 0–4% [121, 122]. Abdominal rectopexy involves fixation of the rectum to the sacrum with sutures or mesh. Equivalent recurrence and functional improvement rates are reported between open and laparoscopic techniques [123]. There are three major procedures discussed: posterior suture fixation, posterior mesh rectal fixation (Wells or Ripstein), or ventral rectal fixation (Orr-Loygue). Rectopexy alone is preferred for patients with fecal incontinence and rectal prolapse. Sigmoid resection performed in conjunction with sutured rectopexy (Frykman-Goldberg) is frequently performed for patients with preoperative constipation and rectal prolapse [124]. Postoperative constipation is a complication reported with rectopexy and is thought to be associated with denervation injuries caused by division of the lateral rectal ligaments [125]. Portier et al. reports that limited rectal dissection and preservation of the lateral ligaments seems to prevent postoperative constipation without increasing the risk of prolapse recurrence [126]. There is no clear predominant treatment of choice and the results of all abdominal procedures are comparable. Surgeon experience and training dictate the technique preference. There are few reports in the literature discussing combined surgical procedures for rectal and genital prolapse and advocating its effectiveness [127, 128]. In our institution, we perform multicompartment prolapse procedures with a surgical team of both a gynecologist/urogynecologist and colorectal surgeon. Preoperative symptoms, patient comorbidites, and established prolapse recurrence rates factor into the decision-making process. The choice of procedure is individualized for each patient.

References

1. Weber A, Abrams P, Brubaker L, et al. The standardization of terminology for researchers in female pelvic floor disorders. Int Urogynecol J Pelvic Floor Dysfunct 2001; 12(3):178–186.
2. Jelovsek J, Barber M, Paraiso M, Walters M. Functional bowel and anorectal disorders in patients with pelvic organ prolapse and incontinence. Am J Obstet Gynecol 2005; 193(6):2105–2111.
3. Kupfer C, Goligher J. One hundred consecutive cases of complete prolapse of the rectum treated by operation. Br J Surg 1970; 57(7):482–487.
4. Peters W, Smith M, Drescher C. Rectal prolapse in women with other defects of pelvic floor support. Am J Obstet Gynecol 2001; 184(7):1488–1494; discussion 1494–1495.
5. Altman D, Zetterstrom J, Schultz I, et al. Pelvic organ prolapse and urinary incontinence in women with surgically managed rectal prolapse prolapse: A population-based case-control study. Dis Colon Rectum 2005; 49:28–35.
6. Nichols C, Ramakrishnan V, Gill E, Hurt W. Anal incontinence in women with and those without pelvic floor disorders. Obstet Gynecol 2005; 106(6):1266–1271.
7. Sultan AH, Kamm MA, Hudson CN et al. Anal sphincter disruption during vaginal delivery. N Engl J Med 1993;329:64–70.
8. Bliss DZ, Fischer LR, Savik K et al. Severity of fecal incontinence in community-living elderly in a health maintenance organization. Res Nurs Health. 2004; 27:162–173.
9. Siproudhis L, Bellisant E, Juguet F, et al. Rectal adaptation to distension in patients with overt rectal prolapse. Br J Surg 1998; 85:1527–1532.
10. Hiltunen KM, Matikainen MJ, Auvinen O, Hietanen P. Clinical and manometric evaluation of anal sphincter function in patients with rectal prolapse. Am J Surg 1986; 151:489–492.
11. Kairaluoma MV, Kellokumpu IH. Epidemiologic aspects of complete rectal prolapse. Scand J Surg 2005; 94:207–210.
12. Weber A, Walters M, Ballard L, et al. Posterior vaginal wall prolapse and bowel function. Am J Obstet Gynecol 1998; 179:1446–1450.
13. Ellerkmann R, Cundiff G, Melik C, et al. Correlation of symptoms with location and severity of pelvic organ prolapse. Am J Obstet Gynecol 2001; 185:1332–1338.
14. Kahn M, Breitkopf C, Valley M, et al. Pelvic organ support study and bowel symptoms: Straining at stool is associated with perineal and anterior vaginal descent in a general gynecologic populations. Am J Obstet Gynecol 2002; 192:1516–1522.
15. da Silva G, Gurland B, Sleemi A, Levy G. Posterior vaginal wall prolapse does not correlate with fecal symptoms or objective measures of anorectal function. Am J Obstet Gynecol 2006; 195(6): 1742–1747.
16. Bump R, Mattiasson A, Bo K, et al. The standardization of terminology of female pelvic organ prolapse and pelvic floor dysfunction. Am J Obstet Gynecol 1996; 175:10–17.
17. Altman D, Lopez A, Kierkegaard J, et al. Assessment of posterior vaginal wall prolapse: Comparison of physical findings to cystodefecoperitoneography. Int Urogynecol J 2005; 16:96–103.
18. Brubaker L, Baker R, Jacquentin B, et al. Pelvic organ prolapse. In: Abrams P, Cardozo L, Khoury S, Wein AJ, eds. 2nd International consultation on

incontinence. Plymouth, UK: Health Publication, 2002:243–265.

19. Strohbelm K. Normal pelvic floor anatomy. Obstet Gynecol Clin North Am 1998; 25:683–705.

20. Leffler KS, Thompson JR, et al. Attachment of the rectal vaginal septum to the pelvic sidewalls Am J Gynecol 2001; 185:41–43.

21. Richardson AC. The anatomic defects in rectocele and enterocele. J Pelvic Surg 1995; 4:214–221.

22. Levi A, Borghi F, Garavoglia M. Development of the anal canal muscles. Dis Colon Rectum 1990; 34:262–266.

23. Lester B, Penninckx F, Kerremans R. The composition of anal basal pressure. An in vivo and in vitro study in man. Int J Colorectal Dis 1989; 4: 118–122.

24. Gibbons CP, Trowbridge EA, Bannister JJ, Read NW. Role of anal cushions in maintaining continence. Lancet 1986; 1:886–887.

25. Rothbarth J, Bemelman W, Meijerink W, et al. What is the impact of fecal incontinence on quality of life? Dis Colon Rectum 2001; 44:67–71.

26. Barber MD, Walters MD, Bump RC. Short forms of two condition-specific quality of life questionnaires for women with pelvic floor disorders (PFDI-20 and PFISQ-7). Am J Obstet Gynecol 2005; 193: 103–113.

27. Rogers RG, Coates KW, Kammerer-Doak DN, et al. A short form of the pelvic organ prolapse/ urinary incontinence sexual questionnaire (PISQ-12). Int Urogynecol J Pelvic Floor Dysfunct 14(3): 164–168.

28. Rao SS, Patel RS. How useful are manometric tests of anorectal functions in the management of defecation disorders? Am J Gastroenterol 1997; 92:469–475.

29. Jorge J, Wexner S. A practical guide to basic anorectal physiology investigations. Contemp Surg 1996; 43:214–224.

30. Ahran P, Faverdin C, Persoz B, et al. Relationship between viscoelastic properties of the rectum and anal pressures in man. J Appl Physio 1976;41:677–704.

31. Rasmussen O. Anorectal function. Dis Colon Rectum 1994; 37:386–403.

32. Hancke E, Schurholz M. Impaired rectal sensation in idiopathic fecal incontinence. Int J Colorectal Dis 1987; 2:146–148.

33. Hill J, Hosker G, Kiff E. Pudendal nerve terminal motor latency measurements: What they do and do not tell us. Br J Surg 2002; 89:1268–1269.

34. Ricciardi R, Mellgren AF, Madoff RD, et al. The utility of pudendal nerve terminal latencies in idiopathic incontinence. Dis Colon Rectum 2006; 49:852–857.

35. Gilliland R, Altomare D, Moreira H, et al. Pudendal neuropathy is predictive of failure following anterior overlapping sphincteroplasty. Dis Colon Rectum 1998; 41:1516–1522.

36. Zetterstrom J, Mellgren A, Madoff R, et al. Perineal body measurements improves evaluation of anterior sphincter lesions during endoanal ultrasonography. Dis Colon Rectum 1998; 41:705–713.

37. Oberwalder M, Thaler K, Baig M, et al. Anal ultrasound and endosonographic measurements of perineal body thickness: A new evaluation for fecal incontinence in females. Surg Endosc 2004; 18:650–654.

38. Sleemi A, Levy G, Gurland B. Correlation between perineal body measurements and anal sphincter defect in patients with fecal Incontinence. Abstract presented at the Society for Gynecologic Surgeons (SGS), 31st Scientific Meeting, California, April 2005.

39. Jorge J, Habr-Gama A, Wexner S. Clinical applications and techniques of cinedefecography. Am J Surg 2001; 182:93–101.

40. Thompson J, Chen A, Pettit P, Bridges M. Incidence of occult rectal prolapse in patients with clinical rectoceles and defecatory dysfunction. Am J Obstet Gynecol 2002; 187:1494–1500.

41. Mellgren A, Johansson C, Dolk A, et al. Enterocele demonstrated by defaecography is associated with other pelvic floor disorders. Int J Colorect Dis 1994; 9:121–124.

42. Matsuoka H, Wexner SD, Desai MB, et al. A comparison between dynamic pelvic magnetic resonance imaging and videoproctography in patients with constipation. Dis Colon Rectum 2001; 44:571–576.

43. Roos F, Weishaupt D, Wildermuth S, et al. Experience of four years with open MR defecography: Pictorial review of anorectal anatomy and disease. RadioGraphics 2002; 22:817–832.

44. Mellgren A, Anzen B, Nilsson BY, et al. Results of rectocele repair: A prospective study. Dis Colon Rectum 1995; 38:7–13.

45. Milley S, Nichols D. A correlative investigation of the human rectovaginal septum. Anat Rec 1969; 163:443–451.

46. Richardson AC. The rectovaginal septum revisited: Its relationship to rectocele and its importance in rectocele repair. Clin Obstet Gynecol 1993; 36: 976–983.

47. Kahn M, Stanton S. Posterior colporrhaphy: Its effects on bowel and sexual function. Br J Gynecol 1997; 104:82–86.

48. Lopez A, Anzen B, Bremmer S, et al. Durability of success after rectocele repair. Int Urogynecol J 2001; 12:97–103.

49. Francis W, Jeffcoate T. Dyspareunia following vaginal operations. J Obstet Gynecol Br Comnwlth 1961; 68:1–10.

50. Singh K, Cortes E, Reid W. Evaluation of the fascial technique for surgical repair of isolated posterior vaginal wall prolapse. Obstet Gynecol 2003; 101:320–324.

51. Maher C, Qatawneh A, Baessler K, Schluter P. Midline rectovaginal fascia plication for repair of rectocele and obstructed defecation. Obstet Gynecol 2004; 104:685–689.

52. Bartolami C, Shetty V, Milavec J, et al. Preparation and evaluation of nonproprietary bilayer skin substitute. Plast Reconstr Surg 1991; 87:1089–1098.

53. Ruiz-Torres A. Cross-linking of collagen depending on age. Gerontology 1978; 24:337–342.

54. Hayflick L. The cell biology of aging. Clin Geriatr Med 1985; 1:15–27.

55. Mays P, McAnulty R, Campa J, et al. Similar age related alterations in collagen metabolism in rat tissues in vivo and fibroblasts in vitro. Biochem Soc Trans 1990; 18:957.

56. Altman D, Mellgren A, Blomgren B, et al. Clinical and histological safety assessment of rectocele repair using collagen mesh. Acta Obstet Gynecol Scand 2004; 83:995–1000.

57. Kohli N, Miklos JR. Dermal graft- augmented rectocele repair. Int Urogynecol J (2003) 14:146–149.

58. Altman D, Zetterstrom J, Mellgren A, et al. A three year prospective assessment of rectocele repair using porcine xenograft. Obstet Gynecol 2006; 107:59–65.

59. Petros P. Vault prolapse11: restoration of dynamic vaginal support by infracoccygeal sacropexy: An axial day case vaginal procedure. Int Urogynecol J 2001; 12:296–303.

60. Salvatore S, Soligo M, Meschia M, et al. Prosthetic surgery for genital prolapse: Functional outcome. Neurourol Urodyn 2002; 21:296–297.

61. de Tayrac R, Picone O, Chauveaud-Lambling A, Fernandez H. A 2 year anatomical and functional assessment of transvaginal rectocele repair using a polypropylene mesh. Int Urogynecol J 2006; 17:100–105.

62. Rosato GO. Rectocele and perineal hernias. In: Beck DE, Wexner SD, eds. Fundamentals of anorectal surgery, Second ed. London: W.B. Saunders Company. 1998:187–197.

63. Tjandra JJ, Ooi BS, Tang CL, et al. Transanal repair of rectocele corrects obstructed defecation if it is not associated with anismus. Dis Colon Rectum 1999; 42:1544–1549.

64. Altomare D, Rinaldi M, Veglia A, et al. Combined perineal and endorectal repair of rectocele by circular stapler: A novel surgical technique. Dis Colon Rectum 2002; 45:1549–1552.

65. Stojkovic S, Balfour L, Burke D, et al. Does the need to self-digitate or the presence of a large or nonemptying rectocele on proctography influence the outcome of transanal rectocele repair? Colorectal Disease 2003; 5:169–172.

66. Nieminen K, Hiltunen K, Laitinen J, et al. Transanal or vaginal approach to rectocele repair; results of prospective randomized study. Neurourol Urodyn 2003; 22:547–548.

67. Kahn M, Stanton S, Kumar D, Fox SD. Posterior colporrhaphy is superior to the transanal repair for treatment of posterior vaginal wall prolapse. Neurourol Urodyn 1999; 18:70–71.

68. Watson S, Loder P, Halligan S, et al. Transperineal repair of symptomatic rectocele with Marlex mesh: A clinical, physiological and radiologic assessment of treatment. J Am Coll Surg 183:257–261.

69. Parker M, Phillips R. Repair of rectocele using Marlex mesh. Ann R Coll Surg Engl 75:193–194.

70. Lyons T, Winer W. Laproscopic rectocele repair using polyglactin mesh. J Am AssocGynecol Laparosc 1997; 4:381–384.

71. Cundiff GW, Harris RL, Coates K, et al. Abdominal sacral colpoperineopexy: A new approach for correction of posterior compartment defects and perineal descent associated with vaginal vault prolapse. Am J Obstet Gynecol 1997; 177:1345–1355.

72. Fox SD, Stanton SL. Vault prolapse and rectocele: Assessment of repair using sacrocolpopexy with mesh interposition. BJOG 2000; 107:1371–1375.

73. Sullivan E, Longaker C, Lee P. Total pelvic mesh repair: A ten-year experience. Dis Colon Rectum 2001; 44:857–863.

74. Hallban J. Operative gynecology. Berlin, Urban and Schwarzenberg, 1932:172.

75. Moschcowitz A. The pathogenesis, anatomy and cure of prolapse of the rectum. Surg Gynecol Obstet 1912; 15:7–14.

76. Webb M, Aronson M, Ferguson L, et al. Posthysterectomy vaginal vault prolapse: Primary repair in 693 patients. Obstet Gynecol 1998; 92: 281–285.

77. Shull B, Bachofen C, Coates K, Kuehl T. A transvaginal approach to repair of apical and other associated sites of pelvic organ prolapse with uterosacral ligaments. Am J Obstet Gynecol 2000; 183: 1365–1374.

78. Karram M, Goldwasser S, Kleeman S, et al. High uterosacral vaginal vault suspension with fascial reconstruction for vaginal repair of enterocele and vaginal vault prolapse. Am J Obstet Gynecol 2001; 185:1339–1343.

79. Richardson A. The anatomic defects in rectocele and enterocele. J Pelvic Surg 1995; 1:214–221.

80. Miklos J, Kohli N, Lucente V, Saye W. Site-specific fascial defects in the diagnosis and surgical management of enterocele. Am J Obstet Gynecol 1998; 179:1418–1423.

81. Cheetham M, Brazzelli M, Norton C, Glazener C. Drug treatment for faecal incontinence in adults. Cochrane Database Syst Rev 2003; 3:1–67.

82. Guillemot F, Bouche B, Gower-Rousseau C, et al. Biofeedback for the treatment of fecal incontinence. Dis Colon Rectum 1994; 38:393–397.

83. Norton C, Cody J, Hosker G. Biofeedback and/or sphincter exercises for the treatment of faecal incontinence in adults. Cochran Database Syst Rev 2006; 3:CD002111.

84. Vaizey C, Kamm M. Injectable bulking agents for treating faecal incontinence. Br J Surg 2005; 92:521–527.

85. Efron J, Corman M, Fleshman J., et al. Safety and effectiveness of temperature controlled radiofrequency delivery to the anal canal (SECCA procedure) for the treatment of fecal incontinence. Dis Colon Rectum 2003; 46:1606–1618.

86. F Nichols C, Gill E, Nguyen T, et al. Anal sphincter injury in women with pelvic floor disorders. Obstet Gynecol. 2004; 104:690–696.

87. Halverson A, Hull T, Paraiso M, Floruta C. Outcome of sphincteroplasty combined with surgery for urinary incontinence and pelvic organ prolapse. Dis Colon Rectum 2001; 44:1421–1426.

88. Steele S, Lee P, Mullenix P, et al. Is there a role for concomitant pelvic floor repair in patients with sphincter defects in the treatment of fecal incontinence. Int J Colorectal Dis 2006; 21:508–514.

89. Fernando R, Sultan A, Kettle C, et al. Methods of repair for obstetric anal sphincter injury. Cochrane Database Syst Rev 2006; 3:CD002866.

90. Fernando R, Sultan A, Kettle C, et al. Repair techniques for obstetric anal sphincter injuries: A randomized controlled trial. Obstet Gynecol 2006; 107(6):1261–1268.

91. Zorcolo L, Covotta L, Bartolo C. Outcome of anterior sphincter repair for obstetric injury: Comparison of early and late results. Dis Colon Rectum 2005; 48:524–531.

92. L Halverson A, Hull T. Long-term outcome of overlapping anal sphincter repair. Dis Colon Rectum 2002; 45:345–348.

93. Chen A, Luchtefeld, Senagore A, et al. Pudendal nerve latency: Does it predict outcome of anal sphincter repair? Dis Colon Rectum 1998; 41:1005–1009.

94. Matsuoka H, Mavrantonis C, Wexner S, et al. Postanal repair for fecal incontinence—Is it worthwhile? Dis Colon Rectum 2000; 43:1561–1567.

95. Rosen HR, Urbarz C, Holzer B, et al. Sacral nerve stimulation as a treatment for fecal incontinence. Gastroenterology 2001; 121:536–541.

96. Malouf AJ, Vaizey CJ, Nicholls RJ et al. Permanent sacral nerve stimulation for fecal incontinence. Ann Surg 2000; 232:143–148.

97. Ganio E, Ratto C, Masin A, et al. Neuromodulation for fecal incontinence: Outcome in 16 patients with definitive implant. The initial Italian sacral neurostimulation group(GINS) experience. Dis Colon Rectum 2001; 44:965–970.

98. Matzel K, Stadelmaier U, Hohenfellner M, et al. Electrical stimulation of sacral spinal nerves for treatment of fecal incontinence. Lancet 1995; 346:1124–1127.

99. Leroi A, Parc Y, Lehur P, et al. Efficacy of sacral nerve stimulation for fecal incontinence Ann Surg 2005; 242:662.

100. Kenefick NJ, Vaizey CJ, Cohen RC, et al. Medium term results of permanent sacral nerve stimulation for fecal incontinence. Br J Surg 2002; 89:896–901.

101. Baeten C, Bailey R, Bakka A, et al. Safety and efficacy of dynamic graciloplasty for fecal incontinence. Dis Colon Rectum 2000; 43:743–751.

102. O'Brien P, Dixon J, Skinner S, et al. A prospective, randomized, controlled clinical trial of placement of the artificial bowel sphincter (acticon neosphincter) for the control of fecal incontinence. Dis Colon Rectum 2004; 47:1852–1860.

103. Mundy L, Merlin T, Maddern G, Hiller J. Systematic review of safety and effectiveness of an artificial bowel sphincter for faecal incontinence. BJS 2004; 91:665–672.

104. Wald A. Outlet dysfunction constipation. Gastroenterology 2001; 4:293–297.

105. Johanson J, Wald A, Tougas G, et al. Effect of tegaserod in chronic constipation: A randomized, double blind, controlled trial. Clin Gastroenterol Hepatol 2004; 2:796–805.

106. Heyman S, Jones K, Scarlett Y, Whitehead W. Biofeedback treatment of constipation a critical review. Dis Colon Rectum 2003; 46:1208–1217.

107. Chiarioni G, Whitehead W, Pezza V, et al. Biofeedback is superior to laxatives for normal transit constipation due to pelvic floor dyssynergia. Gastroenterology 2006; 130:657–664.

108. Hallan R, Williams N, Melling J, et al. Treatment of anismus in intractable constipation with botulinum toxin. Lancet 1988; 24:714–717.

109. Mimura T, Roy AJ, Storrie JB, Kamm MA. Treatment of impaired defecation associated with rectocele by behavioral retraining (biofeedback) DCR 2000; 43:1267–1272.

110. Johnson E, Carlsen E, Mjaland O, Drolsum A. Resection rectopexy for internal rectal intussuscep-

tion reduces constipation and incomplete evacuation of stool. Eur J Surg 2002; 588 (Suppl):51–56.

111. Brown A, Anderson J, McKee R, Finlay I. Surgery for occult rectal prolapse. Colorect Dis 2004; 6: 176–179.

112. Pescatori M, Boffi F, Russo A, Zbar AP. Complication and recurrence after excision of rectal internal mucosal prolapse for obstructed defecation (oral presentation). EACP Annual Meeting, September 17, 2004.

113. Boccasanta P, Venturi M, Stuto A, et al. Stapled transanal rectal resection for outlet obstruction: A prospective, multicenter trial. Dis Colon Rectum 2004; 47:1285–1297.

114. Renzi A, Izzo D, Di Sarno G, et al. Stapled transanal rectal resection to treat obstructed defecation caused by rectal intussusception and rectocele. Int J Colorectal Dis 2006; 21:661–667.

115. L Corman M, Carriero A, Hager T, et al. Consensus conference on stapled transanal rectal resection (STARR) for disordered defaecation. Colorectal Dis 2006; 8:98–101.

116. Ganio E, Masin A, Ratto C, et al. Short term sacral nerve stimulation for functional anorectal and urinary disturbances: Results in 40 patients. Dis Colon Rectum 2001; 44:1261–1267.

117. Keneflick NJ, Nichols RJ, Cohen RG, Kamm MA. Permanent sacral nerve stimulation for treatment of idiopathic constipation. Br J Surg 2002; 89:882–888.

118. Khanduja K, Hardy T, Aguilar P, et al. A new silicone prosthesis in the modified Thiersch operation. Dis Colon Rectum 198; 31:380–383.

119. Agachan F, Reissman P, Pfeifer J, et al. Comparison of three perineal procedures for the treatment of rectal prolapse. South Med J 1997; 90:925–932.

120. Madiba T, Maig M, Wexner S. Surgical management of rectal prolapse. Arch Surg 2005; 140: 63–73.

121. Briel JW, Chouten WR, Boerma MO. Long term results of suture rectopexy in patients with fecal incontinence associated with incomplete rectal prolapse. Dis Colon Rectum 1997; 40:1228–1232.

122. Khanna AK, Misra MK, Kumar K. Simplified sutured sacral rectopexy for complete rectal prolapse in adults. Eur J Surg 1996; 162:143–146.

123. Kariv Y, Delaney C, Casillas S, et al. Long-term outcome after laparoscopic and open surgery for rectal prolapse. Surg Endosc 2006; 20:35–42.

124. Frykman HM, Goldberg SM. The surgical treatment of rectal procidentia. Surg Gynecol Obstet 1969; 129:1225–1230.

125. Mollen RM, Kuijupers HC, van Hoek. Effects of rectal mobilization and lateral ligament division on colonic and anorectal function. Dis Colon Rectum 2000; 43:1283–1287.

126. Portier G, Iovino F, Lazorthes F. Surgery for rectal prolapse: Orr-Loygue ventral rectopexy with limited dissection prevents postoperative induced constipation without increasing recurrence. Dis Colon Rectum 2006; 49:1136–1140.

127. Ayav A, Bresler L, Brunaud L, et al. Surgical management of combined rectal and genital prolapse in young patients: Transabdominal approach. Int J Colorectal Dis 2005; 20:173–179.

128. Dekel A, Rabinerson D, Ben Rafael Z, et al. Concurrent genital and rectal prolapse: Two pathologies-one joint operation. BJOG 2000; 107(1):125–129.

Part VI
Management of Male Incontinence

Chapter 28
Primary Urge Incontinence

Craig V. Comiter

Introduction

Urinary incontinence affects up to 30% of community-dwelling individuals over the age of 65 and up to 50% of nursing home residents [1, 2]. This morbid and costly condition is often responsible for the institutionalization of the frail elderly, as incontinence predisposes to skin breakdown, urinary tract infections, falls, and hip fractures [3]. Furthermore, the patient often succumbs to embarrassment, leading to social isolation and depression [4, 5]. While urgency incontinence (UI) may affect only one third of patients who suffer from the overactive bladder (OAB) syndrome, it is the most common type of incontinence in adults and has an even greater negative impact on quality of life than does stress urinary incontinence (SUI) and OAB [6, 7].

With SUI, there is no effective pharmacotherapy, yet surgical intervention often is minimally invasive, efficacious, and with low morbidity. In contrast, the ideal therapy for UI is not agreed upon. Behavioral modification and biofeedback can be efficacious in mild to moderate cases but are labor-intensive with unproven durability. Multiple pharmacotherapeutic agents are available and approved for OAB and UI, but their expense, limited efficacy, and substantial side effect profile limit their utility, especially in older men on fixed incomes.

UI in older adults involves more than simply the presence of an OAB. Physical function, cognitive function, and medications are important for continence. A substantial proportion of men with UI have a combination of both "storage" and "voiding" symptoms. Although voiding symptoms are most common in older men, storage symptoms are most bothersome (especially UI) and interfere the most with activities of daily life. UI in males, just as in females, usually is related to an inability to store urine due to bladder dysfunction. However, the presence of a potentially obstructing prostate confounds the situation. In women, OAB can be diagnosed based on history, physical examination, and urinalysis, and treatment usually can be initiated with a trial of behavioral modification, pelvic floor exercises, and anitmuscarinic medications. In men with UI, however, consideration must be given to the possibility of an obstructed outlet, which can have a substantial effect on the evaluation and the treatment of UI. Regardless of the etiology, however, the goal of treatment is to alleviate symptoms, prevent clinical deterioration, and improve quality of life.

Nomenclature

In order to best discuss the prevalence, evaluation, treatment, and complications associated with various urinary disorders of storage and emptying, it is important to categorize and properly label the various symptoms, signs, and diagnoses associated with voiding dysfunction. This is best done by utilizing the nomenclature provided by the International Continence Society standardization subcommittee [8].

Symptoms

Storage symptoms are those symptoms experienced during the storage phase of the bladder. Examples of storage symptoms include daytime frequency, nocturia, increased bladder sensation, urgency and UI. Urinary incontinence has been simplified and redefined as "the complaint of any involuntary leakage of urine." Urge urinary *incontinence* is defined as "the complaint of involuntary leakage (of urine) accompanied by or immediately proceeded by urgency." Urgency is recognized by the International Continence Society as "the complaint of a sudden compelling desire to pass urine, which is difficult to defer." Voiding symptoms are experienced during the voiding phase and include complaints of a slow or intermittent stream, hesitancy, straining, split stream, or terminal dribbling. These symptomatic terms are descriptive, should be thought of as the patient's complaints, and should not be used to make a definitive diagnosis.

Signs

Signs are observed by the examiner and are useful to verify and quantify the various lower urinary tract symptoms (LUTS). Urodynamic observations (such as detrusor overactivity, increased bladder sensation, and elevated voiding pressure) are indicated to help explain LUTS, and similar to symptoms do not represent a definitive diagnosis or condition.

Urodynamic observations may help to explain the symptoms but do not represent a definitive diagnosis, disease, or condition. Whether these observations are made during filling cystometry, urethral pressure profilometry, voiding profilometry, or pressure-flow studies, the urodynamics are only useful if they reproduce the patients' symptoms. For example, if a patient complains of urgency and UI, a urodynamic evaluation that reveals poor sensation and absent bladder contraction is not particularly useful in formulating a diagnosis to explain the patient's condition.

Increased bladder sensation is defined as "an early desire to void and/or an early strong desire to void, which occurs at low bladder volume and persists." Bladder compliance is the relationship between changes in bladder volume per change in detrusor pressure. While the International Continence Society does not define normal values for bladder sensation and compliance, at the author's institution the normal male usually tolerates at least 300 cc of water or saline without an uncomfortable urge and demonstrates compliance greater than 30 cc cm^{-1} water pressure. Detrusor overactivity (DO) is a urodynamic observation characterized by involuntary detrusor contractions (either spontaneous or provoked) during filling cystometry and may or may not be associated with incontinence. Although the specific change in pressure may depend on the strength of the bladder contraction and the resistance of the outlet, when the change in detrusor pressure is equivocal, video is often helpful to demonstrate a change in vesicular shape, thereby confirming the unstable bladder contraction. Phasic DO is characterized by an oscillating pressure wave during cystometry, while terminal DO comprises a single involuntary detrusor contraction occurring at capacity, resulting in incontinence. DO can be classified as "neurogenic" when a neurological condition is thought to cause the detrusor overactivity or idiopathic when involuntary detrusor contractions occur in the absence of a defined neurological cause.

Detrusor hyperactivity with impaired contractility (DHIC) occurs when the bladder is overactive (DO) but empties inefficiently. This impaired emptying is associated with diminished detrusor contractile function, of slow velocity, with little detrusor reserve power, and a significant amount of residual urine. DHIC may in fact represent a more advanced stage in the natural history of DO, characterized by deterioration of detrusor contractility [9].

Diagnoses

Bladder outlet obstruction (BOO) is the generic term for obstructed voiding, characterized on urodynamics by increased detrusor pressure and reduced urine flow rate. While no particular voiding pressure at maximum urinary flow rate defines obstruction, various nomograms are useful to define obstructed urination using a model of turbulent flow through a collapsible tube. One must realize that mathematical BOO is not identical to clinical BOO. Since an obstructing prostate and a decompensated bladder often may coexist, BOO should be thought of as a term to describe the relationship between the bladder and the outlet. For example, a weak (decompensated) detrusor may be relatively obstructed by a normal prostate, just as a normal bladder may be obstructed by an overly restrictive or compressive prostate.

Benign prostatic hyperplasia (BPH) often is an inappropriately used term, which actually describes the typical histopathological pattern of increased glandular or stromal growth of the prostate, and increases in prevalence with increasing age (Fig. 28.1). Histology (often seen only following surgery or autopsy) does not correlate well with symptoms, signs, or urodynamics. In fact, only 25–50% of men with histological BPH have bothersome LUTS [10]. Benign prostatic enlargement (BPE) refers to enlargement of the gland due to histological benign prostatic hyperplasia. Benign prostatic obstruction (BPO) is one type of bladder outlet obstruction. BPO is diagnosed when the cause of BOO is known to be related to BPE, due to histological BPH. Urological lore often recognizes these "presumptive diagnostic terms" as definitive. However, proper use of terminology can avoid significant confusion, and along with accurate diagnostic tests can lead to rational treatment of LUTS, potentially avoiding unnecessary and often inefficacious pharmacotherapy and surgery.

Pathophysiology

Normal Storage and Voiding

The ability to eliminate metabolic toxins via liquid waste has gone through millions of years of evolutionary change. However, since passing urine can leave a visual and olfactory footprint, thereby alerting the predator to the recent position of the prey, it is selectively advantageous to the organism to store urine for prolonged periods of time and void episodically [11]. In some species, coaptive evolution has linked micturition with the advantageous behavior of marking a territory or even determining social status and reproductive rights [11].

As passing urine can leave the organism vulnerable, it is necessary for the mature animal to store urine for prolonged periods of time, while voiding only episodically. Storage occurs at low pressure in a compliant bladder (thus preserving renal function), without unstable bladder contractions and without unpleasant sensations. Voiding normally occurs via a reflex contraction of the bladder, coordinated with a relaxed outlet, typically until the bladder is empty.

Normal storage relies on the inhibitory input to the bladder supplied by the sympathetic neurons originating in the thoracic and lumbar spinal segments and the excitatory input to the bladder

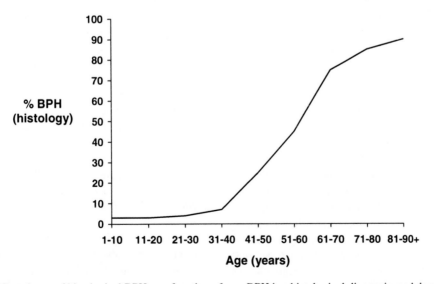

FIG. 28.1. Prevalence of histological BPH as a function of age. BPH is a histological diagnosis, and does not necessarily equate with symptoms, signs, or urodynamic findings

outlet. Together, these efferent pathways contribute to normal storage. The "guarding reflex," which occurs during normal bladder filling, is triggered by bladder afferent nerves that project to the sacral cord, which synapse with interneurons, which in turn activate the urethral external sphincter efferents (via the pudendal nerve); this facilitates urine storage [12].

Normal voiding relies on excitatory efferent input to the bladder. Sacral parasympathetic preganglionic fibers travel in the pelvic nerve and provide the bulk of the excitatory efferent input to the bladder. Preganglionic neurons synapse within the parasympathetic ganglion near the detrusor. The postganglionic neurons (parasympathetic) provide excitation to the smooth muscle of the bladder primarily via acetylcholine release. Acetycholine then attaches to the muscarinic receptors, mediating bladder contraction. The two predominant muscarinic receptors responsible for bladder contraction are the M3 and M2 subtypes. It appears that in the normal bladder, M3 receptor agonism is mostly responsible for the bladder contraction, while M2 agonism plays a secondary role via reversal of β-adrenergic mediated relaxation. However, in the spinal cord-injured rodent [13] and in the rodent with an obstructed bladder [14], M2 activation has been shown to play a more dominant role in mediating bladder contraction.

What makes the bladder unique among the viscera is the conscious control and inhibition over urination. While the immature human relies on reflex voiding, mediated by bladder tension receptors triggering a reflex bladder contraction through the sacral micturition center, the mature human normally has the ability to consciously delay urination until socially appropriate.

Several reflexes assist complete evacuation in the normal state: amplification, in which a weak smooth muscle signal from the bladder can be augmented to ensure an efficient contraction; coordination, whereby the bladder contraction and sphincteric relaxation occur concomitantly until the bladder is empty; and timing, so that volitional voiding can be initiated at different bladder volumes under conditions of varying degrees of urgency. Amplification occurs through a "bladder—bladder" reflex. Bladder afferents synapse with the sacral cord interneurons, which in turn synapse with bladder efferent parasympathetics.

Positive feedback then activates more afferent firing and more reflex efferent activity [15]. Bladder afferents also influence urethral smooth muscle relaxation ("bladder—urethra" reflex), via inhibitory reflexes [16]. The pontine micturition center is responsible for maintaining and coordinating outlet relaxation with the bladder contraction. Taken together, amplification and coordination permit volitional voiding over a wide range of bladder volumes, with varying degrees of urgency.

Urgency and Urge Incontinence

The complex excitatory and inhibitory reflex mechanisms that regulate normal voiding also can be a liability. Various disease processes can lead to the emergence of bladder hyperactivity and incontinence, with loss of volitional control over the micturition reflex. Although most easily thought of as an inability to store urine due to the bladder, it is useful to categorize this pathophysiology according to neurogenic, myogenic, intravesical, and extravesical.

Neurogenic

OAB can result from the loss of the central inhibitory controls via injury/disorder of the brain or suprasacral spinal cord. Examples of brain disorders leading to UI include cerebrovascular accident, Parkinson's disease, and dementia. Disruption of axonal pathways within the spinal cord includes transverse myelitis, traumatic suprasacral myelopathy, cervical spondylosis, and multiple sclerosis [17] (which can affect the brain as well). Other neurological abnormalities include increased afferent nerve input and loss of peripheral inhibition. An example of an abnormal sensitization of bladder afferent input is the emergence of abnormal C-fiber activity. Normally, in the mature adult, bladder sensation is mediated through tension receptors acting via A-delta myelinated neurons. The unmyelinated afferent C-fiber nociceptors are normally quiescent during bladder filling. Various insults can lead the nociceptors to become mechanosensitive with decreased activation thresholds, such as inflammation or outlet obstruction. Inappropriate C-fiber activation can mediate increased neurotransmission to and within the sacral cord, thereby leading to bladder muscle overactivity.

Recent evidence supports a neurogenic etiology of UI due to DO in men with BOO. Nerve growth factor (NGF) levels are elevated in bladders of men with BOO and in men with OAB. It has been demonstrated that specific blockade of NGF prevents neural plasticity and bladder overactivity in experimental models of BOO and OAB [18, 19]. NGF mediates DO by altering the properties of sodium and potassium channels in bladder afferent neurons. Furthermore, NGF upregulates TRPV1 in sensory fibers and brings this receptor from an inactive into an active configuration, further mediating urgency and UI [20, 21].

Myogenic

Changes in the bladder itself, including in the detrusor muscle, also can contribute to UI, either with or without BOO. Interstitial cells have long been known to exist in the ureter, contributing to automatic peristaltic activity, which helps to propel the urine from the renal pelvic to the bladder. Such pacemaker cells also are present in the suburothelial urethra and bladder body. These are electrically active cells, which can communicate via gap junctions and appear to respond to ATP as the main neurotransmitter [22].

In addition, suburothelial spindle cells known as myofibroblasts lie in close apposition with bare nerve endings and communicate with detrusor muscle cells via gap junctions, creating a "functional syncytium." These mechanoreceptors are activated by stretch [23]. Alterations in these cells, as well as increased abutment junctions among detrusor muscle cells which can occur with normal aging, can contribute to increased detrusor activity and UI [24].

Recent evidence supports a myogenic component (in addition to the aforementioned neurogenic component) of DO in men with BOO. Akari et al. [25] demonstrated that epithelial sodium channels (which are expressed in the bladder epithelium) contribute to mechanosensory transduction in the bladder afferent pathways. The expression of the sodium channels is increased in men with BOO and in fact correlates with storage symptoms in men with BOO [26]. In addition, urinary levels of PGE2 were shown to be elevated in men with BOO and normal detrusor contractility compared to those with BOO and detrusor underactivity;

it also was shown that PGE2 levels in the urine were negatively correlated with maximum bladder capacity. In addition, partial denervation of the bladder smooth muscle leads to an increase in the number of spontaneous action potentials [27]. Even in the absence of BOO, normal aging is associated with replacement of the normal intermediate cell junctions with an increase in protrusion junctions and abutment junctions, which allow these spontaneous action potentials to propagate from cell to cell [28].

Intravesical

Occasionally, the cause of UI may be due to an intravesical reversible process. Bladder stones often will present with both storage and voiding symptoms. Stones may be associated with BOO due to prostatic obstruction or may be secondary to nonobstructive urinary stasis. The space-occupying stone lies within the bladder lumen, thereby diminishing functional urinary capacity. In addition, the contact between the stone and the bladder wall can lead to increased afferent stimulation of the bladder, which can contribute to UI. Finally, the BOO associated with bladder stones in turn can lead to the neurogenic and myogenic changes outlined above.

Carcinoma in situ may be associated with irritative storage symptoms, including UI. In men with UI in the absence of voiding symptoms, especially in the presence of microscopic or gross hematuria, cystoscopy and bladder barbotage (and possible bladder biopsy) are indicated to rule out carcinoma in situ.

Acute urinary tract infection also can mediate UI. This should be readily detected by urinalysis and urine culture. One must be aware, however, that bacteriuria is common in older adults and may be coincidentally present in an individual with UI, rather than directly causing the UI. That said, a trial of antibiotics is indicated as an initial treatment in patients with UI and bacteriuria.

Extravesical

There are some factors that may contribute to UI which are separate from (yet often related to) bladder function. In the UUI patient, there often is a component of pelvic floor dysfunction. Volitional pelvic floor muscular contraction provides an inhibitory input (via a sacral cord reflex) to the bladder, suppressing an involuntary detrusor contraction [29]. Thus one patient may be wet with an unstable bladder contraction of 15 cm water, while another may be dry despite an unstable bladder contraction of 40 cm water. The former patient cannot adequately recruit the pelvic floor muscles into a coordinated contraction of appropriate magnitude to suppress the unstable bladder activity. Thus, it is logical that Kegel exercises (when correctly taught and performed) can be so successful in treating UUI. Strengthening the pelvic floor muscles and reestablishing voluntary control over the pelvic floor can help to suppress the detrusor overactivity, hence preventing UUI. SUI also can contribute directly to UI. In patients with stress incontinence, leakage of urine into the proximal urethra can activate urethral afferents and facilitate voiding reflexes, thereby contributing to DO and UI [30].

Additional factors that may contribute to UI in older men are those related to urine production and toileting. Clearly, demented or delirious patients may not have the cognitive faculties to be aware of their environs and may engage in socially inappropriate urination. Restricted mobility also may contribute to UUI. While the man may be aware of his urge to void and may even be able to voluntarily contract his pelvic floor, slow movement or the need for travel assistance can lead the patient to succumb to the unstable bladder contraction. In addition, disorders of urine production can "overwhelm" the bladder. Polydypsia clearly causes polyuria, as may diabetes mellitus, diabetes insipidus, renal concentration defects, and the use of diuretics. If an uninhibited detrusor contraction regularly occurs at a certain bladder volume, consistently challenging the bladder with excess urinary volume will lead to urge incontinence. Similarly, lower extremity edema and congestive heart failure can lead to sudden increases in urine production, especially with the patient in the recumbent position.

Evaluation

The initial evaluation for a man with UI includes a detailed medical history and focused physical examination. History should inquire about LUTS, including both storage symptoms (frequency, nocturia, urgency, incontinence) and voiding symptoms (hesitancy, straining, double voiding, force of stream). Duration, triggering factors, irritants (caffeine, alcohol), and any history of hematuria, dysuria, urinary tract infections, or urinary retention are relevant. Perhaps most important is the patient's perception of his bladder condition and his goals for improvement (eg, stop leaking versus reduce frequency or nocturia, etc.). Associated medical conditions such as heart failure, spinal or prostate surgery, bowel function, and dementia also are important. A detailed list of medications are necessary, especially those medications that may have urinary side effects, such as diuretics, antidepressants, alpha-adrenergic antagonists, beta-adrenergic agonists and antagonists, sedatives, anxiolytics, anticholinergics, and analgesics.

Physical examination should include a general physical examination, with specific observation of gait and mental status, with an evaluation of the patient's mobility and his neurological status. Digital rectal examination is indicated to assess for prostate size (and masses) and to check pelvic floor tone and voluntary squeeze of the pelvic floor muscles. Notation should be made of lower extremity edema (fluid overload) or decreased skin turgor (fluid depletion).

Laboratory evaluation should include urinalysis, looking for blood cells, pus cells, nitrates, crystalluria, and glucosuria. AUA guidelines recommend measurement of serum prostate-specific antigen [31] (coincidental prostate cancer treatment may obviate or affect treatment of BPE), and the Agency for Health Care Policy and Research guidelines suggest gross evaluation of renal function via measurement of serum creatinine [32].

Evaluation also should include measurement of postvoid residual urine volume (PVR). An elevated PVR (which must be considered in the context of voided volume) simply means that the bladder did not contract sufficiently enough during the micturition cycle to overcome the urethral resistance and empty efficiently. An elevated PVR is not diagnostic of BOO, nor does a low PVR exclude BOO. However, in a patient with a high PVR (low voiding efficiency), one should be suspicious of detrusor underactivity and/or BOO. Elevated PVR is only weakly associated with BOO [33]. Similar to measurement of PVR, uroflowmetry can be measured noninvasively, has no risk, yet provides invaluable information. Although low flow can indicate BOO and/or detrusor underactivity, the vast majority of men with a maximum urinary flow rate <10 ml s^{-1} have BOO (up to 88%) [34]. Optional tests include cystoscopy and urine cytology, and are appropriate if one suspects bladder stone or transitional cell carcinoma in situ.

It is often difficult to differentiate patient with BOO, OAB, and/or DHIC based on history and physical examination alone. Only urodynamic evaluation can precisely distinguish among these potential diagnoses. While it may not be necessary to make this distinction in order to introduce behavioral treatment, initiation of pharmacotherapy or surgical treatment is best done once a proper diagnosis is established.

Urodynamics, if indicated, should start with uroflowmetry, followed by measurement of PVR. Filling cystometry is useful to measure bladder sensation, compliance, capacity, and to identify any uninhibited bladder contractions (either spontaneous or provoked). Measurement of abdominal leak point pressure is necessary to rule out intrinsic sphincter deficiency. Pressure-flow study or micturitional urethral pressure profilometry [35] should then follow, in order to assess bladder contractility and to rule out bladder outlet obstruction. Rectal monometry allows the examiner to determine whether abdominal straining is present. Furthermore, the presence of rectal contractions may indicate a subtle neuropathy [36]. Electromyography will help to rule out detrusor-sphincter-dyssynergia, which may be associated with multiple sclerosis or other suprasacral spinal cord pathology, or poor voluntary control of the striated sphincter, which may be present with Parkinson's disease [37]. Finally, fluoroscopy is helpful to assess for bladder trabeculation and to help identify any anatomic abnormalities.

Symptoms and physical findings are not necessarily predictive of urodynamic findings, and therefore often are not sufficient to make a correct diagnosis in and of themselves. DO and BOO are both common in men with LUTS *with or without* and UI [38]. However, while UI strongly correlates with DO, other LUTS do not correlate well with urodynamic findings, such as BOO [39, 40]. While some investigations have shown that the incidence of DO increases with the degree of BOO [40, 41], others do not support such findings [42–44], instead

implying that DO and BOO are concomitant disorders, perhaps each related independently to the aging process. Neither the physical finding of an enlarged prostate nor the sign of elevated PVR are strongly associated with BOO. Approximately 50% of unobstructed older men have an elevated PVR, and 30% of men with BOO have normal PVR [45]. Thus presence of UI with or without DO is not diagnostic of BOO, nor is the presence of voiding symptoms even with an elevated PVR predictive of BOO. This lack of correlation among symptoms, signs, and urodynamic findings also is the case for younger men with LUTS and UUI, who may not be at risk for prostatic obstruction but may be at risk for congenital bladder neck obstruction or urethral stricture disease [46]. Therefore, urodynamics are necessary for the proper evaluation and treatment of complex voiding dysfunction in men with UI when there is diagnostic uncertainty.

In men with suspected neurogenic voiding dysfunction, urodynamic evaluation is even more important prior to instituting treatment. For example, treating a patient with pure neurogenic DO in the *absence* of BOO with deobstructive therapy may clearly risk devastating UI. Similarly, in men with Parkinson's disease and UI who demonstrate a lack of voluntary sphincter control, the risk of postoperative incontinence may be as high as 80% [47]. However, the presence of neurogenic DO should *not* be a contraindication to deobstructing therapy when BOO is present. Table 28.1 summarizes the suggested evaluation of a man with UI.

Management

Behavioral Modification

Behavioral therapy should be offered as an initial treatment, as it is nonmorbid, noninvasive, and often efficacious. In general behavioral modification is associated with a 50% decrease in UI [48]. A trial fluid restriction, caffeine restriction, timed voiding, and pelvic floor exercises poses minimal risk. Behavioral modification requires that the patient understand the basic pathophysiology of UI, namely that the bladder is unable to store a sufficient quantity of urine prior to the involuntary evacuation of that urine. In such patients, fluid intake often is greater than necessary and usually

TABLE 28.1. Evaluation of male with urge incontinence

History
Storage symptoms
Voiding symptoms
Duration
Triggers
Associated symptoms (dysuria)
Medications
Physical examination
General
Digital rectal examination
Bulbocavernosis reflex
Pelvic floor muscle tone
Gait
Mental status
Mobility
Laboratory examination
Urinalysis
Serum prostate specific antigen
Serum creatinine (if concern regarding obstructive uropathy)
Postvoid residual urine volume
Uroflowmetry
Additional urodynamic evaluation (if considering surgical treatment)
Cystometry
Pressure-flow study/micturitional urethral pressure profilometry
Rectal monometry
Electromyography
Abdominal leak point pressure
Cystoscopy/cytology (if suspicious of carcinoma, carcinoma in situ, or bladder stone)

can be safely reduced to 1,000–1,500 ml per day. Contraindications to fluid restriction include recurrent nephrolithiasis, frequent urinary tract infections, and severe constipation. Caffeinated beverages should be eliminated but must be done gradually to avoid precipitating rebound headaches. A trial of timed voiding whereby the patient volitionally empties his bladder prior to a strong sense of urgency (and UI) is recommended. If a diuretic is being taken, it may be best to schedule even more frequent voids (as often as every 30 min) during the time of active diuresis. The final component of conservative management is pelvic floor muscle physiotherapy. The patient's ability to contract the pelvic floor can be evaluated during the rectal examination by prompting the patient to squeeze the examiner's finger with his anal sphincter. Another useful method is to ask the patient to contract the anal sphincter as if he

were holding in gas, but should be reminded not to contract the abdominal or gluteal muscles. For the patient who cannot isolate the pelvic floor muscles, a trial of physical therapy or biofeedback is useful. The goal of physical therapy and biofeedback should be to teach the patient proper pelvic floor exercises, which then can be done on a regular basis at home. Finally, it is useful to remind the patient to contract the pelvic floor when a strong sense of urgency arises, in order to suppress the uninhibited bladder contraction and subsequent internal sphincter relaxation that can mediate UI [49]. When combined with pharmacotherapy, the improvement in UI is greater than with behavioral therapy alone [50].

Pharmacotherapy

More than half of men with BPE also suffer from OAB (urgency, often accompanied by frequency and nocturia, occasionally associated with UI). And it is the OAB symptoms that are often most bothersome. In addition, the majority of men with UI have DO, while the presence of concomitant BOO is less than 50% [51]. Thus the use of pharmacotherapy that targets the prostate in order to treat presumed BOO (such as alpha-adrenergic antagonists and 5-alpha reductase (5AR) inhibitors) is appropriate in less than half of men with UI, while the use of antimuscarinics would be appropriate in the majority of patients.

The use of alpha-adrenergic inhibitors for the treatment of men with LUTS associated with BPE does not adequately treat the UI and other storage symptoms in a substantial proportion of the patients [52]. It is curious why the most common pharmacotherapy for men with UI directed at treating the BOO rather than the UI and DO [53]. Treating the prostate for a process that clearly can be localized to the bladder should no longer serve as first-line treatment. Newer safety and efficacy data regarding the use of antimuscarinics in men with DO even with BOO may help to shift current practice patterns.

Alpha Blockers

UI clearly is related to an inability to store urine due to the bladder and may or may not be associated with prostatic obstruction. However, the most common practice among urologists, internists, and family physicians is to treat the outlet with alpha-adrenergic antagonists [53]. Inhibition of the alpha-adrenergic receptors aims at treating the dynamic component of the obstructing prostatic urethra, by relaxing the smooth muscle of the prostate and bladder neck. Prostatic and bladder neck smooth muscle tone is mediated by alpha-adrenergic receptors [54]. The predominant type of receptor in the prostate and bladder neck (75%) is α_{1a} [54, 55].

There is no doubt that $\alpha 1$-receptor antagonists are efficacious in reducing LUTS and the bother from LUTS in men with BOO [56]. While phenoxybenzamine (nonselective, teratogenic) and prazosin (short-acting, significant risk of hypotension) are no longer recommended as first-line therapy for LUTS associated with BPE, the efficacy of terazosin, doxazosin, tamsulosin, and alfuzosin (long-acting α_1 receptor antagonists) has been proven in prospective, randomized, placebo-controlled trials, mediating significant improvements in symptom scores, QOL indexes, and uroflow. The efficacy of these different medications is comparable among the long-acting agents at appropriate therapeutic doses [57] but are differentiated by their side-effect profile and the requirement for dose titration (Table 28.2). Although more expensive, alfuzosin and tamsulosin are associated with a substantially lower risk of dizziness and hypotension than are doxazosin and terazosin.

Alpha-adrenergic inhibitors do not necessarily deobstruct the obstructed outlet [58] and not all men with LUTS and UUI have concomitant BOO. Alpha-adrenergic antagonists are even successful in symptomatic men *without* BOO [59]. This can be explained by the presence of α_{1d} receptors in the spinal cord, brain, and bladder body, which, if inhibited, can mediate a decrease in storage LUTS [60].

5 Alpha Reductase Inhibitors

The static component of BOO can be treated successfully with 5AR inhibitors, which reduce the volume of the prostate stroma and epithelium by inhibiting the formation of dihydrotestosterone from testosterone. Treatment with this class of medication has been shown to decrease the progression of and complications of LUTS associated with BPE [61]. The incidence of urinary retention and the likelihood of surgery are each reduced by 50% in men with prostate size >30–40 cc, and the prostate volume is reduced by approximately one third in men treated with finasteride (type-2 5AR inhibitor) or dutasteride (type-1 and type-2 5AR inhibitor). Symptomatic improvement is less dramatic and no studies have investigated the specific change in UI in men treated with 5AR inhibitor monotherapy. Certainly, there is no obvious mechanism of action for 5AR inhibitors in men with UI without BOO.

Antimuscarinics

A substantial proportion of men with LUTS have a combination of both storage and voiding symptoms, and accordingly urodynamic evaluation reveals that many men have coexisting DO and BOO. In women, storage symptoms and UI generally are treated with antimuscarinics. However, guidelines from the European Association of Urologists and from the American Urological Association do not mention the therapeutic role of anticholinergic drugs for treating storage symptoms in men [62]. Antimuscarinic therapy for men with LUTS associated with BPE is perceived as a potential risk for urinary retention. However, men with LUTS associated with BPE demonstrate urodynamic BOO only 50% of the time. Therefore, the use of α-blockers and/or 5AR inhibitors may not

TABLE 28.2. Alpha adrenergic antagonists commonly used in men with UI

Agent	Dosing (mg)	Titration to effective dose	Most common side effects (compared to placebo)
Terazosin	1, 2, 5, 10, 20	Yes	Dizziness
Doxazosin	1, 2, 4, 8, 16	Yes	Dizziness
Tamsulosin	0.4, 0.8	No	Ejaculatory dysfunction
Alfuzosin	10	No	Dizziness

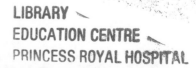

be necessary in approximately half of the men to whom they are prescribed! In addition, 50–75% of men with BPH also have OAB, and it is the OAB symptoms that often are most bothersome [53]. Furthermore, despite the general efficacy of alpha-adrenergic antagonism, the vast majority of men with LUTS associated with BPE continue to have bothersome storage symptoms (OAB) following alpha-blocker treatment. Accordingly, the use of antimuscarinics in men with LUTS and UI recently has been investigated.

The rationale for the use of antimuscarinics in patients with LUTS associated with BPE is consistent with recent views on the mechanism of action of antimuscarinics. No longer are antimuscarinics believed to simply block muscarinic receptors on the detrusor muscle thereby decreasing bladder contractility. Rather, antimuscarinics likely act on the storage phase, during which acetylcholine is released from neuronal and nonneuronal sources, and then act on afferent nerves in the suburothelium and detrusor. Urinary retention should be unlikely, as most antimuscarinic drugs are competitive antagonists. During the (normal) massive release of acetylcholine at the time of voiding, the effects of the antimuscarinic medications decrease, and therefore should not impair bladder contractility and should not lead to urinary retention [63].

Abrams et al. evaluated the safety and efficacy of tolterodine alone versus placebo in men with OAB and BOO [64]. Not only did tolterodine ameliorate the urodynamic storage dysfunction (increase in capacity and increase in volume at unstable contraction), but there were no instances of urinary retention in the tolterodine arm, nor were there important changes in urinary flow, voiding pressure, or PVR. Lee et al. demonstrated that a combination of the antimuscarinic medication propiverine (not currently available in the United States) plus doxazosin provided superior symptomatic relief of the storage symptoms in men with OAB and BOO more than did doxazosin alone [65]. Despite a statistically significant increase in PVR in the group receiving the antimuscarinic medication, there were no instances of urinary retention, and discontinuation rates were the same with or without the antimuscarinic. Athanasopoulos et al. evaluated the combination of tolterodine plus tamsulosin versus tamsulosin alone in men with urodynamically documented DO and BOO [66]. While

both arms demonstrated significant improvement in urinary flow rate and volume at first unstable contraction, only the tolterodine arm demonstrated improvement in QOL. Furthermore, addition of the antimuscarinic did not lower uroflow or elevated PVR. These results suggest that antimuscarinics can be safely administered in men with BOO.

Despite this evidence documenting the safety and efficacy of antimuscarinic medication in men with urodynamically proven BOO, many opinion leaders still recommend "pretreating" the outlet prior to initiating antimuscarinic pharmacotherapy [67, 68]. Based on the growing body of literature documenting the safety and efficacy of antimuscarinics in men with UI with or without BOO, the use of antimuscarinics should become less controversial and more mainstream.

Surgical

Transurethral resection of the prostate (TURP) or other deobstructing surgical procedures such as simple open prostatectomy or laser enucleation/vaporization of the prostate as a therapy for UI should be offered in selected cases when there is a significant degree of prostatic urethral obstruction. The urological literature is replete with studies demonstrating substantially worse outcomes when TURP is performed in patients without BOO who suffer from incontinence due to DO [69].

As DO is present in the majority of men with UI, the purpose of urodynamics is not to demonstrate DO, but rather to assess for the presence and degree of BOO. While BOO is a relative indication for TURP, DO is *not* a contraindication for TURP. In fact, DO and UI are improved or reversed in approximately two thirds of men following deobstructing surgery [70, 71]. It should be noted, however, that the greatest degree of improvement occurs in the most severely obstructed men [72], further strengthening the argument for detailed urodynamic evaluation of men with UI. While DO is necessary for UI, it often is not sufficient to cause incontinence without a concomitant abnormality of cognition or of pelvic floor muscular control. Cognitive impairment should not be, however, a deterrent to surgery, especially in the patient with significant BOO. In the cohort reported by Gormely et al. those with the most improvement also were cognitively impaired [72].

Despite the common perception that most older men with LUTS suffer from prostatic obstruction and that most older men benefit from TURP, symptomatic improvement and overall outcome is significantly worse in patients with DO and without BOO [73]. Postoperatively, UI was more likely to persist in men without clear BOO than in those who were obstructed preoperatively. It appears that persistent UI secondary to DO may be the principle cause of unfavorable outcomes following TURP [74]. In addition, the characterization of DO may help to predict favorable versus unfavorable surgical outcome. Persistent UI after surgery is most likely in those with low-volume DO (capacity <160 (c) and if the unstable bladder contractions are of the phasic rather than the terminal variety [75].

Despite the evidence demonstrating more favorable outcomes for TURP in the setting of urethral obstruction, urodynamic evaluation is recommended as "optional" by the American Urological Association and by the Agency for Health Care Policy and Research guidelines prior to deobstructing surgery. While results are dramatically different in patients with UI who suffer from obstruction versus those without obstruction, TURP occasionally can lead to symptomatic improvement in the latter group through a mechanism of action independent of deobstruction. It is possible that the heat effect on periprostatic nerves secondary to TURP or minimally invasive prostate therapy may mediate improvement in the bladder overactivity [76].

Neuromodulation

Neuromodulation treats UI primarily via *afferent* nerve stimulation/modulation. Afferent stimulation of the pelvic and pudendal nerve fibers results in modulation of voiding and continence reflex pathways in the CNS [77, 78].

Sacral nerve stimulation (SNS) with the InterStim (Medtronic, Minneapolis, MN) relies on transforaminal stimulation of the third sacral root, following surgical implantation of a quadripolar lead and an implantable pulse generator. What makes this a particularly attractive option for the patient with UI refractory to behavioral modification and pharmacotherapy is the minimally invasive nature and the reversibility of the test procedure. Prior to implantation of the pulse generator, the patient is given a 1- to 4-week trial of neuromodulation, using an external pulse generator and a percutaneously implanted quadripolar electrode, which stimulates the third sacral root. The patient may elect placement of the permanent stimulation device only following a successful test stimulation period. The pulse generator is placed in the upper outer quadrant of the buttocks and connected to the preplaced quadripolar lead. Stimulation settings are typically frequency 14 HZ, pulse width 150 ms, and a variable amplitude from 0.1 to 10.5 V. The patient is able to control the amplitude of stimulation, thus achieving an efficacious and comfortable level of nerve stimulation. As the device has been FDA-approved for approximately a decade, there is wide experience with this treatment modality. Long-term efficacy (defined as >50% reduction in incontinence episodes) is generally 60–76% [79, 80].

SNS is thought to work via inhibition of the ascending (afferent) pathway in which the sensory information from the bladder is transmitted via the spinal tract neurons to the pontine micturition center. Sacral nerve stimulation activates specific inhibitory pathways, inhibiting involuntary reflex voiding [78]. Low-stimulation current applied to the A-delta myelinated sacral root fibers selectively excites central inhibitory pathways. These central inhibitory pathways in turn modulate the activity of the somatic nerves traveling through the pelvic nerve, innervating the external urethral sphincter and pelvic floor. Thus, SNS indirectly inhibits the afferent mediated excitatory reflexes by suppressing interneuronal transmission within the sacral cord. However, it does not inhibit the voluntary voiding that occurs via direct descending supraspinal excitatory input to the pelvic parasympathetic neurons [81]. Furthermore, the low-stimulation frequencies do not reach the threshold required to activate the autonomic nerve fibers (ie, direct motor responses), and thus a simultaneous bladder contraction is avoided [82–84].

Alternative methods of neuromodulation include posterior tibial nerve stimulation (PTNS) and pudendal nerve stimulation (PNS). PTNS has been shown to help with both neurogenic and nonneurogenic UI refractory to conservative management, with cure rates of approximately 50% [85, 86], and even higher with the addition of an antimuscarinic medication. [87]. Advanced Bionics Corp. (Velerick, CA) has introduced a leadless, rechargeable, implantable microstimulator, which is percutaneously placed transperineally at the level of the pudendal nerve. PNS is not yet FDA approved; however, the Bion® pudendal nerve stimulator currently is being evaluated in a prospective, randomized, sham-controlled study for the chronic treatment of UI.

Augmentation Cystoplasty

Augmentation cystoplasty, whether performed through a laparotomy or performed laparoscopically [88], is more commonly offered to men with neurogenic voiding dysfunction than to men with nonneurogenic voiding dysfunction. The usual indication is to protect the upper urinary tracts in the setting of diminished bladder compliance, hydronephrosis, recurrent nephrolithiasis, vesicoureteral reflux, or recurrent pyelonephritis. Although less common, augmentation cystoplasty also is efficacious in nonneurogenic refractory UI. Although the majority of men are cured of their UI [89, 90], in the author's experience, approximately 15% of patients have permanent postoperative retention, and therefore must be able to perform clean intermittent self-catheterization.

Intravesical

Botulinum Toxin

Intradetrusor injections of botulinum toxin (BTX) recently have emerged as a viable treatment for UI due to neurogenic and idiopathic DO. The heavy chain of BTX binds to the presynaptic motor terminal and enters the cell by endocytosis. The disulfide bond linking the two BTX chains (heavy chain and light chain) is broken, and the light chain is translocated out of the endocytic vesicle into the cytoplasm. Each serotype of the toxin works by enzymatic cleavage of one or more of the proteins necessary for normal acetylcholine exocytosis. The preferred method of injection is via 5 Fr needle through a rigid cystoscope. Thirty sites are each injected with 1 m of 10 U m^{-1} BTX-A, while the trigone is spared of injection. BTX-A is associated with a cure/improved rate of 85% for both neurogenic and nonneurogenic DO [91, 92]. Improvement is realized immediately following intradetrusor injection and lasts for up to 6 months. The risk of nausea, vomiting, dry mouth, dysphagia, and respiratory muscle weakness appears to be minimal when BTX is used for lower urinary tract dysfunction. Side effects include impaired

bladder sensation and hesitancy and straining of urination, and complications include urinary tract infection and transient urinary retention requiring intermittent catheterization [93]. BTX-B has a shorter duration and higher side effect profile [94].

C-Fiber Desensitization

RTX is a specific ligand of the vanilloid receptor (TRPV1) receptor, a nonselective ion channel abundantly expressed in type-C bladder afferent nerve fibers and in urothelial cells [95–99]. Following RTX binding to TRPV1, bladder C fibers become inactivated through a phenomenon usually known as desensitization during which bladder sensory input is prevented from reaching the spinal cord [100]. Intravesical application of RTX is followed by a prolonged disappearance of TRPV1 immunoreactivity in the bladder [101] and has been shown to reduce frequency, urgency, and UI in patients with neurogenic and nonneurogenic DO [102–105]. In addition, the blockade of bladder C fiber sensory input recently has been investigated as a new strategy to treat storage LUTS (without frank UI) in BPE patients. Dinis et al. demonstrated the efficacy of 50-nM RTX solution in men with BPH-associated storage LUTS, with four of six patients cured of UI and the other two at least 50% improved [106].

A recently published randomized study of RTX versus BTX-A demonstrated efficacy for both agents, but demonstrated superiority of BTX-A over RTX in patients with neurogenic DO [107].

Management of the Failed TURP

Approximately 15–20% of men following TURP have persistent or recurrent voiding symptoms requiring further therapy. Just as symptoms and signs do not correlate well with urodynamic findings prior to TURP, symptoms are unreliable in predicting urodynamic findings (especially BOO versus DO) following TURP. In men with bothersome LUTS post-TURP, only 16–38% demonstrate BOO, while 4–25% will have detrusor underactivity. Sphincteric insufficiency is rare, with a prevalence of only 8%. Approximately 50% of patient with nonneurogenic voiding dysfunction will demonstrate DO, while 76% of those with neurogenic dysfunction will have uninhibited bladder contractions on urodynamics [108, 109]. As the etiology of post-TURP voiding dysfunction varies, urodynamic evaluation is vital for directing rational treatment in the already dissatisfied patient. While surgical relief of obstruction does indeed facilitate symptomatic improvement in the majority of men with UI who demonstrate BOO, persistent DO can be noted in about 30–50% of the patients [52, 110]. The rate of de novo DO has been reported to be at most 10% in patients following prostatectomy [52], thereby suggesting that the prognostic value of DO with regard to the treatment efficacy of TURP may be attributed to the postoperative *persistent* DO. An additional poor prognostic urodynamic indicator is diminished vesical compliance with unstable contractions arising at small capacity (<160 cc). On the other hand, terminal DO at volumes >160 cc is likely to resolve following TURP in the patient with BOO.

The urologist often is faced with the patient who has had multiple deobstructing surgeries. In a study of men who had failed two or more TURPs, urodynamic evaluation revealed DO in 80%, BOO in only 27%, detrusor underactivity in 27%, and sphincteric incompetence in only 20% [72]. Therefore, residual BOO occurs in a minority of patient following TURP, and secondary TURP or incision of a bladder neck contracture is usually not indicated. As DO, BOO, and detrusor underactivity are all common causes of post-TURP voiding dysfunction and UI, urodynamics plays a central role in the diagnostic workup of such patients.

Conclusions

The etiology of UI is substantially more complex than the presence of DO, especially in the geriatric male population. Unstable bladder contractions represent only one of several contributing factors, and therefore a full evaluation is necessary, including history and physical examination, urinalysis, and measurement of uroflow and PVR. Symptoms and signs should not be confused with diagnoses, and if suspicion of any confounding diagnoses, such as BOO, DHIC, or detrusor underactivity remain, then multichannel urodynamics are indicated. Treatment should begin conservatively with behavioral modification and pelvic floor exercises and then should progress to pharmacotherapy. Although treatment of presumed BOO with α_1-adrenergic antagonists with or without 5AR inhibitors is the most common practice, newer data support the safety and efficacy of antimuscarinic medication, even in men with urodynamically proven BOO.

Deobstructing surgery should be offered only to patients with urodynamically proven BOO. Neither cognitive impairment nor neurogenic voiding dysfunction is a contraindication to outlet surgery in the obstructed patient. Nevertheless, surgery should be undertaken cautiously, especially in the patient with Parkinson's disease and a lack of sphincteric control. The patient with refractory urge incontinence following TURP should be reevaluated with urodynamics. Secondary deobstructive surgery is indicated in only 25% of patients, so it should be offered only in the setting of supportive urodynamic findings. Men with persistent incontinence following surgery are much more likely to suffer from DO than from sphincteric incompetence, and they should be offered behavioral modification, pelvic floor physiotherapy, and pharmacotherapy, but may ultimately benefit from neuromodulation, intradetrusor BTX injection, or even augmentation cystoplasty.

References

1. Fantl JA, Newman DK, Colling J, et al. Urinary incontinence in adults: Acute and chronic management. In: Clinical practice guideline. Rockville, Maryland: United States Department of Health and Human Services, No. 2, 1996.
2. Hu TW, Wagner TH, Bentkover, JD, et al. Costs of urinary incontinence and overactive bladder in the United States: A comparative study. Urology 2004, 63:461-65.
3. Hu TW, Wagner TH, Bentkover JD, et al. Estimated economic costs of overactive bladder in the United States. Urology 2003, 61:1123-8.
4. Lukacz ES, Lawrence JM, Burchette RJ, et al. The use of Visual Analog Scale in urogynecologic research: A psychometric evaluation. Am J Obstet Gynecol 2004, 191:165- 70.
5. Heidrich SM, Wells TJ. Effects of urinary incontinence: Psychological well-being and distress in older communitydwelling women. J Gerontol Nurs 2004, 30:47- 54.
6. Grimby A, Milsom I, Molander U, et al. The influence of urinary incontinence on the quality of life of elderly women. Age Ageing 1993 22:82- 9.
7. Liberman JN, Hunt TL, Stewart WF, et al. Health-related quality of life among adults with symptoms of overactive bladder: Results from a U. S. community-based survey. Urology 2001, 57:1044- 50.

8. Abrams P, Cardozo L, Fall M, et al. The standardisation of terminology of lower urinary tract function: Report from the standardisation sub-committee of the International Continence Society. Neurourol Urodyn 2002; 21:167-78.

9. Resnick NM, Yalla SV. Detrusor hyperactivity with impaired contractile function. An unrecognized but common cause of incontinence in elderly patients. JAMA 1987, 257:3076-3081.

10. Ziada A, Rosenblum M, Crawford ED. Benign prostatic hyperplasia: An overview. Urology 1999; 53:1-6.

11. Hinman Jr, F. The art and science of piddling: Voiding habits of man and beast London: Vespasian Pr, 1999.

12. de Groat WC, Vizzard MA, Araki I, et al. Spinal interneurons and preganglionic neurons in sacral autonomc reflex pathways. Prog Brain Res 1996; 107:97- 111.

13. Braverman AS, Ruggieri MR. Hypertrophy changes the muscarinic receptor subtype mediating bladder contraction from M3 toward M2. Am J Physiol Regul Integr Comp Physiol 2003; 285: R701-8.

14. Braverman AS, Doumanian LR, Ruggieri MR. M2 and M3 muscarinic receptor activation of urinary bladder contractile signal transduction. II. Denervated rat bladder. J Pharmacol Exp Ther 2006; 2:875-80.

15. Chancellor MB, Leng W: The mechanism of action of sacral nerve stimulation in the treatment of detrusor overactivity and urinary retention. In: Jonas U, Grunewald V, editors. New perspectives in sacral nerve stimulation for control of lower urinary tract dysfunction. London: Martin Dunitz Ltd, 2002:17-28.

16. MaLossi J, Chai TC. Sacral neuromodulation for the treatment of bladder dysfunction. Cur Urol Rep 2002; 3:61-66.

17. Araki I, Matsui M, Ozawa K, et al. Relationship of bladder dysfunction to lesion site in multiple sclerosis. J Urol 2003; 169:1384-7.

18. Steers WD, Tuttle JB. Mechanism of Disease: The role of nerve growth factor in the pathophysiology of bladder disorders. Nat Clin Pract Urol 2006; 3:101-10.

19. Kim JC, Park EY, Hong SH, et al. Changes of urinary nerve growth factor and prostaglandins in male patients with overactive bladder symptom. Int J Urol 2005; 12:875-80.

20. JiRR, Samad TA, Jin SX, et al. P38 MAPK activation by NGF in primary sensory neurons after inflammation increases TRPV1 levels and maintains heat hyperalgesia. Neuron 2002; 36:57–68

21. Chuang HH, Prescott ED, Kong H, et al.. Bradykinin and nerve growth factor release the capsaicin receptor from PtdIns(4,5)P2-mediated inhibition. Nature 2001; 411:957–62.

22. LagouM, De Vente J, Kirkwood TB, et al. Location of interstitial cells and neurotransmitters in the mouse bladder. BJU Int 2006; 97:1332-7.

23. Kanai A, de Groat W, Birder L, et al. Symposium report on urothelial dysfunction: Pathophysiology and novel therapies. J Urol 2006; 175:1624-9.

24. Elbadawi A, Yalla SV, Resnick NM. Structural basis of geriatric voiding dysfunction. III. Detrusor overactivity. J Urol 1993; 150:1668-80.

25. Araki I, Du S, Kamiyama M, et al. Overexpression of epithelial sodium channels in epithelium of human urinary bladder with outlet obstruction. Urology 2004; 64:1255-60.

26. Kim JC, Park EY, Hong SH, et al. Changes of urinary nerve growth factor and prostaglandins in male patients with overactive bladder symptom. Int J Urol 2005; 12:875-80.

27. Wein AJ, Rackley RR. Overactive bladder: A better understanding of pathophysiology, diagnosis and management. J Urol 2006; 175:S5-10.

28. Elbadawi A, Yalla SV, Resnick NM. Structural basis of geriatric voiding dysfunction. III. Detrusor overactivity. J Urol 1993; 150:1668-80.

29. Andersson KE, Wein AJ. Urethral afferent nerve activity affects the micturition reflex; implication for the relationship between stress incontinence and detrusor instability. Pharmacol Rev 2004; 56:581-631.

30. Jung SY, Fraser MO, Ozawa H, et al. Urethral afferent nerve activity affects the micturition reflex; implication for the relationship between stress incontinence and detrusor instability. J Urol 1999; 162:204-12.

31. Nickel JC, Herschorn S, Corcos J, et al. Canadian guidelines for the management of benign prostatic hyperplasia. Can J Urol 2005; 12:2677-83.

32. McConnell JD, Barry MJ, Bruskewitz RC, et al. Benign prostatic hyperplasia: Diagnosis and treatment. In: Clinical practice guideline. Rockville, MD: Agency for Health Care Policy and Research, 1994.

33. de la Rosette JJ, Witjes WP, Schafer W, et al. Relationships between lower urinary tract symptoms and bladder outlet obstruction: results from the ICS "BPH" study. Neurourol Urodyn 1998; 17:99-108.

34. Poulsen AL, Schou J, Puggaard L, et al. Prostatic enlargement, symptomatology and pressure/flow evaluation: Interrelations in patients with symptomatic BPH. Scand J Urol Neph 1994; 157:67-73

35. Sullivan MP, Comiter CV, Yalla SV. Micturitional urethral pressure profilometry. Urol Clin North Am 1996; 23:263-78.

36. Combs AJ, Nitti VW. Significance of rectal contractions noted on multichannel urodynamics. Neurourol Urodyn 1995; 14:73-80.

37. Staskin DS, Vardi Y, Siroky MB. Post-prostatectomy continence in the Parkinsonian patient: The significance of poor voluntary sphincter control. J Urol 1988; 140:117-8.

38. Diokno AC, Brown MB, Brock BM, et al. Clinical and cystometric characteristics of continent and incontinent noninstitutionalized elderly. J Urol 1988; 140:567-71.

39. Sakakibara R, Hamano S, Uchiyama T, et al. Do BPH patients have neurogenic detrusor dysfunction? A uroneuroloigcal assessment. Urol Int 2005; 74:44-50.

40. Hyman MJ, Groutz A, Blaivas JG. Detrusor instability in men: Correlation of lower urinary tract symptoms with urodynamic findings. J Urol 2001; 166:550-2.

41. Wadie BS, Ebrahim el-HE, Gomha MA. The relationship of detrusor instability and symptoms with objective parameters used for diagnosing bladder outlet obstruction: A prospective study. J Urol 2002; 168:132-4.

42. Rosier PF, de la Rosette JJ, Wikjkstra H, et al. Is detrusor instability in elderly males related to the grade of obstruction. Neurourol Urodyn 1995; 14:625-33.

43. Knutson T, Edlund C, Fall M, Dahlstrand C.BPH with coexisting overactive bladder dysfunction--an everyday urological dilemma. Neurourol Urodyn 2001; 20:237-47.

44. Comiter CV, Schacterle RS, Sullivan MP, et al. Urodynamic risk factors for renal insufficiency in adult men with obstructive and non-obstructive voiding dysfunction. J Urol 1997; 158:181-5.

45. Chatelain C, Denis L, Foo KT, et al. Benign prostatic hyperplasia. Paris, France; The International Consultation on Benign Prosatatic Hyperplasia, 2000.

46. Nitti VW, Lefkowitz G, Ficazzola M, et al. Lower urinary tract symptoms in young men: Videourodynamic findings and correlation with noninvasive measures. J Urol 2002; 168:135-8.

47. Abrams P, Cardozo L, Khoury S, et al. Incontinence: 3rd international consultation on incontinence. Plymouth, United Kingdom: Health Publication Ltd, 2005.

48. Fantl JA, Wyman JF, McClish DK, et al. Efficacy of bladder training in older women with urinary incontinence. JAMA 1991; 265:609-13.

49. Shafik A, Shafik IA. Overactive bladder inhibition in response to pelvic floor muscle exercises. World J Urol 2003; 20:374-7.

50. Burgio KL, Locher JL, Goode PS: Combined behavioral and drug therapy for urge incontinence in older women. J Am Geriatr Soc 2000; 48:370-4.

51. Eckardt MD, van Nenrooij GE, Boon TA. Interactions between prostate volume, filling cystometric estimated parameters, and data from pressure-flow studies in 565 men with lower urinary tract symptoms suggestive of benign prostatic hyperplasia. Neurourol Urodyn 2001; 20:579-90.

52. de Nunzio C, Franco G, Rocchegiani A, et al. The evolution of detrusor overactivity after watchful waiting, medical therapy and surgery in patients with bladder outlet obstruction. J Urol 2003; 169:535-9.

53. Chapple CR, Roehrborn CG. A shifted paradigm for the further understanding, evaluation, and treatment of lower urinary tract symptoms in men: Focus on the bladder. Eur Urol 2006; 49:651-9.

54. Narayan P, Tewari A. A second phase III multicenter placebo controlled study of 2 dosages of modified release tamsulosin in patients with symptoms of benign prostatic hyperplasia. United States 93-01 Study Group. J Urol 1998; 160:1701-6.

55. Goepel M, Wittmann A, Rubben H, et al. Comparison of adrenoceptor subtype expression in procine and human bladder and prostate. Urol Res 1997; 25:199-206.

56. Tiwari A, Krishna NS, Nanda K, et al. Benign prostatic hyperplaisia: An insight into current investigational medical therapies. Expert Opin Investig Drugs 2005; 14:1359-72.

57. Vallancien G. Alpha-blockers in benign prostatic hyperplasia. Urology 1999; 54:773-775.

58. Gleason DM, Bottaccini MR. Effect of terazosin on urine storage and voiding in the aging male with prostatism. Neurourol Urodyn 1994; 13:1-12.

59. Gerber GS, Kim JH, Contreras BA, et al. An observational urodynamic evaluation of men with lower urinary tract symptoms treated with doxazosin. Urology 1996; 47:840-4.

60. Schwinn DA. The role of alpha1-adrenergic receptor subtypes in lower urinary tract symptoms. BJU Int 2001; 88 Suppl 2:27-34.

61. TarterTH, Vaughan ED Jr. Inhibitors of 5alpha-reductase in the treatment of benign prostatic hyperplasia. Curr Pharm Des 2006; 12:775-83.

62. Reynard JM. Does anticholinergic medication have a role for men with lower urinary tract symptoms/benign prostatic hyperplasia either alone or in combination with other agents? Curr Opin Urol 2004; 14:13-16.

63. Andersson KE, Yoshida M. Antimuscarinics and the overactive detrusor—which is the main mechanism of action? Eur Urol 2003; 43: 1-5.

64. Abrams P, Kaplan S, De Koning Gans HJ, et al. Safety and tolerability of tolterodine for the treatment

of overactive bladder in men with bladder outlet obstruction. J Urol 2006; 175:999-1004.

65. Lee KS, Choo MS, Kim DY, et al. Combination treatment with propiverine hydrochloride plus doxazosin controlled release gastrointestinal therapeutic system formulation for overactive bladder and coexisting benign prostatic obstruction: A prospective, randomized, controlled multicenter study. J Urol 2005; 174:1334-8.

66. Athanasopoulos A, Gyftopoulos K, Giannitsas K, et al. Combination treatment with an alpha-blocker plus an anticholinergic for bladder outlet obstruction: A prospective, randomized, controlled study. J Urol 2003; 169:2253-6.

67. Gonzalez RR, Te AE. Overactive bladder and men: Indications for anticholinergics. Curr Urol Rep 2003; 4:429-35.

68. Staskin DR, Dmochowski RR. Future studies of overactive bladder: The need for standardization. Urology 2002; 60(5 Suppl 1):90-3.

69. Machino R, Kakizaki H, Ameda K, et al. Detrusor instability with equivocal obstruction: A predictor of unfavorable symptomatic outcomes after transurethral prostatectomy. Neurourol Urodyn 2002; 21:444-9.

70. Hebjorn S, Andersen JT, Walter S, et al. Detrusor hyperreflexia. A survey on its etiology and treatment. Scand J Urol Nephrol 1976; 10:103-9.

71. Akino H, Gobara M, Okada K. Bladder dysfunction in patients with benign prostatic hyperplasia: Relevance of cystometry as prognostic indicator of the outcome after prostatectomy. IntJ Urol 1996; 3:441-7.

72. Gormley EA, Griffiths DJ, McCracken PN, et al. Effect of transurethral resection of the prostate on detrusor instability and urge incontinence in elderly males. Neurourol Urodyn 1993; 12:445-5373.

73. Abrams PH, Farrar DJ, Turner-Warwick RT, et al. The results of prostatectomy: A symptomatic and urodynamic evaluation analysis of 152 patients. J Urol 1979; 121:640-5.

74. Ameda K, Koyanagi T, Nantani M, et al. The relevance of preoperative cystometrography in patients with benign prostatic hyperplasia: correlating the findings with clinical features and coutcome after prostatectomy. J Urol 1994; 152 :443-7.

75. Kageyama S, Watanabe T, Kurita Y, et al. Can we predict persistent do after TURP? Neurourol and Urodyn 2000; 19:223-240.

76. Sugiyama T, Park YC, Hanai T, et al. Why is transurethral microwave thermotherapy (TUMT) positively effective? Int Urol Nephrol 1998; 30:293-300.

77. Lycklama A, Nijeholt AAB, Groenendijk PM, et al. Clinical and urodynamic assessments of the mode of action of sacral nerve stimulation. In: Jonas U, Grunewald V, editors, New perspectives in sacral nerve stimulation for control of lower urinary tract dysfunction. London: Martin Dunitz Ltd, 2002:43-54.

78. Chancellor MB, Chartier-Kastler EJ: Principles of sacral nerve stimulation (SNS) for the treatment of bladder and urethral sphincter dysfunctions. Neuromodulation 2000; 3:15-26.

79. Abrams P, Blaivas JG, Fowler CJ, et al. The role of neuromodulation in the management of urinary urge incontinence. BJU Int 2003; 91:355-9.

80. Siegel SW, Catanzaro F, Dijkema HE, et al. Long-term results of a multicenter study on sacral nerve stimulation for treatment of urinary urge incontinence, urgency-frequency, and retention. Urology 2000; 56:87-91.

81. Van Kerrebroeck, PEV: The role of electrical stimulation in voiding dysfunction. Eur Urol 1998; 34(suppl 1):27-30.

82. MaLossi J, Chai TC: Sacral neuromodulation for the treatment of bladder dysfunction. Curr Urol Rep 2002; 3:61-66.

83. Van Balken MR, Vergunst H, Bemelmans BLH: The use of electrical devices for the treatment of bladder dysfunction: A review of methods. J Urol 2004; 172:846-51.

84. Grunewald V, Hofner K, Thon WF, et al. Sacral electrical neuromodulation as an alternative treatment option for lower urinary tract dysfunction. Restor Neurol Neurosci 1999; 14:189-193.

85. Vandoninck V, Van Balken MR, Finazzi Agro E, et al. Posterior tibial nerve stimulation in the treatment of urge incontinence. Neururol Urodyn 2003; 22:17-23.

86. van der Pal F, van Balken MR, Heesakkers JP, et al. Correlation between quality of life and voiding variables in patients treated with percutaneous tibial nerve stimulation. BJU Int 2006; 97:113-6.

87. Karademir K, Baykal K, Sen B, et al. A peripheric neuromodulation technique for curing detrusor overactivity: Stoller afferent neurostimulation. Scand J Urol Nephrol 2005; 39:230-3.

88. Rackley RR, Abdelmalak JB. Laparoscopic augmentation cystoplasty. Surgical technique. Urol Clin North Am 2001; 28:663-70.

89. Herschorn S, Hewitt RJ. Patient perspective of long-term outcome of augmentation cystoplasty for neurogenic bladder. Urology 1998; 52:672-8.

90. Albo M, Raz S, Dupont MC. Anteiror flap extraperitoneal cystoplasty. J Urol 1997; 157:2095-8.

91. Schurch B, de Zeze M, Denys P, et al. Botulinum toxin type A is a safe and effective treatment for neurogenic urinary incontinence: Results of a single treatment, randomized, placebo controlled 6-month study. J Urol 2005; 174:196-200.

92. Kuo HC. Clinical effects of suburothelial injection of botulinum A toxin on patients with nonneurogenic detrusor overactivity refractory to anticholinergics. Urology 2005; 66:94-8.

93. Patterson JM, Chapple CR. Botulinum toxin in urinary incontinence. Curr Opin Urol 2006; 16:255-60.

94. Ghei M, Maraj BH, Miller R, et al. Effects of botulinum toxin B on refractory detrusor overactivity: A randomized, double-blind, placebo controlled crossover trial. J Urol 2005; 174:1873-7.

95. Szallasi A, Blumberg PM. Vanilloid (capsaicin) receptors and mechanisms. Pharmacol Rev 1999; 51:159-211.

96. Caterina MJ, Schumacher MA, Tominaga M, et al. The capsaicin receptor: A heat-activated ion channel in the pain pathway. Science 1997; 389:816-24.

97. Yiangou Y, Facer P, Ford A, et al. Capsaicin receptor VR1 and ATP-gated ion channel P2X3 in humanurinary bladder. BJU Int 2001; 87:774-9.

98. Avelino A, Cruz C, Nagy I, et al. Vanilloid receptor type 1expression in the rat urinary tract. Neuroscience 2002; 109:787-98.

99. Birder LA, Kanai AJ, de Groat WC, et al. Vanilloid receptor expression suggests a sensory role for urinary bladder epithelial cells. Proc Natl Acad Sci USA 2001; 98:13396-401.

100. Avelino A, Cruz F, Coimbra A. Intravesical resiniferatoxin desensitizes rat bladder sensory fibres without causing intense noxious excitation. A c-fos study. Eur J Pharmacol 1999; 378:17-22.

101. Apostolidis AN, Brady C, Yiangou Y, et al. Parallel changes in suburothelial vanilloid receptor TRPV1 (VR1) and pan-neuronal marker PGP9.5 immunoreactivity in patients with neurogenic detrusor overactivity (NDO) following intravesical RTX. Eur Urol Suppl 2003; 2:91.

102. Fowler CJ, Jewkes D, McDonald WI, et al. Intravesical capsaicin for neurogenic bladder dysfunction. Lancet 1992; 339:1239.

103. Silva C, Rio ME, Cruz F. Desensitization of bladder sensory fibres by intravesical resiniferatoxin, a capsaicin analogue: Long-term results for the treatment of detrusor hyperreflexia. Eur Urol 2000; 38:444–52.

104. Silva C, Ribeiro MJ, Cruz F. The effect of intravesical resiniferatoxin in patients with idiopathic detrusor instability suggests that involuntary detrusor contractions are triggered by C-fiber input. J Urol 2002; 168:575–9.

105. Kuo H. Effectiveness of intravesical resiniferatoxin for anticholinergics treatment refractory detrusor overactivity due to nonspinal cord lesions. J Urol 2003;170:835–9. 100

106. Dinisa P, Silvaa J, Ribeiroa MJ, et al. Bladder C-fiber desensitization induces a long-lasting improvement of BPH-associated storage LUTS: A pilot study. Eur Urol 2004; 46:88–94.

107. Giannantoni A, Di Stasi SM, Stephen RL, et al. Intravesical resiniferatoxin versus botulinum-A toxin injections for neurogenic detrusor overactivity: A prospective randomized study. J Urol 2004; 172:240-3.

108. Seaman EK, Jacobs BZ, Blaivas JG, et al. Persistence or recurrence of symptoms after transurethral resection of the prostate: A urodynamic assessment. J Urol 1994; 152:935-7.

109. Nitti VW, Kim Y, Combs AJ. Voiding dysfunction following transurethral resection of the prostate: Symptoms and urodynamic findings. J Urol 1997; 157:600-3.

110. Van Venrooij, GE, Van Melick HH, Eckhardt MD, et al. Correlations of urodynamic changes with changes in symptoms and well-being after transurethral resection of the prostate. J Urol 2002; 168:605-9.

Chapter 29
Pharmacotherapy of Male Incontinence

Peter Tsakiris and Jean J.M.C.H. de la Rosette

Introduction

According to EAU Guidelines on Urinary Incontinence [1], the clinical presentations of men with symptoms and history of urinary incontinence may be grouped into four subdivisions: post-micturition dribbling, postprostatectomy incontinence, incontinence with frequency/urgency, and incontinence with a complex history (Fig. 29.1) Postprostatectomy incontinence and incontinence with urgency/frequency are symptoms that are suggestive of stress urinary incontinence (SUI), urgency urinary incontinence (UUI), mixed incontinence, and "overflow" incontinence. The etiology of these conditions mainly is sphincteric incompetence, detrusor overactivity, bladder outlet obstruction (BOO), or detrusor underactivity.

Prevalence estimates of these subtypes vary somewhat. The predominant type of urinary incontinence in men is UUI, while in women it is SUI. The distribution in men is 73% UUI, 19% mixed, and only 8% SUI, as opposed to women where 49% of all cases are SUI [3].

Because UI may cause social isolation, loss of sexual function, or other psychosocial problems [4, 5], it could have significant impact on patients' psychosocial well-being and quality of life (QOL). Studies have shown that patients suffering with UI are more depressed [6, 7], psychologically distressed, emotionally disturbed, and socially isolated [8]. Moreover, compared with continent individuals, those patients with UI also have higher levels of anxiety, lower QOL, and poorer life satisfaction [7]. The severity of UI also is correlated with degrees of mental distress, social restrictions, and restricted activities [4, 5]. As a result, UI has an adverse effect on patients' daily lives and could become a barrier for normal social function.

Current treatments for UI include *behavioral* (e.g., bladder training, fluid manipulation, scheduled toileting, pelvic muscle exercises), *pharmacological*, and *surgical* interventions, used either alone or in combination [9–11]. Behavioral techniques currently are recommended as first-line therapy in the treatment of UI except for overflow incontinence due to BOO. Behavioral interventions usually are relatively inexpensive and easy to implement, but the effectiveness chiefly depends on the patient's adherence [12]. When nonpharmacological interventions have failed, drug therapy can be an option [9].

The goal of this chapter is to present the current status in pharmacotherapy options of male UI by looking into the four main subtypes of male incontinence: urgency, stress, overflow, and postprostatectomy UI.

Urgency Urinary Incontinence

UUI involves a strong, sudden need to urinate immediately followed by a bladder muscle contraction, resulting in an involuntary loss of urine. It is basically a storage problem in which detrusor muscle contracts involuntarily, and often these contractions occur regardless of the amount of urine that is

- post-micturition dribbling

- post-prostatectomy incontinence ⎫   - stress UI   ⎫ → sphincteric incompetence
                                ⎪   - urge UI   ⎬ → overactive detrusor
- incontinence with freq/urgency ⎬   - mixed UI   ⎨ → bladder outlet obstruction
                                ⎪   - overflow UI ⎭ → underactive detrusor
- incontinence with a complex history ⎭

FIG. 29.1. Male incontinence

in the bladder [1]. UUI is a clinical symptom of the overactive bladder syndrome (OAB) characterized by urgency, with or without incontinence, and usually is associated with frequency and nocturia.

UUI in men is most commonly associated with neurogenic bladder or detrusor muscle instability. What characterizes male UI with regard to female is the greater possibility of BOO [due to benign prostatic hyperplasia (BPH), urethral stricture, bladder neck stenosis) in men. This difference between the two genders when dealing with UI in most of the cases causes an increased intravesical pressure, which subsequently causes detrusor overactivity (DO) via partial neurological denervation of the bladder smooth muscle and consequent supersensitivity of muscarinic acetylcholine receptors [13]. Increased bladder outlet resistance also may result in ischemia, increased detrusor collagen content, changes in electrical properties of detrusor smooth muscle cells [14], and reorganization of the spinal micturition reflex [15], all of which are associated with the development of DO in animal models. However, comorbid BOO and DO are not always evidence of a cause-and-effect relationship between these two conditions. OAB symptoms can be caused solely by bladder dysfunction that is independent of prostatic pathology. The observation that many men with OAB symptoms do not have BOO [16] underscores the potential role of bladder dysfunction. The fact that OAB symptoms are not limited to men provides further support for this assertion, bearing in mind that female BOO is extremely uncommon (Fig. 29.2).

In one study of 160 men with lower urinary tract symptoms (LUTS), including UI, urinary frequency, nocturia, or difficulty in voiding, BOO was confirmed in 109 (68%) [17], while Laniado et al. [18] reported that only 48% of men with LUTS had urodynamically confirmed BOO. A study in

- Alzheimer's disease
- Diabetes mellitus
- Multiple sclerosis
- Parkinson's disease
- Ruptured intervertebral disk
- Stroke
- Syphilis
- Traumatic brain or upper spinal-cord injury
- Tumors located in the brain or spinal cord

FIG. 29.2. Disorders associated with neurogenic bladder

the United States suggested that 16% of men with OAB symptoms have UUI [19]. It is a fact, however, that men with UUI have been underrepresented in trials of pharmacotherapy for OAB, although 84% of men with UUI report some degree of symptom bother [20].On a theoretical basis, possible potential sites for pharmacological intervention in the management of UI include the bladder smooth muscle, efferent (motor) nerves, afferent (sensory) nerves, and the central nervous system. The mainstay oral drug class for the medical treatment of incontinence is the antimuscarinics. These are anticholinergic agents that act on motor receptors on peripheral smooth muscle and perhaps on sensory receptors as well. Due to the fact that females seek medical care for UI much more often then males, the vast majority of the studies on medical treatment of incontinence with antimuscarinics have been conducted in females or in mixed gender populations dominated by females, ie, under conditions where the data are driven by the overwhelming female population in those trials.

Since our knowledge on medical incontinence treatment is largely driven by data from females, the assumption that female data can be simply extrapolated to males has been a field of quite intensive investigation. Experimental studies have been published addressing the question whether any gender difference is to be expected for muscarinic antagonists. At the beginning of the past decade, male and female rats were reported to exhibit differential sensitivity to the analgesic effects of the muscarinic agonist pilocarpine [21]. Later on, in the context of overactive bladder, the muscarinic antagonist tolterodine was reported to exhibit markedly gender-dependent effects on number of voids and volume voided per micturition in rats [22]. In line with these findings the estrus cycle was reported to affect the sensitivity of isolated rat bladder strips to muscarinic stimulation [23].

Evidence supporting the lack of gender difference for the sensitivity toward muscarinic stimulation is suggested in studies conducted in mice [24] and cats [25] in vitro. In a study exploring the possibility of gender-based differential regulation of M_2 and M_3 receptors in rats and human urinary bladders [26] the authors reported that none of the parameters of muscarinic responsiveness indicated a differential regulation in male and female rat bladder. Their patient data additionally indicated that gender differences of a clinically relevant magnitude also are absent in humans. They concluded that neither the overall muscarinic responsiveness nor the relative roles of M_2 and M_3 receptors are regulated in a gender-specific manner in the rat urinary bladder. These findings are in accordance with the results from a study on about 2,000 OAB patients in which tolterodine was similarly effective in both genders in vivo [27].

A common concern of physicians in treating male incontinence is that the inhibitory effect of antimuscarinics on detrusor muscle contraction theoretically could aggravate the voiding difficulties or cause urinary retention in men with concomitant BOO. It therefore is evident that the evaluation and management of men with symptoms consistent with OAB requires a thorough and diligent evaluation of the lower urinary tract in order to plan optimal therapeutic intervention. Evaluation is predicated on a complete assessment of voiding dynamics and is best accomplished with urodynamic studies. These studies should provide a complete measurement of filling characteristics, pressure and flow criteria, sphincteric activity, and postvoid residual determination in order to assess the existence and degree of obstruction.

However, as it has been stated in a recent review article, little evidence from clinical trials has supported the concern [28]. In a meta-analysis of randomized controlled trials of antimuscarinics used to treat OAB in female or mixed gender populations, only oxybutynin IR significantly increased the risk of urinary retention compared with placebo [29]. Men with BOO and DO who received tolterodine for 12 weeks demonstrated no change in Q_{max} and a reduction in detrusor pressure at Q_{max}. Tolterodine-treated men demonstrated a statistically significant increase in postvoid residual (PVR) urine volume compared with placebo, but whether this increase was clinically relevant is unclear. In this study, tolterodine was not associated with an increase in acute urinary retention (AUR) which required catheterization [30]. There also was no incidence of AUR among 39 men with BPH and LUTS who received open-label tolterodine extended-release (ER) treatment for 6 months [31]. In a recently published 12-week, randomized, double-blind, active- and placebo-controlled trial conducted at 95 urology clinics in the United States [32], 879 patients were randomly assigned to receive placebo, 4 mg of tolterodine ER, 0.4 mg of tamsulosin, or tolterodine ER plus tamsulosin. Changes in PVR volume, Q_{max}, or incidence of AUR did not differ significantly among the four treatment groups. However, this study did not include patients with PVR volume >200 ml and maximum urinary flow rate <5 ml/s.

Although several antimuscarinics are used to treat OAB, tolterodine has been most extensively investigated for the treatment of male OAB symptoms. Abrams et al. [30] reported a 12-week trial of tolterodine versus placebo in 222 men with frequency, urgency with or without incontinence, urodynamically confirmed DO, and mild to severe obstruction. Exclusions included PVR >40% of cystometric capacity and urinary retention within the preceding 12 months. The typical patient was moderately obstructed with proven DO. Only one episode of AUR was seen in the placebo group, with none in the tolterodine group. However, two patients on tolterodine were withdrawn due to a high PVR (320 ml in one, undefined in the other). There was no difference in the overall incidence of adverse events. Dry mouth was common among the tolterodine-treated patients (24%), but only one patient considered it severe. Urodynamic results showed evidence of fairly small treatment differences due to tolterodine for residual urine +27 ml; voiding efficiency −7%; and bladder contractility index (BCII) −10%. Significant reductions due to tolterodine were seen in detrusor pressure at maximum flow, with a difference between groups of −7 cm H_2O.

In a post hoc analysis study, the researchers assessed the efficacy and tolerability of tolterodine ER for reducing UI episodes in 163 men with OAB and urgency UI [33]. Key exclusion criteria of this study were, among others, the existence of clinically relevant BOO (judged by the investigator and based on patient history) and patients with a mean micturition (void) volume of <200 ml. Reductions in weekly UI episodes after 12 weeks of treatment were significantly greater in the tolterodine ER group than in the placebo group (median % change, 71% vs. 40%, $P < 0.05$). A significantly larger percentage of men receiving tolterodine ER reported an overall benefit of treatment (63% vs. 46%, $P = 0.04$). Except for dry mouth, the incidence of adverse events in men receiving tolterodine ER was low and similar to placebo. One man receiving tolterodine ER had symptoms suggestive of urinary retention, leading to his withdrawal from the study. None of the men had AUR retention requiring catheterization.

In accordance with these, significant reductions in total micturitions and urgency-related micturitions were observed in men with OAB symptoms who received tolterodine ER treatment for a period of 12 weeks [34]. However, all these reports are secondary analyses of subpopulations and not prospective clinical trials. Moreover, all of these studies were underpowered to detect clinically relevant increases in the incidence of a relatively rare event such as AUR, for example, to detect a doubling of AUR incidence.

Combination of Antimuscarinics Plus a_1-Receptor Antagonists

Some small and short-term studies have proposed that antimuscarinics can be safely combined with a_1-receptor antagonists to treat men with OAB symptoms in the presence or absence of BOO. Fifty men with urodynamically confirmed mild or moderate BOO and DO received tamsulosin for 1 week before being randomized to tamsulosin/tolterodine

combination therapy or tamsulosin alone [35]. Group allocation was randomized, but there was no blinding. Significant reductions in maximum detrusor pressure during micturition and maximum involuntary contraction pressure were observed in men who received the combination treatment for 3 months. These patients also demonstrated significantly increased Q_{max} and volume at first involuntary contraction, as well as improvements in a QOL measure. There was no incidence of urinary retention in either treatment group; however, it should be noted that men with severe obstruction (not defined) were specifically excluded. In the randomized, controlled trial by Kaplan et al. [32], patients were treated with placebo, only tolterodine, only tamsulosin, or both tolterodine ER plus tamsulosin for 12 weeks. Patients receiving the combination treatment compared with placebo experienced significant reductions in UUI (−0.88 vs. −0.31, $P = 0.005$), urgency episodes without incontinence (−3.33 vs. −2.54, $P = 0.03$), micturitions per 24 h (−2.54 vs. −1.41, $P < 0.001$), and micturitions per night (−0.59 vs. −0.39, $P = 0.02$). Patients receiving tolterodine ER plus tamsulosin demonstrated significant improvements on the total International Prostate Symptom Score (−8.02 vs. placebo, −6.19, $P = 0.003$) and QOL item (−1.61 vs. −1.17, $P = 0.003$).

The efficacy and tolerability of oxybutynin ER in combination with the a_1-blocker tamsulosin in reducing the irritative and obstructive components of LUTS was evaluated in a multicenter, double-blind trial [36]. Subjects of the trial were required to demonstrate a Q_{max} <8 ml/s and a PVR <150 ml on two occasions in order to qualify. A total of 418 men were randomized. Tamsulosin combined with oxybutynin ER resulted in a significantly greater improvement in total AUA symptom score compared with tamsulosin and placebo after 8 ($P = 0.033$) and 12 ($P = 0.006$) weeks of treatment. Combining active treatments resulted in greater decreases in AUA irritability scores after 4 ($P = 0.008$), 8 ($P < 0.001$), and 12 ($P < 0.001$) weeks. The incidence of an elevated PVR volume >300 ml was 2.9% ($n = 6$) in patients receiving combination therapy and 0.5% ($n = 1$) in patients receiving tamsulosin alone. Incidence of reduced Q_{max} (<5 ml/s) was 3.8% ($n = 8$) and 5.7% ($n = 12$), respectively. No patients developed AUR requiring catheterization.

Lee et al. [37] studied 228 men with urodynamically proven BOO and with frequency and urgency episodes at least daily, in an 8-week, randomized, double-blind, multicenter study. Patients were excluded if the PVR was >30% of cystometric capacity. Monotherapy with doxazosin was compared to combined treatment using doxazosin and propiverine. Symptoms were assessed by the IPSS. The combined treatment group had significant improvement rates with regard to urinary frequency (23.5% vs. 14.3%, $P = 0.004$), average micturition volume (32.3% vs. 19.2%, $P = 0.004$), and storage (41.3% vs. 32.6%, $P = 0.029$. There were no episodes of retention, but two patients in the combined group were withdrawn due to a rise in PVR, and the average PVR increased significantly in the combined group. Dry mouth was significantly more common in the combined group, although less than a third of affected patients left the study. It should be mentioned that the majority of patients studied fell into the equivocal range of obstruction as defined by an AG number [now termed the bladder outlet obstruction index (BOOI)] of 20–40. Furthermore, only 35% of patients had DO. Thus, the typical patient in this study was only mildly obstructed and tended not to have DO.

To date, no studies have evaluated the efficacy of combining antimuscarinics with 5a-reductase inhibitors, and there is no evidence to suggest that this cannot be a safe combination for the treatment of men with BPH and OAB symptoms. When treating male patients with UI and OAB syndromes in general, caution has to be exercised in those with significant PVR, since there is potential for increased risk of infection, further bladder decompensation, or renal insufficiency [38]. Close monitoring is recommended in these patients. At present, we must conclude that the literature is based on pilot studies that use urodynamic criteria for patient selection that do not necessarily represent real-life practice. Some of these studies are not placebo-controlled or are not adequately powered. Additionally, the short duration of the treatment trials (8 and 12 weeks) in the studies necessitates the investigation of anticholinergic treatment for a longer period. Combination therapy with an anticholinergic and an a_1-receptor antagonist in men with OAB and with suspected BOO is an interesting potential direction in pharmacotherapy that requires testing in well-designed clinical trials before it can be recommended for routine clinical use.

Stress Urinary Incontinence

SUI is defined as the involuntary leakage of urine on effort or exertion or on sneezing or coughing [1] and accounts for less than 8% of male urinary incontinence. It is a condition caused by sphincteric incompetence and usually occurs in women, while the most cases in men occur after pelvic surgery and especially prostatectomy. The etiology of sphincteric incompetence in these cases is lesions of autonomic parasympathetic nerves or the urethral sphincter itself.

Progress is significantly slower in the development of drugs for SUI compared to UUI. The main aim of drug treatment of SUI is to increase outflow resistance. Because SUI is a condition usually occurring in women, the studies investigating the effectiveness of pharmacotherapy in men are spare. Additionally, the anatomical differences of the lower urinary tract between males and females are responsible for the different underlying pathophysiological mechanisms of SUI. Consequently, the results from the use of drugs for treatment of female SUI might differ on men (Fig. 29.3).

Currently there is no pharmacological treatment approved for SUI in men. Theoretically, an increase in outflow resistance and therefore beneficial drug effects can be obtained in some patients by use of active a-adrenoceptor agonists and inhibitors of reuptake of noradrenaline and serotonin in adrenergic nerve endings [41, 42].

a-Adrenoceptor agonists have been used for SUI because they are effective at increasing bladder outlet resistance during bladder filling in animal models [43]. They have been found to be effective for SUI in both open-label and controlled clinical trials [41]; nevertheless there is a lack of long-term, randomized, controlled clinical trials. Additionally, the side effects observed where quite serious. Phenylpropanolamine was withdrawn from the US market by the Food and Drug Administration (FDA) because of the risk of hemorrhagic stroke in women [44]. Furthermore, a-adrenoceptor agonists lack exclusive selectivity for urethral a-adrenoceptors and may cause elevated blood pressure, sleep disturbances, nausea, dry mouth, headache, tremor,

Agent	Mechanism
Oxybutinin	Antimuscarinic action
Tolterodine	Target-specific antimuscarinic action rather than subtype-specific
Solifenacin	M3 selective receptor antagonist
Darifenacine	M3 selective receptor antagonist
Trospium	M1-3 antagonist. Does not cross normal blood brain barrier
Propiverine	Anticholinergic and calcium antagonistic actions
Capsaicin analogue agents	Block vanilloid receptors of c-fibers
Calcium channel blockers	Not encouraging results
Potassium channel openers	Not encouraging results
a-adrenergic antagonists	Need further trial
b-adrenergic agonists	Need further trial
Prostaglandin synthesis inhibitors	Need further trial

FIG. 29.3. Pharmacotherapy for male SUI

palpitations, and exacerbation of abnormal cardiac rhythms [45]. Interestingly, an agent that could potentially be useful in managing stress incontinence is clenbuterol, a b-adrenergic antagonist [46]. Although one would expect that such an agent would not be useful for SUI based on its mechanism of action, limited controlled studies have shown that the beneficial effects might result from improvement of the striated or extrinsic sphincteric mechanism. In a study of 72 incontinent men after prostate resection (BPH), clenbuterol improved 76.3% of treated men [47]. However, no drug in these categories has been subjected to rigorous clinical trials, and therefore none has received FDA approval for the treatment of SUI.

Imipramine, a tricyclic antidepressant, was among the first drugs with serotonin [5-hydroxytryptamine (5-HT)] and norepinephrine (NE) reuptake inhibitory action to be investigated for the treatment of SUI that showed some effectiveness in a few studies; however, side effects were considered serious enough to preclude further investigation.

During the last years, new interest has been given to drugs that stimulate sensomotor activity in the external urethral sphincter. Duloxetine is another combined 5-HT–NE reuptake inhibitor [48, 49]. In different double-blind, randomized, placebo-controlled clinical trials, a significant reduction of urinary incontinence and significantly improved incontinence quality of life (I-QOL) for women could be demonstrated [50–53]. Considering the proven effect on the striated sphincter muscles in incontinent women, it is plausible that a similar effect can be reached in men if the nervous structure or the sphincteric apparatus is not totally destroyed. By increasing the neural input the sphincteric activity, it is expected that continence will increase as well.

Data on the effect of duloxetine in men with SUI are still sparse,, and these studies have been published only during the last months [54–56]. Schlenker et al. presented their preliminary results from a pilot study on the off-label use of duloxetine for the treatment of SUI after radical prostatectomy or cystectomy with orthotopic neobladder [54]. Over a 2-year period, 18 patients with SUI postradical prostatectomy or radical cystectomy were treated with 40 mg of duloxetine twice daily. The average number of pads pretreatment was 8 a day. After an average of 9.4 weeks of pharmacotherapy with duloxetine, the average number of pads fell to 4.2 pads/day ($P < 0.0001$). Fifteen of the 18 patients (83.33%) reported improvement of SUI after the use of duloxetine and 7 of 18 patients (39%) were completely dry or used one pad per day at the most for safety reasons. The mean pad use in these patients before duloxetine was 3.9 pads/day. Six patients reported no side effects at all; the majority reported mild side effects such as fatigue ($n = 4$), dry mouth ($n = 3$), nausea ($n = 1$), or insomnia ($n = 1$). Most of the side effects vanished within 4 weeks but six patients (33.3%) discontinued the medication due to adverse events.

In another study, the researchers investigated the impact of duloxetine in urodynamic parameters of 18 men with SUI 12 months after radical prostatectomy [55]. All underwent a pad test to quantify the degree of urine loss and urodynamic evaluation before and after a 3-month duloxetine-treatment period. The intrinsic sphincter was evaluated by abdominal leak point pressure (ALPP) and retrograde leak point pressure (RLPP), and the striated sphincter by maximal urethral closure pressure (MUCP). In their results, they reported an increase in all three parameters and a significant reduction in urine loss. Additionally, after HCl duloxetine treatment there was significant correlation between RLPP and ALPP, while before treatment among all three urodynamic parameters.

Filocamo et al. [56] recently published a prospective, randomized, single-blind study in which they assessed the efficacy and safety of association of duloxetine and rehabilitation compared with rehabilitation alone in men with SUI after radical retropubic prostatectomy (RRP). From a total of 112 men, 92 patients completed the study and ten were removed due to adverse events (nine for duloxetine and one for placebo, discontinuation rates 15.2 and 1.8%, respectively). In their results, there was a significant decrease in pad use in the combined treatment group right after the completion of the 4-month treatment period, 39 patients versus 27 were dry ($P = 0.007$). However, 1 month after planned interruption of duloxetine, they observed a U-turn; 23 patients were completely dry vs. 38 in the rehabilitation alone group ($P = 0.008$). This shift also was observed 2 months later. On trying to explain these results, the authors stated that probably patients treated with duloxetine had less motivation than rehabilitation-only patients to learn to reproduce an adequate pelvic floor muscle precontraction during effort.

These studies suggest a beneficial effect of duloxetine on men with SUI, with drug tolerability, however, appearing to be an important issue. It is evident that larger prospective studies with adequate placebo control and a longer and standardized follow-up are recommended in order to draw more representative conclusions for the effectiveness of duloxetine in men with SUI.

Postprostatectomy Incontinence

The incidence of incontinence following prostatectomy varies between 1 and 15% depending mainly on the procedure used. In late life, preexisting bladder problems may coexist, accounting for the observed underlying pathology. The highest incidence is associated with radical prostatectomy, the incidence of stress incontinence requiring some

treatment varying between 5 and 15% [57]. After transurethral prostatectomy(TURP) or transvesical prostatectomy (TVP), the risk of incontinence is reported to be 0.4–1%. This might increase up to 20–40% following radical retropubic prostatectomy (RRP) [58, 59]. After being cured from some major problems such as voiding difficulties and malignancy, these patients are confronted with the social and hygienic problems brought about by incontinence. The integrity of the striated muscle sphincter is compromised in approximately 25% of incontinent patients [60]. Underlying detrusor instability accounts for the majority of cases either alone or in combination with sphincteric insufficiency. It therefore is evident that proper urodynamic investigation should be followed in order to properly diagnose the primary etiology of incontinence and provide adequate treatment; detrusor instability, sphincteric incompetence, or mixed.

Factors that have been associated with an increased risk of incontinence following prostatectomy are an increased age [61], associated neurological disease, or cognitive impairment [62, 63]. Evidence indicates that surgical technique can play a role, as a decrease in the risk of urinary incontinence is seen when manipulation of the lower urinary tract structures and tissues is limited, stitches in the smooth muscle of the urethra are avoided, and urethral length of at least 2.5 cm is preserved [64, 65]. The relationship between preoperative urine leakage and postoperative continence is less clear because baseline rates can be confounded by the obstructive symptoms of the disease often seen prior to surgery [66]. There is some debate about the influence of prior surgery in more recent series and it appears likely that there is no additional risk attributable to a repeat procedure.

Treatment of postprostatectomy incontinence should be targeted at the underlying pathology where appropriate. The drug options for urge and mixed incontinence are described previously in this chapter. There is good evidence that the incidence of detrusor instability will rise in association with increasing age among the postoperative population and that this will lead to an increase in lower urinary tract symptoms which will require treatment [67]. Periurethral injectable materials also have been used in an attempt to treat stress incontinence in men. The reported results of this intervention have been contradictory and success in the short term is followed by relapse [68, 69]. For patients with persistent stress incontinence following medical management, the implantation of an artificial urethral sphincter is a successful option; more than 70% of men will be either cured or significantly improved following the procedure.

Overflow Incontinence

Overflow incontinence (OI) occurs more often in men than women and it is characterized by large postvoid residual volumes of urine. The underlying pathology could be either an underactive (acontractile) detrusor or BOO. These conditions very often coexist, since BOO can lead to underactive bladder.

Underactive detrusor also can result from chronic urinary tract infection or overdistension of the bladder which can damage stretch receptors in the bladder wall. Radical pelvic surgery and diabetic neuropathy may damage the nerves, causing the same to occur. Drugs like anticholinergics, phenothiazines, antidepressants, narcotics, calcium channel blockers, and antihistamines can give rise to the same effects.

Urodynamic investigation is necessary in order to assess the existence of BOO and treat it initially. Surgery is the treatment of choice if obstruction is present; however, pharmacotherapy treatment with a-adrenergic blockers, eg, tamsulosin, terazosin, or doxazosin, may be beneficial [70]. The 5a-reductase inhibitor, finasteride, has been shown to decrease the symptom score and prostatic volume and to increase the urinary flow rates [71, 72]. Combination of these two agents (a-blocker +5a-reductase inhibitors) does not have additive effects on symptoms but seems more effective than either one as monotherapy in preventing a combined endpoint of clinical progression [70].

OI due to poor contraction of the bladder should be managed by clean intermittent self-catheterization (CISC) every 4 h or scheduled voiding training. If CISC is difficult or not possible for the patient, pharmacotherapy treatment can be used. However, little evidence exists suggesting that drug therapy may be beneficial [73]. In general, detrusor contractility can be enhanced either with parasympathomimetics or with drugs that inactivate cholinesterase, thus maintaining the cholinergic

simulation. Bethanechol chloride, a cholinergic agonist, has been used to stimulate bladder contractions, but has not been proven to be effective over the long term [74–77]. In a prospective study, intravesical prostaglandins were given to 36 patients who had urinary symptoms associated with a poorly functioning detrusor; 67% of these patients were found to be in chronic retention. Using standard urodynamic techniques, 72% showed objective evidence of an immediate improvement in detrusor function and there was prolonged therapeutic benefit in 39%. The authors noted that the results were encouraging for those already receiving oral cholinergic stimulation, with a prolonged reduction in the PVR [78]. Based on that observation, a prospective, randomized, double-blind study was conducted recently, investigating the effectiveness of combining intravesical prostaglandin E_2 (PGE_2) and oral bethanechol chloride in patients with underactive bladder [79]. From the 19 patients studied, 17 were men. Although there was evidence of a pharmacological effect, bethanechol chloride and PGE_2 had a limited therapeutic effect compared with placebo.

Distigmine bromide, an anticholinesterase agent, inactivates cholinesterase, leading to a sustained action of acetylcholine on cholinergic nerve endings, which results in improved detrusor contractions. Distigmine shows clinical efficacy in patients with poor detrusor function, and therefore may be used alternatively in selected cases, as was shown in 14 patients after TURP [80] and in a mixed gender study population [81]. In an interesting study published recently, the authors compared the effectiveness of a cholinergic drug, an a-blocker, and combinations of the two for the treatment of underactive detrusor [82]. One hundred-nineteen patients with underactive bladder were assigned to three groups: the cholinergic group, consisting of 40 patients taking bethanechol chloride (60 mg/day) or distigmine bromide (15 mg/day); the a-blocker group, consisting of 38 patients taking urapidil (60 mg/day); and the combination group, consisting of 41 patients taking both a cholinergic drug and an a-blocker. The effectiveness of each therapy was assessed 4 weeks after initialization of the therapy. The results in average and maximum flow rates and PVP showed a significant increase and decrease, respectively, in the combination group ($P = 0.0004$ and $P = 0.0008$, respectively).

General Conclusions

When pharmacotherapy is selected to treat male UI, physicians must have in mind that there are fewer medical treatment studies on males. Studies of UI have been conducted mostly on female populations, while data from mixed gender studies are clearly driven by the overwhelmingly female population in those studies. This chapter presented the medical treatment options for each type of male UI based on published studies; however, much more research is needed in order to allow evidence-based treatment recommendations.

References

1. EAU Guidelines. Guidelines on urinary incontinence. Update March 2005.
2. Abrams P, Cardozo L, Fall M, et al. Standardisation Sub-Committee of the International Continence Society. The standardisation of terminology in lower urinary tract function: Report from the standardisation sub-committee of the International Continence Society. Urology 2003; 61(1):37–49.
3. Jeffcoate TNA, Francis WJA. Urgency incontinence in the female. Am J Obstet Gynecol 1996; 94: 604–618.
4. Shaw C. A review of the psychosocial predictors of help-seeking behaviour and impact on quality of life in people with urinary incontinence. J Clin Nurs 2001; 10:15–24.
5. Hunskaar S, Sandvik H. One hundred and fifty men with urinary incontinence. III. Psychosocial consequences. Scand J Prim Health Care 1993; 11:193–196.
6. Valvanne J, Juva K, Erkinjuntti T, Tilvis R. Major depression in the elderly: A population study in Helsinki. Int Psychogeriatr 1996; 8:437–443.
7. Herzog AR, Fultz NH, Brock BM, et al. Urinary incontinence and psychological distress among older adults. Psychol Aging 1988; 3:115–121.
8. Bogner HR, Gallo JJ, Sammel MD, et al. Urinary incontinence and psychological distress in community-dwelling older adults. J Am Geriatr Soc 2002; 50:489–495.
9. Couture JA, Valiquette L. Urinary incontinence. Ann Pharmacother 2000; 34:646–655.
10. Wilson L, Brown JS, Shin GP, et al. Annual direct cost of urinary incontinence. Obstet Gynecol 2001; 98:398–406.
11. Gormley EA. Biofeedback and behavioral therapy for the management of female urinary incontinence. Urol Clin North Am 2002; 29:551–557.
12. Vapnek JM. Urinary incontinence. Screening and treatment of urinary dysfunction. Geriatrics 2001; 56:25–29.
13. Sibley GN. The physiological response of the detrusor muscle to experimental bladder outflow obstruction in the pig. Br J Urol 1987; 60:332–336.
14. Abdel-Aziz KF, Lemack GE. Overactive bladder in the male patient: Bladder, outlet, or both? Curr Urol Rep 2002; 3:445–451.
15. Steers W. Pathophysiology of overactive bladder and urge urinary incontinence. Rev Urol 2002; 4:S7–18.
16. Hyman MJ, Groutz A, Blaivas JG. Detrusor instability in men: Correlation of lower urinary tract symptoms with urodynamic findings. J Urol 2001; 166:550–552.
17. Hyman MJ, Groutz A, Blaivas JG. Detrusor instability in men: Correlation of lower urinary tract symptoms with urodynamic findings. J Urol 2001; 166:550–553.
18. Laniado ME, Ockrim JL, Marronaro A, et al. Serum prostate specific antigen to predict the presence of bladder outlet obstruction in men with urinary symptoms. BJU Int 2004; 94:1283–1286.
19. Stewart WF, van Rooyen JB, Cundiff GW, et al. Prevalence and burden of overactive bladder in the United States. World J Urol 2003; 20:327–336.
20. Peters TJ, Donovan JL, Kay HE, et al. The International Continence Society "Benign Prostatic Hyperplasia" Study: The bothersomeness of urinary symptoms. J Urol 1997; 157:885–889.
21. Kiefel JM, Bodnar RJ. Roles of gender and gonadectomy in pilocarpine and clonidine analgesia in rats. Pharmacol Biochem Behav 1992; 41:153–158.
22. Yoshimura Y, Schmidt F, Constantinou CE. Gender specificity of tolterodine on micturition and the diurnal variation of urine production of the conscious rat. BJU Int 2000; 87:879–885.
23. Longhurst PA, Levendusky M. Influence of gender and the oestrous cycle on in vitro contractile responses of the rat urinary bladder to cholinergic stimulation. Br J Pharmacol 2000; 131:177–184.
24. Choppin A. Muscarinic receptors in isolated urinary bladder smooth muscle from different mouse strains. Br J Pharmacol 2002; 137:522–528.
25. An JY, Yun HS, Lee YP, et al. The intracellular pathway of the acetylcholine-induced contraction in cat detrusor muscle cells. Br J Pharmacol 2002; 137:1001–1010.
26. Kories C, Czyborra C, Fetscher C, et al. Gender comparison of muscarinic receptor expression and function in rat and human urinary bladder: Differential regulation of M2 and M3 receptors? Naunyn Schmiedebergs Arch Pharmacol 2003; 367(5):524–531.

27. Michel MC, Schneider T, Krege S, Goepel M. Do gender or age affect the efficacy and safety of tolterodine? J Urol 2002; 168:1027–1031.

28. Chapple C, Roehrborn C. A shifted paradigm for the further understanding, evaluation, and treatment of lower urinary tract symptoms in men: Focus on the bladder. Eur Urol 2006; 49(4):651–659.

29. Chapple C, Khullar V, Gabriel Z, Dooley JA. The effects of antimuscarinic treatments in overactive bladder: A systematic review and meta-analysis. Eur Urol 2005; 48:5–26.

30. Abrams P, Kaplan SA, De Koning Gans HJ, Millard R. Safety and tolerability of tolterodine for the treatment of overactive bladder in men with bladder outlet obstruction. J Urol 2006; 175:999–1004.

31. Kaplan SA, Walmsley K, Te AE. Tolterodine extended release attenuates lower urinary tract symptoms in men with benign prostatic hyperplasia. J Urol 2005; 174:2273–2276.

32. Kaplan SA, Roehrborn CG, Rovner ES, et al. Tolterodine and tamsulosin for treatment of men with lower urinary tract symptoms and overactive bladder: A randomized controlled trial. JAMA 2006; 296(19):2319–2328.

33. Roehrborn CG, Abrams P, Rovner ES, et al. Efficacy and tolerability of tolterodine extended-release in men with overactive bladder and urgency urinary incontinence. BJU Int 2006; 97(5):1003–1006.

34. Marschall-Kehrel D, Abrams P, Guan Z, et al. Gender analysis of data from two 12-week randomized controlled trials of tolterodine: Tolterodine reduces overactive bladder-related nocturnal frequency in men and women with overactive bladder. Eur Urol 2005; 4:61.

35. Athanasopoulos A, Gyftopoulos K, Giannitsas K, et al. Combination treatment with an alpha-blocker plus an anticholinergic for bladder outlet obstruction: a prospective, randomized, controlled study. J Urol 2003; 169:2253–2256.

36. MacDiarmid S, Chen A, Tu Nora et al. Effects of tamsulosin and extended-release oxybutynin on lower urinary tract symptoms in men. American Urological Association Annual Meeting, May, 2006 (Abstract, podium presentation).

37. Lee KS, Choo MS, Kim DY, et al. Combination treatment with propiverine hydrochloride plus doxazosin controlled release gastrointestinal therapeutic system formulation for overactive bladder and coexisting benign prostatic obstruction: A prospective, randomized, controlled multicenter study. J Urol 2005; 174:1334–1338.

38. Larsson G, Hallen B, Nilvebrant L. Tolterodine in the treatment of overactive bladder: Analysis of the pooled phase II efficacy and safety data. Urology 1999; 53:990–998.

39. Diokno AC. Medical management of urinary incontinence. Gastroenterology 2004; 126(1 Suppl 1):S77–81 (review).

40. Dinis P, Silva J, Ribeiro MJ, et al. Bladder C-fiber desensitization induces a long—lasting improvement of BPH-associated storage LUTS: A pilot study. Eur Urol 2004; 46(1):88–93; discussion 93–94.

41. Diokno AC, Taub M. Ephedrine in treatment of urinary incontinence. Urology 1975; 5:624–625.

42. Andersson KE. Current concepts in the treatment of disorders of micturition. Drugs 1998; 35:477–494.

43. Brune ME, O'Neill AB, Gauvin DM, et al. Comparison of alpha 1-adrenoreceptor agonists in canine urethral pressure profilometry and abdominal leak point pressure models. J Urol 2001; 166:1555–1559.

44. Fleming G. The FDA regulation and the risk of stroke. N Engl J Med 2000; 343:1886–1887.

45. Anderson KW, Appell R, Awad S, et al. Pharmacological treatment of urinary incontinence. In: Abrams P, Khoury S, Wein A, eds. Incontinence. Plymouth: Health Publications Ltd, 2002:418–511

46. Yasuda K, Kawabe K, Takimoto Y. Clenbuterol Clinical Research Group. A double blind clinical trial of a b2-adrenergic agonist in stress incontinence. Int Urogynecol J 1993; 4:146–151.

47. Zozikov B, Kunchev SI, Varlev C. Application of clenbuterol in the treatment of urinary incontinence. Int Urol Nephrol 2001; 33:413–416.

48. Wernicke JF, Gahimer J, Yalcin I, et al. Safety and adverse event profile of duloxetine. Expert Opin Drug Saf 2005; 4:987–993.

49. Wong DT, Bymaster FP, Mayle DA, et al. LY248686, a new inhibitor of serotonin and norepinephrine uptake. Neuropsychopharmacology 1993; 8:23–33.

50. Dmochowski RR, Miklos JR, Norton PA, Et al. Duloxetine versus placebo for the treatment of North American women with stress urinary incontinence. J Urol 2003; 170:1259–1263.

51. Norton PA, Zinner NR, Yalcin I, Bump RC. Duloxetine versus placebo in the treatment of stress urinary incontinence. Am J Obstet Gynecol 2002; 187:40–48.

52. Kinchen KS, Obenchain R, Swindle R. Impact of duloxetine on quality of life for women with symptoms of urinary incontinence. Int Urogynecol J Pelvic Floor Dysfunct 2005; 16:337–344.

53. van Kerrebroeck P, Abrams P, Lange R, et al. Duloxetine versus placebo in the treatment of European and Canadian women with stress urinary incontinence. BJOG 2004; 111:249–257.

54. Schlenker B, Gratzke C, Reich O, et al. Preliminary results on the off-label use of duloxetine for the treatment of stress incontinence after radical prostatectomy or cystectomy. Eur Urol 2006; 49(6):1075–1078.

55. Zahariou A, Papaioannou P, Kalogirou G. Is HCl duloxetine effective in the management of urinary stress incontinence after radical prostatectomy? Urol Int 2006; 77:9–12.

56. Filocamo M, Li Marzi V, Del Popolo G, et al. Pharmacologic treatment in postprostatectomy stress urinary incontinence. Eur Urol 2007; 51(6): 1559–1564.

57. Catalona WJ, Basler WJ. Return of erections and urinary continence following nerve sparing radical prostatectomy. J Urol 1987; 138:574–578.

58. Fowler FJ Jr, Barry MJ, Lu-Yao G, et al. Patient reported complications and follow-up treatment after radical prostatectomy. The National Medicare Experience: 1988–1990. Urology 1993; 42(6):622.

59. Murphy GP, Mettlin C, Menck H, et al. National patterns of prostate cancer treatment by radical prostatectomy: Result of a survey by the American College of Surgeons Committee on Cancer. J Urol 1994; 152(5 Pt 2):1817.

60. Fitzpatrick JM, Gardina RA, Worth PHL. The evaluation of 68 patients with post prostatectomy incontinence. Br J Urol 1979; 51:552–555.

61. Steiner MS, Morton RA, Walsh PC. Impact of anatomical radical prostatectomy on urinary incontinence. J Urol 1991; 145:S12–15.

62. Hammerer P, Dieringer J, Schuler J, et al. Urodynamic parameters to predict continence after radical prostatectomy. J Urol 1991; 145:292A.

63. Barkin M, Dolfin D, Herschorn S, et al. Voiding dysfunction in institutionalised elderly men: The influence of previous prostatectomy. J Urol 1983; 130:258–259.

64. Moore K. A review of the anatomy of the male continence mechanism and the cause of urinary incontinence after prostatectomy. J WOCN 1999; 26:86–93.

65. Avant O, Jones J, Beck H, et al. New method to improve treatment outcomes for radical prostatectomy. Urology 2000; 56:658–662.

66. Potosky AL, Legler J, Albertsen PC, et al. Health outcomes after radical prostatectomy or radiotherapy for clinically localized prostate cancer: Results from the Prostate Cancer Outcomes Study (PCOS). J Natl Cancer Inst 2000; 92:1582–1592.

67. Thomas AW, Cannon A, Bartlett E, et al. The natural history of voiding dysfunction in men: The long term follow up of TURP. Br J Urol 1998; 81: (Suppl 4)22.

68. Politano VA. Transurethral polytef injection for post prostatectomy incontinence. Br J Urol 1992; 69:26–28.

69. Deane AM, English P, Hehir M, et al. Teflon injection in stress incontinence. Br J Urol 1985; 57:78–80.

70. Hutchison A, Farmer R, Verhamme K, et al. The efficacy of drugs for the treatment of LUTS/BPH. A study in 6 European countries. Eur Urol 2007; 51(1):207–215.

71. Gormley GJ, Stoner E, Bruskewitz RC, et al. The effect of finasteride in men with benign prostatic hyperplasia: the Finasteride Study Group. N Engl J Med 1992; 327:1185–1191.

72. Rittmaster RS. Finasteride. N Engl J Med 1994; 330:120–125.

73. Barendrecht MM, Oelke M, Laguna MP, Michel MC. Is the use of parasympathomimetics for treating an underactive urinary bladder evidence-based? BJU Int 2007; 99(4):749–752.

74. McDowell BJ, Burgio KL, Dombrowski M, et al. An inter-disciplinary approach to the assessment and behavioral treatment of urinary incontinence in geriatric outpatients. J Am Geriatr Soc 1992; 40:370–374.

75. Light JK, Scott FB. Bethanechol chloride and the traumatic cord bladder. J Urol 1982; 128:852,

76. Awad S. Clinical use of bethanechol. J Urol 1985; 134:523–524.

77. Sonda LP, Gershon C, Diokno AC, Lapides J. Further observations on the cystometric and uroflowmetric effects of bethanechol chloride on the human bladder. J Urol 1979; 122:775–777.

78. Desmond AD, Bultitude MI, Hills NH, Shuttleworth KE. Clinical experience with intravesical prostaglandin E2. A prospective study of 36 patients. Br J Urol 1980; 52:357–366.

79. Hindley RG, Brierly RD, Thomas PJ. Prostaglandin E2 and bethanechol in combination for treating detrusor underactivity. BJU Int 2004; 93(1):89–92.

80. Tanaka Y, Masumori N, Itoh N, et al. Symptomatic and urodynamic improvement by oral distigmine bromide in poor voiders after transurethral resection of the prostate. Urology 2001; 57(2):270–274.

81. Bougas DA, Mitsogiannis IC, Mitropoulos DN, et al. Clinical efficacy of distigmine bromide in the treatment of patients with underactive detrusor. Int Urol Nephrol 2004; 36(4):507–512.

82. Yamanishi T, Yasuda K, Kamai T, et al. Combination of a cholinergic drug and an alpha-blocker is more effective than monotherapy for the treatment of voiding difficulty in patients with underactive detrusor. Int J Urol 2004; 11(2):88–96.

Chapter 30
Treatment for Male Incontinence: Historical Review

Drogo K. Montague

Urinary incontinence is a dreaded complication of prostatectomy affecting men in the prime of their lives and causing considerable distress [1]. Cooney and Horton in 1951 wrote: "It is our impression that most urologists have an attitude of resignation regarding urinary incontinence and seldom attempt operative relief of these patients. Many have called attention to the tremendous increase in the sale of Cunningham clamps since the advent of transurethral prostatectomy, and the difficulty with sphincteric control following perineal prostatectomy is also well known. Even in suprapubic prostatectomy there appears to be an irreducible minimum of these embarrassing complications and probably in due time the retropubic prostatectomist will also ruefully acknowledge his guilt in a certain number of cases" [2]. They describe a rectus fascial bulbous urethral sling placed anterior to the pubis which produced cure in two patients and failed for technical reasons in a third.

For decades urologists struggled with the treatment of postprostatectomy incontinence often with disappointing and nondurable results. A major advance in the treatment of male urinary incontinence was the development of the artificial urinary sphincter (AUS) in 1973 [3]. This review of the history of the treatment of male urinary incontinence will be divided into the preartificial urinary sphincter era and the postartificial urinary sphincter era.

Preartificial Urinary Sphincter Era

Foley Prosthesis

Foley in 1947 described "an artificial sphincter" that consisted of a pneumatic or inflatable incontinence clamp which he implanted around the urethra just distal to the penoscrotal junction. This was connected by tubing to a pump that the patient carried in his "trouser's pocket." This pneumatic device was inflated for continence and deflated for voiding. In this 1947 article the author noted, "Under the writer's direct supervision the artificial sphincter as here described has been used with substantial satisfaction in many cases of enuresis and incontinence" [4]. No further results were given.

Male Slings

There is a long history of the use of slings for the treatment of postprostatectomy urinary incontinence. Because of the renaissance of the male sling in recent years, early results with this treatment modality will be discussed along with more recent experience later in this chapter.

Berry Prosthesis

Berry in 1961 reported his preliminary results with an acrylic or silicone prosthesis that was implanted against the bulbous urethra and fixed with wire sutures to the ascending pubic rami in men who had postprostatectomy urinary incontinence [5]. In an update published 10 years later he reported five major modifications of the original prosthesis: H-type, balloon, rolling pin, spindle, and yolk [6]. The report noted that 66 men underwent a total of 103 procedures. Complications included infection, perineal pain, and sinus formation. The procedure was unsuccessful in 80.6% of the cases. Many early successes subsequently became failures due to gradual loosening of the device.

Engle and Wad reported in 1969 on 15 operations for implantation of the Berry prosthesis [7]. Only five achieved continence and at the time of the report only two of those still had their prosthesis. The authors noted: "Our success rate with the Berry prosthesis is considerably less than that of other authors. Also our complication rate has been high. These considerations have left considerable doubt in our minds as to the real merit of this procedure."

Raney in 1969 also reported his experience with the implantation of this device in eight men [8]. Three patients became continent for a few days, one was partially continent for 2 months, and four never regained control. Raney concluded: "We believe that correction of male urinary incontinence with a prosthesis is perhaps a step in the right direction. The Berry procedure has not fulfilled its expectation, partially because the urinary sphincters and their actions are poorly understood."

Kaufman Procedures and Prosthesis

In an effort to compress the bulbous urethra without foreign bodies or prosthetic devices, Kaufman described a procedure in which he detached both crura along with the ischiocavernosus muscles, crossed them over the bulbocavernosus muscles, and attached them to the opposite pubic rami [9]. In a later publication Kaufman reported that of 28 men treated with this procedure, 9 were cured, 7 were markedly improved, and 12 were failures [10]. In the same paper he reported a modification of this procedure where the crura were mobilized but not detached. The mobilized crura were approximated over the bulbous urethra with a wad of Marlex being placed between the urethra and the crura. He called the first operation the

Kaufman I with the modification being known as the Kaufman II procedure. Using the Kaufman II procedure cure or marked improvement was noted in 7 of 11 men all of whom had been followed for at least 5 months.

In 1973 the Kaufman III operation was described [11]. In this procedure a silicone gel prosthesis was placed against the bulbous urethra and anchored in place by passing straps around the crura. In 30 men with postprostatectomy incontinence who underwent the Kaufman III operation as their first procedure, 14 were cured, 10 were greatly improved, 2 were moderately improved, and 4 were failures. In 17 men who had previous unsuccessful operations for incontinence, the Kaufman III procedure resulted in five cures, four with great improvement, four with moderate improvement, and four failures. In a later report Kaufman modified the Kaufman III procedure by stapling the silicone gel prosthesis straps to the pubic rami [12].

Bladder Neck Reconstruction

Tanagho and Smith described a bladder neck reconstruction in the male for treatment of urinary incontinence [13]. In this procedure they completely separated the bladder neck from the prostate. They then created an anterior bladder wall flap 1 in. wide and 1 in. long. This then was fashioned into a tube over a 16–18F Foley catheter and this tube was approximated to the proximal portion of the prostatic urethra. They reported on the results of 15 operations in which the overall success rate was 50%. They noted that with proper patient selection the success rate was about 80%.

Electronic Implants

Alexander and Rowan in 1968 noted: "It has been shown … that the voluntary (sic) muscles of the pelvic floor are in a state of tonic contraction at rest. In patients with incontinence the function of the pelvic-floor musculature is impaired and the object of an electronic implant is restoration of this function…Continuous electrical stimulation by means of electrodes in proximity to the pudendal nerves is effective in preventing escape of fluid from the urinary bladder" [14]. In this report they describe a passive electronic implant similar to that described by Bradley et al. in 1963 [15]. Methods in use included an implantable electronic implant [16, 17], vaginal pessary, and rectal plugs [18, 19]. Other methods using electrical means were designed to induce bladder evacuation and to enable bladder volume sensing [20].

None of these methods proved to be consistently effective. Gerry W. Timm, PhD, a biomedical engineer, wrote to me in March 2002: "The idea for the sphincter (AUS) was first proposed to me in October 1968 by Dr. Bradley (William E. Bradley, MD, a neurologist) on our return from a discouraging visit to a number of international centers studying electrical stimulation to produce bladder evacuation." Dr. Timm quoted Dr. Bradley as saying, "Why not by-pass the need to know lower urinary tract physiology which is required for producing efficient bladder evacuation and instead devise a mechanical device, such as an electromagnetic clothespin, to occlude the urethra for patients with incontinence?" (personal communication, letter March 13, 2002). This led to not only the description of the electromagnetic clothespin type of occlusive device but also the first concept of a totally implantable hydraulic AUS [21]. This concept was defined further in subsequent publications [20, 22–25].

Postartificial Urinary Sphincter Era

American Medical Systems Artificial Urinary Sphincter

Drs. Gerald W. Timm and William E. Bradley, both from the University of Minnesota, joined F. Brantley Scott, MD, a urologist from the Baylor College of Medicine in Huston, to bring the AUS to the point in its development where it was ready to be implanted in humans [3]. To manufacture and market the AUS along with an offshoot of this device, the inflatable penile prosthesis [26], Drs. Scott, Bradley, and Timm joined forces in 1972 with Robert Buuck, a businessman, to form American Medical Systems (AMS), Minnetonka, MN.

Between 1973 and 1983, the AUS underwent several major design changes (Fig. 30.1) [27, 28]. The first device, the AS 721, was introduced in

1973 (Fig. 30.2). This hydraulic device was constructed of medical-grade silicone elastomer and stainless steel. It consisted of a circumferential cuff that could be implanted around the male or female bladder neck or around the bulbous urethra in the adult male. This was connected by tubing to inflation and deflation bulbs that were implanted in the scrotum or labia majora. These bulbs were connected to a fluid reservoir, which was implanted behind the rectus muscle in the lower abdomen. The device was filled with normal saline or isotonic contrast. Pressure in the sphincter was controlled by a mechanical V4 valve above the deflation pump.

Subsequent design changes led to the AS 742 (Fig. 30.3), which was introduced in 1974. This device incorporated a pressure-regulating balloon (PRB), which instead of the V4 valve determined cuff pressure. The PRB also allowed fluid transfer back into the cuff through a delayed filled resistor, thus eliminating the need for the inflation pump. PRBs were provided in three different pressure ranges: 51–60, 61–70, and 71–80 cm H_2O. Cuffs also were provided in a variety of sizes for both the bladder neck and bulbous urethra.

In 1976 the AS 761 (Fig. 30.4) was introduced. In this model, which is similar to the original AS 721, a PRB was placed between the cuff and V4 pressure valve. With this device the PRB rather than the less reliable V4 valve determined cuff pressure.

In 1979 the AS 791 (Fig. 30.5) was introduced. This device and a variant, the AS 792, were streamlined versions of the AS 742. A problem with the AS 742, AS 791, and AS 792 was that once these devices were implanted and connections were made, the cuff remained inflated at all times except when the patient deflated it for voiding. There was no way to stop the automatic refilling of the cuff.

The device used today (AMS Sphincter 800™) (Fig. 30.6) was introduced in 1983. It works on the same principle as the AS 742, AS 791, and AS 792, but it incorporates a deactivation feature. Following surgical implantation, the surgeon cycles the device to open the cuff; the deactivation button is then pushed, and this prevents refilling of the cuff. Usually 4–6 weeks later, when cuff and pump site swelling have resolved, the device

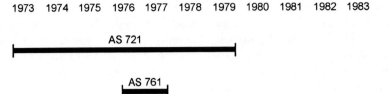

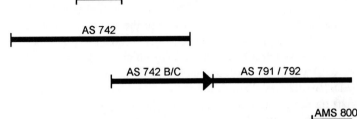

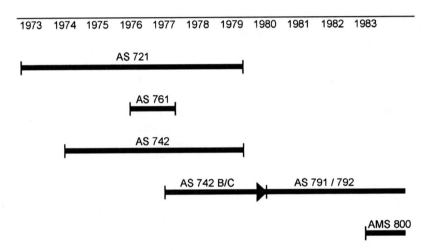

FIG. 30.1. Time line for the five models of American Medical Systems' artificial urinary sphincter (used by permission of American Medical Systems, Minnetonka, MN, USA)

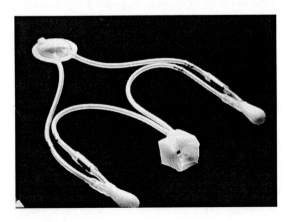

FIG. 30.2. The AS 721

is reactivated by forcibly squeezing the deflation pump. Deactivation can be done again later whenever necessary, for example, if the patient needs an indwelling urethral catheter. This device continues in use today, although there have been numerous modifications to the design of the various components of this device in efforts to increase both effectiveness and longevity. These include a narrow back cuff for the urethra, a smaller 4.0-cm cuff, surface coating for the cuff, kink-resistant tubing, a sutureless connector system, and tubing collars to relieve strain.

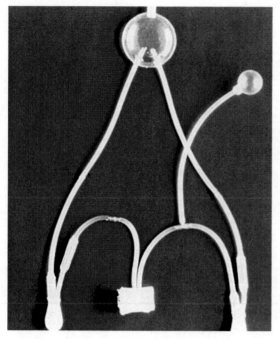

FIG. 30.3. The AS 742

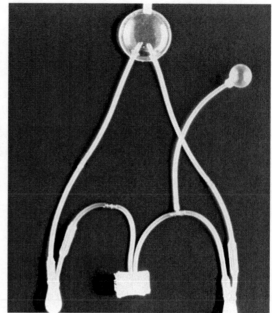

FIG. 30.5. The AS 791

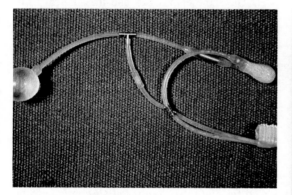

FIG. 30.4. The AS 761

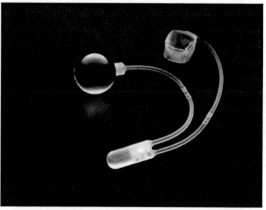

FIG. 30.6. The AMS Sphincter 800™

Rosen Prosthesis

In 1976, 3 years after the introduction of the AUS, Rosen described a three-pronged clamp with two parallel arms on one side and a single arm carrying a balloon that opposed them [29]. The balloon, implanted against the bulbous urethra, was connected by tubing to a scrotal reservoir that could inflate the balloon for continence and deflate it for voiding. Of 16 patients in whom this device was implanted, ten were cured, one was improved, and five failed. Rosen updated his results 2 years later by stating: "Twenty-three patients have been operated on and 18 have been cured. The main complications are device failure and sepsis. The results so far justify a limited optimism that the device has a significant role to play in the management of male urinary incontinence" [30].

Small, in 1980, reported 16 patients in whom the Rosen prosthesis was implanted with follow-up ranging from 2 to 36 months. Eleven of the 16 were reported as being "cured" [31]. Geisy and Barry 1 year later reported less optimistic results [32]. They reported 19 men who had the Rosen device implanted. Follow-up ranged from 9 to 34 months. There were 26 additional operations for balloon leakage, aneurysm, tubing kinks, reservoir malfunction, and urethral erosion. Using life-table actuarial analysis demonstrated that 44% had failed by 6 months and 75% had failed by 12 months. The authors concluded: "Although the simple concept developed by Rosen is an intriguing one and excellent continence can result, the multiple procedures required to achieve satisfactory results leave a great deal of room for product improvement."

In a 1981 report entitled: "Pitfalls of the Rosen anti-incontinence prosthesis," Augspurger reported on 17 male patients who had a Rosen prosthesis implanted. Nine had a functioning device, four had a nonfunctioning prosthesis and were awaiting replacement, and four had had the device removed [33]. Vereecken and associates in 1985 published a paper entitled: "The Rosen prosthesis: A bad experience." In it they noted: "...we implanted 4 Rosen inflatable incontinence prostheses in 4 men with urinary incontinence. Twelve operations were necessary on these 4 patients to assure them to be continent during a total of 43 months. Because of the great number of complications we no longer use the Rosen prostheis" [34].

Collagen Injections

Injections of glutaraldehyde cross-lined bovine collagen have been used to treat postprostatectomy urinary incontinence. More than one injection usually is needed to obtain an initial result and periodic reinjections often are necessary to maintain this result. We summarized the literature concerning collagen injections in the male (Table 30.1) [40].

Male Slings

Uhle in 1957, referring to the earlier work of Cooney and Horton [2], wrote: "This presentation will summarize my experience and thoughts pertaining to the fascial sling placed anterior to the pubis and about the bulbous urethra for the control on urinary incontinence. Ten and one-half years have elapsed since the first case was operated upon. A total of 8 cases form the basis of this report. In 5 cases the aponeurosis of the rectus muscle was used, in 2 cases the fascia lata of the thigh was employed, while the eighth case was subjected to the use of both at different intervals of time. The technique and results of these anteropubic fascial slings which compress the bulbous urethra have been presented....The results were partially effective in fifty per cent of the cases" [41]. The same eight cases and the surgical technique were presented in more detail in a somewhat later publication [42].

Servado in 1974 described six cases of rectus fascial sling around the bulbous urethra and passed retropubically for postprostatectomy urinary incontinence. He noted: "...all regained full continence immediately following the fascial-sling operation. None of them has a residual urine and, therefore, no urinary infection has occurred. There is occasional mild stress incontinence in one case only. The patients have now been followed for one to six years and all continue to be fully continent" [43].

TABLE 30.1. Collagen injection for male incontinencea.

Publication	Dry		Improved	Failed	Mean injections (n)	Mean follow-up (months)
Griebling et al. [35]b	589	152	216	192		5.7–13.3
Martins et al. [36]	46	11	21	14	2.8	26
Sanchez-Ortiz et al. [37]	31	2	9	20	2.6	15
Smith et al. [38]	62	5	24	33	4	29
Klute et al. [39]	20	2	7	11	1	28
Total	748	172 (23)	277 (27)	270 (36)		

Numbers in parentheses are percentagesaUsed by permission by of Elsevier (Urol. 55: 1–4, 2000)bSummary of 13 studies 1989–1996

TABLE 30.2. Summary of recent male sling publications[a].

Publication	n	Mean follow-up (months)	Results (pads per day)	Comments
Castle et al. [46]	38	18	39% 1 pad or less	Bone anchored
Rajpurkar et al. [47]	46	24	37% no pads, 37% 1–2 pads	Bone anchored
Ulrich and Comiter [48]	36	24	67% no pads, 14% 1 pad, 11% 2 pads	Bone anchored
Stern et al. [49]	71	48	Seven slings explanted; results for remaining 64: 68% 1–2 pads, 39% no pads	Three tetrafluoro-ethylene bolster anchored to rectus fascia

[a] From [45]

Pettersson in 1975 reported eight men with postprostatectomy urinary incontinence who were treated with fascia lata bulbous urethral slings passed retropubically. He noted: "Four patients were continent 7–36 months postoperatively. Two patients had stress incontinence and two patients had recidivating incontinence" [44].

There has been a renaissance recently in the use of the male bulbous urethral sling for the treatment of postprostatectomy urinary incontinence. In a recent editorial, we reported that our literature review showed 20 publications from 1997 to 2005 [45]. Only four of these had 20 patients or more with a mean follow-up of at least 1 year, and these four publications are briefly summarized in Table 30.2.

A New Artificial Urinary Sphincter

While there have been numerous modifications to the various components of the AMS Sphincter 800™, its basic design has remained unchanged for more than 20 years. The first commercially available alternative to the AMS Sphincter 800™ was recently announced [50]. This device consists of a newly designed urethral cuff, a scrotal pump-control assembly, and two PRBs. This new device does not have the deactivation feature of the AMS Sphincter 800™; however, it does have a self-sealing port at the bottom of the pump which can be used to add or remove fluid from the system. This new device eliminates the need for tubing connections. Possible advantages of this new AUS are outlined in an accompanying editorial [51]. Eleven patients received this new implant and in two patients the device was removed. In the remaining nine patients there was a reduction in the mean daily leakage volume from 770.6 to 55.1 ml and an overall improvement in the continence index from 54 to 97%.

References

1. Herr HW. Quality of life of incontinent men after radical prostatectomy [see comments]. J Urol 1994; 151(3):652–654.
2. Cooney CJ, Horton GR. An operation for the cure of urinary incontinence in the male. J Urol 1951; 66(4):586–592.
3. Scott FB, Bradley WE, Timm GW. Treatment of urinary incontinence by implantable prosthetic sphincter. Urol 1973; 1(3):252–259.
4. Foley FEB. An artificial sphincter: A new device and operation for control of enuresis and urinary incontinence. J Urol 1947; 58:250–259.
5. Berry JL. A new procedure for correction of urinary incontinence: Preliminary report. J Urol 1961; 85:771.
6. Berry JL, Dahlen CP. Evaluation of a procedure for correction of urinary incontinence in men. J Urol 1971; 105(1):105–106.
7. Engel RM, Wade JC. Experience with the Berry prosthesis. J Urol 1969; 102(1):78–80.
8. Raney AM. Re-evaluation of post-prostatectomy urinary incontinence with the Berry procedure. J Urol 1969; 102(1):81–83.
9. Kaufman JJ. A new operation for male incontinence. Surg Gynecol Obstet 1970; 131(2):295–299.
10. Kaufman JJ. Surgical treatment of post-prostatectomy incontinence: Use of the penile crura to compress the bulbous urethra. J Urol 1972; 107(2):293–297.
11. Kaufman JJ. Treatment of post-prostatectomy urinary incontinence using a silicone gel prosthesis. Br J Urol 1973; 45(6):646–653.
12. Kaufman JJ, Raz S. Passive urethral compression with a silicone gel prosthesis for the treatment of male urinary incontinence. Mayo Clin Proc 1976; 51(6):373.

13. Tanagho EA, Smith DR. Clinical evaluation of a surgical technique for the correction of complete urinary incontinence. J Urol 1972; 107(3):402–411.

14. Alexander S, Rowan D. Electrical control of urinary incontinence by radio implant. A report of 14 patients. Br J Surg 1968; 55(5):358–364.

15. Bradley WE, Chou SN, French LA. Further experience with the radio transmitter receiver unit for the neurogenic bladder. J Neurosurg 1963; 20:953–960.

16. Caldwell KP. The treatment of incontinence by electronic implants. Hunterian lecture delivered at the Royal College of Surgeons of England on 8th December 1966. Ann R Coll Surg Engl 1967; 41(6):447–459.

17. Caldwell KP, Cook PJ, Flack FC, James D. Treatment of post-prostatectomy incontinence by electronic implant. Br J Urol 1968; 40(2):183–186.

18. Glen ES. Effective and safe control of incontinence by the intra-anal plug electrode. Br J Surg 1971; 58(4):249–252.

19. Hopkinson BR. Electrical treatment of incontinence using an external stimulator with intra-anal electrodes. Ann R Coll Surg Engl 1972; 50(2):92–111.

20. Timm GW. Electromechanical restoration of voiding. Vet Clin North Am 1974; 4(3):525–533.

21. Timm GW, Bradley WE. Electronic micturictrion reflex stimulation. Proc 17th Spinal Cord Injury Conference Veterans Administration 1969: 152–157.

22. Timm GW. An implantable incontinence device. J Biomech 1971; 4(3):213–219.

23. Timm GW, Merrill DC, Bradley WE. Intermittent occlusion system. IEEE Trans Biomed Eng 1970; 17(4):352.

24. Timm GW, Frohrib DA, Bradley WE. Genitourinary prosthetics of the present and future. Mayo Clin Proc 1976; 51(6):346–350.

25. Burton JH, Mikulich MA, Timm GW, et al. Development of urethral occlusive techniques for restoration of urinary incontinence. Med Instrum 1977; 11:217–220.

26. Scott FB, Bradley WE, Timm GW. Management of erectile impotence: Use of implantable inflatable prosthesis. Urol 1973; 2:80–82.

27. Montague DK. Evolution of implanted devices for urinary incontinence. Cleve Clin Q 1984; 51(2): 405–409.

28. Montague DK. The Scott–Bradley–Timm artificial urinary sphincters. J Urol 1981; 125(6):796–798.

29. Rosen M. A simple artificial implantable sphincter. Br J Urol 1976; 48(7):675–680.

30. Rosen M. The Rosen inflatable incontinence prosthesis. Urol Clin North Am 1978; 5(2):405–414.

31. Small MP. The Rosen incontinence procedure: A new artificial urinary sphincter for the management of urinary incontinence. J Urol 1980; 123(4): 507–511.

32. Giesy JD, Barry JM, Fuchs EF, Griffith LD. Initial experience with the Rosen incontinence device. J Urol 1981; 125(6):794–795.

33. Augspurger RR. Pitfalls of the Rosen anti-incontinence prosthesis. J Urol 1981; 125(2):201–203.

34. Vereecken RL, Van den Bussche L, Tailly G. The Rosen prosthesis: A bad experience. Urol Int 1985; 40(1):30–32.

35. Griebling TL, Kreder KJ Jr, Williams RD. Transurethral collagen injection for treatment of postprostatectomy urinary incontinence in men. Urol 1997; 49:907–912.

36. Martins FE, Bennett CJ, Dunn M, et al. Adverse prognostic features of collagen injection therapy for urinary incontinence following radical retropubic prostatectomy. J Urol 1997; 158:1745–1749.

37. Sanchez-Ortiz RF, Broderick GA, Chaikin DC, et al. Collagen injection therapy for post-radical retropubic prostatectomy incontinence: Role of valsalva leak point pressure. J Urol 1997; 158:2132–2136.

38. Smith DN, Appell RA, Rackley RR, Winters JC. Collagen injection therapy for post-prostatectomy incontinence. J Urol 1998; 160(2):364–367.

39. Klutke JJ, Subir C, Andriole G, Klutke CG. Long-term results after antegrade collagen injection for stress urinary incontinence following radical retropubic prostatectomy. Urol 1999; 53:974–977.

40. Montague DK, Angermeier KW. Postprostatectomy urinary incontinence: The case for artificial urinary sphincter implantation [editorial]. Urol 2000; 55(1):2–4.

41. Uhle CA. Use of anteropubic fascial sling for treatment of surgical incontinence in the male. J Urol 1957; 77(3):478–484.

42. Uhle CA, Bradley RH Jr. The use of rectus fascia and fascia lata in the sling operation for urinary incontinence in the male. J Urol 1958; 80(2): 132–139.

43. Servadio C. The use of fascial sling for the correction of postprostatectomy incontinence. Isr J Med Sci 1974; 10(6):612–616.

44. Pettersson S. Free fascial sling to correct urinary incontinence after prostatic surgery. Results of eight operated patients. Scand J Urol Nephrol 1975; 9(1):24–27.

45. Montague DK, Angermeier KW. Treatment of postprostatectomy urinary incontinence: The case against the male sling. Nat Clin Pract Urol 2006; 3(6):290–291.

46. Castle EP, Andrews PE, Itano N, et al. The male sling for post-prostatectomy incontinence: Mean follow-up of 18 months. J Urol 2005; 173(5):1657–1660.

47. Rajpurkar AD, Onur R, Singla A. Patient satisfaction and clinical efficacy of the new perineal bone-anchored male sling. Eur Urol 2005; 47(2):237–242; discussion 242.

48. Ullrich NF, Comiter CV. The male sling for stress urinary incontinence: 24-Month follow-up with questionnaire based assessment. J Urol 2004; 172(1):207–209.

49. Stern JA, Clemens JQ, Tiplitsky SI, et al. Long-term results of the bulbourethral sling procedure. J Urol 2005; 173(5):1654–1656.

50. Knight S, Susser J, Craggs M, et al. A new artificial urinary sphincter with conditional occlusion for stress urinary incontinence: Preliminary clinical results. E Urol 2006; 50:574–580.

51. Montague DK. Reflections on a new artificial urinary sphincter. Eur Urol 2006; 50:421–423.

Chapter 31
Treatment for Male Incontinence: Surgical Procedures (Post-TURP/RRP)

Rajeev Kumar and Ajay Nehra

Surgical Anatomy and Innervation of the Sphincter

The last few decades have seen a refined definition of the continence mechanism in the male, which consists of two sphinteric mechanisms, with the *proximal continence* mechanism provided by an intact bladder neck with its smooth muscle, the preprostatic sphincter. This definition has been based primarily on numerous male autopsy and radiological studies. The preprostatic sphincter is a continuous structure that runs from the bladder neck to the bulbar urethra with varying amounts of tissue on the dorsal aspect [1]. This sphincter is responsible for providing resting continence in a normal male (Fig. 31.1). The second sphinteric mechanism – the *distal sphincteric mechanism* – described by Strasser et al. [2], was about 1.5 cm in a study of 14 male specimens, while Myers et al. [3] found this to vary from 1.5 to 2.4 cm, with a mean of 2.0 cm based on MRI imaging studies [4] (Fig. 31.2).

These findings have given rise to numerous controversial issues. Myers suggests that this region, also known as the rhabdosphincter, comprises both striated and smooth muscle components extending from the veru montanum to the bulbar urethra and should be thought of as "sphincteric urethra" rather than membranous urethra, since it encompasses the various elements that provide continence at this level [3]. The smooth muscle component lies internal to the striated muscle and is continuous with the proximal smooth muscle sphincter [1, 3]. External

to this is the striated muscle layer that contains predominantly type I slow-twitch fibers which are adapted to maintain tone over long periods of time, and thus provide resting continence [5]. These muscle fibers apparent even in early fetal development [6] do not surround the urethra and form a horseshoe or omega configuration, are deficient posteriorly, and are bulkiest anteriorly [1, 2]. The fact that the native sphincteric mechanism does not depend on a posterior support may be a reason for relatively poor results of male sling procedures. It is important to note that the levator ani muscles do not form a part of this sphincteric mechanism and are found to be separated from it by a clear layer of connective tissue [1, 7]. The levator ani muscles primarily consist of fast-twitch (type II) fibers that are responsible for the "quick stop" mechanism of urinary control [8], provides the voluntary control to voiding.

The innervation is complex, and debate persists on whether the somatic innervation via the pudendal nerve reaches the sphincter or not. Karam et al. [9] (Fig. 31.3) evaluated ten male human fetuses in order to identify the innervation of the external urethral sphincter. They found the presence of both unmyelinated autonomic and myelinated somatic nerves in the striated sphincter. The unmyelinated nerves entered at the 5 o"clock and 7 o"clock positions, while the myelinated nerves entered the striated fibers of the prostatic capsule at the 9 and 3 o"clock positions. Both sets of nerves existed close to the bladder neck and on the lateral and anterior surfaces of the rectum. At the level of the bladder

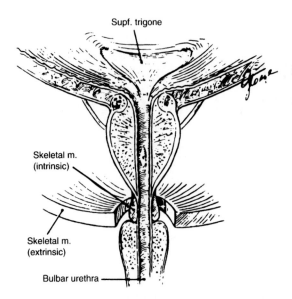

FIG. 31.1. Functional anatomy of the male continence mechanism. The proximal urethral sphincter extends from the bladder neck through the prostatic urethra above the verumontanum. The distal urethral sphincter extends from the prostatic urethra below the verumontanum through the membranous urethra. It includes the rhabdosphincter (intrinsic skeletal and smooth muscle) and extrinsic paraurethral skeletal muscle. Supf., superficial (copywrite with permission)

neck, the fibers were found to be below the pelvic fascia. Studies by Narayan et al. [10] found that the dorsal nerve of the penis also supplied the external sphincter and were 0.3–1.3 cm away from the prostatic apex. These nerves may be sensory and damage to them could lead to abolition of a reflex sphincteric mechanism that may be responsible for continence, particularly during sleep [5].

Prostatectomy, both radical and transurethral, results in a destruction of the proximal smooth muscle sphincteric mechanism. Continence in these patients continues to be maintained through the action of the distal urethral sphincter. Apposition of the mucosal folds of the urethra and resting tone maintained by the smooth muscle and the striated muscle provide resting continence. During periods of stress or during voluntary inhibition of stream, the somatic fibers likely come into play, causing contraction of the type II fibers of the levator ani and also some of the fibers of the striated sphincter. Damage to these fibers and their innervation probably is the prime cause for postprostatectomy stress incontinence [11].

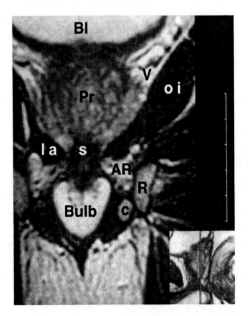
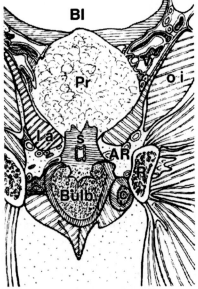

FIG. 31.2. "Sphincteric urethra" might be more appropriate than "membranous urethra." Coronal view through bladder (bl), prostate (Pr), striated urethral sphincter (s), bulb, veins (V), obturator internus (o i), levator ani (l a), anterior recess (AR) of ischioanal fossa, ischiopubic ramus (R), and corpus cavernosum (c). (Sagittal inset for orientation.) (By permission of Mayo Foundation for Medical Education and Research) (copywrite with permission)

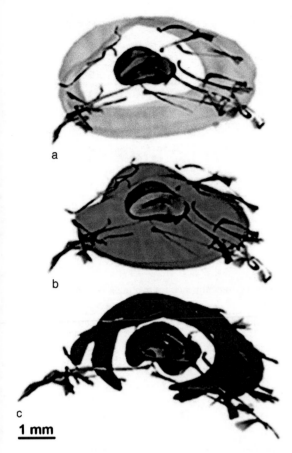

a

b

c

1 mm

FIG. 31.3. Three-dimensional reconstruction of nervous fibers from transverse sections of 36-week-old male fetus (CRL 330 mm). (**a, b**) The unmyelinated nerves (in *yellow*) give branches, which penetrate into the prostate (in *magenta*) and emerge from the verumontanum for innerved the prostate, the smooth muscles, and the submucosa (in *cyan*). (**c**) The striated muscular fibers (in *red*), situated at the anterolateral faces of the prostate, are innerved by myelinated nervous fibers (in *green*) (copywrite with permission)

Pathophysiology of Incontinence

Continence requires the storage of urine within the bladder at low pressures with absence of involuntary contractions, coupled with an outflow resistance that voluntarily can be decreased. Postprostatectomy incontinence (PPI) may be the result of a number of mechanisms acting either alone or in combination. These mechanisms are faulty sphincteric action, bladder dysfunction, or anatomic abnormalities

of vesicourethral anastomosis. The most common type of incontinence seen after radical prostatectomy is stress incontinence. With sudden increases in intra-abdominal pressure and subsequent rise in vesical pressure, the sphincteric resistance would prevent any urine leak during such rises. But a compromised sphincteric function that results from damage following the surgery would not be able to resist this rise in pressure, resulting in a urine leak. Detrusor instability with repeated involuntary contractions may raise the bladder pressure above the sphincteric resistance, resulting in a leak typically present as urgency or urge incontinence. Urge incontinence is more common after transurethral resection than after radical prostatectomy [12]. At times, both mechanisms may be present simultaneously. Overflow incontinence due to an anastomotic stricture results in urinary retention followed by overflow.

Intrinsic Sphincter Deficiency

Following radical prostatectomy, sphincteric deficiency appears to be the most common cause of incontinence [5]. Ficazzola and Nitti [12] evaluated 60 patients with PPI in order to identify the cause of incontinence and correlate symptoms with urodynamic findings (Table 31.1). Stress incontinence was the most commonly found complaint, and intrinsic sphincter deficiency (ISD) was demonstrated in 90% of the patients. Majoros et al. [13] found ISD to be present in 90% of their incontinent patients and the sole finding in 60%. The finding of isolated sphincter deficiency as the most common cause of incontinence has been noted by other authors [14, 12]. However, Groutz et al. [15] performed urodynamic examinations in 83 men referred for PPI at a mean of 2.7 years after surgery. They reported a combination of urodynamic findings with 88% of the patients having ISD (Table 31.2): 33.7% with bladder instability and 20.5% with bladder outlet obstruction. Maintenance of adequate urethral length has been proposed in preventing postoperative incontinence. Rudy et al. [16] found a significant decrease in the mean functional sphincter length from 4.3 to 1.6 cm and believed this to be a significant contribution. Hammerer and Huland [17] found that the mean functional urethral length decreased from 61 mm preoperatively to 25.9 mm postoperatively,

TABLE 31.1. Summary of several contemporary series on post-radical prostatectomy incontinence with regard to sphincter and bladder dysfunctiona.

	N	Sphincter dysfunction		Bladder dysfunction	
		Total (%)	Alone (%)	Total (%)	Alone (%)
Leach et al. (1996)	162	82	40	36	14
Goluboff et al. (1995)	25	60	8	90	40
Chao and Mayo (1995)	74	96	57	43	4
Gudziak et al. (1996)	37	97	NA	NA	3
Desautel et al. (1997)	35	95	59	39	3
Ficazzola and Nitti (1998)	60	90	53	45	3
Winters et al. (1998)	92	98.5	59	29	1.5
Groutz at al. (2000)	83	88	33a	34	4

NA, not applicablea This study considered urodynamic diagnoses of obstruction and impaired contractility so that patients with sphincteric insuffiency and impaired contractility or obstruction without bladder dysfunction are not included in this group

TABLE 31.2. Summary of several series on postprostatectomy incontinence for treatment of benign disease with regard to sphincter and bladder dysfunction.

	N	Sphincter dysfunction		Bladder dysfunction	
		Total (%)	Alone (%)	Total (%)	Alone (%)
Andersen and Nordling (1978)[a]	34	50	21	74	44
Fitzpatrick et al. (1979)[b]	68	79	28	66	16
Yalla et al. (1982)[c]	21	62	52	38	29
Goluboff et al. (1995)	31	20	3	97	77
Leach et al. (1996)[d]	51	78	39	59	20
Nitti et al. (1997)	20	20	20	75	75
Winters et al. (1998)	27	93	44	56	7

Patients underwent transurethral prostatic resection except when otherwise noted
[a] All patients underwent open transvesical prostatectomy
[b] Contains 21 patients who underwent open prostatectomy
[c] Contains five patients who underwent radical prostatectomy, not stratified in data
[d] Contains 14 patients who underwent open prostatectomy

and the maximal urethral pressure declined from 89.6 to 65.2 cm. However, other studies have noted the length to be of no importance; rather, the maximal urethral closure pressure is of prime significance [13, 18]. Following transurethral resection, incontinence more often is urge rather than stress. Sphincteric damage may occur in 3–47% of these patients [19].

Bladder Instability

Bladder instability is a common finding in patients with PPI, both transurethral and radical. In transurethral resections, bladder instability is the most common finding in incontinent patients [19]. Patients undergoing radical prostatectomy may have a number of etiologies for their bladder instability. Hellstrom et al. [20] noted a decreased bladder compliance from 37 to 23 ml following surgery. An incidence of 9–11% of poor compliance also was found by Gomha and Boone [21] and Chao and Mayo [22]. Groutz et al. [15] found detrusor instability in 33.7% of their patients, and this was the sole finding in 3.6%. Impaired contractility also was present in 28.9% of their patients, and most of these patients had a concomitant sphincteric weakness, thus suggesting the lack of outflow resistance is severe enough to allow incontinence even in the presence of a hypocontractile detrusor. A number of men undergoing this surgery may have had preexisting bladder instability. This may have been asymptomatic in the presurgery period and may have arisen from advanced age or associated benign prostatic hyperplasia (BPH) [11]. While evaluating 68 men scheduled for radical prostatectomy before surgery, Majoros et al. [13] found detrusor overactivity (DO) in 23.8% of the patients. In six of the men, DO improved after surgery.

Giannantoni et al. [23] similarly evaluated 49 patients prior to radical prostatectomy and found decreased bladder compliance in 20.4% of patients at baseline. They also noted a de novo decrease in compliance in 18.4% patients and 42.8% of patients had impaired detrusor contractility at baseline. There is evidence that this instability may be due to the outflow obstruction and resolves after radical surgery. Kleinhans et al. [24] reported an improvement in detrusor instability in all but two of their 34.6% patients who had a preoperative unstable bladder. It is important to realize that while bladder instability often is present in these patients, it may not be the primary cause of incontinence and may actually be a coexisting feature with ISD. Patients with severe ISD may have small bladder capacities, which result in falsely decreased bladder compliance values on cystometrograms [12].

Nerve Damage

Denervation of the bladder base and proximal urethra also may result in loss of posterior urethral sensations. John et al. [25] used a catheter-mounted stimulating ring electrode distal to the bladder neck preoperatively and postoperatively in 34 patients undergoing radical prostatectomy. Incontinent patients had a higher sensory threshold than the continent patients. The authors believe that loss of afferent sensory stimuli may lead to a loss of the reflex guarding and result in incontinence. Bladder base denervation also may be responsible for the development of bladder instability in previously stable bladders [20]. John et al. [26] noted a decrease in the trigonal nerve fiber density in post-prostatectomy bladder trigonal biopsies, and the decrease was greater in incontinent patients than in continent patients. They also noted an increase in nerve fiber density in 19 incontinent patients with a greater rise in the subset that regained continence. Earlier studies on bladder biopsies of

patients undergoing pelvic surgery also revealed a decrease in the density of nerve fibers in the trigone with evidence of reinnervation on EMG studies of the sphincter [27]. However, this denervation may not solely be the result of surgery but also may be the result of chronic outflow obstruction. In either case, they provide evidence for bladder dysfunction due to neural damage.

Nerve preservation is considered a standard surgical step in current radical prostatectomy. The primary reason for nerve preservation is maintenance of postoperative erectile function. It is postulated that continence primarily is mediated in the post-surgical patients through the somatic fibers from the pudendal nerve, which are always preserved in radical prostatectomy, and thus cavernosal nerve preservation may not contribute to continence. Majoros et al. found the incontinence rate to be similar in their cases irrespective of the surgical technique [13]. Steiner et al. [28] reviewed 593 of their patients and found the incontinence rate to be similar in both the nerve-sparing and the non-sparing group of patients. Catalona et al. [29] also reported similar findings in their study of 1,870 men followed for a minimum period of 18 months. It is possible that the failure to find a difference in continence rates in these studies is due to the low incidence of incontinence that generally existed in these series. However, there is evidence to suggest that nerve preservation also may help in improving continence.

Burkhard et al. [30] evaluated 536 patients who underwent open radical retropubic prostatectomy and found the incidence of incontinence to be 1.3, 3.4, and 13.7% among patients who underwent bilateral or unilateral nonnerve-sparing surgeries, respectively. The differences were statistically significant. Eastham et al. [31] reviewed their results in 581 patients and found that nerve preservation had a significant beneficial effect in preserving continence. This was evident for even single-nerve preservation, and preserving both bundles further added to the continence. The role of these nerves in preserving continence may be multifactorial. Apart from preserving direct efferent innervation to the sphincter as stated previously [6], they also may be important in providing afferent sensations and mediating a reflex continence mechanism.

Bladder Neck Contracture and Fibrosis

Anastomotic strictures also contribute to the development of incontinence. While Groutz's series [15] found the incidence to be about 20.5%, Chao et al. [22] found this incidence to be 26% among the incontinent patients. They also believed that this scarring may extend down to the level of the sphincter, causing impairment in its normal closure. Ficazzola and Nitti [12] found a similar incidence of anastomotic strictures, while Desautel et al. [14] noted strictures in 67% of their patients. The mechanism of incontinence in obstructed patients is believed to be a combination of overflow and urge incontinence. Continuous outflow obstruction can result in bladder instability, causing urge incontinence, while chronic retention may result in overflow. There also is a possibility of deranged sphincteric function due to extensive postoperative scarring and fibrosis which may prevent normal coaptation of the urethral walls. Groutz et al. [15] talk about this in terms of "decreased urethral compliance." They found urinary flow with the 7 French catheter in situ to be lower by greater than 10 ml s$^-$ in 30% of patients compared to catheter-free flow. Since a 7 French catheter normally should not impede the flow of urine, they believed this to be a manifestation of decreased urethral compliance. They further stated that this could be due to anastomotic strictures, fibrosis, or bladder neck contractures and these are a contributory cause of incontinence.

Patient Evaluation

History and Examination

The history in a patient with PPI should focus on determining the type and severity of incontinence and its impact on the patient's quality of life. Stress urinary incontinence usually has a typical presentation of leakage during periods of mobility or increased abdominal pressure. Patients with a history of stress incontinence usually have a finding of ISD in cystometrograms. This symptom has a positive predictive value of 95% and a negative predictive value of 100% [12]. Urge, however, may not be an accurate predictor of bladder instability. Ficazolla and Nitti [12] found unstable bladders in only 8 of 18 men who complained of

urgency, while of 42 men who did not complain of urgency 8 had bladder instability on urodynamics. The severity of incontinence may be assessed by the number of pads soaked per day or the use of a penile clamp or such devices. The stream of urination and the need for straining may indicate the presence of a stricture or bladder neck contracture. It also is important to evaluate the presurgery continence status of the patient if this has not already been documented in the surgical note. A detailed history of associated comorbidities, particularly stroke, spinal trauma, or other neurological conditions, is important since it may impact the management. The patient's physical dexterity to manage a prosthetic implant also should be assessed. It also is important to assess the erectile function during this visit, since it may require simultaneous management and may have been affected by the incontinence. Finally, the impact on the patient's quality of life and expectations after therapy are to be evaluated in order to determine the therapeutic options.

The goal of the examination is to rule out evident causes for the incontinence. These include the presence of a distended bladder, which would suggest outflow obstruction and overflow incontinence. A brief neurological assessment is recommended to evaluate the perineal innervation and the deep tendon reflexes. A demonstration of urinary leakage using the Valsalva maneuver in patients with stress incontinence may be performed; however, this is not essential in case urodynamic testing is being ordered.

Urodynamics

A complete urodynamic examination is mandatory when evaluating any patient with PPI (Figs. 31.4 and 31.5). The relative frequency of bladder instability among these patients, particularly those who have undergone a transurethral resection, already has been discussed. The history, per se, is an inadequate guide to the presence or severity of bladder instability, and concurrent management of both sphincter deficiency and instability is required in order to achieve optimal results.

A urodynamic assessment may begin with a voiding uroflowmetry and postvoid urine assessment. The patient should be asked to void at the time of a normal desire. An obstructed uroflow pattern will

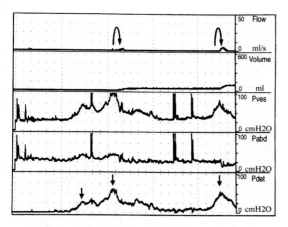

FIG. 31.4. Urodynamic evaluation of a 75-year-old man, 2 years after transurethral prostatic resection, with severe urge incontinence, increased with standing up. Note episodes of detrusor instability (*straight arrows*) on two separate fills. Also, incontinence is noted on flowmeter (*curved arrows*) and volume lost on the volume graft maximum bladder capacity was 88 ml. Patient was tested for stress incontinence on three occasions (simultaneous spikes in abdominal and detrusor pressure), and none was demonstrated. Diagnosis – severe detrusor instability with urge incontinence (copywrite with permission)

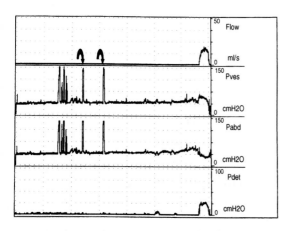

FIG. 31.5. Urodynamic tracing of a 67-year-old man 1 year after radical retropubic prostatectomy with incontinence, which by history is related to increases in abdominal pressure. Patient wears three pads per day. Urodynamics showed loss of urine only during increases in abdominal pressure, with an abdominal leak point pressure of 145 cm H2O (*arrows*). Patient otherwise had a stable and compliant bladder with a capacity of 500 mg. Voiding phase is normal (copy write with permission)

suggest the presence of an anastomotic stricture and the need for a videourodynamic study. The postvoid residual urine assessment should be performed using either an ultrasonogram or bladder catheterization. An ideal urodynamic evaluation includes a videourodynamic study that visualizes the bladder neck and urine leak along with pressure measurements. This allows a clear separation of the relative contributions of bladder instability and sphincteric deficiency to the pathology.

The study is performed using a 7–8 French double-lumen catheter placed in the bladder. One lumen is used to record the vesical pressure, while the other is used to infuse saline or radiographic contrast material. A 7 French diameter catheter normally should not impede the outflow in a patient with a compliant urethra. A second catheter, connected to a pressure transducer, is placed in the rectum to measure the intra-abdominal pressure. The detrusor pressure is calculated after deducting the abdominal pressure from the vesical pressure. A fill rate of 25–50 ml/min⁻ is used. Slower rates may be preferred in patients with severe urgency or documented low bladder capacities, since a faster fill rate can induce uninhibited contractions of the detrusor. The patient's symptoms are recorded during the filling process. Any uninhibited contraction of greater than 15 cm H_2O pressure is considered to be detrusor instability [32]. It also is recommended that incontinence should be documented during the procedure. An unstable contraction, along with a sensation of urgency and associated with urinary leak, is indicative of urge incontinence. In patients with pure stress incontinence, a Valsalva leak point pressure (VLPP) assessment is required. The patient is asked to perform a Valsalva maneuver at various bladder volumes, beginning with about 150 ml. The abdominal pressure at which the urine leaks is designated the VLPP. Failure to demonstrate a leak at 150 ml necessitates a repeat assessment at progressively higher volumes. Some patients with a clear history of stress incontinence may not leak during the study. Such patients may have an anastomotic stricture or the presence of a 7 French catheter which prevents leakage. Such patients should be tested for the VLPP at the end of the study after removal of the urethral catheter; the pressure reading from the rectal catheter is used for pressure recording. At the end of the study, a pressure flow graph is obtained by asking the patient to void of his own volition. The detrusor pressure generated in order to void is compared against standardized nomograms to determine the presence or absence of outflow obstruction. A low pressure voiding is suggestive of a hypocontractile bladder with concomitant sphincteric damage. The video study demonstrates the leak at the time of the recorded event and also may demonstrate the presence or absence of an anastomotic site stricture. A simultaneous urethrogram may be obtained if a stricture is suspected.

While a VLPP routinely is obtained during an urodynamic study for incontinence, its importance in management of the patient or in determining the type of treatment is unclear. Twiss et al. [33] evaluated 29 men 9 months following prostatectomy for stress incontinence. They found the mean VLPP to be 92.8 cm H_2O, and it had an insignificant, weak association with the amount of leakage per day. In contrast to female patients where VLPP is used to grade the degree of incontinence and to determine the type of therapeutic intervention necessary for their management, the authors concluded that VLPP had little bearing on the degree of leakage or determining treatment outcomes in the postprostatectomy-incontinent man. They did agree, however, that a urodynamic study was useful in confirming the presence of stress incontinence and evaluating the presence and severity of bladder instability.

Cystoscopy

We recommend a cystourethroscopic examination in all patients prior to any surgical intervention. Patients with pure bladder instability who are to be managed with oral medications may not need a cystoscopy. However, in all other patients, particularly those scheduled for an artificial genitourinary sphincter, a visual examination confirms the absence of a urethral, anastomotic stricture, or foreign body, which, if present, would need to be treated before the implantation of a sphincter (Fig. 31.6).

Management Strategies

It is widely accepted that PPI is significantly affected by surgical technique of radical prostatectomy, particularly the handling of the dorsal venous

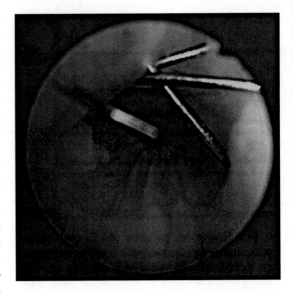

FIG. 31.6. Cystoscopic evaluation of patient following radical retropubic prostatectomy and external beam radiation therapy which reveals bladder neck contracture and multiple surgical clips at the level of the bladder neck

complex, distal urethra, and the bladder neck apart from direct damage to the sphincter. Modifications in the surgical technique to minimize this complication are discussed elsewhere in this text. We will limit ourselves to the management of the problem once it is established.

Conservative/Medical

While the incidence of PPI may be up to 56% in the early postoperative period, continence tends to increase over time. In the early postsurgical period, a trial of conservative therapy is recommended both to improve continence and to help the patient adjust to the problem and achieve social acceptance. Patients need reassurance and support, with regular reviews to assess the degree of improvement. Basic measures to help improve continence are a decrease in fluid intake, minimization of caffeine-based products, and medical management with imipramine [34]. Pelvic floor exercises (PFE) were promoted by Kegel in 1951 in an attempt to enhance urinary control through increase in urethral resistance [35]. PFE along with biofeedback also may be useful in the management of PPI. Various exercises aimed at strengthening the pelvic floor muscles have been devised. These include pelvic musculature contraction while in the supine, standing, and squatting positions; during increased abdominal stress; and with the use of varying groups of muscles. A physical therapist generally is involved in the training during these exercises, and a home-based program then is developed for the patient to continue without supervision. This is supplemented with regular visits with the physical therapist to reinforce the benefit and confirm the adequacy of the technique. A number of studies attest to the beneficial effects of PFE and biofeedback. Filocamo et al. [36] randomized 300 postprostatectomy patients to receive either PFE training or no intervention beginning immediately following catheter removal. The intervention group performed PFE regularly for at least 6 months. All patients underwent an objective and subjective evaluation for continence at regular intervals up to 12 months. At 12 months, the incontinence rate in the nontreated group was 12.1% compared with 1.3% in the treated group. This difference in continence was visible as early as 1 month postsurgery. Biofeedback and PFE may be started even before the surgery. Burgio et al. [37] performed a prospective randomized study to evaluate the benefits of preoperative PFE in 125 men and found training reduced the time to continence and the proportion of patients with severe incontinence at 6 months of follow-up. However, Parekh et al. [38] did not concur in their report wherein, while the return to continence was quicker in the treated group, patients with severe incontinence did not benefit, and there were no significant improvements in the long-term outcomes. A recent Cochrane database review confirms the current doubts about the efficacy of PFE in the management of PPI [39]. Since these exercises do no harm and potentially may benefit the patient, a trial during the phase of conservative management is justifiable.

Surgical Options

Most patients with persistent urinary incontinence after 1 year of prostatectomy will require some form of surgical intervention in order to become dry. Currently used surgical procedures to augment continence are based on devices that often date back to the eighteenth century [40]. The functioning of these devices is based on one of two principles.

The first aims at providing a fixed resistance to urine outflow. This fixed resistance prevents urine leakage during periods of stress but is not enough to occlude the normal micturition process completely. Dynamic resistance devices allow the patient to modulate the resistance manually, lowering it during micturition and raising it during periods of continence.

Penile Clamps

The penile clamp is one of the most rudimentary and earliest devices available for the management of male incontinence. The availability of a penile shaft surrounding the urethra allows the placement of a clamp during periods of activity to prevent incontinence. This clamp can be removed during micturition. Various modifications of the penile clamps are available and continue to serve an important function. However, they are associated with the possibility of local trauma, erosion, and discomfort, and do not have significant patient acceptance. Modifications of this device in order to minimize complications include the Baumrucker clamp that provides an "S" curve to the urethra rather than compressing it at opposing points [41].

Artificial Genitourinary Sphincters

The first artificial urinary sphincter and surgery for its placement was described by Foley in 1947 [42]. This procedure required the isolation of a segment of the urethra with the surrounding corpora spongiosa from the remaining components of the penile shaft. These were then encircled with an inflatable cuff that was connected to an external pump carried in the patient's pocket. The first model of the currently available artificial genitourinary sphincter (AGUS) was described by Scott in 1973 [43]. This device, called the AS-721, was developed by American Medical Systems, Minnetonka, Minnesota. It had four components: an inflatable cuff that was placed around the urethra, a reservoir that contained fluid, and two pumps – one placed in each hemiscrotum to activate or deactivate the pump. Activation of one pump pushed fluid out of the reservoir into the cuff to occlude the urethra. Activating the opposite pump resulted in a flow of fluid in the opposite direction out of the cuff into

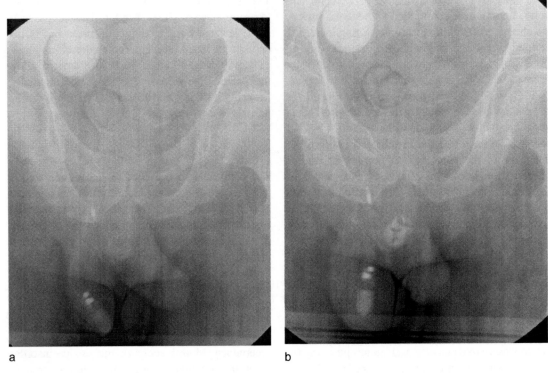

FIG. 31.7. (a) Plain abdominal X-rays 6 weeks following placement of an AGUS revealing the reservoir, the deactivated tandem cuff, and the scrotal activating/deactivating mechanism (b) Plain abdominal X-rays of the same patient revealing the tandem cuff in the inflated state

the reservoir and resulted in subsequent opening of the urethra. Mechanical valves controlled the one-way action of the pumps while the device itself was made of a polyethylene terephthalate polymer. This device and its modifications continued to be in use until the development of the currently available AMS 800 sphincter (Fig. 31.7a, b).

Design

The AMS 800™ AGUS device is the most commonly used prosthesis for the management of PPI. It is a refined version of the original AS-721 device. Unlike the original device, the AMS 800 consists of only three components: the urethral cuff, a pressure-regulating balloon (PRB), and the pump control which has both the activating and deactivating mechanisms in one assembly. The pressure on the urethra is controlled by balloons rather than valves, and the cuff is made of a dip-coated silicone rubber. The cuff is usually 2 cm wide after deflation and is available in a variety of lengths ranging from 4 to 11 cm depending on the size of the urethra and the site of placement. The cuff has clear tubing that is connected to similar clear tubing on the pump. The pump also is made of a silicone elastomer and is placed in the scrotal soft-tissue to allow patient and physician access for activation and deactivation. It consists of a soft lower part and a hard upper part. The hard upper part contains the valves that regulate the direction and flow of fluid while the lower part is mechanically pumped by the patient to drive the fluid. The hard upper part also contains a deactivation button that freezes the function of the pump so that fluid cannot flow in either direction. The pump has two exit tubes, a clear tube that connects to the cuff and a black tube for connection to the PRB.

The PRBsusually are implanted in the prevesical space. They are available in a variety of pressure ranges, and the device is chosen depending on the amount of pressure required at the patient’s cuff. The balloons are connected to the pump using a black connecting tube.

The standard device packaging also includes an accessory kit of materials necessary for an implant. These include a disposable cuff sizer used to estimate the length of the cuff required, special needles for preparing the device components, tubing connection tools, and documentation. Most of the components are disposable and presterilized. However, some components such as the insertion needles or tubing connectors are made of steel and need to be sterilized before each procedure. The implantable components are not resterilizable and must not be reused.

Preparation for Surgical Implant

Since the device is made out of a synthetic polymer, a possibility of allergic reactions to the implanted materials exists, and this needs to be highlighted during patient consent. Prevention of infection is the single-most important precaution during the preparation of the patient and device. Certain steps taken in order to minimize this are prophylactic antibiotics, part preparation only in the operating room, laminar flow, minimal traffic, and strict aseptic surgical scrub and component handling.

Silicone attracts dust and lint. Therefore it is essential to use nonpowdered surgical gloves and totally avoid the use of paper or cloth drapes. These may result in device malfunction and also serve as a nidus for device infection. The device-filling solution usually is a diluted radiopaque contrast material. This must be completely sterile and isotonic. During preparation of the various components before implant, it is important to ensure the egress of all air bubbles, since these can cause an air lock in the pumping mechanism resulting in device malfunction.

Control pump preparation: Both the tubings exiting the pump are dipped in a basin containing the filling solution. The bulb is repeatedly squeezed until all the air inside is expelled through the tubing. While the tubings are kept submerged in the solution, they are clamped with a rubber-shod fine artery clamp.

Pressure-regulating balloon preparation: The PRB is actively filled with the filling solution using a blunt-tipped needle and syringe. The balloon then is squeezed to expel all the air inside and finally aspirated with the syringe and needle to withdraw any remaining air bubbles. This process may be repeated to ensure removal of all air bubbles before the hemostat is applied to the tubing with the balloon in a collapsed state. The balloon is kept in a basin of filling solution until implantation.

Cuff preparation: The cuff is filled with the filling solution using a blunt-tipped needle. It then is squeezed to deflate into the syringe, and any remaining air is aspirated. The cuff is then refilled with 1–5 cc of solution depending on the cuff size so that the cuff is just filled and not over distended. The tubing is then clamped.

Surgical Procedure

The AMS 800 AGUS can be implanted either around the bladder neck or the bulbar urethra. The bulbar urethral implant is the most common procedure and will be described here. There are two basic surgical approaches for implantation of the AGUS. These are the scrotal incision and perineal incision. The choice of procedure depends primarily on the familiarity of the surgeon with each approach. The perineal approach requires two incisions while the transverse scrotal approach requires only one. However, the perineal approach provides a more direct access to the bulbar urethra.

Perineal approach: The patient is placed in a lithotomy position and prepped and draped for both the perineal and suprapubic incisions.

Cuff placement: A Foley catheter is inserted into the urethra to aid in identification. A midline perineal incision is made to expose the bulbocavernosus muscle surrounding the urethral bulb. The space around the muscle is carefully dissected so that the urethral bulb is not denuded of this muscle coat. Anteriorly, the bulb is mobilized bluntly to allow a circumferential placement of a Penrose drain of about 2–3 cm width. A cuff sizer may be used at this time to measure the circumference of the urethra and the length of cuff required. Most such placements require a 4- or 4.5-cm cuff. It should be remembered that the cuff length reflects the outer circumference of the cuff, whereas the direct measurement is closer to the inner circumference of the cuff. Once the cuff has been prepared, it is brought into the operating field and gently placed around the urethra and secured. The "tab" end of the cuff is passed under the urethra and held gently with a mosquito clamp while the cuff is manipulated. The tubing is passed through the designated hole after serial unclamping and clamping of the two hemostats on it so as to avoid entry of any air bubble. The cuff is locked using the tab, and the tubing is positioned to exit lateral to the urethral midline (Fig. 31.8).

PRB placement: A transverse suprapubic incision is made and the rectus fascia is divided. The linea alba is gently spread, and the prevesical space is exposed. Space for the balloon is created using blunt dissection ensuring complete hemostasis. The balloon is placed in this space. A separate incision is made in the rectus fascia below the original incision, and the exit tubing of the PRB is guided out

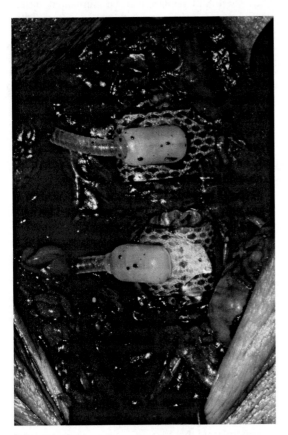

FIG. 31.8. Intraoperative photograph revealing placement of the tandem cuff

through this hole using sequential clamping of two hemostats on the tubing to prevent entry of air bubbles. The balloon is filled with appropriate filling solution, and gentle suprapubic pressure is applied on the balloon region to allow excess fluid to enter the syringe. The tubing is then clamped until its connection with the pump is completed.

Pump placement: Using blunt dissection through the perineal incision, a subdartos pouch is created in the scrotum anterolaterally. The pump placement is on the same side as the PRB placement. The pump is placed into the scrotal pouch with the deactivation button facing outward so that it is palpable. The special introducer needle is passed through the Scarpa's fascia from near the PRB tubing into the perineal incision. It is important to stay lateral to the spermatic cord, which is protected from injury by one of the surgeon's fingers. The black tubing from the pump is attached to the special end of this needle and its hemostats removed. The needle is withdrawn into the suprapubic incision, bringing the tubing from the pump close to the tubing exiting the PRB. The tubing is then connected to the PRB using the supplied connecting device. The white tubing exiting the pump is trimmed and connected to the white tubing exiting the cuff in the perineal incision.

Transverse scrotal approach: Unlike the perineal approach, the patient stays in the supine position with legs gently abducted. An upper transverse scrotal incision is made and kept open using a Scott retractor. The bulb of the urethra is freed from its posterior attachment to the perineal septum and anteriorly from the corpora cavernosa in order to allow circumferential mobilization for placement of the cuff. Cuff measurement and placement is similar to the perineal approach. For placement of the PRB, the surgeon performs a finger dissection of the superficial inguinal ring and then uses a sharp hemostat to pierce the posterior wall of the ring and enter the perivesical space. It is important to ensure that the bladder is empty and the cord is protected by the surgeon's finger. The perivesical space is developed, and the PRB is placed within it. The tubing exits through the external ring, which may be tightened using an absorbable suture. Placement of the pump is identical to that in the perineal approach, and all connections are similarly completed.

Deactivation at completion: Once the components have been connected, the device is tested. The pump is squeezed and released repeatedly to empty the cuff. The pump is allowed to fill partially by waiting for about 15 s before the deactivation button of the pump is pressed, thus leaving it in a deactivated status for 6 weeks.

Results

The quantification of success of therapy is difficult because of the subjective influence of the patient’s attitude and behavior. While a strict definition would mean total absence of any leakage at any time and under any condition, individual perception varies, and some patients may be content with the occasional leak of a few drops while others may be happy wearing one pad a day. Since the aim of therapy is improvement in patient quality of life, various researchers have used different definitions of success. A rationale evaluation would combine both these parameters: an objective evaluation of the amount of leakage or number of pads changed and an assessment of the quality of life.

The number of pads used to define success has varied from none to two pads per day [44, 45]. Litwiller et al. [44] evaluated the results of AGUS implant in 65 patients, 51 postradical prostatectomy, 13 after TURP, and one after open prostatectomy. All patients had severe preoperative incontinence. They defined continence strictly as no leakage and found an initial continent rate of 44%. This declined to 20% over 28 months. However, the majority of patients (90%) reported satisfaction with the surgery, since it helped improve their continence from the preoperative status. Ninety-six percent believed they would recommend the procedure to their friends, and 92% agreed that, in retrospect, they would undergo the procedure again. Gousse et al. [46] reviewed their data on 71 men who had undergone an artificial sphincter implant following radical prostatectomy. At a mean follow-up of 7.7 years, 27% patients used no pads, 32% used one, and 15% used up to three pads per day. Fifty-eight percent of the patients were very satisfied, while another 19% were satisfied with the outcome of their surgery. Hussain et al. [47] recently reviewed the data on AGUS use in postprostatectomy patients. Their own experience with 10 years of follow up had a continence rate of 91%. One of the largest experiences in the use of AGUS for PPI has been reported by Elliot and Barrett [48] from the Mayo Clinic. In a mixed population of patients, they noted a continence rate of 88% at a mean of 6.5 years following surgery. Long-term results of AGUS implant for PPI are not widely available. Fulford et al. [49] reported a 10-year follow-up with implants including a majority for neurogenic bladder dysfunction. The continence rate was over 60%.

Complications

Complications frequently are seen with the use of an AGUS. Most would result in a device replacement. In a study of 36 children operated on over 10 years, Levesque et al. [50] found only 33% required no second surgery and Kryger [51] et al. found only 56% of original devices to be functional. Similarly, high revision and explantation rates have been described in other studies [46]. The common complications necessitating these revisions are infection, erosion, and mechanical failure. All these may present with progressive incontinence.

Infection: As with all prosthetic devices, AGUS are prone to infection. The source of pathogens may be hematogenous, intraoperative introduction through the skin, unsterile instruments, environment, or unrecognized urethral breach. This may manifest early in the form of local signs of inflammation or with an erosion of the device through the urethra. Erosion also may occur later where the etiology may be either infection or pressure necrosis. The use of a strict aseptic operative room procedure is the only preventive measure to avoid this significant problem apart from ensuring sterile urine before surgery. The infection rate may be as high as 14.5% in some series [52], but the average rates are around 4–5% [47]. Infected or eroded devices need removal and the placement of a urethral catheter to allow healing of the urethra. The urethra usually heals well with rare stricture formation.

Urethral atrophy: Atrophy of the urethra may occur either due simply to pressure or as a consequence of infection. It may occur in up to 9% of cases [48] and is manifest as progressive loss of continence, erosion, or the need for increased pumping to void and deflate the cuff. One of the device modifications that have helped decrease the incidence of pressure necrosis is the narrow cuff design. Gousse et al. [46] reported a revision rate of 7 of 42 in the patients with a narrow cuff compared with 18 of 23 with the older design. Similarly, Elliott and Barrett [48] reported a lower failure and revision rate with the narrow cuff design compared with the original sphincter design. Downsizing the cuff also may be an option for the management of urethral atrophy. Saffarian et al. [53] reviewed 17 patients with urethral erosion following a standard AGUS placement. All patients underwent cuff downsizing to a 4-cm cuff within the capsule of the original cuff, and the patient satisfaction rate improved from 15 to 80%.

If the urethral atrophy cannot be managed by a simple downsizing, a tandem-cuff placement may be used. The second or tandem cuff usually is placed distal to the first cuff, but on occasion it may need to be placed more proximally if it is detected that the primary cuff was placed too distally on the urethra. It is advisable to include the bulk of the bulbospongiosus muscle within the cuff to lend it more tissue. Some authors also may prefer to replace the original cuff while placing a tandem cuff, especially if the duration of cuff placement has been greater than 5 years [54]. The two cuffs are joined with a Y connector and connected to the already existing pump and PRB. Dimarco and Elliott [54] found the tandem cuff to be effective in most patients, with 89% of the 19 patients requiring less than three pads per day with an 88% satisfaction rate.

Another option for the management of erosion is the transcorporal cuff placement. Erosion of the urethra often necessitates a more distal placement of the cuff, either the primary cuff or a second tandem cuff. Guralnick et al. [55] describe a procedure whereby the urethra is dissected dorsally through the two corpora cavernosum, maintaining a layer of the tunica albuginea on the urethra. This adds bulk to the urethra and minimizes the risk of dorsal perforation. In their series of 31 patients at a mean of 17 months follow-up, 26 patients had mild or no stress incontinence. None of the cuffs had an erosion or infection. However, there is a risk of inducing erectile dysfunction in a preoperatively potent patient. In this series, only one patient was fully potent preoperatively, and he continued to have normal erections postsurgery.

Mechanical failure: This usually results from an incorrect choice of cuff or balloon or an incorrect surgical procedure. There may be an obstruction to the flow of fluid due to kinks in the tubes. A large cuff may require a greater pressure balloon or cuff downsizing. Most of these complications were seen in the earlier devices and have decreased since the introduction of the narrow cuff design. However, the incidence is still about 3–5% [47]. Improvement in surgeon experience may significantly decrease the incidence of such complications.

Male Sling Procedures

Following the principles of incontinence surgery in females, increasing the urethral outflow resistance by urethral compression was attempted surgically by Kaufman. He described three different procedures including crural crossover, crural approximation, and subsequently the addition of an implantable gel prosthesis [56–58]. These procedures showed early promise and have now been used to devise the male urethral sling procedures. These use synthetic, dermal, or porcine tissue to provide a similar posterior support to the urethra and bladder neck. Jorion et al. [59] described their experience of using the rectus fascia sling in 30 patients where the sling was constructed prophylactically during the radical prostatectomy procedure itself. They reported a 90% continence rate compared with 70% in the group without the sling at 3 months. The results improved to 100 and 93%, respectively, at 12 months.

Schaeffer et al. [60] described a procedure using synthetic material in which three bolsters of Cooley soft vascular graft material or polyethylene terephthalate covered by a polytetrafluoroethylene sleeve were used in 64 men with PPI. A Stamey needle was used to guide a nylon thread from each bolster into the suprapubic area from either side of the bladder neck. With a mean follow up of 22.4 months following a single-sling procedure, 64% of patients were either dry or improved. Twenty-three retightening procedures were performed. They found previous irradiation to be the only significant poor risk factor for success.

Castle et al. [61] reported their results with the use of a synthetic device, the InVance Male Sling System (AMS, Minnetonka, Minnesota). This device consists of a silicone-coated knitted mesh of polyester. The authors used the mesh in combination with a porcine dermis sheet that was placed between the mesh and the bulbar urethra. The mesh is placed through a perineal incision and anchored on either side of the urethra to the undersurface of the pubic bone using three bone anchors on either side. The mesh was tightened by imbricating in the midline. Defining success as wearing one pad or less per day, the authors reported a 39.5% continence rate at 18 months. Only 15.6% patients were completely dry.

The AdVance Male Sling (AMS, Minnetonka, Minnesota) consists of a synthetic mesh (Fig. 31.8) that recently has been introduced. While single- and multicenter trials are ongoing, modifications by the individual surgical group(s) have apparently enhanced the effectiveness of the sling in predominantly mild and moderate incontinence-associated surgical candidates (personal communication). The mesh here is introduced at the level of the bulbar urethra following a perineal incision and brought out at the skin level via proprietary trocars without anchoring the sling (Figs. 31.9 and 31.10). Continence rates of 50% have been reported initially; however, as selection criteria and long-term results are published, we may see an improvement.

Another device based on these principles is the adjustable continence therapy – ProACT (Uromedical, Plymouth, Minnesota). This device consists of two balloons that are inserted paraurethrally to lie on either side of the urethra under the bladder neck to increase its resistance. The balloons contain a titanium port that can be used to increase or decrease the balloon inflation and control the amount of resistance. The balloon insertion is performed through a perineal incision under fluoroscopic guidance with a cystoscopic confirmation of the safety of the urethra and bladder from perforation and correct placement of the balloons. The balloon ports are placed into the scrotum below the dartos fascia to allow percutaneous needle access for inflation and deflation. Trigo-Rocha [62] reported their results following the use of this device in 23 patients with a mean follow up of 22.4 months. Of these patients, 65% were continent at up to one pad soakage level. Patients not satisfied with the results were 35%, and two opted for an AGUS placement. Four patients required revision surgery. There were no major complications.

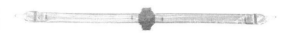

FIG. 31.9. Advance male urethral sling

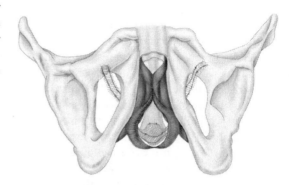

FIG. 31.10. Positioning of the sling following a perineal incision, localization of the sling at the bulbar urethra

All these procedures and devices are relatively new with limited results. Most reported results are of short-term duration and are no better than the AGUS. The main reason for their development seems to be the relatively cheaper cost. Efficacy data and direct comparison with AGUS are still lacking.

Bulking Agents

While the AGUS has proven efficacy in the management of PPI, complications such as infection, erosion, and cost deter some patients from accepting this treatment. The use of an AGUS requires manual dexterity, and its placement requires regional or general anesthesia. These may not be feasible in a subgroup of patients with incontinence who would then require alternative therapy. One of the initially used bulking agents, polytetrafluoroethylene, had good results but was difficult to inject and had reports of migration/granuloma formation at distant sites, which prompted its discontinuation.

Glutaraldehyde cross-linked collagen is FDA approved for treatment of ISD. It has no propensity for migration, induces only a mild local inflammatory reaction, is safe, and does not compromise subsequent therapies if needed. Collagen injections may be deployed through either a retrograde or antegrade route. The retrograde approach is performed using transurethral cystoscopy. For the antegrade approach, a suprapubic cystostomy is performed, and the tract may be dilated to accommodate an Amplatz sheath through which either a nephroscope or cystoscope is introduced to reach the bladder neck. Loughlin et al. [63] described a modified antegrade approach that required a smaller 15.5 French cystoscope instead of a larger dilatation.

In 1998, Smith et al. [64] reported their experience with the use of transurethral collagen injection in 62 men with PPI, 54 after radical prostatectomy, and eight after TURP. At a median follow-up of 29 months, 38.7% were using one pad or less per day while 8.1% became totally dry. The success rate was higher in post-TURP patients than the postradical prostatectomy cases. Percentage of patients who were continent at 1 year was 65%, and they continued to remain so with no further treatment. At 2 years, 42% maintained social continence. A median of four injection procedures were required to achieve social continence. Westney et al. [65] recently reported the long-term outcomes of transurethral collagen injection in 307 men with ISD after therapy for prostate carcinoma and in 15 for BPH. Their mean follow-up was 40 months. Only 17% achieved complete continence with a mean duration of response being 11 months. The overall mean duration of response was 6.3 months. The authors concluded that collagen injections are a good option for short-term therapy in men with PPI.

Rahman et al. [66] reported the combined use of bulking agents with AGUS implantation. Five patients with recurrent incontinence following an AGUS or sling placement underwent a bulking agent injection (Surgisis ES: Cook Urological, Spencer, Indiana) followed by an AGUS placement. The original eroded cuff or sling was removed in all cases. At a mean 11 months of follow-up, all patients reported an improvement in their continence while two were completely dry.

Conclusions

Incontinence following prostatectomy is a significant problem. It is multifactorial with intrinsic sphincter deficiency being the most common cause in radical prostatectomy patients. Complete evaluation is nec-essary to confirm the contribution of various factors to the etiology, and thus tailor the management. A number of patients may improve spontaneously, and definitive therapy should be deferred for about a year postsurgically. AGUS implant provides the best long-term cure rates for the condition. Other modalities of treatment include male slings and bulking agents. Neither has proven long-term results or efficacy superior to the AGUS.

References

1. Yucel S, Baskin LS. An anatomical description of the male and female urethral sphincter complex. J Urol 2004; 171(5):1890–1897.
2. Strasser H, Ninkovic M, Hess M, et al. Anatomic and functional studies of the male and female urethral sphincter. World J Urol. 2000; 18(5):324–329.
3. Myers RP. Practical surgical anatomy for radical prostatectomy. Urol Clin North Am 2001; 28: 473–490.
4. Myers RP, Cahill D, Devine RM, et al. Anatomy of radical prostatectomy as defined by magnetic resonance imaging. J Urol 1998; 159:2148.
5. Heinzer H, Hammerer PG, Huland H. Anatomy and physiology of the male urethral sphincter and its preservation in prostatic surgery. Urol Res. 1999; 27(6):404–408.
6. Ludwikowski B, Oesch Hayward I, et al. The development of the external urethral sphincter in humans. BJU Int 2001; 87(6):565–568.
7. Dorschner W, Biesold M, Schmidt F, Stolzenburg JU. The dispute about the external sphincter and the urogenital diaphragm. J Urol 1999; 162(6): 1942–1945.
8. Gosling JA, Dixon JS, Critchley HO, et al. A comparative study of the human external sphincter and periurethral levator ani muscles. Br J Urol 1981; 53:35.
9. Karam I, Droupy S, Abd-Alsamad I, et al. The precise location and nature of the nerves to the male human urethra: Histological and immunohistochemical studies with three dimensional reconstruction. Eur Urol 2005; 48:858–864.
10. Narayan P, Konety B, Aslam K, et al. Neuroanatomy of the external urethral sphincter: Implications for urinary continence preservation during radical prostate surgery. J Urol 1995; 153:337.
11. Carlson KV, Nitti VW. Prevention and management of incontinence following radical prostatectomy. Urol Clin North Am 2001; 28:595–612.
12. Ficazzola MA, Nitti VW. The etiology of post-radical prostatectomy incontinence and correlation of

symptoms with urodynamic findings. J Urol 1998; 160:1317.

13. Majoros A, Bach D, Keszthelyi A, et al. Urinary incontinence and voiding dysfunction after radical retropubic prostatectomy (prospective urodynamic study). Neurourol Urodyn 2006; 25(1):2–7.

14. Desautel MG, Kapoor R, Badlani GH. Sphincteric incontinence: The primary cause of post-prostatectomy incontinence in patients with prostate cancer. Neurourol Urodynam 1997; 16:153.

15. Groutz A, Blaivas JG, Chaikin DC, et al. The pathophysiology of post-radical prostatectomy incontinence: A clinical and video urodynamic study. J Urol 2000; 163(6):1767–1770.

16. Rudy DC, Woodside JR, Crawford ED. Urodynamic evaluation of incontinence in patients undergoing modified Campbell radical retropubic prostatectomy. A prospective study. J Urol 1984; 132:708.

17. Hammerer P, Huland H. Urodynamic evaluation of changes in urinary control after radical retropubic prostatectomy. J Urol 1997; 157:233–236.

18. Kleinhans B, Gerharz E, Melekos M, et al. Changes of urodynamic findings after radical prostatectomy. Eur Urol 1999; 35:217.

19. Nitti VW, Kim Y, Combs AJ. Voiding dysfunction following transurethral resection of the prostate: Symptoms and urodynamic findings. J Urol. 1997; 157(2):600–603.

20. Hellstrom P, Lukkarinen O, Kontturi M. Urodynamics in radical retropubic prostatectomy. Scand J Urol Nephrol 1989; 23:21.

21. Gomha MA, Boone TB. Voiding patterns in patients with post-prostatectomy incontinence: Urodynamic and demographic analysis. J Urol 2003; 169(5): 1766–1769.

22. Chao R, Mayo ME. Incontinence after radical prostatectomy: Detrusor or sphincter causes. J Urol 1995; 154:16.

23. Giannantoni A, Mearini E, Di Stasi SM, et al. Assessment of bladder and urethral sphincter function before and after radical retropubic prostatectomy. J Urol 2004; 171:1563–1566.

24. Kleinhans B, Gerharz E, Melekos M, et al. Changes of urodynamic findings after radical retropubic prostatectomy. Eur Urol 1999; 35:217–221.

25. John H, Sullivan MP, Bangerter U, et al. Effect of radical prostatectomy on sensory threshold and pressure transmission. J Urol 2000; 163(6):1761–1766.

26. John H, Hauri D, Leuener M, et al. Evidence of trigonal denervation and reinnervation after radical retropubic prostatectomy. J Urol 2001; 165(1): 111–113.

27. Kirby RS, Fowler CJ, Gilpin SA, et al. Bladder muscle biopsy and urethral sphincter EMG in patients with bladder dysfunction after pelvic surgery. J R Soc Med 1986; 79:270–273.

28. Steiner MS, Morton RA, Walsh PC. Impact of anatomical radical prostatectomy on urinary continence. J Urol 1991; 145:512–514.

29. Catalona WJ, Carvalhal GF, Mager DE, Smith DS. Potency, continence and complication rates in 1,870 consecutive radical retropubic prostatectomies. J Urol 1999; 162:433–438.

30. Burkhard FC, Kessler TM, Fleischmann A, et al. Nerve sparing open radical retropubic prostatectomy — does it have an impact on urinary continence? J Urol 2006; 176:189–195.

31. Eastham JA, Kattan MW, Rogers E, et al. Risk factors for urinary incontinence after radical prostatectomy. J Urol 1996; 156:1707–1713.

32. Abrams P, Blaivas JG, Stanton S, et al. The standardization of terminology of lower urinary tract function. Scand J Urol Nephrol 1988; 114(Supp):5.

33. Twiss C, Fleischmann N, Nitti VW. Correlation of abdominal leak point pressure with objective incontinence severity in men with post-radical prostatectomy stress incontinence. Neurourol Urodyn 2005; 24(3):207–210.

34. Walsh PC. Anatomic radical retropubic prostatectomy. Campbell's 8th edn, 2002; vol. 4:3107–3129.

35. Kegel AH. Physiologic therapy for urinary stress incontinence. JAMA 1951; 146:915.

36. Filocamo MT, Marzi VL, Popolo GD, et al. Effectiveness of early pelvic floor rehabilitation treatment for post prostatectomy incontinence. Eur Urol 2005; 48:734–738.

37. Burgio KL, Goode PS, Urban DA, et al. Preoperative biofeedback assisted behavioral training to decrease post-prostatectomy incontinence: a randomized, controlled trial. J Urol 2006; 175:196–201.

38. Parekh AR, Feng MI, Kirages D, et al. The role of pelvic floor exercises on post prostatectomy incontinence. J Urol 2003; 170:130–133.

39. Moore KN, Cody DJ, Glazener CMA. Conservative management for post prostatectomy urinary incontinence. Cochrane Database Syst Rev 2001; 2:CD001843.

40. Madjar S, Raz S, Gousse AE. Fixed and dynamic urethral compression for the treatment of post-prostatectomy urinary incontinence: Is history repeating itself? J Urol 2001; 166:411–415.

41. Baumrucker GO. A new male incontinence clamp. J Urol 1979; 121:201.

42. Foley FEB. An artificial sphincter: A new device and operation for control of enuresis and urinary incontinence. J Urol 1947; 58:250.

43. Scott FB, Bradley We, Timm GW. Treatment of urinary incontinence by implantable prosthetic sphincter. Urology 1973; 1:252.

44. Litwiller SE, Kim KB, Fone PD, et al. Post prostate-ctomy incontinence and the artificial urinary sphinc-ter: A long-term study of patient satisfaction and criteria for success. J Urol 1996; 156:1975–1980.

45. Wang Y, Hadley HR. Experiences with the artificial urinary sphincter in the irradiated patient. J Urol. 1992; 147(3):612–613.

46. Gousse AE, Madjar S, Lambert MM, Fishman IJ. Artificial urinary sphincter for post-radical prosta-tectomy urinary incontinence: Long-term subjective results. J Urol 2001; 166(5):1755–1.

47. Hussain M, Greenwell TJ, Venn SN, Mundy AR. The current role of the artificial urinary sphincter for the treatment of urinary incontinence. J Urol 2005; 174(2):418–424.

48. Elliott DS, Barrett DM. Mayo Clinic long-term analysis of the functional durability of the AMS 800 artificial urinary sphincter: A review of 323 cases. J Urol 1998; 159(4):1206–1208.

49. Fulford SC, Sutton C, Bales G, et al. The fate of the "modern" artificial urinary sphincter with a follow-up of more than 10 years. Br J Urol 1997; 79(5):713–716.

50. Levesque PE, Bauer SB, Atala A, et al. Ten-year experience with the artificial urinary sphincter in children. J Urol 1996; 156(2 Pt 2):625–628.

51. Kryger JV, Spencer Barthold J, Fleming P, Gonzalez R. The outcome of artificial urinary sphincter place-ment after a mean 15-year follow-up in a pediatric population. BJU Int 1999; 83(9):1026–10231.

52. Scott FB. The artificial urinary sphincter. Experience in adults. Urol Clin North Am 1989; 16:105.

53. Saffarian A, Walsh K, Walsh IK, Stone AR. Urethral atrophy after artificial urinary sphincter placement: Is cuff downsizing effective? J Urol 2003; 169:567–569.

54. DiMarco DS, Elliott DS. Tandem cuff artificial urinary sphincter as a salvage procedure following failed primary sphincter placement for the treatment of post-prostatectomy incontinence. J Urol 2003; 170(4 Pt 1):1252–1254.

55. Guralnick ML, Miller E, Toh KL, Webster GD. Trans-corporal artificial urinary sphincter cuff placement in cases requiring revision for erosion and urethral atrophy. J Urol 2002; 167(5):2075–2078.

56. Kaufman JJ. Surgical treatment of post prostatec-tomy incontinence: Use of the penile crura to com-press the bulbous urethra. J Urol 1972; 107:293.

57. Kaufman JJ. Urethral compression operations for the treatment of post prostatectomy incontinence. J Urol 1973; 110:93.

58. Kaufman JJ. Treatment of post prostatectomy incon-tinence using a silicone gel prosthesis.Br J Urol 1973; 45:646.

59. Jorion JL. Rectus fascial sling suspension of the vesicourethral anastomosis after radical prostatec-tomy. J Urol. 1997; 157(3):926–928.

60. Schaeffer AJ, Clemens JQ, Ferrari M, Stamey TA. The male bulbourethral sling procedure for post-radical prostatectomy incontinence. J Urol 1998; 159(5):1510–1515.

61. Castle EP, Andrews PE, Itano N, et al. The male sling for post-prostatectomy incontinence; mean follow up of 18 months. J Urol 2005; 173(5):1657–1660.

62. Trigo-Rocha F, Gomes CM, Pompeo AC, et al. Prospective study evaluating efficacy and safety of adjustable continence therapy (ProACT) for post radical prostatectomy urinary incontinence. Urology 2006; 67(5):965–969.

63. Loughlin KR, Comiter CV. New technique for antegrade collagen injection for post-radical prosta-tectomy stress urinary incontinence. Urology 1999; 53(2):410–411.

64. Smith DN, Appell RA, Rackley RR, Winters JC. Collagen injection therapy for post-prostatectomy incontinence. J Urol 1998; 160(2):364–367.

65. Westney OL, Bevan-Thomas R, Palmer JL, et al. Transurethral collagen injections for male intrinsic sphincter deficiency: University of Texas-Houston experience. J Urol 2005; 174(3):994–997.

66. Rahman NU, Minor TX, Deng D, Lue TF. Combined external urethral bulking and artificial urinary sphincter for urethral atrophy and stress urinary incontinence. BJU Int 2005; 95(6):824–826.

Part VII
Special Situations

Chapter 32
Current Concepts and Treatment Strategies for Genitourinary Fistulas

Gamal M. Ghoniem and Carolyn F. Langford

History of Vesicovaginal Fistula

Vesicovaginal fistula (VVF) is a debilitating condition that has plagued women for thousands of years. The first recorded references of VVF were made in 1550 BC in ancient Egypt. Avincenna, a renowned Arabic physician, was the first person to document the relationship between VVF and obstructed labor, or traumatic delivery, in 1037 [1]. In 1923, Derry examined the earliest case of VVF (2050 BC) in the mummified body of Queen Henherit [2].

James Marion Sims established the foundations of VVF repair in 1852, after a series of experimental surgeries on slaves in Montgomery, Alabama, in 1845. These fundamentals included:

1. Proper exposure with the knee–chest position
2. Use of a weighted vaginal retractor
3. The use of silver wire sutures
4. Tension-free closure of the defect
5. Proper postoperative bladder drainage

Definition and Incidence

Vesicovaginal fistulae are epithelialized or fibrous communications between the bladder and vagina. VVF are relatively uncommon and yet are some of the most socially devastating conditions a patient may experience. Third World countries have a drastically higher prevalence compared to that of developed nations [2]. The true incidence of VVF is unknown but is estimated at 0.3–2% in countries such as the United States (Table 32.1) [3]. Iatrogenic postsurgical VVF are estimated at 81–91% from iatrogenic surgical injury in these patients [1]. In countries such as Nigeria, it has been estimated by the World Health Organization (2001) to occur in 800,000 to 1 million women. Obstetric trauma is by far the most common cause in most Third World countries.

Etiology of Adult VVF

Iatrogenic

Postsurgical VVF accounts for 81–91% of VVF occurrence in developed countries. Hysterectomy is the most common surgery leading to VVF in developed countries with an 80% incidence [4]. The incidence varies with the approach: 1:1000 transabdominal, 0.2:1000 transvaginal, and 2.2:1000 with laparoscopic procedures. The most common sites are superior to the trigone, corresponding to the vaginal cuff [5]. Other gynecological procedures account for up to 11%, including cesarean section and dilation and curettage. Incontinence surgery, formalin injections, and laparoscopy are less reported causes of VVF [6].

Pelvic radiation for malignancy has a 5% incidence of VVF formation, even after many years. The resulting fibrosis with arthritis nodosa and decreased blood supply leads to tissue necrosis, sloughing, and fistula formation.

Noniatrogenic

Obstetric trauma, including obstructed and prolonged second stage labor is the leading cause of
VVF in underdeveloped countries, especially the
South Sahara of Africa. In Western countries, this
encompasses only 5% of all VVF. Pelvic tumor,
pelvic trauma, congenital anomalies, foreign body,
and abscess account for 5% or less of VVF [6, 7].

Presentation

Generally, time to onset is 7–10 days after surgery, but it can range from immediate to 6 weeks.
Postradiation VVF takes months to years to
develop. Usually the patient presents with continuous leakage of urine. This can be mistaken for early
postoperative discharge, leading to more frustra-
tion for the patient and delayed diagnosis. If there
is intra-abdominal urine extravasation, the patient
may present with abdominal pain and ileus.

Diagnosis

The most critical factor in diagnosing a VVF is a
high suspicion. Many times the history and physical will reveal the pathology and sometimes even
the etiology. Review of operative reports indicating technical difficulties encountered, such as
excessive bleeding, tumor endometriosis, previous
surgery, pessary use, elevated creatinine, and obesity will suggest the etiology. A critical part of the
diagnosis is confirmation of urine leakage. This
can be done in a number of ways. At the Cleveland
Clinic Florida, we use the double-dye technique to
help differentiate between vesicovaginal and ureterovaginal fistula (UVF). The patient is brought
to the clinic after taking phenazopyridine. The
nurse instills 100 ml of diluted methylene blue
solution into the bladder, and the catheter is then
removed. A tampon is inserted vaginally and the
patient is asked to come back in 2 h. The tampon is
inspected. If it is stained blue, it is VVF. If stained
orange, it is UFV, and further workup is needed.
Further evaluation includes oral Indigo Carmine
IV or phenazopyridine to detect ureterovaginal
fistula. An intravenous pyelography (IVP) also can
help define anatomical defects. In 25% of VVFs

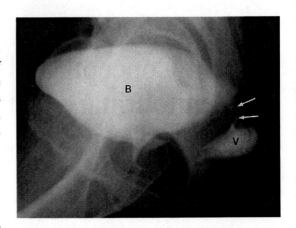

FIG. 32.1. Flouroscopy of vesicovaginal fistula

there will be a hydronephrosis, with 10% having a
concomitant UVF [8].

An antegrade pyelogram also can help define
anatomy using the nephrotomy tube, which may
show filling of the vagina with contrast. Cystoscopy
and vaginoscopy may help determine the site, size,
and number, as well as the location in relation to
ureteral orifices [9, 10]. There may be multiple,
small fistulae in a supratrigonal transverse position
found, especially after aggressive closure of the
vaginal cuff. Biopsy is recommended if there is
a history of malignancy. Flourourodynamic studies can be used to determine bladder compliance,
capacity, and outlet competence. It also allows better identification of fistulae that may otherwise be
missed (Fig. 32.1).

Management

Conservative Treatment

Only in small, clean, nonmalignant VVF may
conservative treatment be attempted. Prolonged
catheter drainage for 3–5 weeks is suggested.
Additionally, anticholinergic medication relaxes
the detrusor muscle and prevents spasm. Topical
estrogens are used routinely in postmenopausal
women to promote healing. Raz et al. as well as
our group, have utilized conservative therapy for
fistulae less than 5 mm, including therapy such as
catheter drainage alone or with electrocautery [1,
3] (Fig. 32.2).

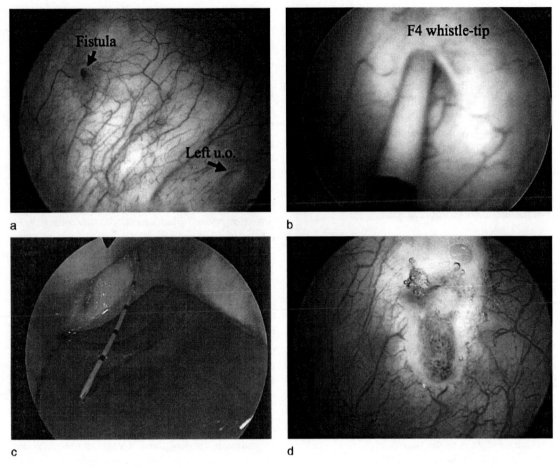

F<small>IG</small>. 32.2. Cystoscopy of a small VVF. (**a**) Supratrigonal lateral VVF. (**b**) F5 ureteric catheter inserted into fistula. (**c**) Vaginoscopy confirming the connection. (**d**) Fulgeration of fistulous tract, followed by 3 weeks bladder drainage and anticholinergics

In the last few years, we have been successful in managing small VVF with catheterization and cystoscopic fulguration with/without fibrin glue injection. In a case report from Osaka, Japan, fibrin glue was used for a 1-mm VVF at the site of recurrent endometrial tumor at the "vaginal stump." They used 1 cc of fibrin glue (Beriplast-P™, Aventis Pharma, LTD) after curetting a small area of tissue around the fistula. They reported maintenance of continence for 26 months. This same patient then developed a second separate fistula, 1.2 mm in size, which was treated in a similar fashion, with continence lasting 33 months [11]. Conservative

treatments, including the use of glue products, report varying degrees of success and are dependent on the cause, size, and location of the fistula. The literature in this area is very limited.

Surgical Repair Considerations

Each case of VVF should be individualized and, as in most surgeries, the first attempt at surgical repair is the best and most likely to succeed. The choice of surgical approach also should be determined by the surgeon's familiarity and skill with the technique.

Surgical Timing

VVF is most likely to heal well when properly diagnosed and repaired close to the time of formation. For example, an uncomplicated posthysterectomy VVF will still have many of the planes evident and is easier to surgically repair than an obstetric fistula. Zimmern observed no increased rate in morbidity or failure in patients with early repair performed only 2 to 3 weeks after injury [12]. Fistulae such as those caused by radiation or obstetrics need time for tissue regeneration prior to repair. In the latter situations, a delayed repair at 3–6 months is more appropriate.

Surgical Approach

Clearly, location of the fistula will dictate the best approach to a VVF repair. The most common site for VVF in the Western world is at the vaginal cuff status postabdominal hysterectomy. The current trend toward a transvaginal approach, even for deep and large fistulae, has been shown to have lower morbidity rates than transabdominal repairs. In addition, the approach to the type of vascularized interposition flap also is determined by how proximal (peritoneal) or distal (Martius) the genitourinary fistula is in the vagina.

Raz et al. evaluated their 10-year data on 207 women with interposition grafts and found that peritoneal tissue is an excellent source for interposition in complex proximal VVF and is at least as successful as Martius grafts in VVF [3]. Evans et al. evaluated the need for interposition grafts in both benign and malignant VVF, which showed a clearly higher success rate with interposition grafts regardless of type or etiology of fistula in the transabdominal approach. The key to success appeared to be related to a quality vascular pedicle in the interposition graft [7].

The approach usually is determined by the surgeon's preference, experience, and also the position of the fistula. The transvaginal approach, which is our personal preference at the Cleveland Clinic Florida, causes less morbidity and can be used for most VVF. The transabdominal approach is best when ureteric reimplantation or augmentation is necessary or if the woman has a deep and/or narrow vagina. The transvesical approach is a less commonly used approach, with higher morbidity.

A *transvaginal approach* for distal fistula requires wide dissection for mobilization. Closure is nonoverlapping layers under no tension. There also must be a method for checking for leaks. We like to use Foley instillation with diluted methylene blue and a clean white laparotomy sponge allowing for precise leakage site identification. If radiation or poor tissue quality is an issue, a Martius graft (in distal) or other biological graft materials have been used to assist in fistula reconstruction. Success rates are reported at 92–96% [1, 3, 13]. A minimum of a three-layer closure is one of the keys to success in treatment of VVF. Layer one is composed of revised bladder mucosa or epithelialized edges of the fistula tract, layer two is imbricated perivesical fascia, and level three is undermined vaginal epithelium or an advancement flap.

We prefer a Latzko procedure, or minicolpocleisis, as our method of choice for high vaginal cuff VVF (Fig. 32.3). In this repair there is no need to excise the fistula, as its margins provide good anchoring for the first-layer of sutures. The damaged vaginal wall is closed in layers over the fistula. The resulting vaginal shortening is nearly negligible and has no sequelae.

The *transabdominal approach* is intraperitoneal with wide mobilization of the bladder. If this technique is chosen, the O'Conor technique is our preferred technique. This allows excellent mobilization of different layers and omental interposition. Success rates are 85–100% [7]. The technique includes:

- Bivalving the bladder in the midline passing the fistula and excising it (O'Conor technique)
- Isolate the bladder in two layers
- Close bladder in two to three layers
- Close vagina in two layers
- Routine use of omental interposition (Fig. 32.4)

The *transvesical approach* is best utilized when the fistula is loculated and the ureteric orifices are cannulated. The fistulous tract must be incised using a scalpel, leaving the vaginal wall intact. The dissection would be carried out circumferentially for 1–2 cm. During closure it is key not to overlap the suture lines and to use both transverse and perpendicular suture lines if possible.

Complications include frequency, urgency, urge incontinence, recurrence, stress urinary incontinence (10–12%), ureteral obstruction, and bowel obstruc-

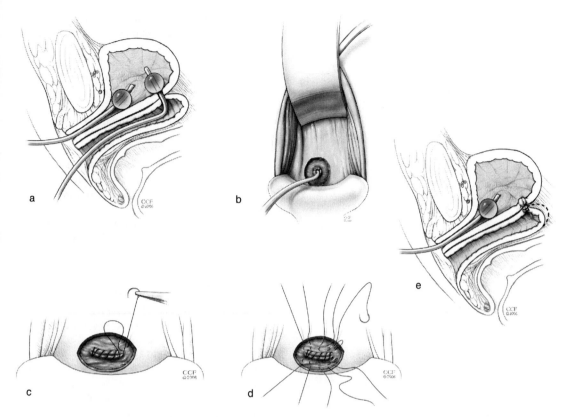

FIG. 32.3. Latzko technique. (**a**) VVF catheterized with small Foley's catheter. (**b**) The vaginal epithelium around the fistula is denuded, leaving the fistula margins. (**c**) Water-tight closure of the fistula. (**d**) Multiple mattress sutures in 2–3 layers. (**e**) Insignificant shortening of the vaginal cuff after complete closure

tion. The only alternative with end-stage bladder and multiple failed surgeries is urinary diversion.

Laparoscopic repair using the O'Conor technique has been reported by Chibber et al. They report the main advantages of a laparoscopic approach are decreased morbidity and recovery time. Maintaining pneumoperitoneum once the fistula is excised is a challenge, and a Foley catheter is used for this purpose. They were successful in 7 of 8 patients. Mean operative time was 220 min [7]. Success rates are reported to be as high as 93% at 26 months [14]. Omental J-flaps also were successfully utilized by other groups, such as Miklos et al. even after transvaginal failures with Latzko procedures [12, 15].

Laparoscopic VVF repair with robotic reconstruction has been reported twice in the Journal of Urology since 2004. Melamud et al. reported a case using the DaVinci™ robot with a total operative time

of 280 min [16]. There was an estimated blood loss of 50 cc with 16-week follow-up revealing cure for a proximal VVF at the cuff posthysterectomy [17]. A second article reporting five cases by Sundaram et al. showed a 100% cure rate at 6 months [14]. Clearly, the robotic repairs will require further evaluation and randomized controlled studies in the future, allowing for better options for VVF patients. The disadvantages to robotic VVF repair are obvious, including increased learning curve, time, expense, and availability as well as surgeon experience.

Large posthysterectomy and postradiation VVFs also can be managed by ileocystoplasty. This technique carries a high rate of morbidity but has proven effective in small groups of women with large VVF. The key to its success is using a well-vascularized portion of ileum, which has not been radiated [18].

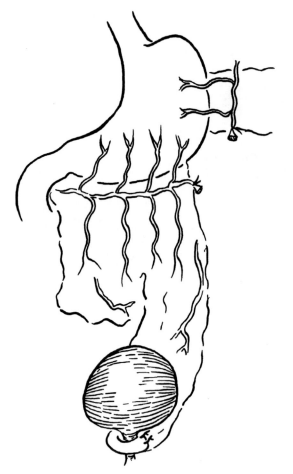

3. Schlunt Eilber K, Kavalier,E, Rodriguez L, et al. Ten-year experience with transvaginal vesicovaginal fistula repair using tissue interposition. J Urol 2003; 169:1033–1036.
4. Tancer, M.L. Observations on prevention and management of vesicovaginal fistula. J Urol 1980; 123:839–840.
5. Harkki-Siren P, Sjoberg J, Tiitinen A. Urinary tract injuries after hysterectomy. Obstet Gynecol 1998; 92 (1):113–118.
6. McKay HA, Hanlon K. Vesicovaginal fistula after cervical carclage: Repair by transurethral suture cystorrhaphy. J Urol 2003; 169:1086–1087.
7. Chibber PJ, Navinchandra Shah H, Jain P. Laparoscopic O'Conor's repair for vesico—vaginal and vesico-uterine fistulae. BJU Int 2005; 96: 183–186.
8. Goodwin WE, Scardino PT. Vesicovaginal and ureterovaginal fistulas: A summary of 25 years experience. J Urol 1980; 123:370–374.
9. Andreoni C, Bruschini H, Truzzi JC, et al. Combined vaginoscopy—cystoscopy: A novel simultaneous approach improving vesicovaginal fistula evaluation. J Urol 2003; 170:2330–2332.
10. Cassio A, Bruschini 1H, Truzzi JC, et al. Combined vaginoscopy—cystoscopy: A novel simultaneous approach improving vesicovaginal fistula evalution. J Urol 2003; 170:2330–2332.
11. Kanaoka Y, Hurai., Ishiko O, et al. Vesicovaginal fistula treated with fibrin glue. Int J Gynecol Obstet 2001; 73:147–149.
12. Zimmern PE, Hadley HR, Staskin DR, Raz S. Genitourinary fistulae. Vaginal approach for repair of vesico-vaginal fistulae. Urol Clin North Am 1985; 12:361.
13. Ghoniem GM. Transvaginal repair of recurrent vesicovaginal fistula utilizing suburethral sling and martius grafts. Video-Urology Times, Vol. 5, Program 4, 1992.
14. Sundaram BM, Kalidasan G, Hemal A. Robotic repair of vesicovaginal fistula: Case series of five patients. Urology 2006; 67:970–973.
15. Miklos JR, Sobolewski C, Lucente V. Laparoscopic management of recurrent vesicovaginal fistula. Int Urogynecol J 1999; 10:116–117.
16. Melamud O, Eicheel B, Turbow B, Shanberg A. Laparoscopic vesicovaginal fistula repair with robotic reconstruction. Urology 2005; 65.(1)
17. Melamud O, Eichel B, Turbow B, et al. Laparoscopic vesicovaginal fistula repair with robotic reconstruction. J Urol 2005; 65:163–166.
18. Tabakov ID, Slavchev BN. Large post-hysterectomy and post-radiation vesicovaginal fistulas: Repair by ileocystoplasty. J Urol 2004; 171:272–274.

FIG. 32.4. Omental interposition

Postoperative Care

Postoperative care is as crucial to the procedure as is the procedure itself. A vaginal pack is placed after surgery until the following morning. Usually, antibiotics are administered for 1–2 weeks post-surgery depending on the length of need for Foley. We recommend anticholinergics until catheters are removed. We will traditionally do a cystogram in 3 weeks, if the suprapubic tube or Foley is out.

References

1. Ghoniem GM, Khater UM. Vesicovaginal fistula, pelvic floor dysfunction. Springer, London, 2006.
2. Riley VJ. Vesicovaginal fistula. EMedicine for WebMD, June 25, 2006.

19. Eilber KS, Rosenblum N, Rodriguez LV. Vesicovaginal fistula: Complex fistulae, female urology, urogynecology, and voiding dysfunction. New York: Marcel Dekker, 2005.

20. Richman MB, Goldman HB. Vesicovaginal fistula: Complex fistulae, female urology, urogynecology, and voiding dysfunction. New York: Marcel Dekker, 2005.

21. Latzko W. Postoperative vesicovaginal fistulas; Genesis and therapy. Anat J Surg 1942; LVIII(2).

22. Sotelo R, Marandolino B M, Garcia-Segui A, et al. Laparoscopic vesicovaginal fistula. J Urol 2005; 173:1615–1618.

23. Dolan LM, Easwaran SP, Hilton P. Congenital vesicovaginal fistula in association with hypoplastic kidney and uterus didelphys. J Urol 2004; 63(1).

Chapter 33
Urologic Consequences of Pelvic Irradiation in Women

Mary M.T. South and George D. Webster

The first reported case of a patient being cured with radiation therapy was in 1899, shortly after the discovery of X-rays and radium in the late 1800s [1]. The intracavitary treatment of cervical cancer was initiated in the early part of the twentieth century, with a significant increase in use noted particularly in the 1920s [1].

The basic concept behind radiation therapy is to minimize the damage to healthy, normal tissue while maximizing destruction of malignant tissue [2]. Radiation changes to tissues may appear obvious soon after exposure, but in most cases the changes are not apparent for long periods of time and may be apparent only at a microscopic level [2]. Long-term effects from radiation exposure, such as urological complications, may not present for several months to years after treatment.

Approximately one third of Americans will face cancer during their lifetime [3]. With an aging population, the gynecologist, as well as the urologist, are going to see an increase in gynecological malignancies and the complications resulting from the treatment of these cancers [3]. Both the malignancy itself, as well as the treatment, can result in urological side effects [3]. Treatment of gynecological malignancies involves chemotherapy, surgery, and irradiation, all of which can lead to both temporary and permanent urological complications [3]. This chapter will focus on the postradiation effects on the female urogenital tract, including primarily the bladder and urethra, and the resulting effects on continence.

Radiation therapy plays a large role in the treatment of pelvic cancers [3]. Cervical cancer is one of the most common types of female cancers that is treated with radiation therapy. The bladder, urethra, and ureters are anatomically situated close to the cervix, predisposing them to the damaging side effects of radiation therapy [3].

Other cancers that are treated with pelvic irradiation include prostate cancer, retroperitoneal or pelvic sarcomas, and other gynecological malignancies including uterine cancers. As one would expect, bladder symptoms are not limited to those patients being treated for cervical cancer with pelvic radiation. A questionnaire was distributed to 202 prostate cancer patients to assess bowel, bladder, and sexual function after pelvic radiotherapy and 4% of patients reported significant bladder symptoms (including urinary incontinence, hematuria, and severe dysuria); although 17% reported daily incontinence, only 2% required usage of pads [4]. A later study done by Nguyen et al. on postradiation prostate cancer patients found an even larger percentage of patients reporting incontinence (30%) but again only 2% required the use of pads [5].

Biological Effects of Radiation

Therapeutic radiology is based on the ability to selectively destroy tissues [2]. Neoplastic cells tend to be more susceptible to the destructive effects of radiation than do surrounding normal tissues, as rapidly proliferating cells are highly radiosensitive [2]. The biological effects seen in irradiated tissue

461

are primarily the result of DNA damage [2]. DNA damage can occur directly from absorption of the radiation into the biological material or indirectly via production of free radicals in the cell, ultimately resulting in cell death [2].

The key to successful destruction of neoplastic cells is the ability to place the radiation in close proximity to the malignancy while at the same time using a dosage that is tolerable to surrounding tissues (ie, for example, the use of brachytherapy in the treatment of cervical cancer) [2]. The uterus and normal tissues of the cervix are relatively tolerant of high doses of radiation; however, other organs, such as sigmoid, rectosigmoid, rectum, and bladder, are less tolerant to exposure to radiation.

Pathological changes noted in tissues after radiation reveal mainly fibrosis and some necrosis. Autopsy in 22 patients who had undergone intraoperative radiotherapy showed histological evidence of fibrosis of the retroperitoneal soft tissues, hypocellularity of the vertebral bone marrow, and perineural fibrosis in the retroperitoneal and pelvic nerve trunks [6]. These autopsies did not uncover a significant amount of radiation-induced changes in blood vessels, intestine, or ureters.

Complications of Pelvic Radiation

Complications from radiation therapy can occur acutely or chronically over a long period of time [3]. Acute complications usually occur during the course of therapy or toward the completion of treatment [3]. Patients may develop symptoms of frequency and dysuria and, on occasion, hematuria [3]. These patients also tend to have an increased frequency of urinary tract infections [3]. Usually these side effects can simply be treated with anticholinergics or antibiotics [3].

Chronic urological radiation complications include vesicovaginal fistula, reduced bladder capacity due to radiation fibrosis, neurogenic bladder, detrusor overactivity, and intrinsic sphincter deficiency (ISD) [3]. Upon review of the literature, severe urological complications can occur anywhere from 2 to 14% after pelvic irradiation [7, 8, 9, 10, 11]. Compared with complications of the rectum or intestines, urological complications tend to occur much later (6.4 vs 2.2 years respectively, $P < 0.0001$) [11]. One study showed a dose-dependent rate of rectal and bladder complications with

delay in symptoms of approximately 22 months for the bladder [10]. A rare long-term complication after pelvic irradiation is bladder cancer. Maier et al. found an increased risk of developing urothelial bladder cancer in a population of 10,709 Austrian women treated with brachytherapy for primary gynecological carcinomas (RR 4.66) [12]. Physicians should have a high index of suspicion for this condition even years after treatment [13].

Another complication of pelvic irradiation, particularly with the use of high-dose-rate brachytherapy, is spontaneous rupture of the urinary bladder, which may not be as rare as once thought and urologists should be aware of this potentially life-threatening event [14].

Wilkinson et al. studied 366 women who received brachytherapy for cervical cancer [9]. Of the 366 women, 60 women with bladder complications were compared with 60 age- and stage-matched controls without symptoms, specifically looking at size of applicators, height of the applicators set above the pubic symphysis, the degree of anteversion or retroversion of the applicator sets, and radiation dosages. Unfortunately, based on their findings, no reliable predictor of bladder complications following brachytherapy was identified. However, it does appear that severe bladder injuries (ie, fistulas) may be more common in patients with stage IIIA and IIIB disease and those receiving high external beam radiation (>5,000rads) [8].

Vesicovaginal Fistula

Fewer than 5% of patients develop vesicovaginal fistula following radiation therapy [3]. Presentation may occur anytime from 6 months to 30 years after completion of treatment [15, 16, 17]. Patients with tumor that is close to the anterior vaginal wall appear to be more predisposed to development of a fistula [3]. In patients with a history of cervical cancer who present with a vesicovaginal fistula, it is important to biopsy the fistula because 50% if these patients have evidence of recurrent disease [18].

Generally speaking vesicovaginal fistula will be diagnosed by physical examination, cystoscopy, and pyridium pad study. Other studies used have included cystography, computed tomography (CT) scan, and Doppler color ultrasound. CT findings consistent with a diagnosis of vesicovaginal fistula include contrast, air, and/or fluid in the vagina. Performing a CT scan also may be beneficial for identifying associated findings such as radiation changes, contiguous pelvic mass, or adherent bowel. These findings may give an indication of the etiology of the fistula, such as recurrent disease, or aid in preparing for surgical repair [19]. Volkmer et al. report on a method of vesicovaginal fistula detection by filling the bladder with a diluted contrast media and using ultrasound to detect a jet phenomenon through the bladder wall into the vagina, revealing the presence of a fistula in 11 of 12 patients studied [20].

Many of the commonly employed methods for repairing vesicovaginal fistula will not be successful in the setting of radiation-damaged tissue. The success rates reported after repair in the irradiated patient range from 40 to 100% compared with 70 to 100% in nonradiated patients [21]. The reduced success rate seen with repair of postirradiated vesicovaginal fistulas is likely due to the poor vascularity of these tissues [22]. In those circumstances where the fistula develops in the early aftermath of radiation treatment, it is recommended that repair be delayed for weeks or months to allow for maturation of the fistulous tract. Vaginal repair of vesicovaginal fistulas, either with a modified Latzko procedure or a layered closure, should be the preferred route in general because the success rates are similar when compared with abdominal repair with fewer complications. Loran et al. report on a modification of the Latzko procedure using a high colpocleisis in 174 postirradiated vesicovaginal fistulas that resulted in spontaneous urination and a return to preirradiated bladder capacities [16].

Eilber et al. found excellent results with vaginal repair of complex vesicovaginal fistulas by using a tissue interposition after reviewing outcomes at their institution over a 10-year period of time on 207 patients [23]. The most common etiology for a fistula in their cohort was hysterectomy (91%), while 4% of their patients had radiation-induced fistulas. Their definition of a complex fistula was any fistula that was either radiation-induced or greater than 2cm in size. Of the 207 patients, tissue interposition was used in 58% of the cases. For proximal fistulas, they employed a peritoneal flap and for distal fistulas they used a Martius flap. In the event the patient had insufficient vaginal epithelium, the authors used a full-thickness labial

flap. The cure rates for the Martius and peritoneal flaps were 97 and 96%, respectively.

Most urologists would prefer an abdominal approach to the repair of postradiation fistula with the rationale that this gives the opportunity to interpose omentum at the repair site and also offers the opportunity to address small bladder capacity by enterocystoplasty and to deal with associated ureteral obstruction. Obviously there is a spectrum of severities of presentation of such cases and the approach must be individualized.

Some postradiation fistula are so complex and severe that they are unable to be reconstructed and urinary diversion may be necessary as the last resort [24]. Mannel et al. reported the use of an ileocecal continent urinary reservoir in patients with a history of pelvic irradiation (6 of the 37 patients had radiation-induced vesicovaginal fistulas while the rest had pelvic exenterations) and found comparable results in these patients compared to nonirradiated patients [25]. A smaller report on four patients describes the use of an interposition ileocystoplasty to repair large postradiation vesicovaginal fistulas. The benefits of this type of repair in the postradiated patients, per the authors, are as follows: (1) wide dissection of the bladder is not necessary; (2) the defect in the bladder is repaired with a well-vascularized (and undamaged) distal ileum; (3) bladder capacity is enlarged; (4) improved quality of life with high probability of spontaneous voiding; and (5) the ability to adapt this procedure in the setting of damaged distal ureters [26].

Leissner et al. suggested that, should urinary diversion be necessary to regain continence in patients with postirradiated vesicovaginal cases, some patients may desire reconstructive surgery to create a neovagina [24]. The authors incorporated the bladder into a neovagina in six patients who had undergone urinary diversion, five of whom were postirradiation. These patients had a mean follow-up of 4.7 years with reported good functional and cosmetic results. Vaginal reconstruction also may be accomplished using enteric segments and by bilateral pedicled rectus or grascilis flaps [22].

Bladder Dysfunction after Pelvic Radiation

In addition to direct damage resulting in fibrosis, radiation may also damage the innervation to the bladder and urthra. Although this was not believed to be the case in the past, several studies have shown that peripheral nerve damage can occur after radiotherapy [27, 28, 29]. Olsen et al. evaluated 161 breast cancer patients for radiation-induced brachial plexopathy [28]. Interestingly, they found that larger fraction size and cytotoxic therapy increased the damage done by radiotherapy and that younger patients were more vulnerable to this type of injury. Chemotherapy administered with radiotherapy may result in further vulnerability of the peripheral nervous system to damage depending on the dose and type of drugs used [30]. As mentioned earlier, radiation therapy works by damaging DNA, and if not repaired results in cell death. Because glial and Schwann cells of the peripheral nervous system have slow reproductive cycles, damage may not become apparent for many months if the original insult was not lethal to the cell. Thus, the complication of neurogenic bladder resulting in bladder dysfunction following radiotherapy may not be immediately apparent [27].

Damage to the peripheral nerves in the pelvis may be difficult to avoid given their close proximity to the structures being irradiated, regardless of the treatment method employed [27]. Tait et al. performed a randomized trial comparing conformal versus conventional pelvic radiotherapy to assess acute toxicity, but they failed to show a difference in urinary symptoms between the two arms [31]. In one large animal model, an intraoperative radiation dose of less than 20Gy was not associated with significant peripheral nerve injury, but all animals receiving 20Gy developed a paresis consistent with nerve injury [32]. A long-term follow-up of this study suggests that the intraoperative radiation dose may be inversely related to time to develop neuropathy (ie, the higher the dose, the sooner neuropathy may present) [33].

Although a large body of evidence supports the concept that peripheral nerve damage results in the neurogenic bladder seen after radiation exposure, bladder hypertonicity also may be due to changes at the neuromuscular junction. Michailov et al. demonstrated that the detrusor muscle's response to acetylcholine is diminished in the postirradiated bladder in rats [34]. In a prior study, the same authors also demonstrated an immediate tonic contraction in the detrusor muscle exposed to radiation [35]. They conclude that both immediate exposure of the detrusor muscle to radiation and long-term

changes in the muscles sensitivity to the neurotransmitter acetylcholine may help to explain the hypertonicity seen in the postirradiated bladder.

Parkin et al. performed urodynamic studies on 40 patients 5–11 years after radiation therapy for cervical cancer [36]. The authors compared these 40 patients to 27 patients prior to treatment. Patients who had undergone radiation therapy had mean volumes at first bladder sensation lower than the mean volumes before treatment. The mean maximum cystometric capacity also was lower in the treatment group. The mean filling detrusor pressure was higher and a significant reduction in the maximal urethral closure pressure and functional profile length was noted in the treatment group. The authors also found detrusor instability to be a common finding in the treatment group and concluded that treatment of these symptoms should be attempted before attributing symptoms to fibrosis. Similar findings were noted by Farquharson et al., who studied 33 patients undergoing pelvic irradiation for cervical cancer, noting reductions in peak urinary flow, volume at first desire to void, cystometric capacity, and bladder compliance specifically in those patients receiving more than 3000rads to the entire bladder from external beam irradiation [37].

Little has been reported on the effects of radiation therapy on bladder function compared with the well-known effects following radical hysterectomy, for example. Farquharson compared urodynamics and symptoms in 30 patients who had undergone radical hysterectomy alone (RH) to 30 patients who had undergone both radical hysterectomy and pelvic irradiation (RH+RT) and 30 patients who had undergone pelvic irradiation alone (RT) [38]. Altered bladder sensation and voiding problems were more frequent after RH or RH+RT than RT ($P=0.002$). Abdominal straining during voiding was noted in 50% of RH patients compared to 10% who had only RT. Fifteen percent of patients had urinary incontinence prior to treatment. Following treatment, the group with the largest percentage of incontinence was the RH+RT group (63%), followed by the RH patients (26%), and then the RT group (23%). Bladder compliance was noted to be reduced in the RT patients, and compared with RH alone the RH+RT group was noted to have a significantly decreased bladder compliance ($P=0.0001$). No difference was found between any of the groups in reference to bladder neck and urethral function. The authors noted that the urinary incontinence seen in the RH+RT group, as well as the decrease in bladder compliance, was related to the bladder dose of external radiation.

Lin et al. assessed the urodynamic findings in patients after radical hysterectomy or pelvic irradiation for cervical cancer and found abnormal findings usually exist before treatment but worsen or new abnormal findings are noted [39]. Detrusor instability or low bladder compliance was seen in 45% of patients treated with pelvic irradiation alone and 80% of patients treated with both pelvic irradiation and radical hysterectomy. Voiding with abdominal strain was noted to be 100% in the radical hysterectomy, pelvic irradiation, and radical hysterectomy plus pelvic irradiation groups, but was noted to be 0% in the control group (stage IB cervical cancer prior to treatment). Finally, the frequency of a positive pad test was noted to be 46% in the pelvic irradiation group but 100% in the group treated with both radical hysterectomy and pelvic irradiation.

Behr et al. evaluated the urodynamics in 104 patients who had undergone primary irradiation for cervical cancer [40]. All patients were found to be incontinent of urine by 2 years after treatment. Sixty percent of those patients appeared to have urge urinary incontinence, which the authors felt to be related to the radiation-induced fibrosis of the bladder (decreased compliance and capacity). The other 40% of the patients were found to have stress incontinence that had already been present prior to irradiation, with an increase in stress incontinence seen only after 6 years or later, which the authors conclude was presumably related to advancing age.

Parkin et al. mailed questionnaires to 66 patients from 5 to 11 years after radiotherapy for cervical carcinoma and found that 45% of these patients had symptoms of urgency and urge incontinence [41]. This study found that voiding dysfunction was less common than bladder overactivity.

Management of Bladder Dysfunction

There is no literature specific to the management of bladder dysfunction following radiation therapy and so the general principles of treatment of bladder overactivity, low bladder compliance, and poor contractility must be followed. Unfortunately, it is these authors' experience that treatments are much less successful when radiation is the underlying etiology. While anticholinergics may improve symptoms in patients with detrusor overactivity, those patients with reduced functional capacity due to low bladder compliance are less likely to be improved significantly. Botox and sacral neuromodulation have been used with success in intractable bladder overactivity of other causes, but there currently is no literature supporting its use in irradiated cases. These uses await further clinical trial. Finally, augmentation enterocystoplasty also has a long history of use to treat intractable bladder overactivity and low compliance, but the literature specific to bladder dysfunction following radiation therapy is scant.

Intrinsic Sphincter Deficiency and Stress Urinary Incontinence after Radiation

A variety of factors determine whether or not a urethra will remain continent in conditions of stress (activity/increased abdominal pressure). One factor is the ability of the urethra to form a tight seal, which requires that it be sufficiently pliable to easily coapt. The irradiated rigid and fibrotic urethra loses this ability [42]. Additionally, in the irradiated pelvis the urethra may become fixed and immobile. The literature provides very little insight into the management of radiation-induced intrinsic sphincter deficiency (ISD) resulting in stress urinary incontinence. No studies have been done looking specifically at the best way to manage these patients other than urinary diversion.

The degree of urethral dysfunction following radiation therapy occurs in a wide spectrum of severities and may be accompanied by a spectrum of associated bladder dysfunctions as discussed above. In its least complex form a patient who previously has undergone radiation therapy in the pelvis develops stress urinary incontinence and has no associated bladder dysfunction (bladder overactivity or poor contractility) and has healthy vaginal tissues and a mobile urethra. Such a patient will likely be dealt with, as would any woman with such symptoms, by a pubovaginal sling and similar outcomes might be anticipated. At the other end of the spectrum is the woman with a fibrotic, nonpliable, immobile, and incompetent urethra that also is associated with a bladder of poor functional capacity, overactivity, low compliance, and poor contractility. Such patients are destined for urinary diversion. Between these two extremes the entire spectrum of combinations of urethral and bladder dysfunction occur, and treatment must be individualized and generally the prognosis for outcome is guarded. The use of periurethral bulking agents is an alternative to the pubovaginal sling, but once again there are no data that comment on outcomes [42]. It is probable that results will be less successful than the already-mediocre results achieved in nonradiated patients.

In these authors' experience the most frequent dilemma is whether or not a pubovaginal sling is appropriate for obvious stress incontinence, and if so what technique and what sling product should be chosen. Certainly when stress incontinence is evident by history, a positive stress test is found on examination, the pad weight is significant, and urodynamics show a low leak point pressure, then a sling is an appropriate treatment. These authors prefer a minimally invasive (midurethral) technique and the choice of synthetic versus biological material might be best based on how much tension the sling requires. Our preference is for a synthetic sling even when the sling is tensioned to be coaptive, but this selection of material in this situation remains controversial. Sling tension is determined primarily by the degree of urethral hypermobility and also by the "rigidity" of the urethra. Most often the "rigid" urethra is not very mobile, and in these circumstances the sling will need to be tensioned to coapt the urethra to be successful, but in doing so invites the problem of urinary retention and increases the risk of urethral erosion. On occasion, particularly when poor contractility is also present, retention and an intermittent self-catheterization program may be the only way to achieve continence. Unfortunately, even in this latter situation, the fact that these patients also often have poor functional bladder capacity because of bladder overactivity or low compliance, their need for self-catheterization may be too frequent to be acceptable.

References

1. Hoskins, ed. Principles and practice of gynecologic oncology, 3rd ed. Phildadelphia: Lippincott Williams & Wilkins; 2000.
2. DiSaia, ed. Clinical gynecologic oncology, 6th ed. St Louis: Mosby; 2002.
3. Walters, ed. Urogynecology and reconstructive pelvic surgery, 2nd ed. St Louis: Mosby; 1999.
4. Crook. Effect of pelvic radiotherapy for prostate cancer on bowel, bladder, and sexual function: The patient’s perspective. Urology1996; 47(3): 387–394.
5. Nguyen. Late effects after radiotherapy for prostate cancer in a randomized dose–response study: Results of a self-assessment questionnaire. Urology1998; 51(6):991–997.
6. SindelarWFHH, RestrepoC, KinsellaTJ. Pathological tissue changes following intraoperative radiotherapy. Am J Clin Oncol1986; 9(6):504–509.
7. WangCJ, LeungSW, ChenHCet-al., High-dose-rate intracavitary brachytherapy (HDR-IC) in treatment of cervical carcinoma: 5-year results and implication of increased low-grade rectal complication on initiation of an HDR-IC fractionation scheme. Int J Rad Oncol Biol Phys1997; 38(2):391–398.
8. Stryker. Bladder and rectal complications following radiotherapy for cervix cancer. Gynecol Oncol1988; 29(1):1–11.
9. Wilkinson. A retrospective study of bladder morbidity in patients receiving intracavitary brachytherapy as all or part of their treatment for cervix cancer. Br J Radiol2003; 76(912):897–903.
10. Orton. Dose dependence of complication rates in cervix cancer radiotherapy. Int J Rad Oncol Biol Phys1986; 12(1):37–44.
11. Fujikawa. High incidence of severe urologic complications following radiotherapy for cervical cancer in Japanese women. Gynecol Oncol2001; 80(1):21–23.
12. Maier. Late urological complications and malignancies after curative radiotherapy for gynecological carcinomas: A retrospective analysis of 10,709 patients. J Urol1997; 158(3):814–817.
13. Kaplan. Bladder cancer after pelvic irradiation for cervical cancer. South Med J1985; 78(9):1068–1070.
14. Fujikawa. Spontaneous rupture of the urinary bladder is not a rare complication of radiotherapy for cervical cancer: Report of six cases. Gynecol Oncol1999; 73(3):439–442.
15. Zoubek. The late occurrence of urinary tract damage in patients successfully treated by radiotherapy for cervical carcinoma. J Urol1989; 141(6):1347–1349.
16. Loran OB-GL, Zaitsev AV, Lipskii VS. High colpocleisis in the treatment of postradiation vesicovaginal fistulas. Urologiia 2000; (4):41–42.

17. Gellrich JHO, Oehischlager S, Wirth MP. Manifestation, latency and management of late urological complications after curative radiotherapy for cervical carcinoma. Onkologie2003; 26(4):334–340.
18. Cushing. Major urologic complications following radium and X-ray therapy for carcinoma of the cervix. Am J Obstet Gynecol1968; 101(6):750–755.
19. Kuhlman. CT evaluation of enterovaginal and vesicovaginal fistulas. J Comput Assist Tomogr1990; 14(3):390–394.
20. Volkmer. Colour Doppler ultrasound in vesicovaginal fistulas. Ultrasound MedBiol2000; 26(5):771–775.
21. AngioliRPM, MuziiL, MendezLet-al., .Guidelines of how to manage vesicovaginal fistula. Crit Rev Oncol Hematol2003; 48(3):295–304.
22. HorchREGG, Schultze-SeemannW. Bilateral pedicled myocutaneous vertical rectus abdominus muscle flaps to close vesicovaginal and pouch-vaginal fistulas with simultaneous vaginal and perineal reconstruction in irradiated pelvic wounds. Urology2002; 60(3):502–507.
23. Eilber KS, et al. Ten-year experience with transvaginal vesicovaginal fistula repair using tissue interposition. J Urol2003; 169(3):1033–1036.
24. Leissner J, et al. Vaginal reconstruction using the bladder and/or rectal walls in patients with radiation-induced fistulas. Gynecol Oncol2000; 78(3):356–360.
25. Mannel RS, et al. Use of ileocecal continent urinary reservoir in patients with previous pelvic irradiation. Gynecol Oncol1995; 59(3):376–378.
26. Tabakov ID, SlavchevBN. Large post-hysterectomy and post-radiation vesicovaginal fistulas: Repair by ileocystoplasty. J Urol2004; 171(1):272–274.
27. Corcos JSE, ed. Textbook of the neurogenic bladder: Adults and children.London: Martin Dunitz; 2004.
28. Olsen NK, et al. Radiation-induced brachial plexopathy: Neurological follow-up in 161 recurrence-free breast cancer patients. International JRad Oncol Biol Phys1993; 26(1):43–49.
29. Johnstone PASWE, O'ConnellPG. Lumbosacral plexopathy secondary to hyperfractionated radiotherapy: A case presentation and literature review. Radiat Oncol Invest Clin Basic Res1993; 1:126–130.
30. Keime G. Neurological complications of radiotherapy and chemotherapy. J Neurol1998; 245(11):695–708.
31. TaitDM, et al. Acute toxicity in pelvic radiotherapy; A randomised trial of conformal versus conventional treatment. Radiother Oncol1997; 42(2):121–136.
32. Kinsella TJ, et al. Threshold dose for peripheral neuropathy following intraoperative radiotherapy (IORT) in a large animal model. Int J Rad Oncol Biol Phys1991; 20(4):697–701.
33. Johnstone PAS, et al. Clinical toxicity of peripheral nerve to intraoperative radiotherapy in a canine model. Int J Rad Oncol Biol Phys1995; 32(4):1031–1034.
34. Michailov MC, et al.. Influence of X-irradiation on the motor activity of rat urinary bladder in vitro and in vivo. Strahlenther Onkol 1991; 167(5):311–318.
35. Michailov MC, et al. Immediate mechanical reactions of isolated human detrusor muscle on x-irradiation. Strahlentherapie1979; 155(4):284–286.
36. Parkin DE, et al.. Urodynamic findings following radiotherapy for cervical carcinoma. Br JUrol1988; 61(3):213–217.
37. Farquharson DI, et al. The short-term effect of pelvic irradiation for gynecologic malignancies on bladder function. Obstet Gynecol 1987; 70(1):81–84.
38. Farquharson DI, et al. The adverse effects of cervical cancer treatment on bladder function. Gynecol Oncol1987; 27(1):15–23.
39. Lin HH, et al. Abnormal urodynamic findings after radical hysterectomy or pelvic irradiation for cervical cancer. Int J Gynecol Obstet 1998; 63(2):169–174.
40. Behr J, et al. Funktionsveranderungen an den unteren Harnwegen nach Bestrahlung des Kollumkarzinoms. Strahlenther Onkol1990; 166(2):135–139.
41. Parkin DE, et al. Long-term bladder symptomatology following radiotherapy for cervical carcinoma. Radiother Oncol1987; 9(3):195–199.
42. Nygaard. Stress urinary incontinence. Obstet Gynecol2004; 104(3):607–620.

Chapter 34
Recurrent Incontinence

Jørgen Nordling

Surgical treatment of urinary incontinence has been excellently described in the previous chapters, including inclusive failure rates and complications. Recurrent incontinence may be seen in as many as 10–40% [1], and although it has decreased considerably during the last years, it still involves a relatively high number of patients and deserves special attention. Recurrent incontinence involves patients with an initially successful operation suffering from reoccurrence of their urinary incontinence but patients with persisting incontinence due to failure of the surgical procedure to correct the initial malfunction sufficiently often are included. All should be handled in the same way since they present with the same basic problem of urinary incontinence and anatomical consequences of previous surgery for urinary stress incontinence.

Recurrent urinary incontinence does not necessarily mean recurrence of the initial type of incontinence, but may be due to a wrong diagnosis up-front or due to the development of a new type of incontinence, which might be but not necessarily is caused by the previous surgery. It is therefore mandatory to do a meticulous evaluation of the patient before embarking on a new treatment.

Evaluation and Treatment of the Female Patient with Recurrent Urinary Incontinence

The evaluation should include [2]:

• General assessment

• Urinary symptom assessment including frequency volume chart and an assessment of quality of life and desire for treatment
• Physical examination, abdominal and pelvic
• Cough test to demonstrate stress incontinence if appropriate
• Urinalysis ± urine culture
• Assessment of voluntary pelvic floor muscle contraction
• Postvoid residual urine assessment

But in the complicated case of the patient with recurrent incontinence, full urodynamic investigation, urethrocystoscopy, voiding cystourethrography, ultrasound, and in the future possibly even MRI should be considered.

Different risk factors have been identified for failure after operations for genuine stress urinary incontinence: (1) incorrect diagnosis, (2) improper selection of surgical therapy or faulty surgical technique, (3) previous bladder neck procedures, which resulted in urethral and anterior vaginal wall scarring and shortening, (4) preoperative low resting urethral closure pressure, (5) preexisting detrusor overactivity, (6) age in association with hypoestrogenism, and (7) denervation attributed to childbirth [3]. Patient evaluation therefore should be able to identify such risk factors in order to allow appropriate decision making.

De novo urgency is a feared complication of surgery for stress urinary incontinence. It is not a rare complication and has been reported in 8% after a modified Burch colposuspension[4] and in 14.5% after a tension-free vaginal tape (TVT) procedure

[5]. In the latter material 11% had both de novo urgency with urinary incontinence and patients were as troubled by this as they had been by their stress incontinence. It is evident that in such cases it is important to direct the treatment against the overactive bladder and not the previous malfunctioning closure mechanism.

Before the introduction of the TVT treatment, it was generally agreed that previous incontinence surgery impaired the chance of a good outcome after repeated surgery. The cure rate declined almost proportionally with the number of previous surgical procedures for incontinence [3, 6]. Different risk factors for failure of repeated surgery like detrusor overactivity on preoperative cystometry, low-pressure urethra, fibrotic urethra, rigid urethra with significant periurethral scarring, negative Q-tip test, and neurogenic incontinence were described by Holschneider et al. [7]. Cure rate in patients without risk factors was 81.6%, while patients with one or more risk factors had a cure rate of only 43.8% ($P = 0.005$). In a retrospective study of Amaya-Obu et al. it was found that cure rates of 77, 73, and 38% were obtained with a two-team sling procedure after one, two, and three, respectively, previous incontinence procedures. The corresponding numbers after a Burch procedure was 81, 25, and 0%. It was concluded that a Burch procedure should be avoided after more than one previous incontinence operation. Also Bidmead et al. reported an 81% cure rate after colposuspension for recurrent incontinence [4].

This picture has changed completely after the introduction of the TVT procedure. The first indication of this change was published by Rardin et al. [8] in a multicenter study, where cure rate was 87% in primary surgery in 157 patients and 85% in the recurrent stress incontinence population of 88 patients. Rezapour and Ulmsten reported a similar success rate of 82% in 34 patients with recurrent incontinence, where actually a further 9% had significant improvement [9]. Others have not the same high cure rate. Liapis reported a cure rate 70% in 33 patients with a better cure rate if patients had sufficient preoperative urethral mobility (90% cure rate) [10].

The TVT procedure also has demonstrated good results after recurrence of incontinence after the TVT procedure itself. In two cases (with persistent incontinence in one and recurrence in one) a repeated TVT cured the patients [11]. A shortening procedure for recurrent or persistent incontinence after TVT was reported by Lo et al. [4] in five patients with persistent incontinence and nine patients with recurrent incontinence. Cure rate was 71.4% after 1 year.

Other treatment modalities such as bulking agents or another type of sling might be tried in the difficult patient with recurrent stress incontinence.

Evaluation and Treatment of the Male Patient with Recurrent Urinary Incontinence

Stress urinary incontinence in the male is almost always due to previous surgery and especially prostatic surgery. The aetiology is however often multifactorial [12] and evaluation must therefore be extensive before at least surgical treatment is attempted. Primary treatment involves conservative treatments like pelvic floor exercise [13] while surgical treatment includes bulking agents [14, 15, 16], slings [17, 18] and the artificial urinary sphincter [19, 20].

In the case of recurrent incontinence the same applies as in females, a proper assessment is necessary to evaluate if the cause of incontinence is due to another type of incontinence or failure of a previous operation. The evaluation therefore involves the following to diagnose a possible detrusor overactivity and/or bladder outlet obstruction:

- Focused history and physical examination
- Urine analysis and culture
- Voiding diary
- Pad test
- Urodynamics

In the case of implanted material filled with contrast medium a plain film of the abdomen will demonstrate whether the system has lost fluid. Cystourethrography might be indicated to demonstrate fistulas, strictures, or urethral diverticula.

Persistent incontinence after bulking agents or slings often will lead to a more invasive procedure and an artificial sphincter will be implanted. Treatment of recurrent urinary incontinence therefore is mainly a matter of handling the failed artificial urinary sphincter [21].

In the case of the failed artificial urinary sphincter, the patient presents with persistent or recurrent incontinence. As in female incontinence the etiology for failures varies but an accurate diagnosis is necessary to handle the problem.

Causes of Persistent or Recurrent Incontinence After Implantation of an Artificial Urinary Sphincter

- Urinary tract infection
- Detrusor overactivity
- Initial selection of incorrect cuff size or balloon pressure
- Urethral atrophy resulting in a too large cuff
- Leakage of fluid from the system
- Cuff erosion
- Device malfunction most often due to valve problems
- Silicone aging
- Urinary tract infection

A simple cystitis is in many cases the cause of recurrent incontinence and treatment of the infection restores normal function. A urine analysis and a culture therefore always is performed before moving on to more sophisticated diagnostic procedures.

Detrusor Overactivity

The male population receiving an artificial sphincter often is elderly because the main indication is postprostatectomy incontinence. Detrusor overactivity is common in this age group and it is often difficult to separate the detrusor and sphincter component of the urinary incontinence. The restoration of continence might reveal an overactive bladder problem in the case with severe stress incontinence previously hidden by the bladder never getting filled. The incidence of overactive bladder also increases with age and de novo urgency incontinence therefore also is a possibility.

Initial Selection of Incorrect Cuff Size or Balloon Pressure or Urethral Atrophy Resulting in a Too Large Cuff

The circumference of the posterior bulbous urethra is difficult to measure because of the surrounding spongious tissue. The best cuff size is 4.0 or 4.5 cm. Larger cuffs will not be able to compress the urethra sufficiently and will result in incomplete closure. With time, the tissue inside the cuff undergoes a considerable atrophy, which also might cause improper urethral closure. If the cuff is too large, it is unable to close completely, and consequently emptying demands more pumps. Normally one to three pumps is sufficient, but if that number increases, it is an indication of a too large cuff. It is possible during urethroscopy to visualize the incomplete cuff closure and at the same time rule out cuff erosion. If possible the cuff should be downsized, but the smallest cuff size is 4 cm, so something else has to be done. Relocation of the cuff either proximally or distally is a possibility in the case of urethral atrophy. Distal positioning may require a transcorporal approach [22]. Another possibility is the implantation of a second cuff [23, 24]. Recently, preliminary good results of using an external urethral bulking agent have been reported [25]

Leakage of Fluid from the System

Leakage might occur at any time and might be caused by trauma or material fatigue. It is most often seen from the cuff, but it might happen any place in the system. If the system has been filled with contrast medium, a plain X-ray will demonstrate a downsizing of the balloon or an empty system. Ultrasound also might be used. The leaking part of the system must be changed and it might be difficult to determine which part is actually leaking. Intraoperative electrical testing might be useful [26], but if in doubt the whole system should be changed.

Cuff Erosion

Infection or pressure often is the cause of cuff erosion. Cuff erosion often presents as recurrent incontinence or pain. It is diagnosed by urethroscopy and demands explantation of the cuff. A 16-Ch urethral catheter is left in place for 3–4 weeks and a new cuff implanted in another location after 3–6 months. In case of severe erosion with circumferential loss of urethra, a urethroplasty at the time of cuff explantation might be necessary [21]. Results after reimplantation is almost as good as after primary implantation, with a success rate of 82% compared to 90% after primary implantation [27].

Device Malfunction Most Often due to Valve Problems or Aging

If by accident blood has come into the system, clots will develop. They might circulate in the system for a while, but when they reach the control unit, valves or connections will become dysfunctional and retention or recurrent incontinence will occur. Inability to pump might be caused by the patient accidentally inactivating the system. The problem is easily solved by reactivation.

The artificial sphincter is made of silicone, a material in many ways similar to glass. It changes with time, loses elasticity, and eventually degrades. This means that the implanted sphincter has a limited lifetime and has to be changed after 10–15 years. Malfunction might appear as recurrent incontinence, pump problems, or leakage.

As with females, bulking agents or slings might be tried if implantation of a urinary sphincter is no longer possible.

Conclusion

Recurrent incontinence in the male and the female demands thorough evaluation in order to make an accurate diagnosis. In the female the introduction of the TVT and related procedures have made handling of recurrent stress incontinence easier, with a high cure rate similar to the primary procedure. In the difficult case, bulking agents or another type of sling might be indicated.

In the male persistent or recurrent incontinence after treatment with less invasive procedures such as bulking agents or slings might be handled by the implantation of an artificial urinary sphincter. If this fails, reimplantation almost always is possible and almost always as successful as primary implantation.

References

1. Bent AE. Management of recurrent genuine stress incontinence. Clin Obstet Gynecol 1990; 33(2): 358–366.
2. Abrams P, Andersson K-E, Brubaker L, et al. Recommendations of the international scientific committee in incontinence. In: Abrams P, Cardozo L, Khoury S, Wein A, eds. Incontinence. Plymouth: Health Publicatons, 2005:1589–1630.
3. Amaye-Obu FA, Drutz HP. Surgical management of recurrent stress urinary incontinence: A 12-year experience. Am J Obstet Gynecol 1999; 181(6):1296–1307.
4. Bidmead J, Cardozo L, McLellan A, et al. A comparison of the objective and subjective outcomes of colposuspension for stress incontinence in women. BJOG 2001; 108(4):408–413.
5. Holmgren C, Nilsson S, Lanner L, Hellberg D. Frequency of de novo urgency in 463 women who had undergone the tension-free vaginal tape (TVT) procedure for genuine stress urinary incontinence – A long-term follow-up. Eur J Obstet Gynecol Reprod Biol 2007; 132(1):121–125.
6. Petrou SP, Frank I. Complications and initial continence rates after a repeat pubovaginal sling procedure for recurrent stress urinary incontinence. J Urol 2001; 165(6 Pt 1):1979–1981.
7. Holschneider CH, Solh S, Lebherz TB, Montz FJ. The modified Pereyra procedure in recurrent stress urinary incontinence: A 15-year review. Obstet Gynecol 1994; 83(4):573–578.
8. Rardin CR, Kohli N, Rosenblatt PL, et-al. Tension-free vaginal tape: Outcomes among women with primary versus recurrent stress urinary incontinence. Obstet Gynecol 2002; 100(5 Pt 1):893–897.
9. Rezapour M, Ulmsten U. Tension-free vaginal tape (TVT) in women with recurrent stress urinary incontinence – A long-term follow up. Int Urogynecol J Pelvic Floor Dysfunct 2001; 12(Suppl 2):S9–S11.
10. Liapis A, Bakas P, Salamalekis E, et-al. Tension-free vaginal tape (TVT) in women with low urethral closure pressure. Eur J Obstet Gynecol Reprod Biol 2004; 116(1):67–70.
11. Riachi L, Kohli N, Miklos J. Repeat tension-free transvaginal tape (TVT) sling for the treatment of recurrent stress urinary incontinence. Int Urogynecol J Pelvic Floor Dysfunct 2002; 13(2):133–135.
12. Andersen JT, Nordling J. Urinary incontinence after transvesical prostatectomy. Urol Int 1978; 33:191–198.
13. Hunter KF, Moore KN, Cody DJ, Glazener CM. Conservative management for postprostatectomy urinary incontinence. Cochrane Database Syst Rev 2004; (2):CD001843.
14. Cespedes RD, Leng WW, McGuire EJ. Collagen injection therapy for postprostatectomy incontinence. Urology 1999; 54(4):597–602.
15. Bugel H, Pfister C, Sibert L,et-al. [Intraurethral macroplastic injections in the treatment of urinary incontinence after prostatic surgery.] Prog Urol 1999; 9(6):1068–1076.

16. Hubner WA, Schlarp OM. Treatment of incontinence after prostatectomy using a new minimally invasive device: Adjustable continence therapy. BJU Int 2005; 96(4):587–594.

17. Ullrich NF, Comiter CV. The male sling for stress urinary incontinence: 24-month follow-up with questionnaire based assessment. J Urol 2004; 172(1):207–209.

18. Ullrich NF, Comiter CV. The male sling for stress urinary incontinence: Urodynamic and subjective assessment. J Urol 2004; 172(1):204–206.

19. Montague DK. The artificial urinary sphincter (AS 800): Experience in 166 consecutive patients. J Urol 1992; 147(2):380–382.

20. Klijn AJ, Hop WC, Mickisch G, et-al. The artificial urinary sphincter in men incontinent after radical prostatectomy: 5 year actuarial adequate function rates. Br J Urol 1998; 82(4):530–533.

21. Webster GD, Sherman ND. Management of male incontinence following artificial urinary sphincter failure. Curr Opin Urol 2005; 15(6):386–390.

22. Guralnick ML, Miller E, Toh KL, Webster GD. Transcorporal artificial urinary sphincter cuff placement in cases requiring revision for erosion and urethral atrophy. J Urol 2002; 167(5):2075–2078.

23. Brito CG, Mulcahy JJ, Mitchell ME, Adams MC. Use of a double cuff AMS800 urinary sphincter for severe stress incontinence. J Urol 1993; 149(2):283–285.

24. DiMarco DS, Elliott DS. Tandem cuff artificial urinary sphincter as a salvage procedure following failed primary sphincter placement for the treatment of post-prostatectomy incontinence. J Urol 2003; 170(4 Pt 1):1252–1254.

25. Rahman NU, Minor TX, Deng D, Lue TF. Combined external urethral bulking and artificial urinary sphincter for urethral atrophy and stress urinary incontinence. BJU Int 2005; 95(6):824–826.

26. Kreder KJ, Webster GD. Evaluation and management of incontinence after implantation of the artificial urinary sphincter. Urol Clin North Am 1991; 18(2):375–381.

27. Raj GV, Peterson AC, Toh KL, Webster GD. Outcomes following revisions and secondary implantation of the artificial urinary sphincter. J Urol 2005; 173(4):1242–1245.

Chapter 35
Multioperated Recurrent Incontinence/Prolapse

Giacomo Novara and Walter Artibani

Introduction

Pelvic organ prolapse (POP) is a major health care problem. It was reported to be present in 50% of parous women [1], with aggregated rates of prolapse surgery estimated to be between 15 and 49 per 10,000 women/years [2]. Olsen et al., reporting data from the Kaiser Permanent Group, a large health maintenance organization with nearly 393,000 members which draws epidemiological data from a service area of more than 2 million people from North America, showed that the lifetime risk of surgery for POP or stress urinary incontinence (SUI) was 11.1% for a woman with an average life expectancy of 79 years [3].

In the United States, each year approximately 300,000 women require inpatient surgery for POP or SUI [4, 5] and about 100,000 more procedures are performed on an outpatient basis [6]. Moreover, Olsen's study highlighted that 29% of the patients experienced surgical failure and required repeated surgical procedures and that the time interval between reoperation decreased with each successive repair [3]. Consequently, each year about 116,000 operations are repeated surgical procedures, showing that the current available treatments for pelvic floor dysfunction are suboptimal [6].

The pathophysiology of recurrent POP and SUI is not clearly understood. Obviously, many risk factors for pelvic floor dysfunction, such as age, parity, obstetrical factors, cognitive impairment, or genetic factors, are unmodifiable and other relevant ones, such as obesity, smoking habits, or lower urinary tract dysfunction, can persist after the primary sur-

gery and can be regarded as possible causes of recurrence [7]. On the other hand, the effect of multiple surgeries and dissections on sphincter function, as well as the chance of neural injuries, can contribute to the occurrence of further pelvic floor dysfunction. Specifically, Kenton et al. showed by the use of urethral electromyography that women with previous continence surgery had more neural injury to their striated urethral sphincter than women without previous surgery after controlling for age and parity [8]. Other studies hypothesized that pudendal neuropathy or lesions to the somatic urethral innervation can be caused during vaginal dissection in case of anterior colporrhaphy, needle suspension, and paravaginal repair [9, 10, 11, 12].

In the treatment of recurrent pelvic floor dysfunction, the available evidence is largely insufficient due to the lack of long-term results from randomized controlled trials. Moreover, most of the low-quality pieces of evidence provide data only at short- or intermediate-term follow-up.

The present review focuses on the currently available data and recommendations on diagnostic workup and treatment of recurrent POP and SUI.

Materials and Methods

We performed a nonsystematic review of the literature. Data were identified by searching MEDLINE database, using both MeSH and free text searches.

With regard to recurrent POP, the MeSH search was conducted using the terms "Prolapse/surgery,"

"Prolapse/therapy," "Uterine Prolapse/surgery," "Uterine Prolapse/therapy," "Rectal Prolapse/surgery," "Rectal Prolapse/therapy," "Visceral Prolapse/surgery," "Visceral Prolapse/therapy" retrieved from the MeSH browser provided by MEDLINE. The free text search employed the following terms through the field "title and abstract" of the records: "pelvic organ prolapse," "rectocele," "cystocele," "anterior vaginal wall prolapse," "posterior vaginal wall prolapse," "vaginal vault prolapse," "colpocele," "hysterocele," "recurr*." The MEDLINE searches were pooled and the following search limits were used: languages ("English"), gender ("Female"), "humans," and publication type ("Clinical Trial, Meta-Analysis, Practice Guideline, Randomized Controlled Trial, Review, "Clinical Trial, Phase III," "Clinical Trial, Phase IV," Consensus Development Conference, "Consensus Development Conference, NIH," Controlled Clinical Trial, Guideline").

Regarding recurrent SUI, the MeSH search was conducted using the terms "Urinary Incontinence, Stress/surgery," "Urinary Incontinence, Stress/therapy." The free text search employed the following terms through the field "title and abstract" of the records: "stress urinary incontinence," "recurr*." Once the searches pooled, the following search limits were used: languages ("English"), gender ("Female"), "humans," and publication type ("Clinical Trial, Meta-Analysis, Practice Guideline, Randomized Controlled Trial, Review, "Clinical Trial, Phase III," "Clinical Trial, Phase IV," Consensus Development Conference, "Consensus Development Conference, NIH," Controlled Clinical Trial, Guideline").

One hundred and two records were identified in the first search and 135 in the second. The full texts of the papers were reviewed by the authors to select the studies for the present purposes. In addition, other significant texts cited in the reference lists of the selected papers as well as the volumes of the Third International Consultation on Incontinence were considered.

Multioperated Recurrent Stress Urinary Incontinence

The available surgical options for recurrent SUI include Burch colposuspension, pubovaginal sling, tension-free vaginal tape (TVT), urethral bulking agents, placement of an artificial urinary sphincter (AUS), and as last resort bladder neck closure with continent catheterizable augmentation.

Burch Colposuspension

Burch colposuspension was the most popular surgical treatment for SUI for decades. However, the development of the integral theory of continence as well as the widespread use of the tension-free slòings, which are less invasive and are followed by a more favorable profile of complications, substantially have limited the current indications for colposuspension. A few papers specifically addressed the use of Burch colposuspension in the setting of recurrent SUI. Table 35.1 summarizes the main clinical data from the available studies on Burch colposuspension in recurrent SUI. In one of

TABLE 35.1. Surgical series using Burch colposuspension in patients with recurrent stress urinary incontinence.

Reference	Cases	Nr. previous anti-SUI procedures	Follow-up (months)	Cure rate (%)	Complication rate (%)
Enzelsberger [13]	36	NR	32–48	86	Postoperative LUTS 11 Postoperative POP 16
Cardozo [14]	52	1.2	9	80	Intraoperative (overall) 5.7 Postoperative LUTS 2
Maher [15]	53	2.1	9	89	Postoperative LUTS 10
Amaye-Obu [16]	26	1.5	NR	Subj. 88 Obj. 69	Postoperative LUTS 8
Bidmead [17]	32	NR	6–12	Obj. 81	Postoperative LUTS 6
Thakar [18]	56	1.2	48	Subj. 80 Obj. 71	Perioperative (overall) 49 Postoperative POP 20

NR, not reported *LUTS*, lower urinary tract symptoms *POP*, pelvic organ prolapse *Subj*,. subjective cure rate *Obj*, objective cure rate

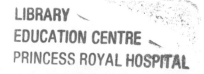

the largest series, Takar et al. analyzed the efficacy of the procedure in 56 patients who previously had undergone a mean of 1.2 surgical procedures for incontinence, mainly Burch colposuspension or anterior colporrhaphy. At a mean follow-up of 48 months, 80% of the patients were subjectively and 71% objectively cured. Stratifying the outcome by the available variables, there was no relationship between failure rate and maximum urethral closure pressure, maximum urethral closure pressure (MUCP) being higher than 20 cm H_2O in all the failed patients. Similarly, age, hysterectomy, parity, body mass index, number, and kind of previous incontinence procedures did not correlate with patients' outcomes. Twelve percent of the patients developed de novo detrusor overactivity but 20% needed further surgery for POP [18]. Similar success rates were provided by Cardozo et al. [14], Maher et al. [15], and Amaye-Obu et al. [16].

Further data come from a comparative study assessing the efficacy of Burch colposuspension and the dura mater pubovaginal sling [13]. Although the study was not randomized, the authors analyzed two small series of patients with similar preoperative characteristics, demonstrating similar success rates (86% for Burch colposuspension vs. 92% for sling) and similar perioperative complications. However, patients undergoing sling procedure had a significantly higher risk of storage (16% vs. 8%) and voiding (13% vs. 3%) symptoms but lower incidence of POP (3% vs. 13%) [13].

However, the limited follow-up of those studies did not allow us to draw a definitive conclusion on the long-term efficacy of Burch procedure, as well as on the related complications. The available literature on Burch colposuspension as primary treatment of SUI indeed clearly showed that cure rates decreased with time and that a percentage of patients as high as 75% can experience lower urinary tract symptoms [19]. Moreover, the patients analyzed in such old reports are quite different from those currently treated for recurrent SUI, due to the declining number of colposuspension performed as primary treatment since the widespread use of TVT.

Pubovaginal Sling

In 1995, De Lancey proposed the hammock hypothesis, suggesting that in the continent patient, the intra-abdominal pressure compresses the urethra against a stable, supporting layer and surgical techniques that reconstruct this supportive layer would effectively cure SUI [20]. Those concepts prompted many urogynecologists to recommend sling procedures to reestablish the hammock mechanism in all cases of SUI. These observations, together with the poor clinical results for patients with internal sphincter deficiency, led to the use of the sling as the most appropriate surgical technique for SUI. Its effectiveness is based on the correction of the hypermobility of the urethra or the coaptation of the mucosa near the bladder neck, promoting a sealing effect with no obstruction of the urethra in situations of increased abdominal pressure [21].

The traditional suburethral sling operation requires a combined abdominal and vaginal approach. Strips of material are tunneled under the urethra. They are attached either to the rectus muscle or the ileopectineal ligaments resulting in a tightening of the sling and increased bladder support every time the woman strains [22].

The materials that have been used for slings may be biological or synthetic. Autologous biological materials include rectus fascia, fascia lata, pubococcygeal muscle, vaginal wall, aponeurosis, and pyramidalis fascia. Exogenous biological materials include fascia and porcine dermis. Synthetic materials include Teflon, Mersilene, Lyodura, polytetrauoroethylene (Gore-Tex), Marlex, Silastic, and polypropylene [22]. Autologous rectus fascia and fascia lata were the most common materials in use until recently and were reported to be associated with high cure rate and low complications [23]. On the other hand, there are several advantages in the use of synthetic slings, such as the reduction in the morbidity of harvesting from a second surgical site, shortened operative time, early postoperative patient recovery, and an unlimited supply of artificial materials [23]. These issues have led to an increase in the number of sling procedures and the use of synthetic material. Although polypropylene meshes had been shown to have low incidence of complications, the use of prosthetic materials raises concerns about the potential occurrence of both sling erosions and infections.

Several papers addressed the use of both autologous and synthetic sling in patients with recurrent SUI. Tables 35.2 and 35.3 summarize the most important studies analyzing the use of autologous (Table 35.2) and synthetic (Table 35.3) sling in

TABLE 35.2. Surgical series using autologous sling in patients with recurrent stress urinary incontinence.

Reference	Material	Cases	Previous anti-SUI procedures	Follow-up (months)	Cure rate (%)	Complication rate (%)
Enzelsberger [13]	Dura mater	36	NR	32–48	92	Postoperative LUTS 29 Postoperative POP 3
Beck [24]	Fascia lata	170	NR	NR	98.2	NR
Breen [25]	Fascia lata	72	2.1	6–38	Subj. 90	UTI 17 CIC 30 Abscess 3
Kaplan [26]	Rectus sheath	43	1.6	23.4	95	Infection 14 CIC 12 LUTS 14
Kane [27]	Rectus sheath anchor sling	13	1.4	26	Subj. 100 Obj. 92	Postoperative LUTS 15
Petrou [28]	Rectus or fascia lata	14	NR	17	Subj. 86 Obj. 50	Abscess 7 Osteitis pubis 7
Juma [29]	Vaginal wall	65	NR	23.9	94	CIC 5.5 LUTS 14.8
Pidutti [30]	Vaginal wall	12	NR	17.3	92[a]	NR
Couillard [31]	Vaginal wall	18	NR	18	100	CIC 6
Kaplan [26]	Vaginal wall	36	1.3	23.4	97	CIC 3 Infection 3 LUTS 8
Raz [32]	Vaginal wall	160	2.8	17	93	Infections 3 Postoperative POP 1 LUTS 5
Litwiller [33]	Vaginal wall	33	1.1	31	74[a]	Hematoma 2 Postoperative POP 3 CIC 12 Dyspareunia 4 Chronic pelvic pain 2
Su [34]	Vaginal wall	23	1	15	Subj. 61 Obj. 35	Epithelial inclusion cysts 13

NR, not reported *LUTS*, lower urinary tract symptoms *POP*, pelvic organ prolapse *Subj.*. subjective cure rate *Obj.*. objective cure rate *CIC*, clean intermittent catheterization *UTI*, urinary tract infection
[a] Cured or improved

TABLE 35.3. Surgical series using prosthetic sling in patients with recurrent stress urinary incontinence.

Reference	Material	Cases	Previous anti-SUI procedures	Follow-up (months)	Cure rate (%)	Complication rate (%)
Morgan [35]	Marlex	281	NR	60	77.4	NR
Amaye-Obu [16]	Marlex	45	1.3	NR	Subj. 89 Obj. 69	CIC 2 Postoperative POP 4 Erosion 2
Morgan [36]	Polypropylene	88	1.6	49.7	85.2	UTI 5.7 CIC 3 Dyspareunia 3 Hematoma 3
Rutman [37]	Polypropylene	69[a]	1.4	60	Subj. 88	Postoperative LUTS 7
Rutman [38]	Polypropylene (spiral sling)	47	2.6	12	68[b]	Postoperative (overall) 1.9 Postoperative LUTS 7

NR, not reported, *LUTS*, lower urinary tract symptoms, *POP*, pelvic organ prolapse, *Subj.* subjective cure rate, *Obj.* objective cure rate, *CIC* clean intermittent catheterization, *UTI* urinary tract infection
[a] Only 52% with recurrent SUI
[b] Cured or improved

patients with recurrent SUI. There is a considerable volume of literature on autologous slings, mainly in the setting of primary anti-incontinence procedure, demonstrating high objective and subjective cure rates (about 85%) at long-term follow-up. However, although more recent studies reported lower figures, long-term voiding dysfunctions can occur in 30% of the patients. On the other hand, both rectus fascia and fascia lata were proved to be safe materials, with only a few cases of erosion being reported [39]. Pubovaginal slings are associated with higher morbidity and longer convalescence compared to other vaginal procedures.

Only a few papers were retrieved that assessed the role of rectus fascia and fascia lata in the setting of recurrent incontinence. Although previous surgery leads to significant scarring around the urethra, rendering tissue planes less recognizable and reoperation somewhat more difficult, those studies reconfirmed the high efficacy of pubovaginal sling procedures, with objective and subjective success rates ranging between 50 and 100%. Similarly, even complication rates, including long-term voiding dysfunction and need for clean intermittent self-catheterization (CISC) (15–30%) were within acceptable ranges (Table 35.3).

Interestingly, even patients who had failed a previous pubovaginal sling can be considered candidates for further similar procedures. Failure of a previous sling can be due to several reasons, including sling material failure, sling suture breakage, poor sling position, and inadequate urethral coaptation due to the sling [28]. However, in the words of Petrou and Frank, it might be difficult to "resist to the temptation to overtighten the sling secondary to the concern that the original sling was tight enough" [28].

Several published papers addressed the efficacy of vaginal wall slings in the setting of recurrent SUI. Compared to the traditional sling procedures, the advantages of the vaginal wall sling procedure were reported to be less tissue dissection, and consequently less neurovascular damage, and simpler surgical procedure with at least the same success rate. In addition, indigenous material is superior to allogenic material, with less infection, rejection, and urethral erosion. Success rates of this technique were reported to range from 74 to 100%.

In the attempt to reduce the morbidity of harvesting fascia, improving effectiveness, and decreasing complications, newer techniques have been described which use different materials. Among these the most popular currently is polypropylene, which has been proven to have long-term efficacy and safety.

Morgan et al., analyzing a series of 88 patients who had previously undergone 1.4 continence procedures, reported success rates as high as 85% at a follow-up of about 50 months [36]. Similar data were provided by Rutman et al. [37]. Interestingly, these studies reported favorable complication rates, with rates of postoperative lower urinary tract symptoms, needs for CISC, and urinary tract infections below 10% [36, 37].

An innovative approach to the surgery for recurrent SUI recently was reported by Rutman et al. [38]. The authors used a spiral polypropylene pubovaginal sling, placed at the level of the proximal urethra. A complete circle of mesh was created around the urethra, folding the sling spirally. The technique was employed as salvage therapy in those patients with multiple failed surgeries and an incompetent "lead pipe" urethra. The authors reported preliminary results on 47 patients who had previously undergone a mean of 2.6 incontinence procedures. At a mean follow-up of 12 months, 65% reported never having symptoms of SUI and 87% reported symptoms of SUI never or less than once weekly. On the UDI-6 questionnaire, 95% reported never or rarely being bothered by SUI. Moreover, the mean number of pads decreased from 6.0 before surgery to 0.9 postoperatively ($P < 0.005$). Those figures were paralleled by a quality of life score related to urinary symptoms, which was as low as 1.4, indicating that patients were between "pleased" and "mostly satisfied." These results, which are encouraging considering the baseline patient characteristics, were associated with low rates of postoperative complication (1.9%) and de novo urge incontinence (7.4%). Moreover, no patients needed CISC or experienced urethral or vaginal erosion [38].

Tension-Free Vaginal Tape

The advent of TVT was a major revolution in the management of SUI, because it offered patients a surgical procedure with reduced morbidity, a low complication rate, and high intermediate-term efficacy [40]. Following the initial encouraging reports of the use of the TVT as a primary treatment of SUI, a few groups attempted its use in patients who had failed previous anti-incontinence surgery. Table 35.4 summarizes the data from the main reports concerning the use of TVT in patients with recurrent SUI. The series with the largest follow-up was reported by Rezapour et al., who pioneered the development of the procedure [41]. The authors assessed 34 patients with recurrent SUI at a mean follow-up of 48 months, showing that 82% of the patients were cured (urinary leakage <10 g/24 h pad test; negative stress test; patients satisfaction >90% at the quality of life evaluation) and a further 9% significantly improved after surgery. Moreover, the authors reported a low complication rate (a single case of bladder perforation in a patient who had been operated on three times with the Marshal–Marchetti–Krantz procedure) and emphasized that there was no significant decline in the results along the follow-up [41].

Similar results were reproduced by other series with shorter follow-up duration [42–47]; the study by Abdel-Hady et al. was the largest one and included 118 cases [47]. The data clearly showed that TVT procedure can be safely and efficaciously performed in patients with recurrent SUI, even outside reference centers. Interestingly, even patients with urethral hypermobility and low Valsalva leak point pressure (VLLP) (<60 cm H_2O) had very high cure rate (86%) [47], while those with reduced urethra mobility (Q-tip test <30°) had unfavorable outcome (failure rate 50%) [46]. Consequently, these findings suggested that patients with recurrent SUI and concomitant urethral hypermobility can be best treated by TVT, in spite of concomitant intrinsic sphincter deficiency. No data are currently available on tension-free trans-obturator tapes in the setting of patients with recurrent SUI.

Bulking Agent Injection

Urethral mucosal coaptation, due to properties of the mucosa as well as to the presence of submucosal vascular cushions and the activity of smooth muscle cells, is considered an important component of the mechanism of urinary continence in women. Failure of this component can play a role in the development of stress incontinence [48]. The injection of bulking agents into the urethral submucosa is designed to create artificial urethral cushions that can improve urethral coaptation, and hence restore continence.

Due to the short length of the female urethra, the technique for administering periurethral bulking agents by injection for treatment of stress incontinence is simple, minimally invasive, and can be performed under local anesthesia, even on an outpatient basis. The agent is injected into the submucosa at two or more sites at the level of the proximal urethra under endoscopic control, which is considered mandatory to allow accurate placement of the substance into the submucosa layer and demonstrate adequate expansion.

Currently no ideal material to inject exists. A urethral bulking agent should be nonimmunogenic and biocompatible, leading to minimal inflammatory and fibrotic response. The particles that make

TABLE 35.4. Surgical series using TVT in patients with recurrent stress urinary incontinence.

Reference	Cases	Previous anti-SUI procedures	Follow-up (months)	Cure rate (%)	Improvement rate (%)	Complication rate (%)
Rezapour [41]	34	1.2	48	82	9	Perioperative (overall) 2.9
Riachi [42]	2	1.5	9.5	100	–	0
Lo [43]	41	1.3	16	82.9	4.8	Perioperative (overall) 9.8 Postoperative LUTS 4.9
Rardin [44]	88	1.3	9.5	85	4.5	Perioperative (overall) 4.5 Postoperative LUTS 5.5
Kuuva [45]	51	1.2	25.3	89.6	6.2	Bladder perforation 5.9 Postoperative LUTS 5.9 Urinary tract infection 5.9
Liapis [46]	33	1.2	20.5	70	6	Urinary retention 9 Urinary tract infection 6
Abdel-Hady [47]	118	NR	6	89	11	NR

NR not reported, *LUTS*, lower urinary tract symptoms

up the agent should be sufficiently large to prevent migration from the site of injection and sufficiently durable to maintain the clinical efficacy over time. The list of currently available agents includes autologous fat, polytetraruroethylene (Polytef™), glutaraldehyde cross-linked bovine collagen (Contigen™), Silicon particles (Macroplastique™), carbon beads (Durasphere™), calcium hydroxylapatite (Coaptite™), ethylene vinyl alcohol copolymer (Uryx™), and several other agents under investiga-

tion in phase II and III trials. The main limitation of the available bulking agents concerns the long-term efficacy, which in almost all the series is suboptimal, due to absorption or migration of the particles from the implant site, leading to the need for repetitions of the procedure.

Several papers have been published assessing the role of bulking agents in SUI (Table 35.5). The largest series, reported by Herschorn et al. in 1996, included 187 patients treated by the injection

TABLE 35.5. Surgical series of injectable bulking agents in patients with stress urinary incontinence.

Reference	Cases	Follow-up (months)	Cured (%)	Cured or improved (%)	Injection sessions
Glutaraldehyde cross-linked collagen					
Eckford [49]	25	3	64	80	1.7
Herschorn [50]	31	8.4	48	90	2
O'Connell [51]	44	NA	45	63	1.5
Monga [52]	29	24	48	68	1.6
Richardson [53]	42	46	40	83	2
Herschorn [54]	187	22	23	75	2.5
Faerber [55]	12	10	83	100	1.25
Kreder [56]	22	NA	40	NA	NA
Smith [57]	94	14	38	67	2.1
Haab [58]	22	7	24	86	1.9
Khullar [59]	21	7	48	57	NA
Cross [60]	139	18	NA	74	NA
Corcos [61]	40	48	30	70	NA
Groutz [62]	63	6.4	13	40	2.1
Winters [63]	58	2	48	79	1.9
Lightner [64]	68	12	NA	69	1.5
Bent [65]	58	12	33	66	NA
Autologous fat					
Santarosa [66]	12	18	NA	57	2.4
Trockman [67]	32	NA	NA	56	1.6
Su [68]	26	12	NA	65.4	1
Haab [58]	45	7	14	43	1.7
Lee [69]	27	3	NA	22	3
Teflon					
Politano [70]	51	6	NA	71	1.8
Lim [71]	28	12	21	75	1
Schulman [72]	56	3	NA	86	1–3
Deane [73]	28	3	NA	61	NA
Osther [74]	26	NA	NA	50	NA
Lockhart [75]	20	NA	NA	90	1.8
Vesey [76]	36	NA	NA	67	1–2
Kiikholma [77]	22	60	NA	18	
Lopez [78]	128	31	54	73	1.5
Herschorn [79]	46	17.9	30.4	71.7	2
Silicone					
Koelbl [80]	32	12	60	NA	1
Barranger [81]	21	31	19	48	NA
Peeker [82]	15	24	68	87	1.3
Tamanini [83]	21	12	57	76	1.4

NA, not available

of glutaraldehyde cross-linked bovine collagen (Contigen™). At a median follow-up of 22 months, only 23% turned out to be cured, although about 50% of them had subjectively improved [54]. Although several series reported significantly higher success rates, the overall methodological quality of the available pieces of evidence was weak, due to study design, short follow-up, inaccurate outcome definitions, and so on [39]. In this context, injection of a bulking agent can be considered a possible option for patients with recurrent SUI mainly because of the limited morbidity, but patients should be informed of the limited long-term efficacy.

Artificial Urinary Sphincter

The last chance to achieve urinary continence maintaining physiological voiding habits is the placement of an AUS, the AMS-800 being the most widespread device. The standard approach to the insertion of the AUS in a female patient requires a suprapubic incision into the preperitoneal space. Once the space of Retzius is developed, the bladder neck is dissected and measured. A fitted cuff is placed around the bladder neck and the pump placed into a pocket created in the labia majora. The reservoir is placed in the standard preperitoneal space behind the rectus abdominis (see Fig. 35.1). Another approach uses a transvaginal incision. The bladder neck can be dissected from

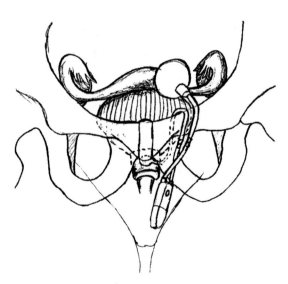

FIG. 35.1. Implanted artificial urinary sphincter in female patients

the anterior vaginal vault and the urethra is circumferentially freed and appropriately sized. Strict antisepsis with copious antibacterial irrigation also should be used during the procedure. By dissecting into the labia through the same vaginal incision the cuff and pump are easily placed but a small infraumbilical incision may be required to place the reservoir [84].Although the overall experience with AUS is far greater in male patients, several series of implanted female patients have been published (Table 35.6). However, in most cases, the patients had incontinence due to different causes, often including neurogenic dysfunction, without any stratification of the data.

As shown in Table 35.6, the reported continence rates were quite high, ranging from 52 to 100%. Although in some series complications were virtually absent, revision rates due to erosions, infections, or mechanical failure were shown to be quite high in most of the experiences. Even in the most recent publications, revision rates ranged from 25 to 50%. In one of the series with a longer follow-up, Petero et al. reported data on 55 patients where 80 AMS-800 had been implanted. Satisfactory continence was achieved in 84% of the patients, with 64% wearing no pad and 7% a single one. Revisions were needed, in fact, in 35% of the patients and 9% required sphincter explantation. The overall median duration of the device was 11.2 ± 1.19 years [98].

When other kinds of incontinence surgery have failed, placement of AUS can be regarded as a very effective procedure in selected cases. The overall cure rates are acceptable, although the risk of complications and need for reoperation increases with follow-up durations and patients should be clearly informed.

Recommendations for Assessment and Treatment of Recurrent Stress Urinary Incontinence

Assessment of the patients with recurrent incontinence has to be as accurate as possible, always including evaluation of quality of life impairment, comprehensive urodynamics, with pressure-flow studies, urethral profilometry, and whenever feasible, videourodynamics to visualize the bladder cycle under fluoroscopy. Although not extensively studied, translabial or introital ultrasound scans are emerging

TABLE 35.6. Surgical series of artificial urinary sphincter in female patients.

Reference	Cases	Cure rate (%)	Complication rate (%)	Revision rate (%)
Scott [85]	139	Socially continent 91 Dry 66	Infection 3 Erosion 4	NR
Light et al. [86]	39	92	Infection 2.5 Erosion 7	54
Donovan [87]	31	68	Erosion 29	32
Diokno [88]	32	91	Dehiscence 3 Pelvic abscess 3	21.8
Abbassian [89]	4	100	0	NR
Appell [90]	34	100	0	8.9
Duncan [91]	29	52	Infection 3.5 Erosion 28	3.5
Webster [92]	25	92	Postoperative death 4 Infection/erosion 0	16
Costa [93]	54	93	Infection 2 Erosion 6	NR
Hadley [94]	18	89	Erosion 11	NR
Stone [95]	54	84	Erosion 6	20
Thomas [96]	18	82	Erosion/infection 28	50
Ngninkeu [97]	4	Socially continent 100 Dry 75	Erosion 0	25
Petero [98]	55	84	Erosion 12	44

NR, not reported

as reliable techniques to evaluate bladder neck position and mobility, as well as the morphology of rhabdosphincter and pelvic floor muscle activity.

Due to the lack of well-performed, randomized, controlled studies the recommendations for treatments of the patients with recurrent SUI have to be based on low-quality evidence only, often an expert's opinion only. The choice among the available surgical options has to be founded on the expectations, wishes, comorbidity and life expectancy of the patients, severity of the stress incontinence, quality of life impairment, kind and number of the previously failed anti-incontinence procedures, and, whenever possible, pathophysiology of the stress recurrent incontinence.In case of patients with mild incontinence, low impact on quality of life, and/or limited life expectancy or significant comorbidity, the most suitable surgical option is likely the injection of a bulking agent, which provides acceptable short-term efficacy but very low perioperative and long-term complication rates. When urethral hypermobility is thought to play a major role in recurrent incontinence, tension-free midurethral slings, such as TVT, can allow quite high success rates with an acceptable risk of inter-

mediate-term complications, even in patients with clues of sphincter deficiency. However, data of the literature do not allow drawing definitive conclusions on the efficacy of a further TVT procedure after failure of previous tension-free midurethral slings and prospective studies are strongly recommended in the field.

Pubovaginal slings are very effective anti-incontinence procedures in the setting of recurrent incontinence, also in patients with intrinsic sphincter deficiency. However, the risk of postoperative lower urinary tract symptoms needing clean intermittent self-catheterization is high and the patients should be clearly aware of such potentially frustrating conditions before surgery.

For the patients who had failed all the above-mentioned surgical solution, AUS is the only chance to preserve micturition and regaining urinary continence. Indeed, the long-term risk of complications needing reoperation can be as high as 50%. Consequently, the patient candidates for placement of an AUS have to be highly motivated, with sufficient mental and manual skill to allow adequate use of the device, ideally with limited comorbidity and, due to the costs, good life expectancy.

G. Novara and W. Artibani

Bladder neck closure with continent catheterizable augmentation has to be considered as the
last resort for the patients who have failed all the
options allowing preservation of the micturition,
including artificial sphincter or unwilling or unfit
for sphincter implantation.

Multioperated Recurrent Prolapse

In case of POP recurrence, repeated prolapse repair,
with or without mesh graft can be performed. In
selected cases, however, colpectomy and colpocleisis can provide a definitive solution to prolapse. As
stated, the available evidence is largely insufficient,
due to the lack of randomized, controlled trials in
patients with recurrent POPs.

Mesh Graft

The ideal prosthetic material should be biocompatible, inert, have minimal allergic or inflammatory
reaction, be sterile, noncarcinogenic, resistant to
infection, and should avoid shrinkage and mechanical stress while being easy to handle and readily
available at a reasonable cost [99]. As to the physical properties of the prosthesis, Amid suggested
a classification based mainly on the porosity and
filament type. Type 1 meshes (Atrium, Marlex,
Prolene and Trelex) have pore size >75 nm, which
allows the infiltration by macrophages, fibroblasts,
collagen fibers, and angiogenesis, reducing the risk
of infection, extrusion, or erosion of the prosthetic
material. Moreover, materials with large pores
have lower stiffness, reducing tissue trauma and
erosive risk. Type II meshes (Gore-Tex), indeed,
are microporous, with pore size is <10 nm, which
presents a barrier to new tissue formation. Type III
meshes (Teflon, Mersilene, SurgiPro) are macroporous materials with multifilamentous or microporous components, while type IV grafts (Silastic,
Cellgard) had submicronic pores [100].

With regard to the mesh in anterior vaginal wall
prolapse repair, Julian and colleagues published an
interesting randomized, controlled trial (RCT) in
which the use of Marlex mesh was assessed in a
cohort of 24 patients with recurrent anterior vaginal
wall prolapse [101]. The authors demonstrated significantly better outcomes in patients where mesh
grafts were used (recurrence rate 0% vs. 34%),

but mesh erosion occurred in 25% of the patients,
requiring surgical excision [101]. Further trials were
subsequently published, mainly in the setting of primary prolapse repair. In 2001, Sand et al. reported
significantly higher objective success rates in the
anterior vaginal wall repair with the use of Vicryl
mesh (75% vs. 57%), without any mesh-related
complication [102]. A nice RCT recently was
published by Gandhi et al., assessing the efficacy
of a patch of cadaveric fascia lata in an adequately
powered cohort of patients with recurrent anterior
vaginal wall prolapse [103]. At a median follow-
up of 13 months, the authors showed similar rates
of prolapse recurrence (21% in the patch group
and 29% in the control group), failing to show any
statistically significant benefit for biological graft
in anterior vaginal repair [103]. However, the short
follow-up time and the lack of reliable data regarding reoperation and complication rates limited the
quality of the evidence. A few large retrospective
surgical series, in fact, reported very high cure rates
(75–100%) associated with acceptable low incidence of infections, erosion, fistula formation, and
other mesh-related complications (0–16%) [104],
supporting the use of synthetic type I mesh graft in
the setting of recurrent cystocele repair.

As with anterior vaginal wall defects, the use
of mesh in the treatment of vaginal vault prolapse
is not adequately established. A landmark RCT
recently was published by Culligan et al., who
compared cadaveric fascia lata and polypropylene mesh in a cohort of 100 patients undergoing
abdominal colposacropexy for posthysterectomy
vaginal vault prolapse. At a median follow-up of 12
months, the authors demonstrated higher success
rates in the mesh arm (91% vs. 68%) [105]. Data
on mesh-related complications were not provided
in the report, but a large review on abdominal colposacropexy reported only 70 cases of mesh erosion out of 2178 procedures (3.4%). In that review,
specifically, cadaveric fascia and Prolene mesh
were followed by very low rates of erosion (0 and
0.5%, respectively) [106]. Those figures, as well
as the failure rates in the surgical series employing
fascia in sacrocolpopexy, might support the use of
polypropylene mesh graft in this setting.

In the context of recurrent posterior vaginal wall
prolapse, the available evidence, based on two
RCT[102, 107], discourages the use of homologous,
autologous, or synthetic meshes in posterior repair.

Obliterative Procedures

This kind of operation is indicated in the case of recurrent or high-stage POP, when operating time has to be kept to the minimum and patients no longer wish to preserve coital function. A total colpocleisis usually refers to the removal of the majority of the vaginal epithelium from within the hymenal ring posteriorly and to within 0.5–2.0 cm of the external urethral meatus anteriorly (Fig. 35.2). In partial colpocleisis, some portion of the vaginal epithelium is left in place, providing drainage tracts for cervical or other upper genital discharge using the technique of LeFort or modifications of LeFort (Fig. 35.3) [108].Several surgical series have been published. Table 35.7 summarizes the data from the contemporary series of partial and total colpocleisis. As shown in Table 35.7, prolapse recurrence rates after colpocleisis are very low, below 10%, and complication rates are quite favorable. However, in some series certain major

complications, such as vesical injury, ureteral occlusion, and sepsis, have been reported.

Conclusions

Recurrent SUI and POP are clinical conditions that represent a considerable challenge for both patients and physicians. The patients require a complete preoperative assessment. Urinary tract imaging always should be performed, including ultrasonography, voiding cystourethrography, or, ideally, MRI, which was proven to have significant accuracy in the assessment of both pelvic organs and the pelvic floor structures. In the meantime, urodynamics or, better, videourodynamics should be performed in each case, aimed at assessing

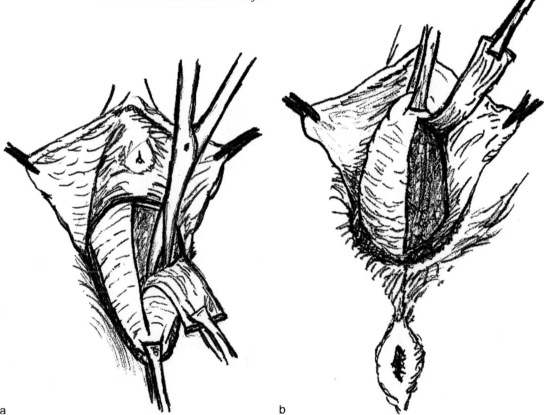

a   b

FIG. 35.2. Schematic representation of total colpectomy. (**a, b**) The vagina is circumscribed by an incision at the site of the hymen and marked into quadrants, which is removed by sharp dissection. (**c**) Purse string sutures are placed. (**d**) The sutures are tied. (**e**) A perineorrhaphy may complete the operation

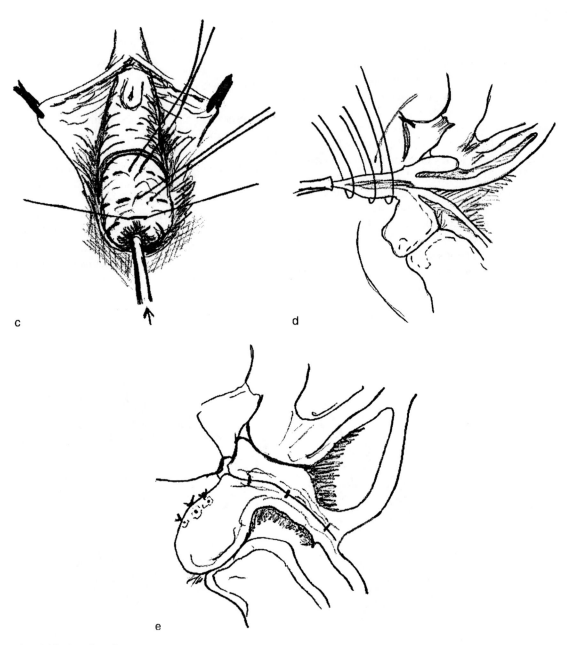

Fig. 35.2. (continued)

the presence of detrusor overactivity, intrinsic sphincter deficiency, and all the characteristics of the voiding pattern, as well as the impact of prolapse on the lower urinary tract function.Several surgical options are currently available for the treatment of recurrent stress incontinence, pubovaginal sling, TVTs, and bulking agents being the most frequently used approaches. Despite the limited availability of randomized controlled trials and even nonrandomized controlled studies to provide an evidence-based approach for this type of patient, the published data clearly suggest that those procedures can be safely and efficaciously used, although TVTs and bulking agents are by far less invasive than the other procedures. The roles of AUS and, as a last resort, bladder neck closure

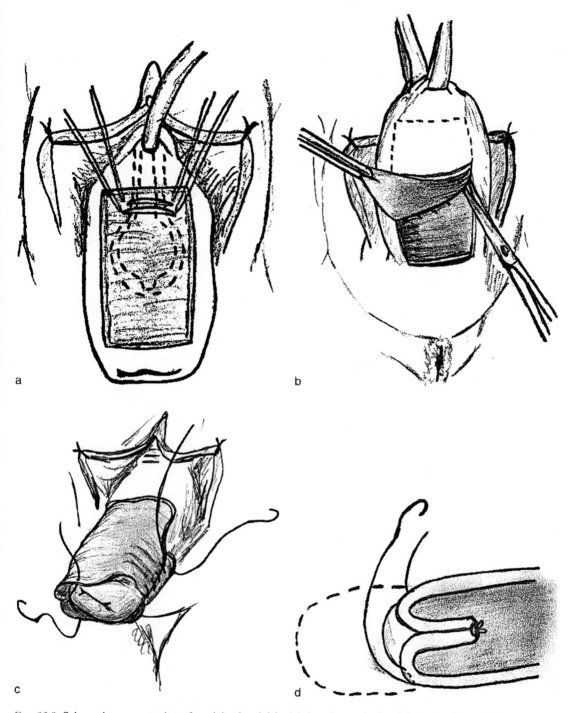

FIG. 35.3. Schematic representation of partial colpocleisis. (**a**) Anterior vaginal wall is removed and plication stitches are placed at the bladder neck. (**b**) Posterior vaginal wall is removed. (**c, d**) Edges of anterior and posterior vaginal walls are sewn to invert uterus and vagina

TABLE 35.7. Contemporary series of colpocleisis.

Reference	Cases	Follow-up (months)	Cure rate (%)	Complication rates (%)
Langmade [109]	102	12–144	100	Sepsis 1
Denehy [110]	20	4–40	95	UTI 15
DeLancey [111]	33	35	97	UTI 6
Cespedes [112]	38	24	100	0
Harmanli [113]	41	28.7	100	Vesical injury 2 Late rectal bleeding 10
Von Pechmann [114]	62	12	97	Transfusion 22 Ureteral occlusion 4
Moore [115]	30	19	90	0
Fitzgerald [116]	64	2–56	97	Vaginal hematomata 3 One postoperative death due to multisystem organ failure (1.5)
Glavind [117]	42	46	90	0

NA, not available, *UTI*, urinary tract infections

and continent catheterizable augmentation are limited to those patients who have failed all the other options and who have significant quality of life impairment due to urinary problems.

The data available on recurrent POP are even more limited. Further repair with mesh augmentation is the most common option, with partial or total colpocleisis limited to frail patients not wishing to preserve coital function.

References

1. Beck RP, McCormick S, Nordstrom L. A 25-year experience with 519 anterior colporrhaphy procedures. Obstet Gynecol 1991; 78(6):1011–1018.
2. Hunskaar S, Burgio K, Ckark A, et al. Epidemiology of urinary (UI) and faecal incontinence. In: Abrams P, Cardozo L, Khoury S, Wein A, eds. Incontinence, 3rd International Consultation on Incontinence. Plymouth: Health Publication 2005:255–312.
3. Olsen AL, Smith VJ, Bergstrom JO, et al. Epidemiology of surgically managed pelvic organ prolapse and urinary incontinence. Obstet Gynecol 1997; 89:501–506.
4. Boyles SH, Weber AM, Meyn L. Procedures for pelvic organ prolapse in the United States, 1979–1997. Am J Obstet Gynecol 2003; 188:108–115.
5. Boyles SH, Weber AM, Meyn L. Procedures for urinary incontinence in the United States, 1979–1997. Am J Obstet Gynecol 2003; 189:70–75.
6. DeLancey JOL. The hidden epidemic of pelvic floor dysfunction: Achievable goals for improved prevention and treatment. Am J Obstet Gynecol 2005; 192:1488–1495.
7. Hunskaar S, Bugio K, Clark A, et al. Epidemiology of urinary and faecal incontinence and pelvic organ prolapse. In: Abrams P, Cardozo L, Khoury S, Wein A, eds. Incontinence. Plymouth: Health Publication 2005:255–312.
8. Kenton K, Mahajan S, FitzGerald MP, et al. Recurrent stress incontinence is associated with decreased neuromuscular function in the striated urethral sphincter. Am J Obstet Gynecol 2006; 194:1434–1437.
9. Ball J, Teichman J, Sharkey F, et al. Terminal distribution to the urethra and bladder neck: Considerations in the management of stress urinary incontinence. J Urol 1997; 158:827–829.
10. Borirakchanyavat S, Aboseif S, Carroll P, et al. Continence mechanisms of the isolated female urethra: An anatomical study of the intrapelvic somatic nerves. J Urol 1997; 158:822–826.
11. Benson J, McClellan E. The effect of vaginal dissection on the pudendal nerve. Obstet Gynecol 1993; 82:387–389.
12. Zivkovic F, Tamussino K, Ralph G, et al. Long-term effects of vaginal dissection on the innervation of the striated urethral sphincter. Obstet Gynecol 1996; 87:257–260.
13. Enzelsberger H, Helmer H, Schatten C. Comparison of Burch and Lyodura sling procedures for repair of unsuccessful incontinence surgery. Obstet Gynecol 1996; 88:251–256.
14. Cardozo L, Hextall A, Bailey J, et al. Colposuspension after previous failed incontinence surgery: A prospective observational study. BJOG 1999; 106:340–344.
15. Maher C, Dwyer P, Carey P, et al. The Burch colposuspension for recurrent urinary stress incontinence following retropubic continence surgery. BJOG 1999; 106:719–724.

16. Amaye-Obu FA, Drutz HP. Surgical management of recurrent stress urinary incontinence: A 12-year experience. Am J Obstet Gynecol 1999; 181: 1296–1309.

17. Bidmead J, Cardozo L, McLellan A, et al. A comparison of the objective and subjective outcomes of colposuspension for stress incontinence in women. BJOG 2001; 108:408–413.

18. Thakar R, Stanton S, Prodigalidad L, et al. Secondary colposuspension: Results of a prospective study from a tertiary referral centre. BJOG 2002; 109:1115–1120.

19. Kjølhede P. Long-term efficacy of Burch colposuspension: A 14-year follow-up study. Acta Obstet Gynecol Scand 2005; 84:767–772.

20. De Lancey JOL. Structural support of the urethra as it relates to stress urinary incontinence: The hummock hypothesis. Am J Obstet Gynecol 1994; 170:1713–1714.

21. Rodrigues P, Hering F, Meler A, et al. Pubo-fascial versus vaginal sling operation for the treatment of stress urinary incontinence: A prospective study. Neurourol Urod 2004; 23:627–631.

22. Bezerra CA, Bruschini H, Cody DJ. Traditional suburethral sling operations for urinary incontinence in women. Cochrane Database Syst Rev 2005, Issue 3:CD001754.

23. Bhargava S, Chapple CR. Rising awareness of the complications of synthetic slings. Curr Opin Urol 2004; 14:317–321.

24. Beck RP, McCormick S, Nordstrom L. The fascia lata sling procedure for treating recurrent genuine stress incontinence of urine. Obstet Gynecol 1988; 72(5):699–703.

25. Breen JM, Geer BE, May GE. The fascia lata suburethral sling urinary stress incontinence for treating recurrent urinary stress incontinence. Am J Obstet Gynecol 1997; 177:1363–1366.

26. Kaplan SA, Santarosa RP, Te AE. Comparison of fascial and vaginal wall slings in the management of intrinsic sphincter deficiency. Urology 1996; 47:885–889.

27. Kane L, Chung T, Latrie H, et al. The pubofascial anchor sling procedure for recurrent genuine urinary stress incontinence. BJU Int 1999; 83:1010–1014.

28. Petrou SP, Frank I. Complications and initial continence rates after a repeat pubovaginal sling procedure for recurrent stress urinary incontinence. J Urol 2001; 165:1979–1981.

29. Juma S, Little NA, Raz S. Vaginal wall sling: Four years later. Urology 1992; 39(5):424–428.

30. Pidutti RW, Gorge SW, Morales A. Correction of recurrent stress urinary incontinence by needle urethropexy with a vaginal wall sling. BJU 1994; 73(4):418–422.

31. Couillard DR, Deckard-Janatpour KA, Stone AR. The vaginal wall sling: A compressive suspension procedure for recurrent incontinence in elderly patients. Urology 1994; 43(2):203–208.

32. Traz S, Stothers L, Young GP, et al. Vaginal wall sling for anatomical incontinence and intrinsic sphincter dysfunction: Efficacy and outcome analysis. J Urol 1996; 156(1):166–170.

33. Litwiller SE, Nelson RE, Fone PD, et al. Vaginal wall sling: Long-term outcome analysis of factors contributing to patient satisfaction and surgical success. J Urol 1997; 157(4):1279–1282.

34. Su TH, Huang JP, Wang YL, et al. Is modified in situ vaginal wall sling operation the treatment of choice for recurrent genuine stress incontinence? J Urol 1999; 162:2073–2077.

35. Morgan JE, Farrow GA, Stewart FE. The Marlex sling operation for the treatment of recurrent stress urinary incontinence: A 16-year review. Am J Obstet Gynecol 1985; 151(2):224–226.

36. Morgan JE, Heritz DM, Stewart FE, et al. The polypropylene pubovaginal sling for the treatment of recurrent stress urinary incontinence. J Urol 1995; 154(3):1013–1014.

37. Rutman MP, Itano N, Deng D, et al. Long-term durability of the distal urethral polypropylene sling procedure for stress urinary incontinence: Minimum 5-year follow-up of surgical outcome and satisfaction determined by patient reported questionnaires. J Urol 2006; 175:610–613.

38. Rutman MP, Deng DY, Shah SM, et al. Spiral sling salvage anti-incontinence surgery in female patients with a nonfunctional urethra: technique and initial results. J Urol 2006; 175:1794–1799.

39. Smith ARB, Daneshgari F, Dmochowski R, et al. Surgery for urinary incontinence in women. In: Abrams P, Cardozo L, Khoury S, Wein A, eds. Incontinence. Plymouth: Health Publication 2005:1297–1370.

40. Cody J, Wyness L, Wallace S, et al. Systematic review of the clinical effectiveness and cost-effectiveness of tension-free vaginal tape for treatment of urinary stress incontinence. Health Tech Assess 2003; 7(21).

41. Rezapour M, Ulmsten U. Tension-free vaginal tape (TVT) in women with recurrent stress urinary incontinence – a long-term follow up. Int Urogynecol J 2001; (Suppl 2):S9–11.

42. Riachi L, Kohli N, Miklos J. Repeat tension-free transvaginal tape (TVT) sling for the treatment of recurrent stress urinary incontinence. Int Urogynecol J (2002); 13:133–135.

43. Lo TS, Horng SG, Chang CL, et al. Tension-free vaginal tape procedure after previous failure in incontinence surgery. Urology 2002; 60:57–61.

44. Rardin CR, Kohli N, Rosenblatt PL, et al. Tension-free vaginal tape: outcomes among women with primary versus recurrent stress urinary incontinence. Obstet Gynecol 2002; 100:893–897.

45. Kuuva N, Nilsson CG. Tension-free vaginal tape procedure: an effective minimally invasive operation for the treatment of recurrent stress urinary incontinence? Gynecol Obstet Invest 2003; 56:93–98.

46. Liapis A, Bakas P, Lazaris D, et al. Tension-free vaginal tape in the management of recurrent stress incontinence. Arch Gynecol Obstet 2004; 269:205–207.

47. Abdel-Hady E, Constantine G. Outcome of the use of tension-free vaginal tape in women with mixed urinary incontinence, previous failed surgery, or low Valsala pressure. J Obstet Gynecol Res 2005; 31(1):38–42.

48. Pickard R, Reaper J, Wyness L, et al. Periurethral injection therapy for urinary incontinence in women. Cochrane Database Syst Rev 2003; Issue 2:CD003881.

49. Eckford SD, Abrams P. Para-urethral collagen implantation for female stress incontinence. Br J Urol 1991; 68(6):586–589.

50. Herschorn S, Radomski SB, Steele DJ. Early experience with intraurethral collagen injections for urinary incontinence. J Urol 1992; 148(6):17971800.

51. O'Connell HE, McGuire EJ, Aboseif S, et al. Transurethral collagen therapy in women. J Urol 1995; 154(4):1463–1465.

52. Monga AK, Robinson D, Stanton SL. Periurethral collagen injections for genuine stress incontinence: A 2-year follow-up. Br J Urol 1995; 76(2):156–160.

53. Richardson TD, Kennelly MJ, Faerber GJ. Endoscopic injection of glutaraldehyde cross-linked collagen for the treatment of intrinsic sphincter deficiency in women. Urology 1995; 46(3):378–381.

54. Herschorn S, Steele DJ, Radomski SB. Follow-up of intraurethral collagen for female stress urinary incontinence. J Urol 1996; 156(4):1305–1309.

55. Faerber GJ. Endoscopic collagen injection therapy in elderly women with type I stress urinary incontinence. J Urol 1996; 155(2):512–514.

56. Kreder KJ, Austin JC. Treatment of stress urinary incontinence in women with urethral hypermobility and intrinsic sphincter deficiency. J Urol 1996; 156(6):1995–1998.

57. Smith DN, Appell RA, Winters JC, et al. Collagen injection therapy for female intrinsic sphincteric deficiency. J Urol 1997; 157(4):1275–1278.

58. Haab F, Zimmern PE, Leach GE. Urinary stress incontinence due to intrinsic sphincteric deficiency: Experience with fat and collagen periurethral injections. J Urol 1997; 157(4):1283–1286.

59. Khullar V, Cardozo LD, Abbott D, et al. GAX collagen in the treatment of urinary incontinence in elderly women: A two year follow up. Br J Obstet Gynaecol 1997; 104(1):96–99.

60. Cross CA, English SF, Cespedes RD, et al. A followup on transurethral collagen injection therapy for urinary incontinence. J Urol 1998; 159(1):106–108.

61. Corcos J, Fournier C. Periurethral collagen injection for the treatment of female stress urinary incontinence: 4-year follow-up results. Urology 1999; 54(5):815–818.

62. Groutz A, Blaivas JG, Kesler SS, et al. Outcome results of transurethral collagen injection for female stress incontinence: Assessment by urinary incontinence score. J Urol 2000; 164(6):2006–2009.

63. Winters JC, Chiverton A, Scarpero HM, et al. Collagen injection therapy in elderly women: Long-term results and patient satisfaction. Urology 2000; 55(6):856–861.

64. Lightner D, Calvosa C, Andersen R, et al. A new injectable bulking agent for treatment of stress urinary incontinence: Results of a multicenter, randomized, controlled, double-blind study of Durasphere. Urology 2001; 58(1):12–15.

65. Bent AE, Tutrone RT, McLennan MT, et al. Treatment of intrinsic sphincter deficiency using autologous ear chondrocytes as a bulking agent. Neurourol Urodyn 2001; 20(2):157–165.

66. Santarosa RP, Blaivas JG. Periurethral injection of autologous fat for the treatment of sphincteric incontinence. J Urol 1994; 151(3):607–611.

67. Trockman BA, Leach GE. Surgical treatment of intrinsic urethral dysfunction: Injectables (fat). Urol Clin North Am 1995; 22(3):665–671.

68. Su TH, Wang KG, Hsu CY, et al. Periurethral fat injection in the treatment of recurrent genuine stress incontinence. J Urol 1998; 159(2):411–414.

69. Lee PE, Kung RC, Drutz HP. Periurethral autologous fat injection as treatment for female stress urinary incontinence: A randomized double-blind controlled trial. J Urol 2001; 165(1):153–158.

70. Politano VA. Periurethral polytetrafluoroethylene injection for urinary incontinence. J Urol 1982; 127(3):439–442.

71. Lim KB, Ball AJ, Feneley RC. Periurethral Teflon injection: A simple treatment for urinary incontinence. Br J Urol 1983; 55(2):208–210.

72. Schulman CC, Simon J, Wespes E, et al. Endoscopic injection of Teflon for female urinary incontinence. Eur Urol 1983; 9(4):246–247.

73. Deane AM, English P, Hehir M, et al. Teflon injection in stress incontinence. Br J Urol 1985; 57(1):78–80.

74. Osther PJ, Rohl H. Female urinary stress incontinence treated with Teflon injections. Acta Obstet Gynecol Scand 1987; 66(4):333–335.

75. Lockhart JL, Walker RD, Vorstman B, et al. Periurethral polytetrafluoroethylene injection following urethral reconstruction in female patients with urinary incontinence. J Urol 1988; 140(1):51–52.

76. Vesey SG, Rivett A, O'Boyle PJ. Teflon injection in female stress incontinence. Effect on urethral pressure profile and flow rate. Br J Urol 1988; 62(1):39–41.

77. Kiilholma P, Makinen J. Disappointing effect of endoscopic Teflon injection for female stress incontinence. Eur Urol 1991; 20(3):197–199.

78. Lopez AE, Padron OF, Patsias G, et al. Transurethral polytetrafluoroethylene injection in female patients with urinary continence. J Urol 1993; 150(3): 856–858.

79. Herschorn S, Glazer AA. Early experience with small volume periurethral polytetrafluoroethylene for female stress urinary incontinence. J Urol 2000; 163(6):1838–1842.

80. Koelbl H, Saz V, Doerfler D, et al. Transurethral injection of silicone microimplants for intrinsic urethral sphincter deficiency. Obstet Gynecol 1998; 92(3):332–336.

81. Barranger E, Fritel X, Kadoch O, et al. Results of transurethral injection of silicone micro-implants for females with intrinsic sphincter deficiency. J Urol 2000; 164(5):1619–1622.

82. Peeker R, Edlund C, Wennberg AL, et al. The treatment of sphincter incontinence with periurethral silicone implants (macroplastique). Scand J Urol Nephrol 2002; 36(3):194–198.

83. Tamanini JT, D'Ancona CA, Tadini V, et al. Macroplastique implantation system for the treatment of female stress urinary incontinence. J Urol 2003; 169(6):2229–2233.

84. Kowalczyk JJ, Mulcahy JJ. Use of the artificial urinary sphincter in women. Int Urogynecol J 2000; 11:176–179.

85. Scott FB. The use of the artificial sphincter in the treatment of urinary incontinence in the female patient. Urol Clin N Am 1985; 12:305–315.

86. Light JK, Scott FB. Management of urinary incontinence in women with the artificial urinary sphincter. J Urol 1985; 134:476–478.

87. Donovan MG, Barrett DM, Furlow WL. Use of the artificial urinary sphincter in the management of severe incontinence in females. Surg Gynecol Obstet 1985; 161:17–20.

88. Diokno AC, Hollander JB, Alderson TP. Artificial urinary sphincter for recurrent female urinary incontinence: Indications and results. J Urol 1987; 138:778–780.

89. Abbassian A. A new operation for insertion of the artificial urinary sphincter. J Urol 1988; 140: 512–513.

90. Appell RA. Techniques and results in the implantation of the artificial urinary sphincter in women with type III stress urinary incontinence by a vaginal approach. Neurourol Urodyn 1988; 7:613–618.

91. Duncan HJ, Nurse DE, Mundy AR. Role of the artificial urinary sphincter in the treatment of stress incontinence in women. Br J Urol 1992; 69:141–143.

92. Webster GD, Perez LM, Khoury JM, et al. Management of type III stress urinary incontinence using artificial urinary sphincter. Urology 1992; 39:499–503.

93. Costa P, Mottet N, Le Pellec L, et al. Artificial urinary sphincter AMS 800 in operated and unoperated women with type III incontinence. J Urol 1994; 151 (part 2):477A, abstract 1000.

94. Hadley R, Loisides P, Dickinson M. Long-term follow-up (2–5 years) of transvaginally placed artificial urinary sphincters by an experienced surgeon. J Urol 1995; 153(part 2):432A, abstract 816.

95. Stone KT, Diokno AC, Mitchell BA. Just how effective is the AMS 800 artificial urinary sphincter? Results of long-term follow-up in females. J Urol 1995; 153(part 2):433A, abstract 817.

96. Thomas K, Venn SN, Mundy AR. Outcome of the artificial urinary sphincter in female patients. J Urol 2002; 167:1720–1722.

97. Ngninkeu BN, van Heugen G, di Gregorio M, et al. Laparoscopic artificial urinary sphincter in women for type III incontinence: Preliminary results. Eur Urol 2005; 47:793–797.

98. Petero VG, Diokno AC. Comparison of the long-term outcomes between incontinent men and women treated with artificial urinary sphincter. J Urol 2006; 175:605–609.

99. Birch C. The use of prosthetics in pelvic reconstructive Surgery. Best Pract Res Clin Obstet Gynaecol 2005; 19(6):979–991.

100. Amid PK. Classification of biomaterials and their related complication in abdominal wall surgery. Hernia 1997; 1:15–21.

101. Julian TM. The efficacy of Marlex mesh in the repair of severe, recurrent vaginal prolapse of the anterior midvaginal wall. Am J Obstet Gynecol 1996; 175:1472–1475.

102. Sand PK, Koduri S, Lobel RW, et al. Prospective randomized trial of polyglactin 910 mesh to prevent recurrence of cystoceles and rectoceles. Am J Obstet Gynecol 2001; 184(7):1357–1364.

103. Gandhi S, Goldberg RP, Kwon C, et al. A prospective randomized trial using solvent dehydrated fascia lata for the prevention of recurrent anterior vaginal wall prolapse. Am J Obstet Gynecol 2005; 192(5):1649–1654.

104. Brubaker L, Bump R, Fynes M, et al. Surgery for pelvic organ prolapse. In: Abrams P, Cardozo L, Khoury S, Wein A, eds. Incontinence, 3rd International Consultation on Incontinence. Plymouth: Health Publication, 2005:1371–1402.

105. Culligan PJ, Blackwell L, Goldsmith LJ, et al. A randomized controlled trial comparing fascia lata and synthetic mesh for sacral colpopexy. Obstet Gynecol 2005; 106(1):29–37.

106. Nygaard IE, McCreery R, Brubaker L, et al. Abdominal sacrocolpopexy: A comprehensive review. Obstet Gynecol 2004; 104:805–823.

107. Gandhi S, Kwon C, Goldberg R, et al. Does fascia lata graft decrease recurrent posterior vaginal wall prolapse (abstract 86). Int Urogynecol J Pelvic Floor Dysfunct 2003; 14 (Suppl 1):S26.

108. FitzGerald MP, Richter HE, Siddique S, et al. Colpocleisis: A review. Int Urogynecol J Pelvic Floor Dysfunct. 2006; 17(3):261–271.

109. Langmade CF, Oliver JA. Partial colpocleisis. Am J Obstet Gynecol 1986; 154:1200–1205.

110. Denehy TR, Choe JY, Gregori CA, et al. Modified LeFort partial colpocleisis with Kelly urethral plication and posterior colpoperineoplasty in the medically compromised elderly: A comparison with vaginal hysterectomy, anterior colporrhaphy, and posterior colpoperineoplasty. Am J Obstet Gynecol 1995; 173:1697–1701.

111. DeLancey JO, Morley GW. Total colpocleisis for vaginal eversion. Am J Obstet Gynecol 1997; 176:1228–1232.

112. Cespedes RD, Winters JC, Ferguson KH. Colpocleisis for the treatment of vaginal vault prolapse. Tech Urol 2001; 7(2):152–160.

113. Harmanli OH, Dandolu V, Chatwani AJ, et al. Total colpocleisis for severe pelvic organ prolapse. J Reprod Med 2003; 48(9):703–706.

114. von Pechmann WS, Mutone M, Fyffe J, et al. Total colpocleisis with high levator plication for the treatment of advanced pelvic organ prolapse. Am J Obstet Gynecol 2003; 189(1):121–126.

115. Moore RD, Miklos JR. Colpocleisis and tension-free vaginal tape sling for severe uterine and vaginal prolapse and stress urinary incontinence under local anesthesia. J Am Assoc Gynecol Laparosc 2003; 10(2):276–280.

116. FitzGerald MP, Brubaker L. Colpocleisis and urinary incontinence. Am J Obstet Gynecol 2003; 189(5):1241–1244.

117. Glavind K, Kempf L. Colpectomy or Le Fort colpocleisis – a good option in selected elderly patients. Int Urogynecol J Pelvic Floor Dysfunct 2005; 16(1):48–51.

Chapter 36
Voiding Dysfunction after Female Anti-Incontinence Surgery

Priya Padmanabhan and Victor W. Nitti

Introduction

Stress urinary incontinence (SUI) affects a large population of adult women. Not surprisingly, over 200 surgical procedures have been described for its treatment. Procedures to treat SUI have evolved which probably cause less voiding dysfunction. An increase in the number of procedures preformed probably has made up for this possible reduction in incidence. When lower urinary tract symptoms (LUTS) replace stress incontinence, patients may be more distressed than at initial presentation. This leaves the clinician with a challenging task of deciding on the timing and type of anti-incontinence procedure to use in the treatment of a patient's troublesome LUTS. The most important factor in preventing obstruction is the understanding that surgical treatment of SUI works by restoring support to the urethrovesical junction and/or improving coaptation of the urethra in intrinsic sphincter dysfunction (ISD), not by changing the position of the urethra. Obstruction often goes undiagnosed. With the recent widespread use of synthetic midurethral slings such as the tension-free vaginal tape (TVT) and transobturator tape (TOT), expedient diagnosis and treatment of bladder outlet obstruction (BOO) is advantageous. This chapter covers the incidence and etiology of postsurgical obstruction, the diagnostic evaluation, management options, and outcomes of surgical interventions.

Incidence of Obstruction after SUI Surgery

The true incidence of iatrogenic obstruction and voiding dysfunction after incontinence surgery is unknown. Variability in reported rates may be due to a variety of factors, such as underdiagnosis and loss to follow-up. Obstruction may go undiagnosed if it is not severe enough to cause urinary retention. For example, an obstructed patient may experience detrusor overactivity with normal emptying. Also, some patients will seek second opinions regarding their surgical outcome. This leaves most series on obstruction after incontinence surgery lacking in the total number of patients undergoing surgery from which the obstructed patients were derived [1]. In 1997, the American Urological Association SUI Clinical Guideline Panel conducted a meta-analysis of surgical procedures for the treatment of SUI. They showed that the reported incidence of urinary retention for more than 4 weeks postoperatively was 3–7% (median CI 5%) for retropubic suspension, 4–8% (median CI 5%) for transvaginal suspensions, and 6–11% (CI 8%) for sling procedures. The incidence of permanent retention was not known, but the panel's opinion was that it was less than 5% for all procedures [2]. Morgan et al. reported on a large pubovaginal sling series with a de novo urgency rate of 23% and de novo urge urinary incontinence (UUI) rate of 5%. There was a 74% resolution of UUI (concomitant anterior colporrhaphy may have contributed, $P = 0.07$) and 92% returned to normal voiding one month postoperatively [3].

Dunn et al. performed an extensive literature review to determine the incidence of "voiding dysfunction" after incontinence procedures performed from 1966 to 2001. All available information were retrospective collections, case reports, or case cohort series. Rates of voiding dysfunction varied from 4 to 22% following Burch colposuspension, 5–20% following Marshall–Marchetti–Krantz (MMK) urethropexy, 4–10% following pubovaginal sling, 5–7% after needle suspension, and 2–4% following TVT. It is inferred that a large number of patients with voiding dysfunction in these series were obstructed [4].

The introduction of new techniques such as the midurethral synthetic slings (done by a retropubic or transobturator approach) has reduced the incidence of postoperative obstruction, but it still remains an issue. Reported rates of urinary retention after TVT have ranged from 1.4 to 9% [55, 6, 7, 8, 9, 10, 11] and 2–4% in other studies [12]. Delorme et al. created the TOT to avoid known vascular, bowel, and bladder complication. They reported on 1-year results, noting that 3% of patients developed obstructive voiding disorders. Only one patient in this group had persistent obstructive symptoms [13]. Two series evaluated the results after treatment with a TOT for SUI. Costa et al. reported 4% of their patients to have postoperative voiding disorders, with five of seven patients recovering normal micturition by 1-year follow-up. De novo UUI was observed in only 5% of their patients with the symptoms of urgency and UUI disappearing in 56.3 and 48.3% of patients, respectively [14]. Deval et al. performed a longitudinal study on 129 consecutive women and assessed voiding function at 1, 6, and 12 months postoperatively. Only 1.5% of women developed urinary retention, but 5.4% had voiding difficulties (residual volume >150 ml) requiring clean intermittent catheterization (CIC) for 4.2 ± 2 days. Postoperative urinary tract infections and de novo urgency were diagnosed in 5.4 and 9.3% of patients, respectively, and 34.2% of the 70 women with preoperative urge symptoms had persistent urgency postoperatively [15].

Etiology

Surgical procedures for the correction of SUI are designed to provide urethrovesical junction support and/or improve urethral coaptation in the cases of ISD. Retropubic cystourethropexy and colposuspension, transvaginal bladder neck suspension, and sling procedures all have been utilized to achieve this. Midurethral synthetic slings by both the retropubic and transobturator approaches appear to work by causing a dynamic kinking of the urethra with stress, and thus can be effective without stopping hypermobility [16, 17, 18, 19]. The voiding dysfunction that develops from iatrogenic outlet obstruction is related to obstruction, detrusor overactivity, or impaired detrusor contractility. The risk of iatrogenic obstruction usually relates to technical factors, ie, placement and tension of sutures or sling material. In a retropubic urethropexy, sutures placed too medially (close to the urethra) can cause urethral deviation or periurethral scarring. Sutures placed too distally may cause kinking with obstruction and an inadequately supported bladder neck/proximal urethra with potentially continued SUI. If retropubic sutures are tied too tightly, excessively elevating the bladder neck toward the pubic bone, "hypersuspension" or overcorrection of the urethrovesical angle may occur. However, in most cases, hypersuspension is not evident on physical examination. In placement of a bladder neck, suburethral, or midurethral sling, it is excessive tension on the sling under or around the bladder neck or urethra that is responsible for obstruction. Excessive tension on a midurethral synthetic sling can result in rolling of the sling into a tight band.

Additional factors affecting a patient's ability to empty after anti-incontinence surgery include preoperative voiding dysfunction and prolapse that was either uncorrected at time of surgery or occurred postoperatively. Prolapse of sufficient size may kink or angulate and externally compress the urethra. It is very important to examine and rule out apical, anterior, and posterior prolapse as an etiology of urethral obstruction. Impaired detrusor contractility, a condition that is present preoperatively, may manifest symptomatically with even a "relative obstruction" when urethral resistance is increased by an anti-incontinence surgery. These should be warned of the possibility of postoperative voiding dysfunction. Learned voiding dysfunction (dysfunctional voiding) or failure of relaxation of the striated urethral sphincter may affect emptying after surgery [20]. A patient who habitually voids by abdominal straining may have difficulty emptying after incontinence surgery. Patient education and biofeedback can be helpful, but when the problem persists, botulinum A toxin injection into the urethral sphincter has been successful [21].

Presentation

The most obvious symptom of obstruction is complete/partial urinary retention or inability to void continuously or slow stream with or without intermittency. Instead, some women will present with predominate storage symptoms, ie, frequency, urgency, and urge incontinence, with or without voiding symptoms. The prevalence of various symptoms varies tremendously among authors. Some report on cohorts with only obstructive symptoms or retention, while others have shown the true variability of voiding dysfunction secondary to obstruction. Carr and Webster reviewed the presenting symptoms of 51 women who underwent urethrolysis [22]. They observed the following symptoms/signs: storage (irritative) symptoms (75%), voiding (obstructive) symptoms (61%), de novo urgency (55%), need for CIC (40%), persistent retention (24%), recurrent urinary tract infections (UTIs) (8%), and painful voiding (8%). Obviously storage and voiding symptoms and retention can coexist in any combination. Therefore, in evaluating a patient who presents with de novo voiding and/or storage symptoms and recurrent UTIs, obstruction must be entertained. In our experience, early presentations of obstruction, ie, within the first 3 months after surgery, tends be more weighted toward retention and obstructive voiding symptoms.

Risk Factors for Postoperative Voiding Dysfunction

In counseling patients preoperatively, it would be useful to know which patients are at risk for postoperative voiding dysfunction. As expected, this question does not have a definite answer. Urodynamic studies have investigated multiple factors to determine which may be predictive. Miller et al. noted that women undergoing an allograft pubovaginal sling who voided with no or minimal detrusor pressure (19%) had a significantly increased risk of postoperative retention. In contrast, no patient with a detrusor contraction developed retention postoperatively. Valsalva voiding did not affect the incidence of postoperative retention [23]. Weinberger and Ostergard studied 108 women undergoing synthetic suburethral slings and found that the absence of detrusor contractions predicted delayed returns to normal voiding. Valsalva voiding had no association with voiding dysfunction [24]. Bhatia and Bergman noted that women who void with Valsalva maneuver (intra-abdominal pressure greater than 10 cm H_2O during voiding and a detrusor pressure less than 15 cm) were at a 12 times greater risk of needing prolonged catheterization in a series of Burch cystourethropexies [25]. Others showed that patients reporting preoperative Valsalva voiding or detrusor hypocontractility are more likely to report de novo urgency [26]. Wang and Chen found that patients with preoperative dysfunctional voiding [maximum free flow (NIQmax) less than 12 ml s^{-1} and detrusor pressure at maximum flow (Pdet@Qmax) of greater than or equal to 20 cm H_2O] were more likely to have a lower objective cure rate and lower quality of life scores after TVT than those with normal pressure–flow voiding dynamics [27]. More recently, Kawashima et al. evaluated the preoperative urodynamic findings predicting postoperative voiding difficulties in 14 women after a TVT [28]. Although there was a paucity of data, they noted that a peak detrusor pressure (Pdetmax) × average flow rate (Qavg) was a good marker for potential detrusor contractility, and a low Pdetmax × Qavg predicted significantly increased postvoid residual after the TVT. No patients voided without a detrusor contraction preoperatively [28]. The association of low voiding detrusor pressures and Valsalva voiding with subsequent voiding dysfunction has not been seen in several other studies [29, 30]. While urodynamic studies are useful in evaluating voiding dynamics of incontinent women, low detrusor pressures or Valsalva voiding preoperatively should not per se exclude patients from anti-incontinence procedures.

To date, data are lacking on risk factors for voiding dysfunction when an anti-incontinence procedure is performed with surgery for pelvic organ prolapse. Sokol et al. noted that among 267 women (66% having concurrent prolapse repair), there was no significant difference in median days to voiding and rate of urinary retention based on prolapse repair status. Yet, increasing age, decreasing body mass index (BMI), and postoperative UTI were independent predictors of time to adequate voiding. Only previous history of incontinence surgery was an independent predictor of urinary retention [31].

Diagnostic Evaluation

Transient voiding dysfunction and urinary retention are frequent and expected after any type of anti-incontinence surgery. This is the rationale behind concomitant placement of suprapubic tubes or teaching CIC preoperatively. After traditional pubovaginal sling (and variants) or colposuspension, most women will begin voiding sufficiently within a few days to weeks, while others may take longer to resume normal voiding. Storage symptoms, such as urgency, frequency, and urge incontinence often are more refractory than retention because they can be related to bladder changes and may take months to resolve. Traditionally, evaluation of urinary retention or severe storage symptoms after pubovaginal sling, colposuspension, and needle suspension has been delayed for up to 3 months depending on symptoms and their degree of bother. This time frame is arbitrary, and has been predicated on the fact that most data in the literature are based on a waiting period of 3 months to ensure adequate time for obstruction to resolve. After 3 months, there is a low probability that persistent retention will resolve without intervention. Recently, some surgeons, including ourselves, have advocated earlier intervention in cases of complete retention and severe symptoms; however, few data on outcomes and recurrence of stress incontinence are available. Few studies have focused on outcomes with respect to waiting a longer period of time before intervention. While it seems intuitive that longer-standing symptoms (especially detrusor overactivity) will be less likely to respond to relief of obstruction, this has not been proven conclusively. Leng et al. conducted a retrospective review of 15 women who underwent urethrolysis and found that patients with persistent symptoms postoperatively (53%) had a significantly longer time for surgery to intervention than those who had no symptoms (47%) [32]. Mean time to urethrolysis was 31.25 ± 21.94 months versus 9 ± 10.1 months, respectively. However, the large overlap, small sample size, and the fact that more patients in the successful group had urinary retention (5/7 vs. 3/8) makes it difficult to make definitive conclusions. In our practice, we do not exclude obstructed patients from intervention based on the duration of their obstruction.

The waiting period advocated for obstruction and retention for more traditional anti-incontinence procedures has been largely abandoned for TVT and other midurethral synthetic slings. In these cases, quicker intervention is suggested when obstruction is suspected [5, 7, 33, 34]. Due to the immobility of the polypropylene mesh and the tremendous ingrowth of fibroelastic tissue at 1–2 weeks, patients with severe symptoms or urinary retention are less likely to improve after this time period.

History and Physical Examination

A focused history and physical exam is the first step in diagnostic evaluation of a patient with voiding dysfunction after incontinence surgery. Key points in the history include patient's preoperative voiding status and symptoms and the temporal relationship of the LUTS to the surgery. The type of anti-incontinence procedure performed and the number and type of other procedures done also are important. Urodynamic data, such as uroflow and pressure flow studies from before incontinence surgery, are useful if available. If patients are straining to void (perhaps by habit), they should be instructed to discontinue this behavior, since incontinence procedures are designed to prevent the flow of urine with abdominal straining. Finally, it is important to determine whether the symptoms of SUI persist.

The most obvious presenting symptom of obstruction after incontinence surgery is inability to void or intermittent/partial urinary retention. Patients also may experience voiding (obstructive) symptoms including slow or interrupted stream and straining to void. Storage (irritative) symptoms of urinary frequency, urgency, and urge incontinence which persist after surgery also may be a sign of obstruction even if emptying is complete.

Physical examination may show overcorrection or hypersuspension where the urethra and urethral meatus appear to be pulled up toward the pubic bone and "fixed," making the angle of the urethra more vertical than normal. When severe, this usually is quite obvious, but can be confirmed by a Q-tip test. Not all obstructed patients appear to be overcorrected. It is important to assess for cystocele and other forms of prolapse, which may cause obstruction (due to a kinking of the urethra). The patient also should be examined for persistent urethral hypermobility and SUI.

Urodynamics

Recent interest in female BOO has resulted in publication of several unique proposals of urodynamic criteria for the diagnosis of female BOO. Chassagne et al. used the cutoff values of Pdet@Qmax of more than 20 cm H_2O and maximum flow rate (Qmax) of less than 15 ml s^{-1} to define obstruction [35]. In 2000, Lemack and Zimmern revised these values to a cutoff of Qmax of 11 ml s^{-1} or less and Pdet@Qmax of 21 cm H_2O or more [36]. The same group made another update with criteria published in 2004, using a small group of controls, elevating the Pdet@Qmax cutoff to 25 cm H_2O [37]. We have used videourodynamic criteria to diagnose BOO. Obstruction is defined as radiographic evidence of an obstruction between the bladder neck and distal urethra in the presence of a sustained detrusor contraction of any magnitude during voiding, with less emphasis on strict pressure–flow criteria [38]. Blaivas and Groutz realized the possibility of test-induced catheter obstruction and designed a nomogram based on the Qmax and the Pdet@Qmax [39]. Although each urodynamic definition has merit, further investigation should provide clarity of when to use which criteria [40].

The diagnosis of obstruction in women after incontinence surgery can be particularly difficult to make urodynamically. In cases of urinary retention and incomplete emptying, urodynamic studies may not be necessary before intervention, particularly if preoperative contractility and emptying are known to be normal. However, in cases of de novo or worsened storage symptoms,

including urge incontinence without a significantly elevated postvoid residual urine volume (PVR), a formal urodynamic evaluation is preferred. Many women with suspected obstruction after incontinence surgery do not generate a significant contraction on UDS but are still obstructed. Outcomes of surgical intervention in such cases are identical to those women with classic high-pressure, low-flow dynamics.

There are no consistent preoperative or urodynamic parameters that predict success or failure of urethrolysis. Foster and McGuire found that patients with detrusor overactivity had a higher rate of failure, but later studies found this not to be the case [41]. Nitti and Raz found that as the postvoid residual increased, so did the failure; but others have not confirmed this correlation [42]. Carr and Webster found that the only parameter predictive of success was no prior urethrolysis [22]. In the study by Nitti and Raz, four women who failed to generate a contraction during UDS testing had a successful urethrolysis. They also reported that UDS findings in patients considered failures after transvaginal urethrolysis failed to elucidate the reason for their continued voiding dysfunction [42]. Due to the limitation of UDS in evaluation of these patients, the temporal relationship of surgery to the onset of symptoms is relied on as an indicator of obstruction. If a patient fails to resume voiding or improve significantly, then continued obstruction is suspected.

Classic high-pressure, low-flow voiding dynamics do confirm the diagnosis of obstruction, but are far from a consistent finding. Urodynamics do yield important information regarding instability, impaired compliance, bladder capacity, and voiding characteristics. Based on our experience, videourodynamics offer an advantage over simple urodynamics in this patient population, because of the ability to simultaneously image the bladder outlet. It must be emphasized that the best selection criteria for intervention for suspected postincontinence surgery obstruction is a temporal relationship between surgery and onset of voiding symptoms. The utility of urodynamics in the postincontinence surgery female patient may be considered as follows: (1) For the patient in retention, UDS can provide valuable information (eg, detrusor overactivity or significantly impaired compliance, the latter being an absolute indication for intervention) and can confirm diagnosis of obstruction but should not exclude the patient from urethrolysis, even with impaired contractility or lack of a detrusor contraction. (2) For the patient with storage symptoms with normal emptying, urodynamics can diagnose obstruction and equally as importantly rule out obstruction. It can help to provide a specific diagnosis that is useful in directing therapy, especially if obstruction cannot be ruled out.

Cystourethroscopy and Imaging

Cystoscopic evaluation of the urethra may show scarring, narrowing, occlusion, kinking, or deviation of the urethra. These findings are especially helpful when UDS are equivocal. The urethra and bladder should be carefully inspected for eroded sutures or sling material and the presence of a fistula. This is facilitated by a rigid scope with a 0–30° lens and little or no beak to allow for complete distention of the urethra. In case intervention is anticipated, cystoscopy should be performed either before surgery or prior to incision. Radiographic imaging may be done independently of UDS. A standing cystogram in the anterior–posterior, oblique, and lateral positions, with and without straining, can assess the degree of bladder and urethral prolapse and displacement or distortion of the bladder. A voiding cystourethrogram can assess the bladder, bladder neck, and urethra during voiding to determine narrowing, kinking, or deviation. While not mandatory, imaging can be extremely useful in equivocal cases.

Management of Iatrogenic Obstruction

Conservative Treatment

Treatment of obstruction and its timing usually are dictated by the degree of bother of symptoms. In some cases an obstructed patient opts for conservative management, including CIC. This is a reasonable option for women not bothered by catheterization or who prefer this option to repeat surgery and risk of recurrent SUI. Most women eventually choose definitive treatment, but chronic CIC is an option in select cases. Patients who are emptying well but have significant storage symptoms from iatrogenic obstruction may be initially treated with pharmacotherapy, ie, anticholinergics, or pelvic floor physiotherapy. In our experience, these measures are not usually successful when obstruction exists, but can be considered before surgery. The role of urethral dilation in iatrogenic obstruction secondary to pubovaginal sling and colposuspension is unclear. Karram et al. did report an 82% cure or improved rate with urethral dilation using a Walther sound performed within 2–6 weeks of TVT insertion for 28 patients with varying amounts of postoperative voiding dysfunction [33]. Two additional groups highlighted the role of urethral dilation in management antiincontinence obstruction. Paick et al. studied 247 women with a minimum of 6 months follow-up after TVT placement [43]. They performed urethral dilation (once or twice) with downward push in the immediate postoperative period and noted resolution of voiding dysfunction in 85% (23 of 27 patients; 14 with retention, 12 with poor urinary flow, and 2 with dysuria). Mishra et al. performed urethral dilation on 3 of 52 cases who had retention 3 months following TVT. Two of the three patients voided effectively after urethral dilation [44]. In this series, the postoperative retention rate is significantly higher (23%) than published data. In all three studies, the use of urethral dilation was uncontrolled and ideally a randomized trial is necessary to prove its efficacy. While many practitioners report anecdotal success, no randomized trials exist in peer-reviewed literature. It is our opinion that urethral dilation is of limited utility and if used too aggressively, it may be detrimental. There are concerns about the potentially traumatic nature of dilation, which could induce scarring of the urethra.

When conservative measures in a symptomatic patient fail, definitive surgical therapy by either formal urethrolysis (transvaginal or retropubic) or sling incision may be required. In addition, there is growing experience with manipulation of midurethral synthetic slings in the early postoperative period.

Surgical Intervention

When voiding dysfunction secondary to obstruction exists beyond a proper waiting period (refer to

Diagnostic Evaluation section), surgical intervention is indicated. The success rate for various procedures ranges from 67 to 100% (see Table 36.1) and is independent of the particular procedure chosen. One procedure is not superior to another, excluding independent factors, ie, surgeon experience; however, some procedures are potentially less morbid with quicker recovery. There have not been any consistent predictors for success identified. Individual series have cited certain factors that are associated with success or failure, but different series have not identified the same factors. For example, Carr and Webster found that the only predictors of success were no prior urethrolysis and omental interposition [22]. Nitti and Raz found that the postvoid residual increased as did the risk of failure [42]. Foster and McGuire noted that patients with detrusor overactivity had a higher rate of failure [41]. This was not confirmed in a later study [45]. Several studies failed to show correlation between urodynamic findings and the likelihood of successful voiding after urethrolysis [41, 42, 46]. Furthermore, outcomes of urethrolysis of women with demonstrable detrusor contraction on UDS (with normal void prior to incontinence surgery) are equivalent to women with classic findings of obstruction.

With all surgical interventions for obstruction, there is an inherent risk of recurrent stress incontinence. In general, the risk is approximately 15%, but reported rates vary from 0 to 39% (see Table 36.1). Segal et al. compared the efficacy of retropubic urethrolysis (10/44 with retropubic urethropexy, laparoscopic bone anchor urethropexy, bladder neck needle suspension, pubovaginal sling), vaginal urethrolysis (20/44 with retropubic urethropexy, bone anchor sling, protegen sling, pubovaginal sling, and Stamey needle suspension), and sling incision (14/44 with TVT) in treating postoperative voiding dysfunction of 44 women after anti-incontinence surgery and reported the SUI recurrence rates of each [47]. All patients were at least 6 weeks post anti-incontinence surgery. Of all the risk factors evaluated for recurrent SUI after urethrolysis, only postmenopausal status and previous hysterectomy were significant. They showed a trend based on type of surgical procedure chosen. SUI was 4.3 times more likely after a TVT takedown, while it was almost 75% less likely after a retropubic urethrolysis. Either the sign of

SUI on simple cystometry or UDS diagnosis was found postoperatively in 63.6% of sling incision, 46.7% of vaginal urethrolysis patients, and 25% of retropubic urethrolysis patients [47]. Starkman et al. conducted a retrospective review of 19 patients to evaluate persistent voiding dysfunction and recurrent SUI after surgical excision of an eroded synthetic midurethral sling at mean of 10.1 months postoperative [48]. This represents a special population with the added complication of erosion or extrusion. Sling excision was accomplished by a vaginal, retropubic, or combined surgical approach. They reported complete cure in only 21 and 42% with recurrent SUI. Five of the patients underwent simultaneous pubovaginal sling, none of whom had recurrent SUI. The worst outcomes noted in this study are most likely due to the intense inflammatory reaction associated with mesh erosion. Residual irritative symptoms (frequency, urgency, UUI) may be an issue for many patients following surgical intervention for obstruction. Goldman et al. suggested that postincision residual irritative symptoms are related to a longer interval between initial surgery and takedown [49].

While some have recommended concomitant anti-incontinence procedures at the same time as the procedure to relieve obstruction [42], others have argued that this is not necessary. Currently we do not routinely perform a repeat anti-incontinence procedure. We believe that in the majority of cases, patients are so disturbed by the symptoms caused by obstruction that relieving them must be the primary goal. If SUI does recur, it can be treated separately with a urethral bulking agent or even a repeat surgical procedure in the future.

Surgical techniques usually are tailored toward individual scenarios and previous surgeries. For example, in certain cases where the incontinence procedure causing obstruction was a retropubic suspension, a retropubic urethrolysis approach may be used to cut sutures and free retropubic adhesions. For transvaginal sling procedures, transvaginal sling lysis alone or formal urethrolysis usually can be performed successfully with less patient morbidity and quicker convalescence. A transvaginal suprameatal approach also may be done; however, we rarely use this. With more common use of the TVT or synthetic midurethral slings, sling-loosening techniques and incision alone may be performed in the clinic setting with

TABLE 36.1. Summary of series on urethrolysis and sling incision/loosening for the treatment of obstruction after incontinence surgery.

Reference	No	Type of urethrolysis	Success[a]	Recurrent SUI[b] (%)
Zimmern et al. [61]	13	Transvaginal	92%	N/A
Foster and McGuire [41]	48	Transvaginal	53%	0
Nitti and Raz [42]	42	Transvaginal	71%	0
Cross et al. [45]	39	Transvaginal	72%	3
Goldman et al. [59]	32	Transvaginal	84%	19
Carey et al. [58]	23	Transvaginal with Martius flap	87%	16
Petrou et al. [53]	32	Suprameatal	67%	3
Webster and Kreder [41]	15	Retropubic	93%	13
Petrou and Young [60]	12	Retropubic	83%	25
Carr and Webster [22]	54	Mixed	78%	14
Amundsen et al. [53]	32	Transvaginal and sling incision	94% retention 67% urge sx	9
Nitti et al. [54]	19	Sling incision	84%	17
Goldman [49]	14	Sling incision	93%	21
Klutke et al. [5]	17	TVT incision or loosening	100%	6
Rardin et al. [7]	23	TVT incision	100% retention 30% urge sx cured 70% urge sx improved	39 (2/3 less SUI than pre-TVT)
Segal et al. [47]	44	Retropubic (10) and vaginal urethrolysis (20), sling incision (14)	32% urge sx cured 73% obstructive sxcured	25–63.6
Long et al. [50]	7	Lateral TVT incision	86%	14
Thiel et al. [55]	13	Sling incision	92%	8

[a]Success is usually defined as cure or significant improvement in presenting symptoms (resumption of normal bladder emptying for patients in retention, and resolution symptoms for patients with obstructive symptoms or frequency, urgency or urge incontinence). In some series success for specific sx (symptoms) is noted
[b]Recurrent SUI is defined as percentage of patients without SUI before urethrolysis who experienced SUI after urethrolysis

local anesthesia in the early postoperative period, prior to the occurrence of significant scarring. The decision of which procedure to perform is based on multiple factors, including the incontinence procedure performed, associated complications, surgeon comfort, and patient preferences.

Midurethral Sling Loosening or Incision

In women with postoperative urinary retention after midurethral synthetic sling, some surgeons, including ourselves, advocate early intervention, within 7–14 days. With midurethral synthetic slings, the vast majority of patients are able to empty fairly normally within 72 h. Early intervention allows one to perform a minimally invasive procedure under local anesthesia in the office or outpatient setting if appropriate. The anterior vaginal wall is infiltrated with local anesthetic and the suture used to close the

vaginal wall is opened. The synthetic sling is easily visualized and hooked with a right-angle clamp (or Metzenbaum scissors dilator). Spreading of the right-angle clamp or downward traction on the tape usually will loosen it 1–2 cm [5]. This usually is possible if intervention is done within 10 days of sling placement. Thereafter, tissue ingrowth may prevent loosening of the sling, in which case, we recommend cutting it in the midline. The incision then is closed and the patient then may attempt to void.

Loosening or cutting of TVT has had excellent results [5, 7, 33, 34, 50]. In the two largest series of 17 and 23 patients [5, 7], there was restoration of normal voiding and emptying in all patients postincision, while storage symptoms were partially relieved in 70% and completely relieved in 30%. Klutke et al. reported resolution of obstruction in all 17 patients, while recurrent SUI occurred in one patient [5]. Rardin and associates found that impaired bladder emptying resolved in 100% of 23 patients with 61% remaining continent, 26% with partial recurrence, and 13% with complete recurrence of SUI [7].

In cases of voiding difficulty or dysfunction beyond 4–6 weeks, the lysis of the TVT sling is better performed in the operating room because of tissue ingrowth. Scarring and patient discomfort are factors to consider, as more extensive dissection may be needed to identify and cut the sling. The technique described below for sling incision is applicable to midurethral slings.

Transvaginal Sling Incision

The transvaginal incision of the pubovaginal sling (autologous, allograft, xenograft, or synthetic) rather than formal urethrolysis may limit morbidity, potential soft tissue and nerve injury, and fibrosis from surgical dissection. Notably, sling incision alone may effectively eliminate obstruction with similar results to formal urethrolysis. In 1995, Ghoniem described a technique of incising the sling in the midline using a free vaginal epithelial interposition graft sutured to each cut end of the pubovaginal sling, theoretically keeping it intact to theoretically reduce the risk of postoperative stress incontinence [51]. Over time, this technique has evolved and interposition no longer is routinely used [49, 52, 53, 54].

Our technique starts with cystoscopy to assess the urethra and rule out erosion or urethral injury. An inverted U or midline incision is made to expose the area of the bladder neck and proximal urethra [54]. As the vaginal flap is dissected off, the sling should be identified above the periurethral fascia. The sling may be encased in scar tissue, and thus require careful dissection of the scar to identify the sling. If the sling has significant tension on it, it may be especially difficult to identify. Insertion of a cystoscope or sound into the urethra with upward deflection may help to expose the bladder neck and isolate the sling. Once the sling is isolated, it should be separated from the underlying periurethral fascia with sharp or blunt dissection. This dissection is facilitated by grasping the sling with an Allis clamp on either side of the midline and exerting downward pressure. Care should be taken to avoid injury to the bladder and urethra by beginning dissection distally, identifying normal urethra, then proceeding more proximally until the plane between the sling and urethra is identified. A right-angle clamp can be placed between the urethra, periurethral fascia, and the sling, enabling lifting of the sling. The sling then is cut in the midline (Fig. 36.1a). Alternatively, if scarring is dense and the plane between the sling and periurethral fascia cannot be developed, the sling can be isolated laterally to the midline, off of the urethra. The edges of the sling are mobilized off of the periurethral fascia to (not through) the endopelvic fascia (Fig. 36.1b). In cases of extreme tension, the ends of the sling may retract back into the retropubic space after incision, but more often the sling stays secure to allow this mobilization. Lateral support is preserved because the retropubic space is not entered and the urethra is not freed from the under surface of the pubic bone. The ends of the sling can be left in situ or excised. We typically excise synthetic material and leave autograph and allograft in place. If there is any concern about urethral injury, cystourethroscopy should be done. In cases of autologous or biological materials, when the sling cannot be clearly identified, formal transvaginal urethrolysis should be done (see below).

TVT and other midurethral slings can be isolated and incised in a similar manner. Unlike autologous and biological slings, it is imperative to identify the sling and cut it. Conversion to urethrolysis without specifically cutting the sling may fail to relieve obstruction. Usually the sling is easily found, but identification can be aided by palpation of the sling or using a sound or cystoscope in the urethra with upward deflection as described above. Sometimes, identification can be difficult especially in cases where the sling rolls onto itself and creates a tight narrow band. In such cases, patience and careful dissection to isolate the sling is required. Sometimes it is necessary to retract the portion of the urethra distal to the sling distally and the portion of the urethra proximal to the sling proximally to find the tight narrow band. In many cases, after the midurethral sling is cut, it retracts away from the urethra. At the surgeon's discretion, segmental resection of the suburethral portion of the sling may be done. Our experience with sling incision has shown results equivalent to formal urethrolysis. The success of the procedure has been reported, ranging from 84 to 93.5% with 8–21% recurrent SUI rate [49, 53, 54, 55]. If the sling incision is

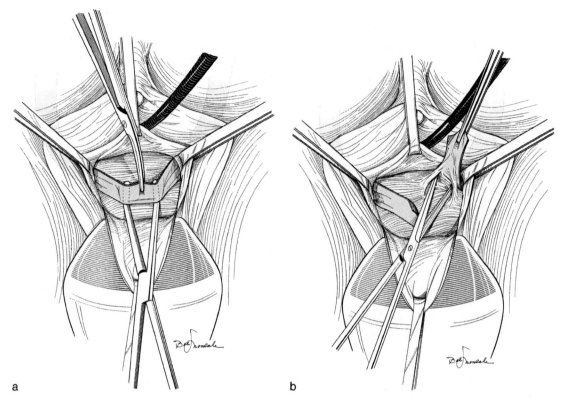

a   b

FIG. 36.1. Transvaginal sling incision. (**a**) After an inverted U or midline incision, the sling is isolated in the midline and incised. A right angle clamp may be placed between the sling and the periurethral fascia to avoid injury to the urethra. (**b**) The sling is freed from the undersurface of the urethra toward the endopelvic fascia. Ends may be excised or left in situ (from [54])

not successful in relieving obstruction, formal urethrolysis may be done.

Transvaginal Urethrolysis

Formal urethrolysis may be accomplished through a retropubic or a transvaginal approach. Both methods have shown equivalent success rates and rates of recurrent SUI, although most series include patients who are obstructed from a number of different anti-incontinence surgeries. The type of urethrolysis chosen will depend on several factors including patient presentation, type of incontinence procedure performed, failed prior urethrolysis, and surgeon preference. It has been our practice to perform transvaginal urethrolysis as a primary operation and a retropubic urethrolysis as a secondary operation. We prefer the transvaginal technique because of its ease and the reduced morbidity and

recovery time afforded by avoiding an abdominal procedure. However, there are times when a retropubic approach may be the best primary procedure: for example, when vaginal anatomy precludes a transvaginal approach; in cases where the original anti-incontinence surgery was associated with bladder perforation, fistula, or other operative complication; when there is a synthetic sling that must be removed; or in cases where the patient wishes to avoid a vaginal incision.

All urethrolysis procedures begin with a thorough endoscopic examination of the urethra, bladder neck, and bladder. Urethroscopy may show scarring, narrowing, occlusion, kinking, or deviation of the urethra. Eroded sutures or sling material or evidence of a fistula should be excluded. A rigid cystoscope with a 0 to 30° lens and little or no beak to allow for complete distention of the urethra is ideal for female urethroscopy. Also, it is common to find that the urethra and/or urethrovesical junction are fixed and there is a lack of mobility when moving the cystoscope up and down. After urethrolysis, mobility should be restored.

The most commonly used transvaginal technique originally was described by Leach and Raz [56]. A midline or inverted U incision approximately 3 cm long is made in the anterior vaginal wall. A midline incision should extend from the midurethra to 1–2 cm proximal to the bladder neck. In the case of an inverted U, the apex should be located half way between the bladder neck and urethral meatus and the lateral wing should extend proximal to the bladder neck. With either incision, lateral dissection is performed along the glistening surface of the periurethral fascia to the pubic bone. The retropubic space is entered sharply by perforating the attachment of the endopelvic fascia to the obturator fascia (Fig. 36.2a). The urethra is dissected bluntly and sharply off of the undersurface of the pubic bone and completely freed proximally to the bladder neck. Sharp dissection usually is required here (Fig. 36.2b). The urethra should be completely freed proximally to the bladder neck so that the index finger can be placed between the urethra and the symphysis pubis. Attachments to the undersurface of the pubic bone are sharply incised or swept down with the index finger retropubically. We recently have found that placement of a Penrose drain around the urethra (after initial mobilization, a right-angle clamp is placed between the pubic bone and the urethra, which allows for its placement) aids in visualization and sharp dissection of all retropubic attachments (Fig. 36.3) [57]. The index finger then may be placed completely around the urethra between the pubic bone. When urethrolysis is finished, there should be complete mobility of the urethra which can be tested with up and down movement of an intraurethral sound or cystoscope. Once this is achieved, the vaginal wall is closed with absorbable sutures. Prior to closure, endoscopic examination is preformed to rule out urethral or bladder injury. In cases of extensive urethrolysis, it is a good idea to assess ureteral integrity by giving intravenous Indigo Carmine prior to endoscopy and assessing ureteral efflux. Success rates with transvaginal urethrolysis vary from 53 to 93% (see Table 36.1).

Carey et al. reported the use of a Martius labial fat pad flap with transvaginal urethrolysis with

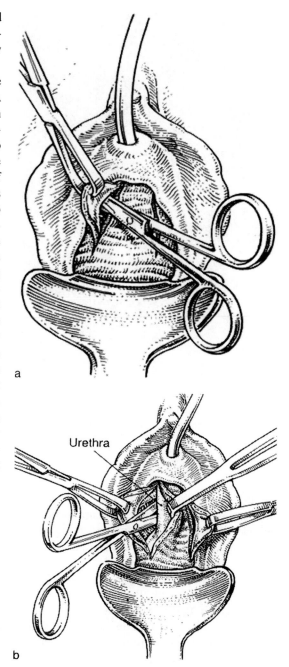

Fig. 36.2. Transvaginal urethrolysis. (**a**) An inverted U incision in the anterior vaginal wall and entrance into the retropubic space. (**b**) The urethra is sharply dissected off of the undersurface of the pubic bone. The endopelvic fascia, periurethral fascia, and vaginal wall are retracted medially to expose the urethra in the retropubic space (from [42])

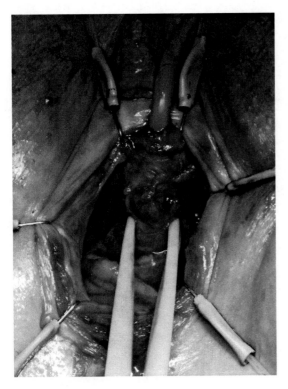

FIG. 36.3. Intraoperative photo after completed urethrolysis. A Penrose drain has been placed around the urethra, isolating it from the pubic bone (from [57])

increase the risk of persistent obstruction, and since most patients are distraught about obstruction, we feel it is best to take care of that problem and deal with recurrent SUI at a later time should it occur. Rates of recurrent SUI after resuspension vary between 0 and 19% when resuspension is not performed [22, 41, 45, 58, 59]. Many of these patients may be salvaged with transurethral bulking agents should stress incontinence recur. Goldman et al. reported a 66% response rate to collagen in women with recurrent stress incontinence after transvaginal urethrolysis [59]. In addition, the option for repeat surgery for SUI at a later date exists. It is important to discuss the pros and cons of resuspension and the treatment of recurrent stress incontinence with patients preoperatively, as this could affect the decision to resuspend or not.

A variant of transvaginal urethrolysis is the suprameatal approach described by Petrou and colleagues [60]. We have found this to have quite limited applicability. A theoretical advantage of this technique is that lateral perforation of the urethropelvic ligament is not needed, minimizing the chance of recurrent urethral hypermobility and subsequent incontinence. An inverted U incision is made around the top of the urethral meatus (approximately 1 cm away) between the 3 and 9 o'clock positions. Using sharp dissection, a plane is developed above the urethra. Then with a combination of sharp and blunt dissection the urethra, vesical neck, and bladder are freed from the pubic and pelvic attachments anteriorly and laterally. The index finger then may be passed into the retropubic space, and with a sweeping motion from medial to lateral, further freeing may be performed. If obstruction is caused by a pubovaginal sling, the lateral wings of the sling may be cut. Likewise, if the obstruction is caused by suspension sutures, these may be cut. As with transvaginal urethrolysis, a Martius flap may be placed. The authors reported a 65% success rate for retention, 67% success for urgency symptoms, and a 3% recurrent SUI rate [60]. This approach may be beneficial if dissection between the urethra and pubic bone is excessively difficult. It may be particularly applicable for cases of repeat transvaginal urethrolysis (after a failed prior urethrolysis) or when scarring is particularly dense.

success in 87% of patients [58]. The Martius flap may decrease the risk of recurrent fibrosis, provide some urethral support, and a future sling may be placed outside the fat pad, decreasing the risk of urethral injury. We reserve it for select cases (eg, repeat urethrolysis, extensive fibrosis). We usually divide the robust fat pad flap midway along its longitudinal axis and wrap the flap around the urethra effectually supporting the undersurface and retropubic surface of the urethra.

In select cases (eg, extensive mobilization or stress incontinence coexisting with obstruction) it may be desirable to resupport the urethra at the time of urethrolysis. Resuspension or pubovaginal sling may be done. Currently our practice is to consider a resuspension or sling only if the patient has stress incontinence prior to urethrolysis or if support structures are severely compromised during urethrolysis. Resuspension does

Retropubic Urethrolysis

Retropubic approaches to urethrolysis may be the preferred method under circumstances which include surgeon experience/familiarity with vaginal anatomy, inadequate vaginal access, original incontinence surgery, or urethrolysis associated with bladder perforation, fistula, or synthetic sling removal, and when the patient desires to avoid another vaginal incision. Complicated cases that have failed prior extensive transvaginal urethrolysis also may be performed retropubically. Previous retropubic surgery such as the MMK still may be managed transvaginally, as shown by Zimmern [61].

The technique of retropubic urethrolysis has been described by Webster and Kreder (Fig. 36.4) [46]. It may be accomplished through a Pfannensteil or low midline incision. The rectus fascia and muscle are opened in midline to the level of the pubic symphysis. After exposing the retropubic space, all prevesical and retropubic adhesions are sharply incised. Complications can be avoided by keeping the tips of the scissors against the pubic symphysis during sharp dissection. The object is to restore complete mobility to the anterior vaginal wall, allowing free movement of the vesicourethral unit.

The urethra and urethrovesical junction are dissected off of the pubic bone, without separating them from the anterior vaginal wall. The boundaries of the vagina in relation to the urethrovesical junction are identified by placement of the surgeon's nondominant hand in the vagina. Alternatively, a sponge stick or similar instrument may be used. Some degree of sharp dissection lateral to the urethra usually is required. In cases of severe scarring, it may be necessary to mobilize laterally as far as the ischial tuberosities. As a result, one is often left with a paravaginal defect. In cases where a paravaginal defect is created as a result of urethral mobilization, the defects should be repaired by reapproximating the paravaginal fascia to the fascia of the obturator internus along the arcus tendineous. The paravaginal repair sutures are left untied. Finally, the peritoneum is opened with a small incision and an omental flap is mobilized. The flap then is placed between the pubic bone and the urethra and secured to the underside of the pubic bone with a 2–0 polyglycolic acid (PGA) suture. The omentum fills the dead space and helps to prevent recurrent adhesion. The paravaginal repair sutures then are tied and the abdomen is closed. Cystoscopy is performed to rule out urethral injury and confirm efflux of Indigo Carmine from the ureteral orifices.

Webster and Kreder reported successful outcomes in 93% of 15 women undergoing retropubic urethrolysis and obturator shelf repair [46]. In another series of 12 women, Petrou and Young reported resolution of obstruction in ten patients with new-onset stress incontinence in 18% of the women [62]. Carr and Webster reported complete or significant resolution of symptoms in 86% of patients with retropubic urethrolysis [22].

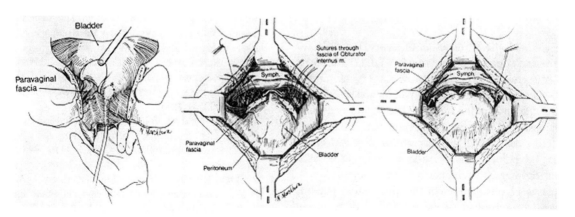

FIG. 36.4. Retropubic urethrolysis. The urethra and urethrovesical junction are dissected off of the pubic bone, without separating them from the anterior vaginal wall with sharp dissection. A paravaginal defect repair is then performed (from [46])

Failed Urethrolysis

Failure of urethrolysis may be due to persistent or recurrent obstruction, detrusor overactivity, impaired detrusor contractility, or learned voiding dysfunction. Recurrent obstruction may result from periurethral fibrosis and scarring or intrinsic damage to the urethra that has occurred as a result of the urethrolysis surgery. We believe that inadequate dissection and lysis of the urethra probably represents the most common reason for failure of initial urethrolysis. When obstruction persists, it is reasonable to attempt a repeat urethrolysis. We have found this to be effective in relieving urinary retention, but not as effective in treating persistent storage symptoms. We have reported on the efficacy of repeat urethrolysis in 24 women who failed initial urethrolysis and remained in urinary retention [63]. Both transvaginal and retropubic approaches were chosen depending on the clinical situation. Obstruction was cured in 92%, but storage symptoms completely resolved in only 12% and were improved and required medication in 69%. SUI recurred in 18%. These data clearly support aggressive repeat urethrolysis in the face of initial failure, at least for retention and incomplete emptying. In general, if an aggressive transvaginal urethrolysis fails, then a retropubic approach may be considered. In cases where it is unknown how aggressive the initial transvaginal procedure was or whether only a sling incision was done, then a repeat transvaginal approach may be appropriate.

Conclusions

Even with the introduction of newer, less invasive anti-incontinence procedures (TVT, TOT), urethral obstruction after incontinence surgery remains a bothersome problem for the patient and a challenging dilemma for the surgeon. The diagnosis usually is based on signs and symptoms, but urodynamic definitions of BOO, cystourethroscopy, and imaging are helpful. The decision to intervene is based on the degree of bother and the clinician's suspicion of obstruction. In this discussion, patients must be informed of the possibility of recurrent SUI and residual or de novo irritative symptoms with surgical treatment of obstruction. Fortunately, the various surgical options are highly successful at restoring efficient voiding. Continued effort will be directed at identifying improved methods of diagnosis and treatment of anti-incontinence procedure obstruction and associated irritative voiding symptoms.

References

1. Rosenblum N, Nitti VW. Post-urethral suspension obstruction. Curr Opin Urol 2001; 11:411–416.
2. Leach GE, Dmochowski RR, Appell RA, et-al. Female stress urinary incontinence clinical guidelines panel summary report on surgical management of female stress urinary incontinence. The American Urological Association. J Urol 1997; 158: 875–880.
3. Morgan TO, Westney OL, McGuire EJ. Pubovaginal sling: 4-year outcome analysis and quality of life assessment. J Urol 2000; 163: 1845–1848.
4. Dunn JS, Bent AE, Ellerkman RM, et-al.. Voiding dysfunction after stress incontinence: Literature and survey results. Int Urogynecol J 2004; 15:25–31.
5. Klutke C, Siegel S, Carlin B, et-al.. Urinary retention after tension-free vaginal tape procedure: Incidence and treatment. Urology 2001; 58:697–701.
6. Niemczyk, Klutke JJ, Carlin BI, et-al. United States experience with tension-free vaginal tape procedure for urinary stress incontinence: Assessment of safety and tolerability. Tech Urol 2001; 7:261–265.
7. Rardin CR, Rosenblatt PL, Kohli N, et-al.. Release of tension-free vaginal tape for the treatment of refractory postoperative voiding dysfunction. Obstet Gynecol 2002; 100:898–902.
8. Sander P, Moller LM, Rudnicki PM, et-al.. Does the tension-free vaginal tape procedure affect the voiding phase? Pressre-flow studies before and 1 year after surgery. BJU Int 2002; 89:694–698.
9. Tamussino K, Hanzal E, Kolle D, et-al.. The Austrian tension-free vaginal tape registry. Int Urogynecol J 2001; 12 (Suppl 2):S28–S29.
10. Kuuva N, Nilsson CG. A nationwide analysis of complications associated with the tension-free vaginal tape (TVT) procedure. Acta Obstet Gynecol Scand 2002; 81:72–77.
11. Moran PA, Ward KL, Johnson D, et-al.. Tension-free vaginal tape for primary genuine stress incontinence: A two centre follow-up study. BJU Int 2000; 86:39–42.
12. Rackley RR, Abdelmalak JB, Tchetgen MB, et-al.. Tension-free vaginal tape and percutaneous vaginal tape sling procedures. Tech Urol 2001; 7(2): 90–100.
13. Delorme E, Droupe S, Tayrac R, et-al.. Transobturator tape (Uratape): A new minimally invasive procedure

to treat female urinary incontinence. Eur Urol 2004; 45:203–207.

14. Costa P, Grise P, Droupy S, et-al.. Surgical treatment of female stress urinary incontinence with a trans-obturator-tape (TOT) Uratape: Short term results of a prospective multicentric study. Eur Urol 2004; 46:102–107.

15. Deval B, Ferchaux J, Berry R, et-al.. Objective and subjective cure rates after trans-obturator tape (OBTAPE) treatment of female urinary incontinence. Eur Urol 2006; 49:373–377.

16. Atherton MJ, Stanton SL. A comparison of bladder neck movement and elevation after tension-free vaginal tape and colposuspension. BJOG 2000; 107:1366–1370.

17. Sarlos D, Kuronen M, Schaer GN. How does tension-free vaginal tape correct stress incontinence? Investigation by perineal ultrasound. Int Urogynecol J 2003; 14:395–398.

18. Lo TS, Horng SG, Liang CC, et-al.. Ultrasound assessment of mid-urethra tape at three-year follow-up after tension-free vaginal tape procedure. Urology 2004; 63:671–675.

19. Minaglia S, Ozel B, Hurtado E, et-al.. Effect of transobturator tape procedure on proximal urethral mobility. Urology 2005; 65(1):55–59.

20. FitzGerald MP, Brubaker L. The etiology of urinary retention after surgery for genuine stress incontinence. Neurourol Urodyn 2001; 20:13–21.

21. Smith CP, O'Leary M, Erickson J, et-al.. Botulinum toxin urethral sphincter injection resolves urinary retention after pubovaginal sling operation. Int Urogynecol J 2002; 13:185–186.

22. Carr LK, Webster GD. Voiding dysfunction following incontinence surgery; diagnosis and treatment with retropubic or vaginal urethrolysis. J Urol 1997; 157:821–823.

23. Miller EA, Amundsen CL, Toh KL, et-al.. Preoperative urodynamic evaluation may predict voiding dysfunction in women undergoing pubovaginal sling. J Urol 2003; 169:2234–2237.

24. Weinberger MW, Ostergard DR. Postoperative catheterization, urinary retention and permanent voiding dysfunction in women undergoing pubovaginal sling. Obstetand Gynecol 1996; 87:50–54.

25. Bhatia NN, Bergman A. Urodynamic predictability of voiding following incontinence surgery. Obstet Gynecol 1984; 63:85–91.

26. Gateau T, Faramarzi-Roques R, Le Norman L, et-al.. Clinical and urodynamic repercussions after TVT procedure and how to diminish patient complaints. Eur Urol 2003; 44:372–376.

27. Wang AC, Chen MC. The correlation between preoperative voiding mechanism and surgical outcome of the tension-free vaginal tape procedure, with reference to quality of life. BJU Int 2003; 91:502–506.

28. Kawashima H, Kouzo H, Okada N, et-al.. The importance of studying pressure-flow for predicting postoperative voiding difficulties in women with stress urinary incontinence: A preliminary study that correlates low Pdet × Qave with postoperative residual urine. Urol Res 2004; 32:84–88.

29. Kobak WH, Walters MD, Piedmonte MR. Determinants of voiding after three types of incontinence surgery: A multivariable analysis. Obstet Gynecol 2001; 97:86–91.

30. McLennan MT, Melick CF, Bent AE. Clinical and urodynamic predictors of delayed voiding after fascia lata suburethral sling. Obstet Gynecol 1998; 92:608–612.

31. Sokol AI, Jelovsek JE, Walters MD, et-al.. Incidence and predictors of prolonged urinary retention after TVT with and without concurrent prolapse surgery. Am J Obstet Gynecol 2005; 192:1537–1543.

32. Leng WW, Davies BJ, Tarin T, et-al.. Delayed treatment of bladder outlet obstruction after sling surgery: Association with irreversible bladder dysfunction. J Urol 2004; 172:1379–1381.

33. Karram MM, Segal JL, Vassallo BJ, Kleeman SD. Complications and untoward effects of the tension-free vaginal tape procedure. Obstet Gynecol 2003; 101:929–932.

34. Croak AJ, Schulte V, Peron S, et-al.. Transvaginal tape lysis for urinary obstruction after tension-free vaginal tape placement. J Urol 2003; 169:2238–2241.

35. Chassagne S, Bernier PA, Haab F, et-al.. Proposed cutoff values to define bladder outlet obstruction in women. Urology 1998; 51:408–411.

36. Lemack GE, Zimmern PE. Pressure flow analysis may aid in identifying women with outflow obstruction. J Urol 2000; 163:1823–1828.

37. Defreitas GA, Zimmern PE, Lemack GE, Shariat SF. Refining diagnosis of anatomic female bladder outlet obstruction: Comparison of pressure-flow study parameters in clinically obstructed women with those of normal controls. Urology 2004; 64:675–681.

38. Nitti VW, Tu LM, Gitlin J. Diagnosing bladder outlet obstruction in women. J Urol 1999; 161:1535–1540.

39. Blaivas JG, Groutz A. Bladder outlet obstruction nomogram for women with lower urinary tract symptomatology. Neurourol Urodyn 2000; 19:553–556.

40. Akikwala TV, Fleischman N, Nitti VW. Comparison of diagnostic criteria for female bladder outlet obstruction. J Urol 2006; 176:2093–2097.

41. Foster HE, McGuire EJ. Management of urethral obstruction with transvaginal urethrolysis. J Urol 1993; 150:1448–1451.

42. Nitti VW, Raz S. Obstruction following anti-incontinence procedures: Diagnosis and treatment with transvaginal urethrolysis. J Urol 1994; 152:93–98.

43. Paick J, Hyeon JK, Shin JW, et-al.. Complications associated with the tension-free vaginal tape procedure: The Korean experience. Int Urogynecol J 2005; 16:215–219.

44. Mishra VC, Mishra N, Karim OM, et-al.. Voiding dysfunction after tension-free vaginal tape: A conservative approach is often successful. Int Urogynecol J 2005; 16:210–214.

45. Cross CA, Cespedes RD, English SF, McGuire EJ. Transvaginal urethrolysis for urethral obstruction after anti-incontinence surgery. J Urol 1998; 159:1199–1121.

46. Webster GD, Kreder KJ. Voiding dysfunction following cystourethropexy: Its evaluation and management. J Urol 1990; 144:670–673.

47. Segal J, Steele AC, Vassallo BJ, et-al.. Various surgical approaches to treat voiding dysfunction following anti-incontinence surgery. Int Urogynecol J 2006; 17:372–377.

48. Starkman JS, Wolter C, Gomelsky A, et-al.. Voiding dysfunction following removal of eroded synthetic mid urethral slings. J Urol 2006; 176:1040–1044.

49. Goldman HB. Simple sling incision for the treatment of iatrogenic urethral obstruction. Urology 2003; 62:714–718.

50. Long C, Lo T, Liu C, et-al.. Lateral excision of tension-free vaginal tape for the treatment of iatrogenic urethral obstruction. Obstet Gynecol 2004; 104:1270–1274.

51. Ghoniem GM, Elgamasy AN. Simplified surgical approach to bladder outlet obstruction following pubovaginal sling. J Urol 1995; 154:181–183.

52. Kusuda L. Simple release of pubovaginal sling. Urology 2001; 57:358–359.

53. Amundsen CL, Guralnick ML, Webster GD. Variations in strategy for the treatment of urethral obstruction after a pubovaginal sling procedure. J Urol 2000; 164:434–437.

54. Nitti VW, Carlson KV, Blaivas JG, Dmochowski RR. Early results of pubovaginal sling lysis by midline sling incision Urology 2002; 59:47–52.

55. Thiel DD, Pettit PDM, McCllelan WT, et-al.. Long-term urinary continence rates after simple sling incision for relief of urinary retention following fasca lata pubovaginal slings. J Urol 2005; 174(5): 1878–1881.

56. Leach GE, Raz S. Modified Pereyra bladder neck suspension after previously failed anti-incontinence surgery. Surgical technique and results with long-term follow-up. Urology 1984; 23:359–362.

57. Huckabay C, Nitti VW. Diagnosis and treatment of obstruction following incontinence surgery: Urethrolysis and other techniques. In: Cardoza L, Stastkin D, eds. Textbook of female urology and urogynecology, 2nd edn. Oxford, UK, Isis Medical Media, 2006:981–995.

58. Carey JM, Chon JK, Leach GE. Urethrolysis with Martius labial fat pad graft for iatrogenic bladder outlet obstruction. Urology 2003; 61:21–25.

59. Goldman HB, Rackley RR, Appell RA. The efficacy of urethrolysis without re-suspension for iatrogenic urethral obstruction. J Urol 1999; 161:196–199.

60. Petrou SP, Brown JA, Blaivas G. Suprameatal transvaginal urethrolysis. J Urol 1999; 161: 1268–1271.

61. Zimmern PE, Hadley HR, Leach GE, Raz S. Female urethral obstruction after Marshall–Marchetti–Krantz operation. J Urol 1987; 138:517–520.

62. Petrou SP, Young PR. Rate of recurrent stress urinary incontinence after retropubic urethrolysis. J Urol 2002; 167:513–615.

63. Scarpero HM, Dmochowski RR, Nitti VW. Repeat urethrolysis after failed urethrolysis for iatrogenic obstruction. J Urol 2003; 169:1013–1016.

Part VIII
Social Aspects of Incontinence

Chapter 37
Economic Impact of Stress Urinary Incontinence and Prolapse: Conservative, Medical, and Surgical Treatments

Lynn Stothers

Introduction

Much of the literature on stress urinary incontinence (SUI) and pelvic organ prolapse briefly mentions costs or cost effectiveness, but few actually involve formal cost analysis [1, 2, 3, 4]. There are several relevant types of cost analysis, from the simple to the very sophisticated:

- *Cost of illness analysis* (COI) typically quantifies the burden of medical expenses (direct costs) and the resulting value of lost productivity (indirect costs) attributable to a specific condition such as an illness or injury [5].
- *Cost effectiveness analysis* (CEA) measures the costs and consequences of two or more diagnostic or treatment pathways related to a single common effect or health outcome. It then summarizes the results in ratios that demonstrate the cost of achieving a unit of health effect for different types of patients and for variations of the intervention [6].
- *Cost utility analysis* (CUA) is a form of CEA in which particular attention is paid to the quality of health outcome related to treatment. In CUA, health effects are expressed in terms of quality-adjusted life years (QALYs) [7]. A QALY is a measure of health outcome that assigns to a given period of time a weighting that corresponds to the health-related quality of life during that period, and then aggregates these weights across time periods. The QALY is important because it considers both quantity and quality of life.

- *Cost benefit analysis* estimates the net social benefit of an intervention by comparing the benefit of the intervention with the cost, with all benefits and costs measured in dollars [7]. Health outcomes are converted into monetary values using "willingness to pay" (the value an individual would pay for reduction in illness severity) or "risk of death" or "human capital" methods (an individual's value to society based on productivity or future wages) [4, 8].

SUI and Costs

Research into SUI usually is limited to women, because they are the most commonly affected. Very little has been done to study the economic burden of SUI in men, although postprostatectomy stress incontinence occurs in up to 20% of patients. This makes it difficult to determine the actual combined costs of male and female SUI to society.

Comparison of costs for conservative, medical, and surgical treatment of SUI also is hampered by a lack of harmonization in defining SUI, standardization of survey methods and validation criteria, and outcome measures [9, 10]. In addition, studies on incontinence often combine SUI with overactive bladder and urge incontinence, making it difficult to isolate costs specifically related to SUI.

Direct costs of SUI are those borne by both the health sector and by individual patients and their families. Direct health sector costs ideally should include supplies, equipment, and health professionals for

511

both inpatient and outpatient services. Direct costs carried by the patient range from medications and protective devices such as pads and diapers to treatments ranging from pelvic floor muscle training (PFMT), bladder training, electrical stimulation, vaginal or urethral devices, to drugs and surgery. The costs of pads and protective undergarments are the most commonly compared direct cost in the SUI literature, but the costs of these products vary widely, and information about the actual product and cost often is not provided in the description of the study. For example, in chart reviews, if the patient reports using three pads per day, it is not known whether they use three small liners which typically cost a few cents each or a sophisticated undergarment which may cost as much as a few dollars per garment.

Indirect costs include lost earnings for both the patient and family or friends who provide care for the affected person. Age and working status are particularly important with respect to indirect costs. For example, since the prevalence of urinary incontinence increases dramatically with age, the working status of the 60+ age group is of particular importance.

Intangible costs include the monetary value of pain, suffering, and anxiety from the disease in question. Intangible costs are difficult to determine in most cases, and are generally the least well measured in the literature.

Costs vary to some extent by year, region, practice patterns in the area, and country. For the sake of simplicity, all costs from the literature discussed subsequently have been converted to US$ 2006.

The Economic Burden of SUI

There are few recent European or North American studies on the economic burden of SUI, which includes both direct costs such as surgical procedures and hospital stay and indirect costs, such as lost productivity. Even when studies are published, it is difficult to generalize costs from one jurisdiction to another due to the different health care system models. Payne estimates the overall cost of urinary incontinence to the American economy to be $16 billion dollars annually, but does not differentiate the costs of SUI from other forms of incontinence [11].

In 2002, Birnbaum, Leong, and Kabra estimated the lifetime medical costs of cardiovascular disease, diabetes, and SUI in women under and over 65 in the United States. For women under 65, annual medical costs were extrapolated from claims from a large employer ($n > 100,000$) with locations throughout the United States and a wide range of job positions. For women 65 years of age and older, calculations were based on the estimate for those <65 years of age, combined with published government statistics. The incremental lifetime medical cost (the difference between the total medical costs of patients with SUI compared to those of controls without the condition) was $58,000 for SUI, compared to $233,000 for diabetes and $423,000 for cardiovascular disease. Incremental medical costs for women treated for SUI increase significantly as women age, from $3,300 annually to $15,000 annually. A woman with SUI has total lifetime medical costs 1.8 times greater than the costs of a similar woman without SUI [12].

The Birnbaum team continued their research in this area with a 2004 claims data analysis (using the same employer database) of the cost of SUI. Using an incremental cost-of-illness model (which controls for comorbid conditions and patient demographics) patients with SUI had direct costs that were 134% more than those for their controls and indirect costs that were 163% more than those for controls. Surgical treatment widened the gap substantially between patients and controls – for patients who received surgical treatment for their SUI, annual direct medical costs (in the year of treatment) were 206% higher than for controls. The authors estimated that the annual average direct medical costs of SUI for 1 year (1998) were $5,642 and the indirect workplace costs were $4,208 per patient [13].

Turner et al. estimated the prevalence and costs of clinically significant urine storage conditions including leakage, urgency, frequency, and nocturia in community-dwelling men and women ≥40 years of age. Prevalence estimates were based on responses from 23,000 questionnaires mailed to a randomly selected sample, and costs were based on home interviews of 613 individuals with urine storage conditions and 523 controls. Total annual cost to the United Kingdom's National Health Service was estimated to be just over $1 billion (1999/2000 prices) ($568 million and $437 million, for men and women, respectively). This was approximately 1.1% of National Health Service spending for the 1999/2000 fiscal year. Individuals reported bearing a substantial cost as well – $55 million and $334 million, for men and women, respectively. In addition, intangible costs, based on willingness to pay as an indicator of the value of alleviating symptoms were estimated to be an additional $1.25 billion ($564 million and $690 million, for men and women, respectively). Costs associated specifically with SUI were not separated out in this study. Interestingly, cost of treatment was greater for males, while individual and indirect costs were greater for females [14]. O'Sullivan et al. found that it was more costly and often more time consuming to treat women with mild compared to moderate SUI [15] (see Table 37.1).

Diagnostic Testing

Two preoperative testing strategies for women with pelvic organ prolapse and SUI symptoms were compared using predicted success rate (cure of urinary incontinence) and cost-effectiveness of treatment as outcomes. According to Weber et al., "the outcome of importance for a test is not merely diagnostic accuracy. For testing to be worthwhile, it must be accompanied by a clinically important improvement in outcome (effectiveness of treatment)" [16]. A decision–analytic approach was used to compare basic office evaluation and urodynamic testing for accuracy in assignment of diagnoses of urinary incontinence for women with SUI symptoms. Based on published data used to predict the probability of outcomes (cure rate of SUI and need for retreatment), the success of treatment and

costs were calculated to assess cost-effectiveness. Basic office evaluation and urodynamic testing had the same cure rate (96%) after initial and secondary treatment. The average cost of treatment was lower for basic office evaluation than urodynamic testing ($4,959 vs. $5,302, respectively). The cost of achieving a single additional cure was achieved by urodynamic testing at a cost of $328,601 relative to basic office evaluation. The only scenario in which basic office evaluation was more cost-effective than urodynamic testing was unlikely because it required that detrusor instability occur in less than 8% or the cost of urodynamic testing was less than $103 [16]. For example, Lemack and Zimmern reported the 2000 Medicare reimbursement for urodynamic studies to be $214.82 [17].

To minimize diagnostic costs, Lemack and Zimmern conducted a retrospective study to determine whether previous surgical history for incontinence and a validated lower urinary tract symptom questionnaire would have identified those who needed urodynamic testing before surgery for SUI. No single test, including physical examination, history, voiding diaries, and validated questionnaires, proved adequate for diagnosing incontinence and in particular in differentiating SUI from detrusor instability. However, the authors reported a response of "2" or "3" to question 3 on the UDI-6 (ie, leakage related to physical activity or straining was moderately or greatly bothersome) combined with a history of previous surgery correctly identified 91% of critical diagnoses while reducing costs substantially. Using this approach in their population of 172 consecutive women who completed the UDI-6 and underwent urodynamic testing, the costs of testing would have been $7,089.06 with a total cost savings of $29,859.98 [17].

TABLE 37.1. Cost of treating and achieving objective versus subjective cure of stress urinary incontinence in mildly and moderately incontinent women.

	Median cost of treatment	Cost to achieve an objective pad test cure	Cost to achieve a subjective cure
Mildly incontinent	$99.52	$98.15	$91.04
Moderately incontinent	$84.65	$74.49	$72.98
Wilcoxon P value	$P = 0.21$	$P = 0.13$	$P = 0.11$

From [15]

Conservative Management

The annual cost of protective devices and related costs such as laundry often are borne as out-of-pocket expenses by those suffering from SUI, although some jurisdictions, such as Germany, reimburse some of these expenses [18]. The cost of diagnosis and treatment with drugs and diapers for SUI for women over 40 in Italy was estimated to be $221.87 [19]. A 1998 study in the United Kingdom showed the preoperative cost of protective pads and towels before surgery to be $7.11/month (mean $15.89), although 15% of women spent over $37/month while others used self-made pads or towels and had zero cost appointed to them for the purpose of the study. After surgery for SUI, median costs dropped sharply to $2.49 (mean $5.48) per month [20].

Pharmaceutical Management

The pharmaceuticals used in the treatment of SUI historically have been available over the counter in many countries as treatment for colds and flu. They include the α-adrenoceptor agonists, some of which have now been removed from the market in certain countries due to serious side effects. Because they are not prescription drugs, information on costs related to these medications often is not captured in studies.

Brunenberg et al. used a Markov model to examine the cost-effectiveness of duloxetine alone and duloxetine (Eli Lily and Company, brand names Cymbalta/Yentreve, Xeristar, or Ariclaim) after inadequate response to PFMT in women aged ≥50 years with SUI. Duloxetine, a serotonin and norepinephrine reuptake inhibitor used primarily for major depressive disorders, has been shown in a small number of studies to improve the quality of life of women with SUI. It is approved for use in Europe but is not FDA approved for this use in the United States. According to their model, PFMT would cost $0.04 per incontinence episode avoided compared to no treatment. Duloxetine taken when PFMT has failed would cost $4.85 per incontinence episode avoided. PFMT had a high probability of being more cost-effective up to $4.64 per incontinence episode avoided. Beyond that point, duloxetine after failed PFMT had the highest cost-effectiveness probability, but would require

society to pay an additional $4.88 to avoid a single incontinence episode [21].

Surgical Management

It was estimated that, in 1991, the direct cost of surgical and other procedures for the treatment of SUI in the United States was $0.5 billion. Although this number has likely grown substantially, the growing population and trend toward more surgical management of SUI is likely offset by more cost-effective procedures [22]. Where possible this section is organized from least to most invasive.

Cost of Illness Analysis

COI has been performed for a variety of individual and comparative surgical approaches. Cost analysis does not allow a comparison of cost-effectiveness among procedures because it does not compare success rates and the costs associated with reoperation.

Bulking Agents

Berman and Kreder compared the cost of endoscopic transurethral collagen injection and fascia lata sling cystourethropexy for the treatment of intrinsic sphincter deficiency, type III genuine SUI (Table 37.2). Immediate costs for fascia lata procedures were an average of $10,381 ± 1,440 compared to $4,996 ± 885 for collagen. However, this does not take into consideration cost-effectiveness. At follow-up (mean 14.9 months for cystourethropexy and 21.3 months for collagen injection), cystourethropexy had better outcome in terms of continence rate (71.4 and 26.7%, respectively) and a lower reoperation rate (one secondary operation for the entire cystourethropexy group versus an average of 1.6 collagen injections per patient in the collagen group). Morbidity was higher in the cystourethropexy group. CEA was not performed, but the authors concluded that the sling procedure was likely more cost-effective due to the higher success rate with fewer reoperations [23].

Maher et al. compared pubovaginal sling versus transurethral Macroplastique™ (Uroplasty, Minnesota, USA) in terms of hospital stay, operating room costs, and the cost of the disposable

TABLE 37.2. Average costs for individual procedures and percentages of total costs for fascia lata sling cystourethropexy versus collagen injection.

Economic parameters	Fascia lata (n = 14)	Collagen (n = 14)
Hospital room	$1,132 ± 306 (11)	$0 (0)
Supply	$398 ± 122 (4)	$63 ± 44 (1.3)
Pharmacy	$492 ± 267 (5)	$112 ± 82 (2.2)
Radiology	$2.8 ± 10.4 (< 1)	$85 ± 163 (1.7)
Collagen	$0 (0)	$1,974 ± 412 (40)
Operating room	$3,706 ± 694 (36)	$643 ± 245 (13)
Postoperative care	$1,233 ± 441 (12)	$627 ± 215 (13)
Laboratory	$63 ± 121 (< 1)	$107 ± 91(2)
Total hospital cost	$7,004 ± 1,185 (68)	$3,883 ± 822 (78)
Physician fee	$3,378 ± 807 (33)	$1,112 ± 130 (22)
Total costs	$10,381 ± 1,440	$4,996 ± 885

Mean US dollars ± standard deviation (percent). From [23]

Macroplastique. The average cost per patient for Macroplastique (including reoperations) ($3,378.55) was significantly greater than the cost for the sling ($2,680.24) (P ≤ 0.0001) [24]. A detailed cost breakdown was not provided.

The authors of a Cochrane review on periurethral injection of bulking agents for treatment of SUI identified the need for cost-effectiveness studies before any specific recommendation could be made [25].

Laparoscopic Procedures

Walter et al. retrospectively analyzed chart data on patients undergoing laparoscopic (n = 76) or open (n = 143) Burch retropubic urethropexy for SUI. Mean hospital charges were $9,900 (SD ± $2,400) for laparoscopic procedures compared to $9,400 (SD ± $2,100) for open procedures. Given the sample size, the 5% difference in costs was not considered statistically significant [26]. In contrast to studies that show stand-alone laparoscopic procedures to be more cost-effective than open procedures [16, 23, 24, 27, 28, 29, 30, 31, 32, 33, 34], the authors concluded that there is no cost advantage to the laparoscopic approach when concurrent transvaginal repairs are required to correct a coexisting pelvic organ prolapse.

In a Cochrane review of laparoscopic colposuspension, the laparoscopic approach was found to be more costly than the open procedure [35]. Kohli et al. found that the higher surgical costs were

not offset by shorter length of stay in a retrospective chart review of 21 women undergoing open Burch colposuspension versus 17 undergoing the same procedure laparoscopically. The laparoscopic group had significantly longer operative time (110 vs 66 min, P < 0.01), resulting in increased operating room charges ($3,479 vs $2,138 respectively, P < 0.001). Mean length of stay was 1.3 days in the laparoscopic group versus 2.1 days for the open group (P < 0.005), incurring accommodation costs of $4,960 versus $4,079, respectively (P < 0.01). Some of the higher operating rooms costs for the laparoscopic group could be attributed to the use of disposable rather than reusable equipment. In contrast, Loveridge et al. reported no significant difference in overall costs in a retrospective COI of laparoscopic (n = 26) versus open colposuspension (n = 23). The authors concluded that higher surgical costs were offset by shorter length of stay (P = 0.533). However, not all surgical costs (eg, nursing time in the operating room) were considered, and the mean difference in costs (the only cost data presented) does not support this conclusion. In addition, the length of stay reported for these procedures is not representative of current practice in North America [36].

Slings and Burch Procedures

Quievy et al. compared the tension-free vaginal tape (TVT) (n = 21) to Burch open colposuspension (n = 17). Costs included medical devices, drugs, laboratory procedures, operating time, hospital stay, and duration of postoperative follow-up. The Burch cost $5,125.47 compared to $2,133.71 for TVT. The difference in cost was attributed to shorter operating room times and hospital stay [34].

Cost-Effectiveness

Subak et al. critiqued research on new gynecologic procedures and found that many studies do not adhere to basic recommended analytic guidelines for CEA [4]. According to the authors, "many of these studies described their research methodology as 'cost-effectiveness analysis' but either failed to include an evaluation of effectiveness or failed to combine cost and effectiveness into a single summary measure (ie, cost per life-year gained). In addition, many articles stated in their conclusions that one intervention was more 'cost-effective' than an alternative intervention without performing a CEA." In addition, they found studies that compared effectiveness and costs of two or more procedures without combining the measures to perform a formal CEA. The authors encouraged investigators to be more precise in their use of the term "cost-effective."

Persson et al. conducted a cost-effectiveness study comparing laparoscopic colposuspension with TVT in 79 women presenting for evaluation of SUI symptoms in terms of direct costs to the hospital owner (the county) and included perioperative and postoperative hospital care and outpatient medical care (Table 37.3). TVT was significantly more expensive to perform than laparoscopic colposuspension. Sensitivity analysis showed that surgical time and anesthesia were the areas of greatest difference. The high investment costs of the TVT kit outweighed the longer surgical time

TABLE 37.3. Total costs to the county in US$ for laparoscopic colposuspension versus TVT procedure.

Economic parameters	Laparoscopic colposuspension (n = 32)	TVT (n = 38)
Basic costs[a] ($0.73 min−1)	$92.97	$69.86
Anesthesia costs[a] ($4.19 min−1)	$491.65	$325.18
Surgical costs[a] ($0.75 min−1)	$45.56	$32.93
Surgical materials[b]	$130.18	$544.59
Hospital care[c]	$797.94	$726.34
Depreciation of video equipment	$22.97	$0.00
Depreciation of laparoscopic instruments	$22.21	$0.00
Outpatient visits to a physician ($74.41 per visit) or a nurse ($29.61 per visit)	$21.83	$14.94
Average total cost per procedure[d]	$1,625.71	$1,714.24
Total costs including reoperations	$1,678.11	$1,867.28

From [31]. Note: Original costs presented in 2001 Euros, converted to 2006 US dollars
[a]Mean times are multiplied with the specific costs per minute
[b]Includes drapes, gloves, gowns, packing, and sterilization of instruments
[c]Includes costs for postoperative analgesics
[d]$P < 0.01$

for laparoscopic colposuspension. The authors suggest that differences might have been less if performed by other researchers with more expertise in the TVT procedure, as the surgical time was 44.9 min compared to 29 min reported by Ulmsten et al. [32] and a median time of 22 min reported by Nilsson and Kuuva [31, 33].

Kung et al. evaluated cost-effectiveness of open versus laparoscopic Burch procedure. Costs included professional fees, diagnostic tests, capital and disposable equipment, hospital stay, and indirect costs. Costs of laparoscopic Burch repair were significantly less than for the open procedure ($2,398 vs $5,692), primarily due to the shorter length of hospital stay associated with the laparoscopic procedure (3.6 days vs 11.2 days, considerably longer than routinely seen in North America) [37]. Buller and Cundiff converted the length of stay costs to standard North American practice (1 day vs 2–3 days) and concluded that the laparoscopic procedure was still less expensive than the open procedure ($666.11 vs $1,016.42–$1,524.64, respectively) [38]. According to Subak et al., the original study met eight of the ten principles for performing CEA, but would have been more informative if follow-up had been longer than 1–2 years, since life expectancy following surgery is far greater [4].

Cost Utility

In a large, multicenter, randomized controlled trial, Manca et al. employed a cost-utility analysis with health outcomes expressed as QALYs. Costs for operating room, hospital, follow-up, complications, reoperations, and further treatments to 6 months following surgery were considered. TVT resulted in a mean cost saving per patient of US$451 (95% CI $373–$633) compared with colposuspension while generating a mean improvement in health outcomes of 0.01 (95% CI –0.01 to 0.03). The probability of TVT being, on average, less costly than colposuspension was 100%. The probability of TVT being more cost-effective than colposuspension was 94.6% if the decision maker was willing to pay $55,700 per additional QALY. The higher operating room costs associated with TVT were offset by a shorter hospital stay [30].

Cody et al. performed a systematic review of 82 published studies on the effectiveness and

TABLE 37.4. Costs of TVT compared to other treatment modalities for SUI.

	Costs[a]	Costs after 5-year follow-up[a]
TVT	$2,101	$2,818–$2,940
Colposuspension	$2,484	$3,120–$3,652
Traditional slings	$2,528	$3,071–$3,600
Laparoscopic colposuspension	$2,484	Not available
Injectable agents	$2,461	Not available

From [10]

[a]Operating room, inpatient, and outpatient costs

cost-effectiveness of TVT for the treatment of SUI. Their findings are summarized in Table 37.4.

In terms of cost utility, compared to open colposuspension, TVT had a lower mean cost ($503) and the same or more QALYs (+0.00048). The likelihood of TVT being considered cost-effective was 100% if decision makers were unwilling to pay for an additional QALY, and 95% if they were prepared to pay up to $37,745 for an additional QALY. TVT was more likely to be considered cost-effective than other surgical procedures if one can assume the following: traditional slings have the same effectiveness as open colposuspension and also are more costly, laparoscopic colposuspension has the same or lower effectiveness as open colposuspension and similar costs, and injectable agents are less effective than TVT but cost more [10].

Conservative versus Surgical Management of SUI in Women

Ramsey et al. used a Markov cohort simulation to calculate expected costs for behavioral therapy, medications, and surgery for the treatment of SUI in elderly women. Decision trees were created for each treatment, incorporating treatment efficacy rates stated in the Agency for Health Policy and Research guideline for urinary incontinence. Two representative, plausible scenarios were used: (1) initial treatment with behavioral therapy and (2) treatment of behavioral therapy failures with medication (phenylpropanolamine plus estrogen) and initial treatment with medication and treatment of medication failures with surgery (needle suspension) (see Fig. 37.1 for the decision tree) [39].

Ten-year expected costs per patient, in 1994 dollars, from lowest to highest, were $25,388 for needle suspension surgery, $52,021 for phenylpropanolamine (no longer available in some countries due to serious side effects) and estrogen, $68,924 for behavioral therapy, and $86,726 for untreated incontinence. Behavioral and pharmacological therapies were less costly only if life expectancy was less than 3.5 years. Significant factors were the likelihood of a patient entering a nursing home, the cost of nursing home care, and the long-term relapse rate after surgery. On the basis of data from the urinary incontinence guideline, the authors concluded that early surgical intervention was the least costly treatment for chronic stress incontinence in elderly women. Unfortunately, the study was performed in 1996 and predates many of the more recent and cost-effective advances in surgical treatment of SUI. However, the lower cost and higher success rates of some of the newer surgical procedures would likely strengthen this conclusion [39].

A retrospective analysis of the direct cost of SUI among women in a Medicaid population was performed using data derived from a four-state Medicaid claims database (MarketScan, Medicaid, Medstat, Inc.). The database included inpatient, outpatient, outpatient prescription drugs, and long-term care claims of approximately 8 million Medicaid recipients from 1999 to 2002. During the study period, 13,672 women were newly diagnosed with SUI. Of these, only 13% were treated surgically, usually with a sling procedure. Mean direct costs for SUI-related care were $795, with a significant difference between surgically and nonsurgically managed patients ($3,258 vs $424, respectively, $P < 0.001$) [40].

Conservative versus Surgical Management of SUI in Men

Brown et al. compared the cost of pads and drip collectors with outpatient transurethral collagen injection or placement of an artificial genitourinary sphincter (AGUS) over a 10-year period (see Table 37.5). Conservative management with pads or drip collectors was significantly less expensive than collagen or AGUS, while treatment with

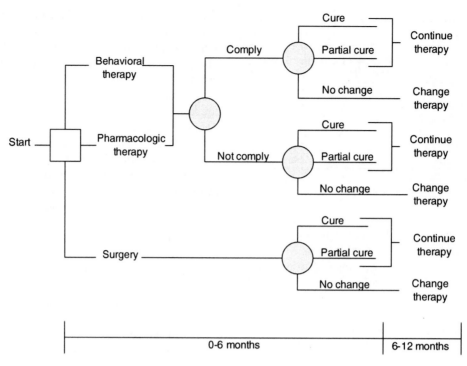

F<small>IG</small>. 37.1. Decision tree representing the Agency for Health Care Policy and Research urinary incontinence treatment options and outcomes. From [39]

T<small>ABLE</small> 37.5. Cost comparison of maintenance and surgical treatment of postprostatectomy incontinence in 1998 US dollars.

Therapy	Cost/item	Pads/day	Items/10 years	Cost/10 years
Depends undergarments	$0.52	5	18,263	$9,497
Active style pads	$0.52	5	18,263	$9,497
Entrust undergarments	$0.99	5	18,263	$18,080
Conveen drip collectors	$1.05	5	18,263	$19,176
Collagen + 0 pads/day	$4,300	0	4	$17,200
Collagen + 2 pads/day	$4,300	2	4	$20,999
AGUS × 1 + 0 pads/day	$15,400	0	1	$15,400
AGUS × 1 + 2 pads/day	$15,400	2	1	$19,199
AGUS × 2 + 0 pads/day	$15,400	0	2	$30,800
AGUS × 2 + 2 pads/day	$15,400	2	2	$34,599

Collagen = transurethral collagen injection, AGUS = artificial genitourinary sphincter. From [41]

AGUS was comparable to three or more collagen injections or the continued use of pads after collagen injection. However, the authors suggest that "when the benefit of urinary continence is considered, however, transurethral injection of collagen or AGUS placement often becomes the preferred treatment" [41].

Conclusion

In this era of rising health care costs, procedures need to be justified not only for their clinical effectiveness, but for their cost impact. In order to understand the cost implications of any new procedure, modeling under various clinical scenarios can be helpful to determine the place of each procedure in the clinical decision tree. Access to certain financial information from individuals, institutions, and insurance companies is necessary to produce realistic cost analyses.

References

1. Cammu H, Van Nylen M. Pelvic floor exercises versus vaginal weigh cones in genuine stress incontinence. Eur J Obstet Gynecol Reprod Biol 1998;77(1):89–93.
2. Diokno AC, Dimaculangan RR, Lim EU, Steinert BW. Office based criteria for predicting type II stress incontinence without further evaluation studies. J Urol 1999;161:1263–1267.
3. Schall CH, Costa RP, Sala FC, Vanni AP, Cortez JP. Longitudinal urethral sling with prepubic and retropubic fixation for male urinary incontinence. Int Braz J Urol 2004;30:307–312.
4. Subak LL, Caughey AB. Measuring cost-effectiveness of surgical procedures. Clin Obstet Gynecol 2000;43(3):551–560.
5. Finkelstein E, Corso P. Cost-of-illness analyses for policy making: A cautionary tale of use and misuse. Expert Rev Pharmacoeconomics Outcomes Res 2003;3(4):367–369.
6. Russell LB, Gold MR, Siegel JE, Daniels N, Weinstein MC. The role of cost-effectiveness analysis in health and medicine. JAMA 1996;276(14):1172–1177.
7. Gallin JI. Principles and practices of clinical research. Academic Press, New York, 2002.
8. Chang RW, Pellisier JM, Hazen GB. A cost-effectiveness analysis of total hip arthroplasty for osteoarthritis of the hip. JAMA 1996;275(11):858–865.
9. Hampel C, Artibani W, Espuna Pons M, Haab F, Jackson S, Romero J, Gavart S, Papanicolaou S. Understanding the burden of stress urinary incontinence in Europe: A qualitative review of the literature. Eur Urol 2004;46(1):15–27.
10. Cody J, Wyness L, Wallace S, Glazener C, Kilonzo M, Stearns S, McCormack K, Vale L, Grant A. Systematic review of the clinical effectiveness and cost-effectiveness of tension-free vaginal tape for treatment of urinary stress incontinence. Health Tech Assess 2003;7(21):182–189.
11. Payne CK. Epidemiology, pathophysiology, and evaluation of urinary incontinence and overactive bladder. Urology 1998;51(2A Suppl):3–10.
12. Birnbaum H, Leong S, Kabra A. Lifetime medical costs for women: Cardiovascular disease, diabetes, and stress urinary incontinence. Women's Health Issues 2003;13:204–213.
13. Birnbaum HG, Leong SA, Oster EF, Kinchen K, Sun P. Cost of stress urinary incontinence. A claims analysis. Pharmacoeconomics 2004;22(2):95–105.
14. Turner DA, Shaw C, McGrother CW, Dallosso HM, Cooper NJ. The cost of clinically significant urinary storage symptoms for community dwelling adults in the UK. BJU Int 2004;93(9):1246–1252.
15. O'Sullivan R, Simons A, Prashar S, Anderson P, Louey M, Moore KH. Is objective cure of mild undifferentiated incontinence more readily achieved than that of moderate incontinence: Costs and 2-year outcome. Int Urogynecol J Pelvic Floor Dysfunct 2003;14(3):193–198.
16. Weber AM, Walters MD. Cost-effectiveness of urodynamic testing before surgery for women with pelvic organ prolapse and stress urinary incontinence. Am J Obstet Gynecol 2000;183:1338–1347.
17. Lemack GE, Zimmern PE. Identifying patients who require urodynamic testing before surgery for stress incontinence based on questionnaire information and surgical history. Urology 2000;55:506–511.
18. Jung U. Hilfsmittelversorgung von Patienten mit Harninkontinenz. Kontinenz 1993;2:210–213.
19. Tediosi F, Parazzini F, Bortolotti A, Garattini L. The cost of urinary incontinence in Italian women. A cross-sectional study. Pharmacoeconomics 2000; 17(1):71–76.
20. Black NA, Bowling A. Impact of surgery for stress incontinence on the social lives of women. Br J Obstet Gynaecol 1998;105(6):605–612.
21. Brunenberg DEM, Joore MA, Veraart CPWM, Berghmans BCM, van der Vaart CH, Severens JL. Economic evaluation of duloxetine for the treatment of women with stress urinary incontinence: A Markov model comparing pharmacotherapy with pelvic floor muscle training. Clin Ther 2006;28(4):604–618.
22. Korn AP, Learman LA. Operations for stress urinary incontinence in the United States, 1988–1992. Urology 1996;48(4):609–612.
23. Berman CJ, Kreder KJ. Comparative cost analysis of collagen injection and fascia lata sling cystourethropexy for the treatment of type III incontinence in women. J Urol 1997;157:122–124.
24. Maher CF, O'Reilly BA, Dwyer PL, Carey MP, Cornish A, Schluter P. Pubovaginal sling versus transurethral Macroplastique for stress urinary incontinence and intrinsic sphincter deficiency: A prospective randomised controlled trial. Br J Obstet Gynaecol 2005;112(6):797–801.
25. Pickard R, Reaper J, Wyness L, Cody DJ, McClinton S, N'Dow, J. Periurethral injection therapy for urinary incontinenc in women. Cochrane Database Syst Rev 2003;(2):CD003881.

26. Walter AJ, Morse AN, Hammer RA, Hentz JG, Magrina JF, Cornelia JL, Magtibay PM. Laparoscopic versus open Burch retropubic urethropexy: Comparison of morbidity and costs when performed with concurrent vaginal prolapse repairs. Am J Obstet Gynecol 2002;186:723–728.

27. Saidi MH, Gallagher MS, Skop IP, Saidi JA, Sadler RR, Diaz KC. Extraperitoneal laparoscopic colposuspension: Short-term cure rate, complications, and duration of hospital stay in comparison with Burch colposuspension. Obstet Gynecol 1998;92:619–621.

28. Kohli N, Jacobs PA, Sze FH, Roat TW, Karram MM. Open compared with laparoscopic approach to Burch colposuspension: A cost analysis. Obstet Gynecol 1997;90:411–415.

29. Das S. Comparative outcome analysis of laparoscopic colposuspension, abdominal colposuspension and vaginal needle suspension for female urinary incontinence. J Urol 1998;160:368–371.

30. Manca A, Sculpher MJ, Ward K, Hilton P. A cost-utility analysis of tension-free vaginal tape versus colposuspension for primary urodynamic stress incontinence. Br J Obstet Gynaecol 2003;11:255–262.

31. Persson J, Teleman P, Eten-Bergquist C, Wolner-Hanssen P. Cost-analyses based on a prospective, randomized study comparing laparoscopic colposuspension with a tension-free vaginal tape procedure. Acta Obstet Gynecol Scand 2002;81:1066–1073.

32. Ulmsten U, Henriksson L, Johnsson P, Vahos G. An ambulatory surgical procedure under local anesthesia for treatment of female urinary incontinence. Int Urogynecol J 1996;7:81–86.

33. Nillson CG, Kuuva N. The tension-free vaginal tape procedure is successful in the majority of women with indications for surgical treatment of urinary stress incontinence. Br J Obstet Gynaecol 2001;108:414–419.

34. Quievy A, Couturier F, Prudhon C, Abram F, Al Salti R, Ansieau JP. Economic comparison of 2 surgical techniques for the treatment of stress urinary incontinence in women: Burch's technique versus the TVT technique. Prog Urol 2001;11(2):347–353.

35. Dean N, Ellis G, Wilson P, Herbison G. Laparoscopic colposuspension for urinary incontinence in women. Cochrane Database Syst Rev 2006;3:CD002239.

36. Loveridge K, Malouf A, Kennedy C, Edgington A, Lam A. Laparoscopic colposuspension. Is it cost-effective? Surg Endosc 1997;11(7):762–765.

37. Kung RC, Lie K, Lee P, Drutz HP. The cost-effectiveness of laparoscopic versus abdominal Burch procedures in women with urinary stress incontinence. J Am Assoc Gynecol Laparosc 1996;3(4):537–544.

38. Buller JL, Cundiff GW. Laparoscopic surgeries for urinary incontinence. A critique of new gynaecologic surgical procedures. Clin Obstet Gynecol 2000;43(3):604–618.

39. Ramsey SWT, Bavendam T. Estimated costs of treating stress urinary incontinence in elderly women according to the AHCPR clinical practice guidelines. Am J Manag Care 1996;2:147–154.

40. Kinchen KS, Long S, Chang S, Girts TK, Pantos B. The direct cost of stress urinary incontinence among women in a Medicaid population. Am J Obstet Gynecol 2005;193:1936–1944.

41. Brown JA, Elliott DS, Barrett DM. Postprostatectomy urinary incontinence: A comparison of the cost of conservative versus surgical management. Urology 1998;51(5):715–720.

Chapter 38
Community Awareness and Education

Diane K. Newman

Urinary incontinence (UI) is a significant health issue affecting children, women, and men of all ages, resulting in physical, social, quality of life, and economic implications for the individual, their caregivers, and the community. Despite the high prevalence of UI, it is consistently underdiagnosed and undertreated, since only one of four women with symptoms of UI and the related overactive bladder (OAB) seeks clinical help [1–3]. A contributing factor is the "stigma" surrounding bladder control problems and the fact that patients have many misconceptions about these conditions and they lack knowledge and understanding about causes and treatments, thus preventing them from seeking care [4]. It is believed that raising awareness in the community can improve help-seeking behavior for men and women with UI. This chapter will explore the barriers to seeking solutions to UI and what has been accomplished worldwide in the area of community awareness.

Barriers to Help-Seeking Behavior

UI usually comes to a health care provider's (HCP) attention only when the patient complains of specific symptoms and in most cases not often [5]. Recent research has reported that only from 13 to 54% of women and 29 to 48% of men with symptoms initiated conversation with a physician about incontinence or OAB symptoms [2, 6, 7]. It is not uncommon for women of all ages to wait from 1 to 3 years before seeking help [8]. According to Mason [9], following childbirth, only 16% of women with stress UI sought help for their symptoms at 8 weeks and only 25% sought help at 1 year postpartum. Those who seek treatment tend to have more significant symptoms that are increasing and causing more personal distress or impact on physical activities [2, 10].

Most are unaware of available treatment while others have low expectations from treatment. A national survey [11] of women with symptoms of OAB indicated that over 50% wait longer than a year (mean = 3.1 years) before seeking treatment. Reasons cited included not feeling that the problem was important enough to bother with, not being asked about symptoms by a HCP, not wanting to take medications or undergo surgery, and feeling that symptoms were something to just live with. This survey also identified the problem with current treatment, in this case, drug therapy for OAB. Women revealed dissatisfaction with current therapies for OAB because of bothersome adverse effects, inconvenient dosing schedules, and lack of efficacy. Many women in this study felt that the ratio of benefits to undesirable aspects of current OAB therapies was unacceptable. They expressed the desire for new treatments that are more effective and convenient and that offer reduced potential for adverse effects such as dryness.

To many, urine leakage, urgency, and frequency are minor problems that can be self-managed and do not require medical intervention. HCPs may dismiss bladder control problems as not worthy of investigation and treatment [12]. Unless specifically addressed by providers, most patients are too embarrassed by their symptom of urine leakage to seek medical help [13]. Even patients reporting with associated symptoms such as urgency and frequency may still be too embarrassed to mention urinary leakage. Consequently, while patients with severe symptomatology inevitably seek treatment, the majority of patients with mild or moderate symptoms of UI often are overlooked [14]. Patients often are unaware that there are effective behavioral and pharmacological therapies that can significantly reduce and even eliminate their symptoms.

What does appear to be major components of help-seeking behavior are the person's beliefs, perceptions, and emotions. Common myths or "urban legends" prevail. Older people may think UI is part of the normal aging process, something to be accepted and managed independently [6, 7]. In a study by Hannestad [15], women reported misconceptions about UI including beliefs that it is inevitable with aging, is too embarrassing to discuss, and that they should just learn to cope.

This lack of help-seeking behavior has been seen in many countries. Great Britain has a government-supported health care system allowing the elderly access to a primary care provider on a routine basis. However, Horrocks [7] found that in a survey of older persons who had UI (39%), only 15% has accessed services specifically for UI. This study found that participant's attitudes about incontinence correlated with attitudes about aging and beliefs about the cause of incontinence: they "normalized" the incontinence as a consequence of aging and as being inevitable. When UI is viewed as normal aging, it negates its cause as a medical condition, thus one that does not need medical intervention [16]. HCPs may be contributing unconsciously to this by their own attitudes and reduced expectations of improvement.

Women are more concerned with the hygienic effects of urine leakage, which may cause embarrassment and shame, so they conceal the problem from family members and friends. Therefore, instead of seeking medical advice, people turn to self-care practices such as restricting fluid intake, carrying containers for voiding whenever the "urge" occurs, crossing legs, avoiding travel outside the home, and practicing daily routines such as "toilet mapping." The use of absorbent pads and products (eg, disposable underwear, adult briefs) are common and often are reported as the initial self-management strategy for over 75% of women with UI [17]. Men, though, avoid use of pads, which they consider for women's use only [7]. The gender of the provider also may be a barrier to seeking treatment, as women may not be comfortable speaking with a male physician.

Overcoming the "Stigmatization" of Incontinence

Triggers for help-seeking behavior are complex and multifactorial and are beyond the scope of this chapter to review here. With a chronic problem like UI, it is important to understand what triggers the patient to consult with a HCP. Incontinence and bodily functions remain taboo in many cultures. Many people also do not consider themselves "incontinent," as this has a negative connotation or is not well understood. In a series of in-depth interviews with 28 young and middle-aged women with UI, it was found that incontinence was considered a taboo, making it difficult to seek professional help or even to focus on and think clearly about [18]. Some reacted with apathy; others were always on the brink of taking action. Many worked hard to maintain "normalcy" and hide the problem. For some there was defensive denial or they subordinated the problem to other priorities.

Bladder continence is an adjustment to the social norm, especially in Western cultures, which have developed acceptable rules and behavior for bladder emptying [19]. Bladder control is a skill that is socially acquired during childhood by toilet training and compliance often is achieved through shame and embarrassment. Children quickly learn that "wetting" themselves is unacceptable and "bad." If incontinence occurs in adulthood, persons revive those childhood beliefs and begin to internalize their condition, causing a decrease in self-esteem and feelings of not being "normal" [4].

The National Association For Continence (NAFC), a public advocacy organization in the United States, has conducted several public surveys over the past two decades [20]. A 2000 survey examined bathroom-related attitudes and behaviors and their relationship to bladder control problems.

Some respondents found the bathroom to be a personal place; a haven to seek refuge. Bathroom activities reported by respondents included reading in the bathroom (53%), contemplation of serious things (47%,) talking on the telephone (33%), and among the 30- to 39-year-old respondents, 27% reported making love in the bathroom. Others felt it symbolized incarceration because of the preoccupation with the need to be near one at all times because of bladder control problems. Older respondents felt that the bathroom is a "private" place and only 25% were comfortable using bathrooms outside their home, which may impact the use of public facilities and the ability to participate in social interaction.

One of the barriers to help-seeking behavior may be misunderstanding of terminology. It has been suggested that when promoting awareness of bladder control disorders, simple language and terminology (eg, bladder health, bladder control, OAB) should be used [21]. The word "incontinence" itself carries stigma, and most individuals with this symptom resist being labeled with this term or even with a problem, such as the loss of bladder control. Mass marketing for OAB medications has demonstrated the effectiveness of terminology in helping to destigmatize incontinence or bladder control problems to the public.

Newman [22] conducted a mail survey that noted that respondents were comfortable (51%) using the terms *overactive bladder* and *incontinence* when discussing this condition. When provided with additional terms, 39% said they were very comfortable with *loss of bladder control*, 33% with *leaks*, 26% with *accident,* and 23% with *incident.* Only one fourth (23%) of respondents said they were not "very comfortable" using any of the terms listed above when discussing their condition/situation. However, this survey was conducted on customers of a mail order medical supply company who were over the age of 65 and probably were more educated about managing incontinence.

Increasing Continence Awareness

Because UI affects millions of men and women of all ages, public health services and private sectors should be encouraged to conduct mass public education regarding the basic physiology of bladder

control, especially to dispel the many myths that are prevalent in the community regarding the diagnosis and treatment of UI and OAB [6]. Currently, there is little evidence-based research about public education to promote continence awareness in the community. Building awareness among the general public has been difficult and fragmented and it is difficult to assess the impact of any one health-promotion initiative, as there are many interacting variables and individuals obtain information from many sources. A promotion program for raising awareness must consider several aspects:

- *Target population*: The prevalence of UI and the lack of knowledge about incontinence are sufficient to justify a health-promotion program without segmentation by age or gender [21].
- *Target issues*: A promotion program should identify the issues that warrant promotion effort as well as barriers to promotion. Issues such as lack of willingness or readiness to seek treatment prevent people from seeking help [23].
- *Content of promotional material*: Any type of advertisement that deals with incontinence, even advertising campaigns for incontinence absorbent products, can have a positive impact on lessening taboos about talking about incontinence. This increased willingness to discuss urinary incontinence can be followed by advice on effective methods of coping with incontinence [24]. A media campaign should use multiple channels (eg, print media and radio) to ensure the broadest coverage [25]. A second channel would be specialized age and health publications. A third channel is the use of posters and brochures placed in physician's offices, hospitals, senior center, pharmacies, and churches. A final channel is direct presentations to the public, such as at senior centers. Another source of information is provided on the internet through websites that provide useful information on incontinence, what it is, and how it can be managed, treated, and cured [26–28]. Table 38.1 lists the top incontinence-related websites on Google.
- *Channels of communication*: Self-interest may be a motivator for public education. HCPs may launch campaigns to increase practice revenues. In Australia, medical entrepreneurs advertised widely in the press to promote urodynamic centers and in so doing stimulated the inception of

TABLE 38.1. Websites: Top five websites on urinary incontinence (Google search).

Website	Sponsor
http://www.incontinence.org/	American Urology Association Foundation for Urologic Disease, USA
http://www.nafc.org/	National Association for Continence, USA
http://www.incontinet.com/	Dr John Perry, USA – focused on pelvic floor disorders and biofeedback
http://www.uib.no/isf/people/inkter.htm	Dr Hogne Sonvik, Department of Public Health and Primary Health Care, University of Bergen, Norway
http://www.seekwellness.com/incontinence	Ms Diane Newman, Nurse Continence Specialist, Division of Urology, University of Pennsylvania, USA

the Australian Urodynamic Society. Such profit-motivated initiatives also may have the effect of raising the profile of incontinence as a health issue, to the benefit of all. Manufacturers often fund public campaigns in order to sell their products. Direct advertising raises public awareness to advance sales and to serve a commercial advantage. Continence-based public advocacy organizations may consider partnering with industry to reach a wider, general public audience. Increased exposure in the media, especially print and television media, has positively influenced attitudes, beliefs, and knowledge about incontinence [7]. Regardless of motivation, care should be taken to avoid raising public expectations beyond what the services or products can deliver.

• *Outcome assessment*: Prior to implementing a UI awareness campaign, it is important to identify outcome variables that will evaluate its effectiveness.

In many cultures, one of the best vehicles to reaching the public is through an informed journalist who uses a "media hook," an interesting story that will take priority over other news on the television, radio, or newspaper. A study of Chinese women by Yu et al. [29] reported that 16% of women who sought help did so because of advice from public media. Having a spokesperson with the problem or finding a celebrity who is willing to speak for the cause can help. This has been used repeatedly in the United States by drug and product manufacturers who have used Hollywood actresses (Debbie Reynolds, June Allyson) and Olympic sports figures (Mary Lou Retton) to get out the message to the public about UI or OAB. These individuals can act as "influence leaders." Using the media to disseminate information in the form of public

service announcements has been used extensively in the United States to promote AIDS awareness and in antismoking campaigns. In 2001, the NAFC produced and disseminated public service announcements to 380 media markets in the United States for the purpose of promoting continence awareness.

Television and print advertisements for OAB drugs have helped to destigmatize the condition by showing that it happens to normal individuals and by giving it a culturally accepted name in a society that places a high value on being active. Being "over" active does not conjure the same negative attribute as being "incontinent." HCP have noticed an increase in patients seeking treatment for their "overactive bladder symptoms" as a result of the drug advertising campaigns.

Telephone help-lines provide an opportunity for individuals suffering from UI to obtain information and advice without having to go through embarrassment of a face-to face meeting with a HCP.

Gartley [30] notes that one of the best ways to promote awareness and encourage people to seek help is through education about the bladder and incontinence. Through education, people become empowered and realize they are not alone and help is available. The United States-based Simon Foundation for Continence, of which Cheryle Gartley is the founder, has proposed a "bladder health mobile" to promote continence. It is hoped that this traveling exhibit would elevate the stature of bladder-related conditions, remove the stigma surrounding incontinence, and provide public awareness and education at the community level. It is not known whether this project will be successful in increasing awareness and driving more sufferers to seek treatment.

Also, a greater effort in the medical and nursing community must be made to educate physicians and nurses of the need to be proactive in identifying and treating these conditions. In 2007, the US National Institutes of Health (NIH) hosted a state-of-the-science conference on fecal and urinary incontinence and explore strategies to improve the identification and screening of persons at risk for developing fecal and urinary incontinence [38].

The Role of Patient Advocacy Continence Organizations

Professionals (eg, urologists, urogynecologists, gynecologists, primary care physicians, nurses) and professional organizations have been instrumental in promoting awareness of continence in all care settings. The International Continence Society established the Continence Promotion Committee (CPC) to promote education, services, and public awareness about incontinence throughout the world and to facilitate communication, exchange of information, and partnerships between continence organizations, health care professionals, governments, and industry [31]. The

CPC's multinational and multidisciplinary representation aims to identify broad issues through an international forum that can facilitate translation at the local and national level. In the past 15 years, national organizations (50 organizations in 36 countries) have been formed under various auspices to tackle issues pertaining to incontinence awareness, education, and promotion [24]. Table 38.2 is a list of countries that have national organizations, the organization names, and websites. While each organization is unique in its mandate, what they have in common is their commitment to improve the status for persons with incontinence.

Each year at the International Continence Society's annual meeting, the CPC has held workshops pertaining to various themes that have a broad national focus such as prevention, general practitioner education, and promotional strategies. Its relevance, as is the case with each of the national organizations, is to recognize the interface between continence management and continence awareness and promotion. The role of national organization is even more relevant because of the underreporting of the problem [31]. The CPC is planning to increase community awareness through the hosting of "public forums" at the time of the International Continence Society annual meeting.

TABLE 38.2. National continence organizations

Australia
Continence Foundation of Australia Ltd: http://www.continence.org.au/
Austria
Medizinische Geseelschaft fur Inkontinenhlife Osterreich: http://www.inkontinenz.at
Belgium
U-Control vzw (Belgian Association for Incontinence): http://www.sosincontinence.org/
Brazil
Brazilian Foundation for Continence Promotion: seabrarios@uol.com.br
Canada
The Canadian Continence Foundation: http://www.continence-fdn.ca
China
Hong Kong Continence Society: emfleung@ha.org.hk
Colombia
Colombian Continence Society, http://www.urologiacali.com Czechoslovakia
Czech Republic Inco Forum http://www.inco-forum.cz
Denmark
Kontinensoreningen (The Danish Association of Incontinent People), www.kontinens.dk/
Danish Continence Association
Email: info@kontinens.dk
France
Feemes pour Toujourns
Email: francoise.kremer@femsante.com
Web: www.femsante.com

(continued)

TABLE 38.2. (continued)

Germany
Gsellschaft fur Inkontinenzhilfe e.V. (GIH), http://www.gih.de
Hungary
Inko Forum: http://www.inkoforum.hu
India
Indian Continence Foundation:
http://www.indiancontinencefoundation.org
Indonesia
Indonesian Continence Society: urogyn@centrin.net.id
Ireland
Continence Foundation of Ireland http://www.continence.ie/
Israel
National Center for Continence: ig054@hotmail.com
Italy
Fondazione Italiana Continenza (The Italian Continence Foundation), http://www.continenza-italia.org
Associazione Italiana Donne Medico (AIDM): http://www.donnemedico.org
The Federazione Italiana Incontinenti (FINCO): finco@finco.org
Japan
Japan Continence Action Society: http://www.jcas.org

Korea
Korea Continence Foundation: http://www.kocon.or.kr
Malaysia
Continence Foundation: lohcs@medicine.med.um.edu.my
Netherlands
Pelvic Floor Netherlands: http://www.pelvicfloor.nl
Pelvic Floor Patients Foundation (SBP): http://www.bekkenbodem.net
Vereniging Nederlandse Incontinentie, Verpleegkundigen (VNIV): http://www.vnic.nl
New Zealand
New Zealand Continence Association: http://www.continence.org.nz
Norway
NORFUS (Norwegian Society for Patients with Urologic Diseases, www.siralf@sensewave.com
Philippines
Continence Foundation of the Philippines: (http://www.mela@info.com.ph)
Poland
NTM (INCO) Forum (The Polish Continence Organisation): http://www.ntm.pl
Singapore
Society for Continence: http://www.sfcs.org.sg
Spain
Associacion Nacional de Ostomizados e Incontinentes (ANOI): http://www.coalicion.org
Sweden
Swedish Urotherapists: birgtha.lindehall@vgregion.se
Sinoba: http://www.sinoba.se
Taiwan
Taiwan Continence Society: http://www.tcs.org.tw
Thailand
Thai Continence Society
Email: ravkc@mahidol.ac.th
United Kingdom
Association For Continence (ACA): http://www.aca.uk.com/
The Continence Foundation, UK: http://www.continence-foundation.org.uk
Incontact, http://www.incontact.org
Enuresis Resource and Information Centre (ERIC): http://www.eric.org.uk
United States
American Urologic Association Foundation: http://www.afud.org
International Foundation for Functional Gastrointestinal Disorders, http://www.aboutincontinence.org/
Interstitial Cystitis Association, Web: http://www.ica.org
National Association For Continence: http://www.nafc.org
Simon Foundation for Continence: http://www.simonfoundation.org

Examples of Community Awareness Programs

There are very few published reports of community awareness for continence. The Continence Promotion, Prevention, Education, and Organization committee of the International Consultation on Incontinence published the results of a 2003 survey from 24 organizations in 19 countries (67.7% response rate) [24]. Organizations have identified education about incontinence as the most important method to decrease the perceived stigma associated with the disorder. A successful method to educate persons has been through public awareness campaigns, health promotion projects, or health fairs. Examples of the programs are found in Table 38.3 and some are detailed here.

In the United States, the Oklahoma State Health Department developed "Dry Anticipations," which was a community demonstration prowject that included a curriculum on UI for small groups of elderly women [25]. This project had three components: an educational intervention with physicians, an educational campaign for the general public, and a test of behavioral treatments for older women. It was implemented by contracting with six sites in Oklahoma using a train-the-trainer model. A train-the-trainer approach, in which a project prepares a group of instructors to deliver an educational intervention to members of a target

TABLE 38.3. Examples of national continence organizations initiatives.

Australia – Helpline promotion
Belgium – GP and incontinence
Canada – Incontinence awareness month
Hong Kong – Continence promotion
Indonesia – GP seminars
India – Public awareness exhibition
Japan – Let's talk and think about continence
Korea – Incontinence awareness campaign
New Zealand – National bladder awareness week
Poland – National billboard campaign
Singapore – Women's health issues & healthy aging
Taiwan – A dry and comfortable spring
UK, Continence Foundation – Continence awareness week
UK, ERIC – Bed-wetting awareness in schools
UK, Incontact – Healthy bladder campaign
USA, IFFGD – Irritable bowel syndrome (IBS) awareness month
USA, SFC – Stigma in healthcare
USA, NAFC – Women's forum on lifelong bladder health

population, is a useful method when one wishes to introduce an intervention into existing agencies or ongoing social settings [32, 33].

The New Zealand Continence Foundation (NZCA) undertakes annual public awareness campaigns by supporting an annual "continence awareness" week, held the first week of September. The NZCA felt that terminology was important to public initiatives and initially branded "Dry Pants Day," an unpopular title so the name was changed to "Life without Limits – Continence Awareness." The NZCA has experience with public meetings organized by continence professional staff in their area and through small interest groups such as community groups (eg, Parkinson's, aging concerns, Alzheimer's, arthritis, etc.), and national awareness campaign events. The NZCA also conducts "public expos and shows" with HCPs to counteract embarrassment and to encourage people to seek professional help.

Western Australian municipal governments have provided funding through development grants that allow for the planning, implementation, and evaluation of continence health promotion seminars targeted at citizens in these areas. The most recent health promotion, called "Simply Busting," was community continence health promotion and education sessions. Participants also are provided with information on further support and management options. Local HCPs including medical centers, pharmacies, and physiotherapy practices, community service organizations, seniors groups, disability and aged care providers, and local sporting and recreation centers are asked to display flyers and posters. Evaluations are conducted immediately afterward and outcome evaluations are conducted at 3 and 12 months after the session. The majority of participants indicate they intend to make changes to their lifestyle as a result of attending the session. These changes include increasing fluid intake, decreasing caffeine consumption, doing pelvic floor muscle exercises, and seeking help from a health care professional.

The NAFC has hosted public forums in certain communities. At an event in 2006, NAFC partnered with a nationally recognized health care center (Duke University Medical Center) to multiply resources. This was especially helpful in reducing costs of advertisement of the forum. They also used government experts and celebrities to increase exposure and credibility of the forum.

In Great Britain, 2003 saw the launch of the "healthy bladder campaign" by the patient advocacy group INCONTACT. The purpose of the healthy bladder campaign was to raise awareness through the media and provide information through booklets and its website (http://www.incontact. org). Since 2003, ten regional and national newspapers, lifestyle and consumer magazines, and health care publications have been targeted, along with 14 regional radio stations. This coverage has resulted in extensive dissemination of the healthy bladder booklet and generated 46,000 hits on the INCONTACT website.

The interventions that best reach the public and trigger the desired behavior seem to vary between countries and cultures. The Japan Continence Action Society held a "toll-free telephone clinic" and callers were asked how they heard about the line. Sixty-five percent replied from a newspaper, 26% from television, and 8% from a poster. A Great Britain campaign found that newspapers were by far the most common source of information, followed by radio [34].

The Singapore Continence Foundation has held an "Incontinence Awareness Day" in the city's biggest shopping mall, which highlighted different types of incontinence, symptoms, and available treatment options. A disc jockey was trained on UI and was the host of the show. This was a very successful program that attracted 2,500 persons. Participants were asked to complete a quiz to determine if learning occurred and prizes were awarded. From the answers on the quiz, participants felt that aging causes incontinence and nobody can avoid this problem, so it was an opportunity to change/correct the common myth that aging causes incontinence.

Evaluating the Effectiveness of Public Awareness Campaigns

It is important to assess whether efforts to educate the public have the desired effect and to define the criteria by which to judge "success." Measures of success could include the number of media "impressions" through newspaper, television, or radio; the number of people who sought help; or the numbers who were actually helped. The mes-sage should be crafted to encourage and motivate the desired action. A questionnaire survey of callers 3 months after phoning the Continence Foundation of the United Kingdom help line during National Continence Week in 1994, found that callers appreciated the information but did not necessarily act on it [34].

In France, the effect of health education was evaluated in a randomized study in sheltered accommodations for the elderly [35]. Twenty centers were randomized to a single 1-h health information meeting or control group. During a 30-min talk, a nurse encouraged people to visit a doctor if they had urinary problems. A questionnaire 3 months later found that the experimental group was much more likely to have had treatment if they were incontinent (41% vs 13% controls) and 82% said that they had received some information about incontinence in the previous 3 months (compared to 22% controls).

A health promotion project called "Dry Expectations" was developed and implemented in six ethnically diverse, predominantly minority, and inner-city senior centers in the United States [36]. The program was designed to address an older population. The project consisted of three phases: orientation and training of key staff members/peer educators at the centers (train-the-trainer model); educating seniors through four 1-h weekly sessions involving visual aids and completion of bladder records and quizzes; and follow-up sessions with senior staff/peer educators to reinforce the previous training. The program was very well received by the participants, and roughly 80% felt they had more control over their bladder by the end of the last session.

This project recently was expanded to determine the health promotion needs of senior citizens concerning bladder control issues [21]. Focus groups of older adults attending health seminars in an urban, community setting were conducted. The primary objective of the project was to determine the understanding of older adults in the areas of general health and their beliefs surrounding the problem of UI. The 81 participants were predominantly African-American women representing all socioeconomic levels. Seniors expressed confusion when asked if "overactive bladder, bladder control issues, and urinary incontinence" were the same condition. Most seniors said they felt comfortable about discussing bladder control issues, but most admitted that their doctor had never asked them nor had they raised the issue. However, they did discuss UI with family members and friends and they were aware that many persons with whom they socialized might have a problem with UI. The majority of seniors answered "no cure" when asked if treatments were successful.

Australian "Continence Awareness" Success

The most successful country in promoting community awareness for continence has been Australia, which has promoted communitywide programs while evaluating their effectiveness [37]. The Australian National Continence National Continence Management Strategy was established in 1998 by the Australian Government Department of Health and Ageing to provide funding (initial funding of $15.4 million over 4 years) to research and service development initiatives aimed at prevention and treatment of this significant problem. Four major priorities were identified: public awareness, education, and information; prevention and health promotion; quality of service; and research. An additional $16 million were approved in 2003 to focus on the implementation of projects on prevention, community education, and improved management of incontinence by primary HCPs, and within community care and residential care facilities. Each funded project is independently evaluated or has built-in outcome measures. The goals of the National Continence National Continence Management Strategy are as follows:

1. Incorporate evidence-based research to promote awareness and encourage prevention, early intervention, and help-seeking behavior with a focus on meeting the needs and access issues of all population groups.
2. Formulate strategies for effective management of awareness-raising activities, ensuring that the roles of both state and federal governments are included.
3. Increase the capacity of all service providers (including consumers and carers as "first-line" service providers) to provide continence promotion and advice. Plan awareness-raising campaigns in conjunction with service providers in order to anticipate and provide appropriate resources to meet increase demand.
4. Ensure mechanisms are in place to measure the impact and cost effectiveness of awareness-raising activities. Establish standard measurements and reporting processes that will identify the changing level of awareness of continence issues within the community.
5. Promote initiatives such as the National Continence Helpline and National Public Toilet Map and ensure that community-focused access points are readily available. Identify opportunities to promote cross-fertilization of all initiatives and evaluate outcomes.
6. Focus national awareness and promotion campaigns on encouraging target groups to access continence-related information; take up prevention and early intervention messages; be prompted to seek help and access links to continence services.
7. Consider the diversity of cultural, linguistic, and ability levels in Australian communities in the development of current and future continence information materials.

Among the various consumer projects is the "public toilet map" – a national mapping of toilets to assist travel for persons with incontinence that will show information about opening hours and disability access, http://www.toiletmap.gov.au.

The National Continence Helpline was established to provide prompt, confidential, and professional advice for people with incontinence, their care givers, and organizations with an interest in continence management. It also provides printed information and educational material to Helpline clients about continence management and to support appropriate referral. As of December 2005, the number of calls to the Helpline had risen to an annual rate of almost 18,000 calls per annum or an average of 1.487 calls per month. A patient satisfaction survey undertaken in September 2005 found a 93% ($n = 51$) response rate for overall satisfaction with the service provided. Eighty-eight percent ($n = 35$) of applicable respondents indicated that the call to the Helpline had provided them with encouragement and empowerment to seek further help by responding to the referral information provided to them. Changes to the survey processes are being implemented with greater emphasis placed on assessing outcomes for callers to the Helpline. Initial funding for the Helpline also included specific funding for printing and promotions to raise community awareness and promote the Helpline.

An early intervention project specifically targeted mothers of young children under 2 years and encouraged a call to action through a continence awareness narrowcast program using convenience advertising with posters and "take away" information. Over 1,000 display points, either a poster or a poster and cardholder, were placed in baby change rooms of selected community health centers, shopping centers, cinemas, and hospitals with maternal health facilities throughout Australia. The results indicated that in excess of 12,000 brochures were taken from these display points during the project period. An evaluation of the project was undertaken using intercept interviews in shopping centers and Maternal Health Care clinics. The results indicated that the respondents recognized the materials used and viewed them positively. Unprompted recall was low but on prompting the recognition rate rose to over 85%. The findings also indicated that respondents saw the initiative as an awareness-raising communication rather than a call for action.

Conclusion

Continence promotion involves informing and educating the public and health care professionals that incontinence is not inevitable or shameful, but is treatable or at least manageable. Taboos about mentioning disorders of the bladder gradually are lifting in most cultures. Two decades ago it was almost impossible to have a discussion about urinary incontinence in the media. Today, in most countries, national "continence" organizations are promoting awareness in communities. Many countries have run national or local public awareness campaigns. Many also have confidential help lines, which can be accessed anonymously. The world wide web provides a convenient source of health information for a growing number of consumers. Continence awareness is growing but there is more needed to increase the numbers of persons seeking treatment.

References

1. Herzog AR, Fultz NH, Normolle DP, Brock BM, Diokno AC. Methods used to manage urinary incontinence by older adults in the community. J Am Geriatr Soc 1998;37(4):339–347.
2. Kinchen KS, Burgio K, Diokno AC, Fultz NH, Bump R, Obenchain R. Factors associated with women's decisions to seek treatment for urinary incontinence. J Womens Health 2003;12(7):687–698.
3. Roberts RO, Jacobsen SJ, Rhodes T, et-al. Urinary incontinence in a community based cohort: Prevalence and healthcare-seeking behavior. J Am Geriatr Soc 1998;46:467–472.
4. Garcia JA, Crocker J, Wyman JF. Breaking the cycle of stigmatization. J Wound Ostomy Continence Nurs 2005;32(1):38–52.
5. Hagglund D, Walker-Engstrom M, Larsson G, Leppert J. Reasons why women with long-term urinary incontinence do not seek professional help: A cross-sectional population-based cohort study. Int Urogynecol J Pelvic Floor Dysfunct 2003;14:296–304.
6. Diokno AC, Sand PK, Macdiarmid S, Shah R, Armstrong RB. Perceptions and behaviours of women with bladder control problems. Fam Pract 2006;23:568–577.
7. Horrocks S, Somerset M, Stoddart H, Peters TJ. What prevents older people from seeking treatment for urinary incontinence? A qualitative exploration of barriers to the use of community continence services. Fam Pract 2004;21:689–696.
8. Koch LH. Help-seeking behaviors of women with urinary incontinence: An integrative literature review. J Midwifery Womens Health 2006;51(6):e39–e44.
9. Mason L, Glen S, Walton I, Hughes C. Women's reluctance to seek help for stress incontinence during pregnancy and following childbirth. Midwifery 2001;17:212–221.
10. Teunissen D, van Weel C, Lagro-Janssen T. Urinary incontinence in older people living in the community: Examining help-seeking behaviour. Br J General Pract 2005;55:776–782.
11. Dmochowski R, Newman DK. Impact of overactive bladder on women in the United States: results of a national survey. Curr Med Res Opin 2007;23(1):65–76.
12. Newman DK. Managing and treating urinary incontinence, 2nd ed. Edition. Health Professions Press, Baltimore, MD, 2008:19–28.
13. Fantl JA, Newman DK, Colling J, et al. Urinary incontinence in adults: Acute and chronic management clinical practice guideline, No. 2, Update. Rockville, MD: US Department of Health and Human Services. Public Health Service, Agency

for Health Care Policy and Research, AHCPR Publication No. 96–0682. March 1996.

14. Brittain KR, Perry S, Williams K. Triggers that prompt people with urinary symptoms to seek help. Br J Nurs 2001;19(2):74–85.

15. Hannestead YS, Rortveit G, Hunskaar S. Help-seeking and associated factors in female urinary incontinence (The Norweigan EPINCONT study: Epidemiology of Incontinence in the County of Nord-Trondelag). Scan J Prim Health Care 2002;51:801–804.

16. Bush TA, Castellucci DT, Phillips C. Exploring women's beliefs regarding urinary incontinence. Urol Nurs 2001;21(3):211–218.

17. Subak LL, Brown JS, Kraus SR, Brubaker L, Lin F, Richter HE, Bradley CS, Grady D. The "costs" of urinary incontinence for women. Obstet Gynecol 2006;107(4):908–916.

18. Ashworth PD, Hagan MT. The meaning of incontinence: A qualitative study of non-geriatric urinary incontinence sufferers. J Adv Nurs 1993;18:1415–1423.

19. Norton C. Nurses, bowel continence, stigma and taboos. J Wound Ostomy Continence Nurs 2004;31(2):85–94.

20. Muller N. What Americans know and how they are affected by bladder control problems: Highlights of a recent national consumer survey. Urol Nurs 2005;25(2):109–115.

21. Palmer MH, Newman DK. Bladder control educational needs of older adults. J Gerontol Nurs 2006;32(1):28–32.

22. Newman DK. Report of a mail survey of women with bladder control disorders. Urol Nurs 2004;24(6):499–507.

23. McFall SL, Yerkes AM. Targets, messages, and channels for educational intervention on urinary incontinence. J Appl Gerontol 1998;17:403–418.

24. Newman DK, Denis L, Gruenwald I, Ee CH, Millard R, Roberts R, Sampselle C, Williams K. Promotion, education and organization for continence care. In: Abrams P, Cardozo L, Khoury S, Wein A, eds.. Incontinence, proceedings from the 3rd international consultation on incontinence. Plymouth UK: Health Publication 2005;35–72.

25. McFall SL, Yerkes AM, Belzer JA, et al. Urinary incontinence and quality of life in older women: A community demonstration in Oklahoma. Fam Commun Health 1994;17:64–75.

26. Boyington AR, Dougherty MC, Yuan-Mei Liao. Analysis of interactive continence health information on the web. J Wound Ostomy Continence Nurs 2003;30(5):280–286.

27. Diering C, Palmer MH. Professional information about urinary incontinence on the world wide web: Is it timely? Is it accurate? J Wound Ostomy Continence Nurs 2001;27(6):1–9.

28. Sandvik H. Health information and interaction on the internet: A survey of female urinary incontinence. Br Med J 1999;319:29–32.

29. Yu H, Wong W, Chen J, Chic W. Quality of life and treatment seeking in Chinese women with urinary incontinence. Qual Life Res 2003;12:327–333.

30. Gartley, C. Bringing Mohammed to the mountain; educating the community for continence. Urol Nurs 2006;26(5):387–393.

31. Fonda D, Newman DK. Tackling the stigma of incontinence – Promoting continence worldwide. In: Cardozo L, Staskin D, eds. Textbook of female urology and urogynecology. 2nd edn. United Kingdom Isis Medical Media, 2006:75–80.

32. McFall SL, Yerkes AM, Cowan LD. Overcomes of a small group educational intervention for urinary incontinence, Health-related quality of life. J Aging Health 2000a;12(3):301–317.

33. McFall SL, Yerkes AM, Cowan LD. Overcomes of a small group educational intervention for urinary incontinence, episodes of incontinence and other urinary symptoms. J Aging Health 2000b;12(3)250–267.

34. Norton C, Brown J, Thomas E. Continence: A phone call away. Nurs Stand 1995;9:22–23.

35. Beguin AM, Combes T, Lutzler P, et-al.. Health education improves older subjects' attitudes toward urinary incontinence and access to care: A randomised study in sheltered accommodation centers for the aged (letter). JAGS 1997;45:391–392.

36. Newman DK, Wallace J, Blackwood N. Promoting healthy bladder habits for seniors. Ostomy Wound Manage 1996;42:18–28.

37. Byles JE, Chiarelli P, Hacker AH, et-al.. An evaluation of three community-based projects to improve care for incontinence. Int Urogynecol J Pelvic Floor Dysfunct 2005;16(1):29–38.

38. Shamliyan T, Wyman J, Bliss DZ, Kane RL, Wilt TJ. Prevention of urinary and fecal incontinence in adults. Evid Rep Technol Assess (Full Rep). 2007 Dec; (161):1–379.

Index

Lightning Source UK Ltd.
Milton Keynes UK
173853UK00001B/17/P